N!

F

AF

Retinal Degenerations

Editors

Robert E. Anderson, Ph.D., M.D.
Professor
Departments of Ophthalmology, Biochemistry, and Physiology
and Molecular Biophysics
Division of Neuroscience
Cullen Eye Institute
Baylor College of Medicine
Houston, Texas

Joe G. Hollyfield, Ph.D.
Professor
Departments of Ophthalmology, Biochemistry, and Physiology
and Molecular Biophysics
Division of Neuroscience
Cullen Eye Institute
Baylor College of Medicine
Houston, Texas

Matthew M. LaVail, Ph.D.
Professor
Departments of Anatomy and Ophthalmology
University of California
San Francisco, California

CRC Press
Boca Raton Ann Arbor Boston London

Library of Congress Cataloging-in-Publication Data

Retinal degenerations / editors, Robert E. Anderson, Joe G.
Hollyfield, Matthew M. LaVail.
     p. cm.
    "Proceedings of the Stockholm Symposium on Retinal Degenerations
held in Stockholm, Sweden, July 24-27, 1990, as a satellite meeting
of the IX International Congress of Eye Research, held in Helsinki,
Finland"—Pref.
  Includes bibliographical references and index.
  ISBN 0-8493-0178-5
    1. Retina—Diseases—Congresses. 2. Retina—Diseases-
-Histopathology—Congresses. 3. Retina—Diseases—Pathophysiology-
-Congresses. 4. Retina—Diseases—Molecular aspects—Congresses.
I. Anderson, Robert E. (Robert Eugene) II. Hollyfield, Joe G.
III. LaVail, Matthew M. IV. Stockholm Symposium on Retinal
Degenerations (1990) V. International Congress of Eye Research (9th
: 1990 : Helsinki, Finland)
    [DNLM: 1. Light—adverse effects—congresses. 2. Photoreceptors-
-pathology—congresses. 3. Pigment Epithelium of Eye-
-transplantation—congresses. 4. Retina—transplantation-
-congresses. 5. Retinal Degeneration—congresses. WW 270 R43828
1990]
RE551.R4715 1991
617.7'3—dc20
DNLM/DLC
for Library of Congress

91-13543
CIP

Direct all inquiries to CRC Press, Inc., 2000 Corporate Blvd., N.W., Boca Raton, Florida 33431.

© 1991 by CRC Press, Inc.

International Standard Book Number 0-8493-0178-5

Library of Congress Card Number 91-13543
Printed in the United States

PREFACE

Inherited and acquired retinal degenerations are among the most debilitating diseases known to mankind because they rob an otherwise healthy individual of the precious gift of sight. Although considerable effort has been put forth over the last two decades to determine the molecular etiology of retinal degenerations, only in recent years have fundamental discoveries been made that may lead to the prevention and possible cure of these devastating eye diseases. At the Sixth International Congress of Eye Research meeting in Alicante, Spain (1984), we organized a symposium on retinal degenerations. The success of this meeting and subsequent publication prompted us to organize satellite meetings on retinal degenerations for ISER Congresses held in 1986 (Nagoya) and 1988 (San Francisco) and to publish the proceedings, along with other invited papers.

This volume is the fourth in a series on retinal degenerations and contains proceedings of the Stockholm Symposium on Retinal Degenerations held in Stockholm, Sweden, July 24 to 27, 1990, as a satellite meeting of the IX International Congress of Eye Research, held in Helsinki, Finland. Most of the participants submitted chapters for this book, as did a number of other individuals who work in this area but were unable to attend the symposium.

The Stockholm Symposium on Retinal Degenerations was held at the Grand Hôtel Saltsjöbaden on the western shore of the Baltic Sea. This majestic setting provided an atmosphere that contributed immensely to the success of the Symposium. The choice of this hotel was made by our local co-organizer, Professor Sven Erik G. Nilsson, Chairman of Ophthalmology at the University of Linköping. Without his strong support, this meeting would not have been possible. He was actively involved in all phases of the planning and was especially successful in raising funds to help defray the cost of the meeting. We are most grateful to Dr. Nilsson and are pleased to dedicate this publication to him. Also, we are grateful to members of Dr. Nilsson's staff who assisted in all phases of planning and execution of this symposium: Dr. Ulla Nilsson, Mrs. Ann-Margret Svensson, Dr. Ola Textorius, Dr. Sven Jarkman, Dr. Anders Wrigstad, and Mrs. Barbo Swenson.

The meeting received strong financial support from several organizations. We are happy to acknowledge support of the National Retinitis Foundation Fighting Blindness, Inc., Baltimore, Maryland; the National Institutes of Health, Bethesda, Maryland; The Swedish Federation of the Visually Handicapped; the Crown Princess Margareta's Foundation for the Visually Handicapped; the Swedish Ministry of Education and Cultural Affairs; the Stockholm City and Stockholm County Councils; Merck, Sharp, and Dohme (Sweden) Co.; Alcon Pharmaceuticals Nordic Co.; Cyanamid International/Lederle Laboratories; and the Department of Ophthalmology, University of Linköping, Sweden.

Finally, we wish to thank Janice Wilson for assistance above and beyond the call of duty in all phases of this effort, from preparing most of the correspondence related to the meeting to editing many of the manuscripts.

Robert E. Anderson
Joe G. Hollyfield
Matthew M. LaVail

THE EDITORS

Robert E. Anderson, Ph.D., M.D., is Professor of Ophthalmology, Biochemistry, and Neuroscience at Baylor College of Medicine, Houston, Texas. He received his Ph.D. degree in Biochemistry (1968) from Texas A&M University and was a postdoctoral fellow at Oak Ridge Associated Universities (1968). At Baylor, he was appointed Assistant Professor in 1969, Associate Professor in 1976, and Professor in 1981. While a faculty member at Baylor, he attended medical school and received his M.D. in 1975.

Dr. Anderson has published extensively in the areas of lipid metabolism in the retina and the biochemistry of retinal degenerations. He has edited five books, four on retinal degenerations and one on biochemistry of the eye.

Dr. Anderson has received the Sam and Bertha Brochstein Award for Outstanding Achievement in Retina Research from the Retina Research Foundation (1980), the Dolly Green Award (1982) and Senior Scientific Investigator Award (1990) from Research to Prevent Blindness, Inc., and an Award for Outstanding Contributions to Vision Research from the Alcon Research Institute (1985). He has served on the editorial board of *Investigative Ophthalmology and Visual Science* and is currently on the editorial boards of the *Journal of Neuroscience Research* and *Current Eye Research*. Dr. Anderson has received grants from the National Institutes of Health, the Retina Research Foundation, the Retinitis Pigmentosa Foundation Fighting Blindness, and Research to Prevent Blindness, Inc. He has been an active participant in the program committees of the Association for Research in Vision and Ophthalmology and has served on the Vision Research Program Committee and the Board of Scientific Counselors of the National Eye Institute. Currently, he is on the Faculty of the Basic and Clinical Science Series of the American Academy of Ophthalmology and is a Councillor for the International Society for Eye Research.

Joe G. Hollyfield, Ph.D., is Professor of Ophthalmology and Neuroscience at Baylor College of Medicine. He received his Ph.D. degree in Zoology (1966) from the University of Texas at Austin and was a postdoctoral fellow at the Hubrecht Laboratory in Utrecht, The Netherlands. He was appointed Assistant Professor of Anatomy assigned to Ophthalmology at Columbia University College of Physicians and Surgeons in New York City in 1969 and was promoted to Associate Professor in 1975. In 1977, he moved to the Cullen Eye Institute, Baylor College of Medicine, where he was promoted to Professor in 1979.

Dr. Hollyfield has published more than 100 papers in the area of cell and developmental biology of the retina and pigment epithelium in both normal and retinal degenerative tissues. He has edited five books, four on retinal degenerations and one on the structure of the eye.

Dr. Hollyfield has received the Marjorie W. Margolin Prize (1981) and the Sam and Bertha Brochstein Award (1985) from the Retina Research Foundation, the Olga Keith Wiess Distinguished Scholars' Award (1981) and a Senior Scientific Investigator Award (1988) from Research to Prevent Blindness, Inc., an Award for Outstanding Contributions to Vision Research from the Alcon Research Institute (1987), and the Distinguished Alumni Award (1991) from Hendrix College, Conway, Arkansas. He has previously served on the editorial boards of *Vision Research* and *Survey of Ophthalmology*. He is currently Retina Section Editor of *Experimental Eye Research*. He has received grants from the National Institutes of Health, the Retina Research Foundation, Fight for Sight, Inc., the Retinitis Pigmentosa Foundation Fighting Blindness, and Research to Prevent Blindness, Inc. Dr. Hollyfield has been active in the Association for Research in Vision and Ophthalmology as a past member of the Program Committee and a current member of the Board of Trustees. He is also the current President and fromer Secretary of the International Society of Eye Research.

Matthew M. LaVail, Ph.D., is Professor of Anatomy and Ophthalmology and Vice-Chairman of Anatomy at the University of California at San Francisco School of Medicine. He received his Ph.D. degree in Anatomy (1969) from the University of Texas Medical Branch in Galveston and was subsequently a postdoctoral fellow at Harvard Medical School. Dr. LaVail was appointed Assistant Professor of Neurology-Neuropathology at Harvard Medical School in 1973. In 1976, he moved to UCSF, where he was appointed Associate Professor of Anatomy. He was appointed to his current position in 1982, and in 1988, he also became director of the Retinitis Pigmentosa Research Center at UCSF.

Dr. LaVail has published extensively in the research areas of photoreceptor-retinal pigment epithelial cell interactions, retinal development, circadian events in the retina, genetics of pigmentation and ocular abnormalities, inherited retinal degenerations, and light-induced retinal degeneration. He is the author of more than 70 research publications and has edited four books on inherited and environmentally induced retinal degenerations.

Dr. LaVail has received the Fight for Sight Citation (1976), the Sundial Award from the Retina Foundation (1976), the Friedenwald Award from the Association for Research in Vision and Ophthalmology (1981), a Senior Scientific Investigator Award from Research to Prevent Blindness, Inc. (1988), a MERIT Award from the National Eye Institute (1989), and Award for Outstanding Contributions to Vision Research from the Alcon Research Institute (1990), and the Award of Merit from the Retina Research Foundation (1990). He has served on the editoral board of *Investigative Ophthalmology and Visual Science* and is currently on the editorial board of *Experimental Eye Research*. Dr. LaVail has been an active participant in the program committees of the Association for Research in Vision and Ophthalmology and the International Society for Eye Research, and he is currently Vice-President of the International Society for Eye Research.

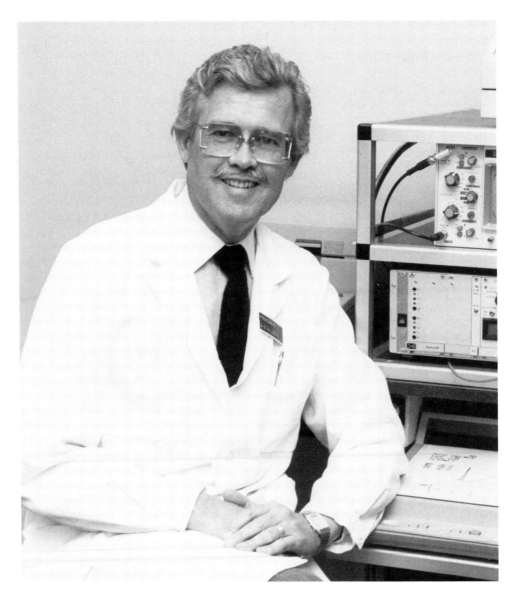

Dedicated to

Sven Erik G. Nilsson, M.D., Ph.D.
Professor and Chairman, Department of Ophthalmology
University of Linköping, Linköping, Sweden

for his early understanding
of the origin of the photoreceptor outer segment,
his lifetime of contributions to basic and clinical visual science,
and his efforts in organizing the
Stockholm Symposium on Retinal Degenerations

TABLE OF CONTENTS

Section V: Molecular Biology of Retinal Degenerations

SECTION I

ANIMAL MODELS OF RETINAL DEGENERATION

The recent successes in identifying precisely the molecular defects in humans and animals with inherited retinal degenerations result directly from the work of a large number of investigators who developed and characterized animal models of inherited retinal degenerations. Through the efforts of these researchers, vertebrate and invertebrate models of retinal degeneration have now been studied in great detail.

The first paper of this section discusses the rationale for using animal models to study human retinal degenerations. Other papers discuss the development of photoreceptor cells in the *rds* mouse and differentiation of *rd* and *rds* retinas in organ culture. A canine form of congenital stationary night blindness is described, which appears to be a suitable model for the human disease. Also described is the Abyssinian cat, in which retinal degeneration begins after the photoreceptors have developed normally and which appears to be an excellent model for human retinitis pigmentosa. The gene defect has now been bred into a mixed breed cat, which should facilitate the use of this model for laboratory investigations. The last chapter in this section is a comprehensive review of an invertebrate with retinal degeneration, the fruitfly *Drosophila*.

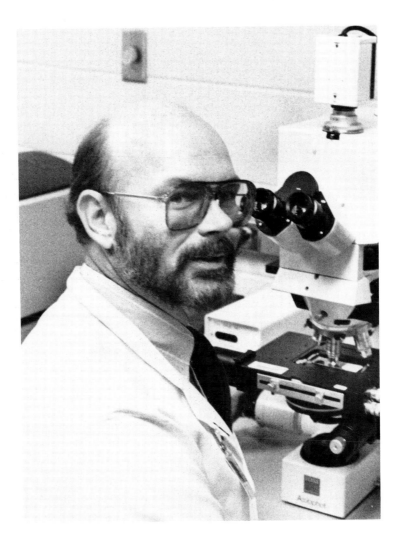

Robert J. Ulshafer, Ph.D.   1949-1990

We were deeply saddened by the untimely death of our colleague and friend, Robert J. Ulshafer, only a few short weeks after he attended the Stockholm Symposium on Retinal Degenerations. Bob was an active participant in each of the three previous symposia on retinal degenerations and was a contributor to all the proceedings publications. As one of the invited speakers at the Stockholm meeting, Bob presented an overview of the work from his laboratory on a mutant strain of Rhode Island Red chickens with retinal degeneration and he planned to contribute a chapter on the same topic to this volume. In lieu of his chapter, we are including the following bibliography which lists all of Bob's publications describing the developmental and cell biology of the *rd* chicken. We are pleased to acknowledge his contributions to the field of retinal degenerations.

The Editors

Publications of R. J. Ulshafer on the *rd* chicken

Ulshafer, R.J., C.B. Allen, W.W. Dawson and E.D. Wolf (1984). Hereditary retinal degeneration in Rhode Island Red chickens: ERG and histology. Exp. Eye Res. 39:123-135.

Ulshafer, R.J. and C.B. Allen (1984). SEM of the retina of an animal model of hereditary retinal degeneration. Scanning Electron Microscopy 2:841-848.

Ulshafer, R.J. (1985). Avian models of hereditary retinal degeneration. In: Retinal Degeneration: Contemporary Experimental and Clinical Studies; LaVail, Hollyfield and Anderson, Eds., Alan R. Liss, Inc., pp. 321-337.

Ulshafer, R.J. and C.B. Allen (1985). Hereditary retinal degeneration in the Rhode Island Red chicken: Ultrastructural observations. Exp. Eye Res. 40:865-877.

Ulshafer, R.J. and C.B. Allen (1985). Ultrastructural observations on the retinal pigment epithelium of congenitally blind chickens. Exp. Eye Res. 4:1009-1021.

Allen, C.B., R.J. Ulshafer, E.A. Ellis and J.C. Woodard (1987). SEM analysis of intraocular ossification in advanced retinal disease. Scanning Microsc. 1:233-239.

Kelley, K.C., R.J. Ulshafer and E.A. Ellis (1987). Intraocular ossification in the *rd* chicken. Avian Pathology. 16:189-192.

Bridges, C.D.B., R.A. Alvarez, S.-L. Fong, G.I. Liou and R.J. Ulshafer (1987). Rhodopsin, vitamin A, and interstitial retinol-binding protein in the *rd* chick. Invest. Ophthalmol. Vis. Sci. 28:613-617.

Spoerri, P.E., K.C. Kelly, C.B. Allen and R.J. Ulshafer (1987). Conditioned medium-mediated photoreceptor differentiation in retinal cultures from embryonic *rd* chickens. Eur. J. Cell Biol. 44:105-111.

Ulshafer, R.J., and E.M. Meyer (1987). Studies on putative neurotransmitters in an animal model of hereditary blindness. In: Degenerative Retinal Disorders: Clinical and Laboratory Investigations, Hollyfield, Anderson and LaVail, eds., Alan R. Liss, Inc., New York, p. 407-422.

Ulshafer, R.J. and M.B. Heaton (1989). Axonal transport and central visual projections of ganglion cells in congenitally blind chickens. Curr. eye Res. 8:321-326.

Semple-Rowland, S.L. and R.J. Ulshafer (1989). Analysis of proteins in developing *rd* chick retina using two-dimensional gel electrophoresis. Exp. Eye Res. 49:665-675.

Ulshafer, R.J., W.W. Hauswirth and A. Van der Langerijt (1989). EM immunocytochemical localization of rhodopsin and IRBP during retinal development. Proc. EM Soc. Am. p. 800-801.

Dawson, W.W., R.J. Ulshafer, R. Parmer and N.R. Lee (1990). Receptor potentials in the normal and retinal degenerate (*rd*) chicks. Clin. Vision. Sci. 5:285-292.

Ulshafer, R.J., E.L. Clausnitzer, D.M. Sherry, A. Szel, and P. Rohlich (1990). Immunocytochemical identification of outer segment proteins in the *rd* chickens. Exp. Eye Res. 51:209-216.

Ulshafer, R.J., D.M. Sherry, R. Dawson and D.R. Wallace (1990). Excitatory amino acid involvement in retinal degeneration. Brain Res. 531:350-354.

A ROLE FOR ANIMALS IN UNMASKING THE CELLULAR BIOLOGY OF INHERITED RETINAL DEGENERATION

RICHARD N. LOLLEY AND REHWA H. LEE

DEPARTMENT OF ANATOMY AND CELL BIOLOGY, AND JULES STEIN EYE INSTITUTE, UNIVERSITY OF CALIFORNIA, LOS ANGELES 90024; DEVELOPMENTAL NEUROLOGY LABORATORY, VETERANS ADMINISTRATION MEDICAL CENTER, SEPULVEDA, CA   91343

I. INTRODUCTION

The study of inherited disorders has advanced significantly during the past decade, with animal models of inherited blindness providing the substrate for intellectual and technical advancement. The period has been charged with excitement for several concurrent events have come to fruition in the past half decade. The mechanisms in normal photoreceptors that absorb light and trigger a coded message (phototransduction) for the brain to interpret were identified and characterized extensively.[1,2,3] It was found that all vertebrate photoreceptors have retained during evolution the same format for phototransduction as that in human rod and cones, making animal studies relevant to the human condition.[4,5] Cellular biology and, more recently, molecular biology have provided the ability to identify tissue-specific proteins, allowing the characterization of several unique photoreceptor proteins. Animal models for RP are finally giving up their secrets, thanks, to the powerful genetic probes that are available from the study of normal, photoreceptor-specific proteins. We can take a moment to celebrate and to place this information in its proper perspective. Then, we must again move on toward our ultimate goal, which is the prevention of photoreceptor dysfunction and death. Identification and characterization of a defective gene is only the first step in the prevention of blindness. Now, we must probe the biological mechanisms which initiate the degenerative process and cell death? Unraveling this puzzle is a major challenge and it should be our dedicated goal in the 1990's.

II. RESEARCH ADVANCES IN RETINAL DEGENERATION ARE DEPENDENT UPON PROGRESS IN UNDERSTANDING THE NORMAL ACTIVITIES OF PHOTORECEPTORS.

Vertebrate photoreceptors have a unique morphology which is designed for the trapping of photons and for the transmission of signals to post-synaptic neurons. Photoreceptor cells also possess mechanisms which were highly conserved during the evolutionary process. From the retina of dogs, cats, chickens, rats or mice may come a finding which is immediately transposable to the human retina and thereby have some relevance to understanding human ocular diseases. Moreover, a genetic or acquired lesion which impairs photoreceptor function and initiates cell death in one species may have the same effect in another mammalian species. This belief is the touchstone of our search for animal models of Retinitis Pigmentosa. Almost every animal species contain members with retinal degeneration which will be informative to some type of Retinitis Pigmentosa or a related condition. Finding these animals, characterizing their genetic lesion and effecting prevention of the disease is our creed.

There has been a fascination with inherited retinal degenerations for many years, but description of the primary genetic defect has remained elusive because insight into the molecular mechanisms of photoreceptor function were missing. The rd disorder of mice is a case in point. Beginning in the late 1950s, Werner Noell[6] investigated for a decade the phenomena of inherited photoreceptor degeneration in rd mice and he arrived ultimately at the idea that the photoreceptor cells failed in the process of terminal differentiation. He was correct! However, he could not go further. Our laboratory took up the gauntlet in the late 1960s and soon found that a deficiency in a phosphodiesterase activity is responsible for the accumulation of cyclic GMP in affected rd photoreceptors.[7] Still, like Werner Noell, we were at a loss to understand either a role for cyclic GMP in photoreceptor activities or its role in the degenerative process.

The past decade has seen the flowering of vision research. Dramatic progress has been made in understanding some of the basic mechanisms of rod and cone photoreceptor cells. Perhaps, the most gratifying achievement for vision was the charting of photo-transduction. It firmly established that cyclic GMP is the intracellular effector that regulates ion channels of the photoreceptor plasmalemma, modulating the influx of sodium and calcium into the cell and controlling membrane polarization.

It appears that all vertebrate photoreceptors use a comparable light-triggered cascade for photo-transduction.[2] Light pulls the trigger by activating rhodopsin to catalyze a series of reactions that culminate in the hydrolysis of cyclic GMP and with the closure of ion channels in the plasmalemma of the photoreceptor outer segment

(Figure 1). There is a linear flow of information from rhodopsin to the cGMP-dependent channels, with signal amplification occurring in two stages along the cascade.

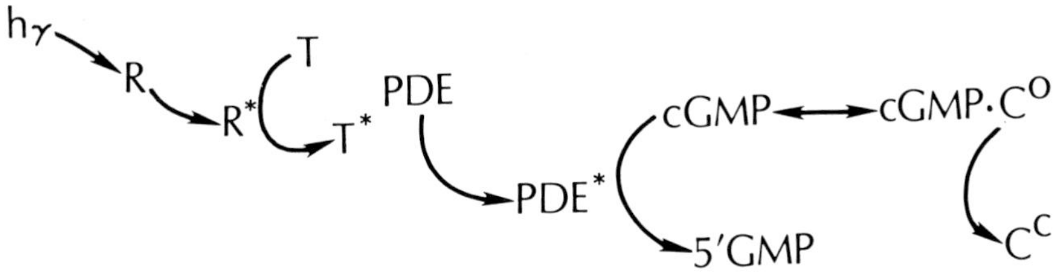

Figure 1:   Light-activation of the phototransduction cascade in vertebrate photoreceptors.   A cascade of reactions is triggered when light (hv) is absorbed by rhodopsin (R) in a rod outer segment.   Photolyzed rhodopsin (R*) then catalyzes the activation of hundreds of transducin (T -> T*) molecules, with each T* binding to a phosphodiesterase (PDE) enzyme and activating it (PDE*) to hydrolyze thousands of cGMP molecules. In the presence of cGMP the channel remains open (C°), but as the intracellular concentration of cGMP is decreased by PDE* the cation channels close (C^c) and the photoreceptor cell becomes hyperpolarized.

When rhodopsin absorbs light, its chromophore is isomerized to <u>all-trans</u> retinal and the protein undergoes conformation changes which expose binding sites for the GTP-binding protein, transducin.[8] Transducin is a heterotrimeric complex containing an alpha, beta and gamma subunit.[9] The alpha subunit contains a guanosine nucleotide binding domain which is occupied usually by GDP, but interactions of transducin with bleached rhodopsin catalyze an exchange of GDP for GTP.   Thus armed with GTP, alpha subunit dissociates from the tightly joined, beta,gamma subunits and from the rod outer segment membrane.   GTP-alpha transducin then interacts with an inactive phosphodiesterase complex that is composed of an alpha,beta and two gamma subunits.[10,11,12] The alpha,beta subunits are tightly coupled and they are believed to contain the catalytic site of the enzyme, with the gamma subunits inhibiting their activity.   The binding of GTP-alpha transducin to the gamma subunit of the phosphodiesterase relieves these inhibitory constraints, releasing the hydrolytic potential of the enzyme.   The activated phosphodiesterase will hydrolyze cyclic GMP at a high rate which is limited only by the availability of substrate through diffusion. The phosphodiesterase remains active until the GTP which occupies the guanosine nucleotide binding domain of alpha transducin is hydrolyzed by the intrinsic GTPase activity of this subunit; upon GTP hydrolysis the gamma-PDE subunit is released to again complex with the phosphodiesterase complex and inhibit enzyme activity. The fall in cyclic GMP that results from light-triggered phosphodiesterase activation is sensed by cation channels of the plasmalemma which are specialized cyclic GMP-binding proteins.[13] The concentration of cyclic GMP is monitored constantly by the dynamics of the binding reaction so that high levels of cyclic GMP (darkness) hold the pore formed by the channel proteins in an open conformation, allowing the influx of sodium and calcium; low levels of cyclic GMP (light) close the channel, blocking cation passage and causing membrane hyperpolarized.[14]

The photo-transduction cascade, as outlined, represents only the activation phase of a photon response for there are mechanisms for down-regulation of the cascade, resynthesis of cyclic GMP, dephosphorylation of opsin and regeneration of 11-cis retinal. Each of these events are important in the restoration of the dark state. They most likely will contribute also to some form of Retinitis Pigmentosa for many, if not all, of the proteins involved are probably specific to photoreceptor cells. The cascade and its associated proteins are the foundation of our current knowledge of photo-transduction and they provided a background for evaluating the types of inherited retinal degeneration in humans and animals.

III. KNOWING A PRIMARY GENETIC LESION IN AN ANIMAL DISORDER OPENS OPPORTUNITIES FOR INVESTIGATING THE CELL BIOLOGY OF PHOTORECEPTOR CELLS.

There is much to be discovered about rod and cone photoreceptors that is masked by our ignorance. Each time we strip away another layer of ignorance, we are challenged with new questions that carry us deeper into the cell biology of the photoreceptor cell. The elegant morphology of rod photoreceptors is an outward expression of metabolic and functional compartmentation within the cell. For a photoreceptor to remain viable, this compartmentation of activities may need to be preserved.

The integrity of the rod outer segment is apparently essential for the continued viability of rod photoreceptors. When rod outer segments fail to form in the rds mouse disorder the photoreceptor cells soon begin to degenerate (15). The rds gene encodes an abnormal form of peripherin that contains an insert of apparently retroviral origin.[16,17] It is conceived that peripherin acts normally in the formation of rod outer segment disks and that this process is disrupted in the rds mutant. The impact of this failed process on the homeostatic mechanisms of developing rod photoreceptors is unknown, but it offers an excellent opportunity for mapping the cellular events that lead to the death and degeneration of the rds photoreceptors.

Even seemingly innocuous changes in the primary structure of rhodopsin appear sufficient to cause photoreceptor degeneration. Individuals with one form of autosomal dominant RP have been shown to possess amino acid substitutions in rhodopsin.[18] Some are located near the N-terminus where the protein protrudes into the intra-discal space. It is possible that these structural defects in rhodopsin disrupt the integrity of the disk membrane or they alter the tertiary organization of rhodopsin so that it is ineffectual in phototransduction. In the rd mouse disorder, a candidate gene for the defect has been identified which encodes the beta subunit of the phosphodiesterase enzyme. It is conceivable that an abnormality in the synthesis or structure of the beta subunit will prevent the rd photoreceptors from forming a phosphodiesterase complex that can hydrolyze cyclic GMP.[19,20] Autosomal dominant RP and the rd and rds animal disorders together suggest that a defect in the phototransduction cascade can initiate the degenerative process and the continued viability of rod photoreceptors requires both the structural and functional integrity of the rod outer segment.

The flow of information from a defective gene product to the ultimate mechanism that triggers cell degeneration is not usually apparent. In autosomal dominant RP and the rds mouse disorder, components of this pathway are totally unknown, but, in the rd mouse disorder, the high levels of cyclic GMP that accumulate prior to the onset of degeneration are perhaps instrumental in the rapid degenerative process. In support of this idea are the observations that drugs which elevate cyclic GMP levels in xenopus or human retinas cause photoreceptor degeneration. By what means does cyclic GMP exert its toxicity?

From the known role of cyclic GMP in photoreceptors and other tissues, an accumulation of cyclic GMP could drive a variety of systems, each of which could impact on other cellular activities. The effect of cyclic GMP is usually expressed through its interactions with cyclic GMP-binding proteins. Whereas there are probably many such proteins in rod photoreceptors, only three classes have been studied in any depth. The light-dependent channel of the rod outer segment binds cyclic GMP and elevated levels of the cyclic nucleotide in rd photoreceptors should predicable recruit above normal numbers of open channels and a corresponding higher influx of cations. Even though the degenerating rd photoreceptors do not appear to swell,[6] an inordinate drain of energy by the ion pumps which regulate cellular volume could compromise photoreceptor viability.

In normal photoreceptor cells, most of the intracellular cyclic GMP is bound, with the concentration of free cyclic GMP regulated near 5 uM.[21] Much of the intracellular pool of cyclic GMP is believed to be bound to non-catalytic sites on the cascade phosphodiesterase enzyme.[22] In the rd disorder, a defective beta subunit of the phosphodiesterase complex could alter the ratio of free to bound cyclic GMP so that the concentration of free cyclic GMP is markedly elevated. The availability of free cyclic GMP could then be important in the disease process because the soluble pool interacts with and regulates the activity of specific protein kinases. Whereas there is apparently little cyclic GMP-kinase in rod photoreceptors, the cyclic nucleotide can modulate the activity of protein kinase A, particularly at concentrations estimated for rd photoreceptors.[23] This would drive the phosphorylation of possibly numerous proteins,[24,25] e.g. phosducin and alter their respective function within the structure or function of the affected cells. The possible paths that radiate from the accumulation of cyclic GMP in rd photoreceptors is finite and amenable to investigation. Such studies could provide insight into the cause of cell death and into the mechanisms that support the metabolism or renewal of normal rod photoreceptors.

IV. MANY ANIMAL MODELS OF INHERITED RETINAL DEGENERATION ARE NEEDED TO MATCH THE DIVERSITY OF HUMAN RETINITIS PIGMENTOSA.

Inherited blindness is a severe handicap for all living creatures and the possibility exists that a variety of photoreceptor or RPE defects can trigger the degenerative process. It is imperative that animal models be developed that mimic closely the many forms of RP and related disorders. They are essential because we need to systematically define each pathological condition, identify the genetic defect and devise methods for prevention of the degenerative process. This information will rapidly be disseminated for what once occurred in isolation now is known quickly through the world. Moreover, modern technology is capable of transferring the information gleaned from animal models directly to patients in the clinic. In vision research we are fortunate in that laboratory findings are integrated rapidly into state-of-the-art clinical practice.

Cellular and molecular biology hold the promise of preventing human blindness, if not in our generation then in the generations to follow. To ensure that the promise is fulfilled, we need to scour the world for preferably small animals with inherited forms of retinal degeneration. We cannot have too many! However, finding the animals is not easy and resolving the cytopathology and biochemistry is often slow and tedious. We who are active in vision research are building a catalog of how photoreceptors function and how they fail when genetic lesions disrupt normal functional activities. We are paving the way for improving genetic counseling, understanding what initiates photoreceptor cell death and constructing the genetic information that is needed for the prevention of blindness.

Animals with inherited blindness are the substrates of our intellectual and academic life and for many of us they have provided an intellectually stimulating career. Each new type of inherited blindness holds a treasure-chest of invaluable information that must be harvested through careful and pains-taking work. We are the hands through which a plighted citizenry can find hope. We have delivered in the past and our future looks brighter than ever. Since caution is our professional norm, we move one step at a time. With persistence, each animal disorder will give up its secrets. We will find that these mutant animals are valuable both to the study of RP and to investigations of normal photoreceptor activities. Any animal with inherited blindness is valuable and should be investigated because we are not so rich in knowledge that a potential surrogate for the human condition can be rejected.

V. REFERENCES

1. Stryer, L., Cyclic GMP cascade of vision. Ann. Rev. Neurosci. 9, 87, 1986.
2.   Hurley, J. B., Molecular properties of the cGMP cascade of vertebrate photoreceptors. Ann. Rev. Physiol. 49, 793, 1987.
3. Lolley, R. N. and Lee, R. H., Cyclic GMP and photoreceptor function. FASEB J. 4, 3001, 1990.
4.   Lerea, C.L., Somers, D. E., Hurley, J.B., Klock, I. B., Bunt-Milam, A. H., Identification of specific transducin alpha-subunit in retinal rod and cone photoreceptors. Science 234, 77, 1986.
5.   Gillespie, P. G., and Beavo, J. A., Characterization of a bovine cone photoreceptor phosphodiesterase purified by cyclic GMP-sepharose chromatography. J. Biol. Chem. 263, 8133, 1988.
6. Noell, W. K., Aspects of experimental and hereditary retinal degeneration. in Biochemistry of the retina, (Ed. Graymore, C. N.), Academic press: New York, 1965, 51.
7.   Farber, D. and Lolley, R., Enzymic basis for cyclic GMP accumulation in degenerative photoreceptor cells of mouse retina. J. Cyclic Nucleotide Res. 2, 139, 1976.
8. Fung, B., Hurley, J. and Stryer, L., Flow of information in the light-triggered cyclic nucleotide cascade of vision. Proc. Natl. Acad. Sci. USA, 78, 152, 1981.
9. Fung, B., Characterization of transducin from bovine retinal rod outer segments. J. Biol. Chem. 258, 10495, 1983.
10.   Baehr, W., Devlin, M. J., Applebury, M. L., Isolation and characterization of cGMP phosphodiesterase from bovine rod outer segments. J. Biol. Chem. 254, 11669, 1979.
11.   Hurley, J. B. and Stryer, L., Purification and characterization of gamma regulatory subunit of the cyclic GMP phosphodiesterase from retinal rod outer segments J. Biol. Chem. 257, 11094, 1982.
12. Wensel, T. G., and Stryer, L., Activation mechanism of retinal rod cyclic GMP phosphodiesterase from bovine rod outer segments Biochemistry 29, 2155, 1990.
13. Cook, N, J., Hanke, W. and Kaupp, U. B., Identification, purification, and functional reconstitution of the cyclic GMP-dependent channel from rod photoreceptors. Proc. Natl. Acad. U.S.A. 84, 585, 1987.
15. Sanyal, S., De Buiter, A. and Hawkins, R., Development and degeneration of retina in rds mutant mice: light microscopy. J. Comp. Neurol. 194, 193, 1980.
16. Travis, G. H., Brennan, M. B., Danielson, P. E., Kozak, C. A. and Sutcliffe, J. G., Identification of a photoreceptor specific mRNA encoded by the gene responsible for retinal degeneration slow (rds). Science, 338, 70, 1989.
17. Connell, G. J. and Molday, R. S., Molecular cloning, primary structure and orientation of the vertebrate photoreceptor cell protein peripherin in rod outer segment disk membrane. Biochemistry 29, 4691, 1990.

18. Dryja, T.P., McGee, T. L., Reichel, E., Hahn, L. B., Cowley, G. S., Yandell, D. W., Sandberg, M. A., and Berson, E. L., A point mutation of the rhodopsin gene in one form of retinitis pigmentosa. Nature, 343, 364, 1990.

19. Bowes, C., Danciger, M., Kozak, C. A., and Farber, D. B., Isolation of a candidate cDNA for the gene causing retinal degeneration in the rd mouse. Proc. Natl. Acad. Sci. 86, 9722, 1989.

20. Lee, R., Navon, S., Brown, B., Fung, B. and Lolley, R., Characterization of a phosphodiesterase-immunoreactive polypeptide from rod photoreceptors of developing rd mouse retinas. Invest. Ophthalmol. Visual Sci. 29, 1021, 1988.

21. Haynes, L., Kay, A. R., and Yau, K.-W., Single cyclic GMP-activated channel activity in excised patches of rod outer segment membrane. Nature 321, 66, 1986.

22. Charbonneau, H., Prusti, R., LeTrong, H., Sonnenburg, W. K., Mullaney, P. J., Walsh, K. A., and Beavo, J. A., Identification of a noncatalytic cGMP-binding domain conserved in both the cGMP-stimulated and photoreceptor cyclic nucleotide phosphodiesterase. Proc. Natl. Acad. Sci. 87, 288, 1990.

23. Walter, U., Cyclic GMP-regulated enzymes and their possible physiological functions. Adv. Cyclic Nucleotide Protein Phosphorylation Res. 17, 249, 1984.

24. Lee, R., Lieberman, B. and Lolley, R., A novel complex from bovine visual cells of a 33,000-dalton phosphoprotein with ß- and τ-Transducin: purification and subunit structure. Biochemistry, 26, 3983, 1987.

25. Lee, R. H., Brown, B. M., and Lolley, R. N., Protein kinase A phosphorylates retinal phosducin on serine 73, in situ. J. Biol. Chem. 265, 15860, 1990.

FUNCTIONAL DIFFERENTIATION OF OUTER SEGMENTS AND PHOTORECEPTOR CELL
DEATH IN THE RETINA OF <u>rds</u> MUTANT MICE

S. Sanyal[1], H.G. Jansen[1], G. Aguirre[2], T. van Veen[3], R.M. Broekhuyse[4]
and W.J. de Grip[4]

[1]Department of Anatomy, Erasmus University, Rotterdam,
The Netherlands
[2]Section of Medical Genetics, University of Pennsylvania,
School of Veterinary Medicine, Philadelphia, Pa, U.S.A.
[3]Department of Zoology, University of Lund, Lund, Sweden
[4]Departments of Biochemistry and Ophthalmology, University of
Nijmegen, Nijmegen, The Netherlands

I. INTRODUCTION

Three distinct facets of structural changes are recognized in the
retina of mice afflicted by the retinal degeneration slow <u>(rds)</u>[1] gene
from the early postnatal period on. First, the anomalous development of
the photoreceptor cells, more specifically, the maldevelopment of the
receptor outer segments (ROS).[2,3] Second is the slow death of the
photoreceptor cells which, despite the early expression of the genetic
defect, starts somewhat later and progresses over almost the entire
life span of the individuals.[4] Finally, the dose dependent expression
of the <u>rds</u> gene in the heterozygous (<u>rds</u>/+) mice allows formation of
the ROS, which however, appear morphologically abnormal, and results in
delayed and slower death of the photoreceptor cells with eventually
only partial loss in the terminal state of the disease.[5]

Previous studies on the cellular changes in the mutant retina,
including retina from chimaeric mice,[6-8] have shown the photoreceptor
cells to be the primary target of the gene and, further, that the gene
acts within the photoreceptor cells. Recent molecular biological
studies have achieved spectacular success in identifying a
photoreceptor cell specific mRNA which is defective in the mutant and
the relevant gene has been cloned and sequenced.[9] The resulting protein
has been shown to be a key component in the assembly of the ROS discs,
and a malfunction of this protein has been suggested to be the primary
molecular defect[10] underlying the spectrum of phenotypic changes and
eventual death of the photoreceptor cells.

As the photoreceptor cells in the mutant retina have a long
survival period and cell death is sporadic, it is obviously apparent
that the consequence of the genetic defect is not immediately lethal.
This observation leads to two immediate questions. First, what is the
exact cause of photoreceptor cell death and second, what is the
functional status of the photoreceptor cells for as long as these cells
are surviving? While no definite information has become available so
far, that can answer the first question and that problem remains in the
realm of speculation. Various observations from a number of

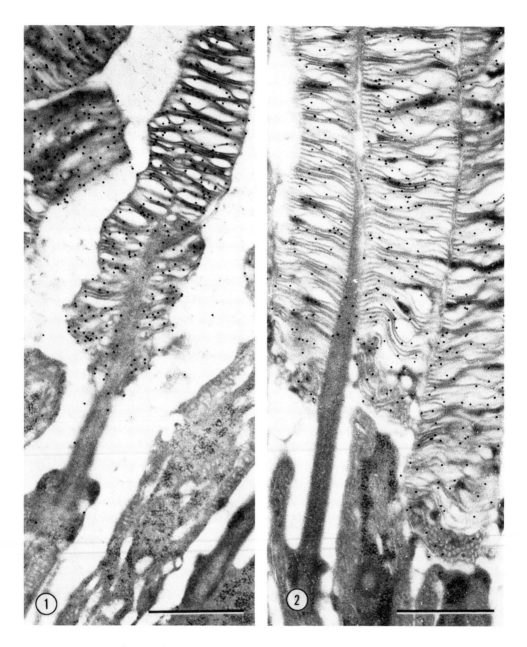

Figure 1. Electron micrograph showing immunohistochemical localization of (rhod)opsin labelled by protein A-gold in the photoreceptor outer segments of the normal retina of adult BALB/c mouse. Bar=1μm.

Figure 2. Similar preparation showing immunogold labelling of S-antigen in the normal retina of BALB/c mouse. Bar=1μm.

All immunohistochemical observations were based on light adapted eyes. Ultrathin sections of retinas fixed in aldehyde mixture and embedded in Lowicryl KM4 were processed by the immuno-Gold procedure using antibodies raised against the bovine proteins.

laboratories show that the different elements representing photoreceptive functions are at least minimally present in the photoreceptor cells of the mutants. Indeed, affected individuals, both homozygous and heterozygous, show a measurable visual capability lasting to varying degrees over the prolonged period of the disease process.

In this chapter we review the available information on the development of the mutant phenotype in the afflicted mice, with special reference to the functional differentiation of the ROS. We compare the ultrastructural changes, cellular localization of such photoreceptor cell specific proteins as opsin, the primary molecular site of photoreception, and S-antigen, also known as 48kDa protein or arrestin that has been identified as an essential intermediary in the process of phototransduction.[11-13] We further examine the photoreceptor status of the surviving cells in the course of the prolonged period of degeneration by comparing the time course of the photoreceptor cell loss and the changes in the retinal contents of opsin and S-antigen. Finally, in the light of these data, we discuss the applicability of the rds mutant mice as a model system for Retinitis Pigmentosa (RP).

II. DEVELOPMENT OF THE MUTANT PHENOTYPE

In mice the major part of retinal development, in particular the differentiation of the photoreceptor cells, occurs during the first two weeks of the postnatal life. In the neonatal retina some of the photoreceptor cells have developed rudiments of inner segments but some of the cells are also still proliferating. S-antigen is already present at this early stage and shows a perikaryal localization.[14] During the first 4 to 5 postnatal days, the inner segments grow rapidly in length and a prominent axonemal structure - a cilium surrounded by plasma membrane - emerges at the receptor end. Both S-antigen[15] and opsin[16-18] are regularly localized along the ciliary plasma membrane. No difference between the normal and the mutant retinas is detectable at this stage, either in ultrastructure or in histochemical localization of the two photoreceptor specific proteins. Then stacks of ROS discs, first somewhat irregularly oriented and then orderly piled up in the characteristic form of ROS, develop in the normal retina and show uniformly positive reaction for opsin (Figure 1) and S-antigen (Figure 2). During this period little progress beyond the axonemal structure is recorded in the homozygous mutant retina. In the absence of ROS discs some membrane bound vesicles of variable size and structural complexity are formed and extruded in the subretinal space.[3,19] These membranous elements show an immunoreaction pattern for opsin (Figure 3,4) and S-antigen (Figure 7) that is identical to the normal ROS discs. These are considered as structural equivalents of ROS disc membrane and are most profusely observed at 2-3 weeks, but at later stages are present in a much reduced frequency. This differential turnover of membranous elements in the homozygous mutant retina can be a counterpart of the differential rate of membrane assembly in the normal retina prevailing at the earlier formative stages of ROS development[20]. These membranous extrusions are removed by the phagocytic activity of the pigment epithelium and also possibly by macrophages which are present in the subretinal space of the rds/rds

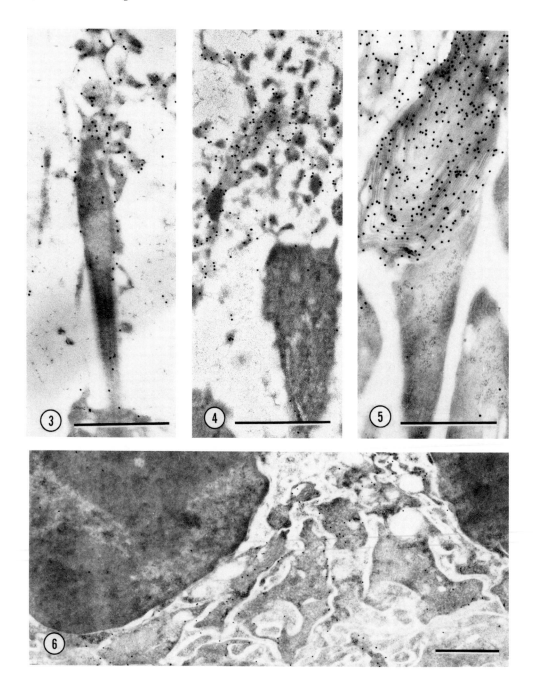

Figures 3-6. Immunogold labelling of opsin sites in the retina of
<u>rds</u> mutant mice. In the absence of true ROS in the homozygous <u>rds</u>
retina opsin is detected over the ciliary plasma membrane (Figure 3)
and extruded membranous vesicles (Figure 4) and also over the plasma
membrane around the perikarya and the terminals (Figure 6). In the
heterozygotes ROS discs develop abnormal form (Figure 5) but labelling
intensity appears normal. Bar=1μm.

retina. One distinguishing feature of the immunoreaction pattern in the homozygous mutant retina is the persistent presence of opsin over the plasma membrane in the perikaryal and the terminal region of the cell (Figure 6) and of S-antigen in the inner segments (Figure 7) as well as perikaryal and terminal cytoplasm.

In the retina of the heterozygous (rds/+) mice disc membranes are formed but instead of developing into an elongated ROS these round up in large whorls of continuous membranes. These also show identical immunoreaction for opsin (Figure 5) and S-antigen as in normal ROS. The total length of the ROS layer in the rds/+ retina is less than in the normal and the anomalous form is a permanent feature of the heterozygous phenotype. Autoradiographic data have further shown that the photoreceptor cells in the rds/+ mice also have an altered pattern of ROS-assembly. In addition, disc shedding is abnormal in the rds/+ retina in that the phagosomes in the pigment epithelium are much larger, show a different pattern of turnover and a differential sensitivity to changes in the light regimen.[21,22]

The development of the rest of the photoreceptor cells in the homozygous and heterozygous mutant retinas follows in normal sequence so that the perikaryal differentiation of the rods and cones is completely similar to normal. The terminals of the rods and cones and the characteristic synaptic contacts have also been shown to be morphologically normal.

In spite of the gross abnormality or near absence of the ROS, some functional capability of the retina in the homozygous mutant mice has been demonstrated by flash evoked ERG.[23] Compared to normal mice, the mutant has a much higher detection tresshold, but this is not surprising in view of the low opsin content (see below). All available evidence thus suggests that the defective gene does not affect differentiation of the photoreceptors, but only impairs outer segment assembly. How does this relate to the subsequent gradual cell death?

III. TIME COURSE OF PHOTORECEPTOR CELL LOSS

In the retina of the rds mutant mice selective loss of photoreceptor cells results in the gradual reduction in the thickness of the outer nuclear layer (ONL) which consists exclusively of the perikarya of the rods and cones. Comparison of the thicknesses of the ONL of the three genotypes - +/+, rds/rds and rds/+ - at different ages has given a reliable idea as to the time of beginning of photoreceptor cell death and the rate of its progression (Figure 8). Differential counts of rods and cones have been used to assess the differential susceptibility of these two receptor types.

In the retina of homozygous muatant mice, both albino 020/A and pigmented C3H strains, a significant reduction in the thickness of the ONL appears to start from the age of 2 or 3 weeks; the decline is initially relatively faster and from the age of about 2-3 months photoreceptor cell death proceeds very slowly. During this phase of the slow progression of the disease a significant difference is recorded between the albino and the pigmented strains. In the albino 020/Ards/rds mice the ONL has completely disappeared from the peripheral retina around the age of 9 months and from the central retina around 12 months. In the pigmented C3Hrds/rds mice, complete

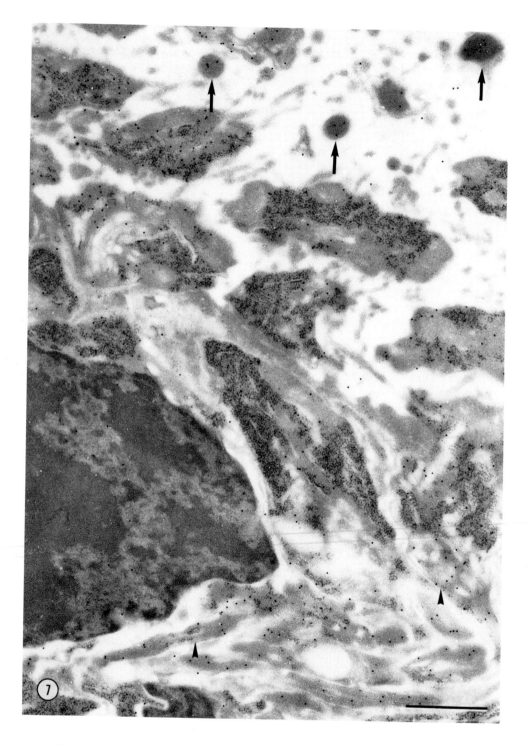

Figure 7. Immunogold labelling of S-antigen in the retina of homozygous <u>rds</u> mutant mice is seen over the membranous vesicles (arrow), inner segments and perikaryal cytoplasm (arrowheads). Bar=1μm.

disappearance of the ONL is registered after about 3-6 months later than in the albinos.[24] Part of the protection comes presumably from the presence of melanin in the various ocular tissues and appears to be more effective in the peripheral retina; however, some strain specific metabolic differences can also have a contributory role in this difference. Also, some individual variation has been observed in both groups.

In the retina of heterozygous mutant mice, death of photoreceptor cells is marked by a clear reduction in the thickness of the ONL, and appears to start from around 2 months. That is later than in the homozygotes. Rate of degeneration in the heterozygous retina is also much slower than in the homozygotes and eventually results in only a partial reduction of the ONL, 3 to 4 rows of outer nuclei being still present in the old animals (Figure 9).

The retina in mice is considered to be rod dominated; only about 3% of the outer nuclei are of the cone type as judged by the difference in nuclear morphology. During the early phase of somewhat rapid photoreceptor cell loss, the frequency of the cones is comparable to that of the normal retina of the same age (Table 1), indicating that

TABLE 1

Changes in the frequency of cone perikarya(%) within the receptor cell population (rods and cones) in the albino BALB/c+/+, 020/Ards/rds and F_1rds/+ mice

Strain genotype	Age in months	Central retina Mean	S.E.M.	Peripheral retina Mean	S.E.M.
BALB/c+/+[a]	2	3.1	0.3	2.4	0.1
	3	3.5	0.1	2.8	0.1
	6	3.9	0.1	2.9	0.3
	9	4.1	0.3	2.7	0.3
	12	4.1	0.3	3.2	0.5
020/Ards/rds[a]	2	3.0	0.4	3.4	0.4
	3	3.3	0.3	4.4	0.3
	6	3.4	0.2	4.2	0.5
	9	5.5	1.0	7.6	0.1
F_1rds/+[b]	2	3.7	0.2	3.0	0.1
	3	3.6	0.0	3.0	0.1
	6	4.3	0.3	3.9	0.5
	9	4.7	0.2	3.4	0.1
	12	7.2	0.5	5.9	0.4

[a]Sanyal, et. al.[4]
[b]Hawkins, et. al.[5]

the lethal effect of the rds gene is identical for the two receptor types. During the later phase of slow photoreceptor cell loss, however, a small but significant increase of the frequency of the cones is observed, indicating that the rods are slightly more susceptible to later degenerative changes than the cones. But the increase in the frequency of the cones is rather small and in both homozygous and heterozygous mutants, the surviving photoreceptor cells uptill the terminal stage of the disease overwhelmingly represent rods. This is different from the retina of homozygous <u>rd</u> mutant mice, where a differential effect of the gene results, in the later stage of the disease, in a single row of outer nuclei, which almost exclusively represent cones.[25]

IV. OPSIN AND S-ANTIGEN CHANGES

It has been reported earlier that rhodopsin, as measured by a light sensitive peak at 500 nm by absorption spectrophotometry, is undetectable in the homozygous <u>rds</u> mutant mice.[2] Subsequent studies using an enzyme-linked immunoassay[26,27] have shown that opsin is present in the mutant retinas though at a much reduced level. Cellular levels of opsin mRNA have been shown to be similar in the homozygous mutant and normal retinas,[9,28] suggesting that the differences in protein content must arise at the post-transcriptional level. Immunohistochemical observations, as described above, show that cellular localization of both opsin and S-antigen are comparable in the normal and mutant retinas at the earliest stages of photoreceptor cell differentiation, prior to the time of ROS development. The subsequent differences in the level of these two photoreceptor specific proteins, that emerge between the normal and the homozygous and heterozygous mutant retinas, can be seen as the result of maldevelopment of ROS and progressive and differential loss of photoreceptor cells. Table 2 shows

TABLE 2
Comparison of opsin and S-antigen contents of eyes from normal,
homozygous and heterozygous <u>rds</u> mutant mice[a]

Strain genotype	Opsin[b] (nmol/eye)	S-antigen[c] (nmol/eye)	Remarks phenotype
Balb/c+/+	0.38 ±0.01	0.36±0.04	albino
020/A<u>rds/rds</u>	0.010±0.001	0.17±0.02	albino
020/AxBalb/c<u>rds</u>/+	0.19 ±0.04	0.40±0.04	albino
C3H+/+	0.49 ±0.05	0.38±0.02	pigmented
C3Hrds/rds	0.014±0.003	0.20±0.01	pigmented
C3H<u>rds</u>/+xC3H+/+	0.27 ±0.03	0.38±0.02	pigmented

[a]Maximum contents attained at the age of 3-8 weeks.
[b]Schalken et al.,[26,27]
[c]Broekhuyse, De Grip and Sanyal, unpublished. Determination of the values[29] were based on a molecular weight of 45kDa[30].

the maximum average content of opsin and S-antigen per eye of normal and affected individuals for the ages of 3-8 weeks. The amount of opsin in the homozygous mutant eye which has already suffered some cell loss in that period is about 3% of that of the normal. In the heterozygotes, which have not yet suffered any detectable cell loss by then, the amount of opsin is about half of normal. The animals of the pigmented C3H strain are seen to have significantly higher levels of

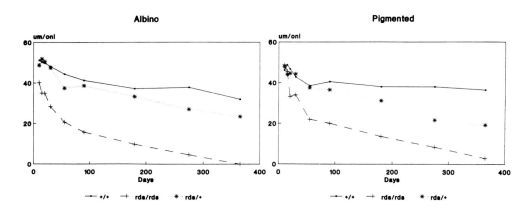

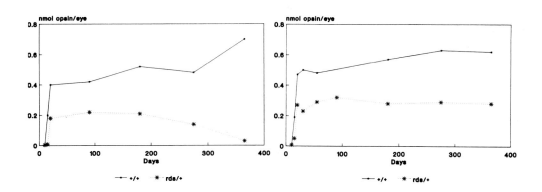

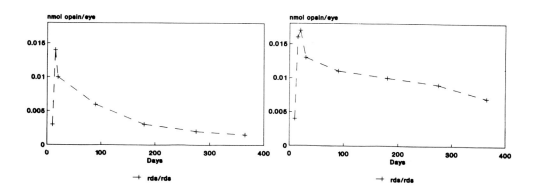

Figure 8. Comparison of the rate of photoreceptor cell loss and changes in the amounts of opsin in the albino and pigmented normal +/+, rds/rds and rds/+ mice. Top: changes in the thickness of the outer nuclear layer (μm/onl) in the central retina. Middle and bottom: changing amounts of opsin (nmol/eye) in the +/+ and rds/+ mice and in the rds/rds mice.

opsin than in the corresponding genotypes of the albino animals. The amounts of S-antigen immunoreactivity in the normal retina of BALB/c and C3H mice are similar and are of equimolar proportion to that of opsin in the BALB/c eye. In the eye of both the pigmented and albino heterozygous mutants, the S-antigen level is similar to normal and thus significantly higher than that of opsin. In the eyes of the homozygous mutants the S-antigen level is stronger reduced in comparison to that in the normal retina but the amounts are much higher than that of opsin. Therefore it appears that S-antigen is more strongly retained intracellularly in the mutant retinas than opsin. This better preservation of S-antigen agrees with the observation that this soluble component normally resides to large proportion in the inner segment.[12] The quite different ratio of opsin to S-antigen in the mutant retina suggests that the desensitization kinetics of the light signal, which partly depends on this ratio, might be affected. This could result in a more rapid decay of the photoreceptor potential in the mutant.

The reduction in the level of opsin in the albino and pigmented homozygous and heterozygous mutant eyes is shown in Figure 8. In general, the reduction in the level of opsin parallels that of photoreceptor cell loss, pigmented animals showing a higher opsin level than their albino counterparts. Particularly noticeable is the consistently higher level of opsin in the pigmented rds/rds mice in comparison to that of the albino rds/rds mice. The increased opsin level at the oldest age of the albino normal mice and the low level in the rds/+ albino mice appear to be out of proportion with the amounts of photoreceptor cell present in the retina at this age. The cause of this discrepancy is not clear but individual differences which prevail in relatively older animals could be a contributory factor. The levels of S-antigen immunoreactivity in the different groups, although better preserved than opsin, show a comparable age dependent reduction (data not shown).

V. STABILITY OF THE ALTERED PHENOTYPE

As mentioned above the slow and continuous death of the photoreceptor cells results in a gradual cell reduction, and in the homozygous mutants, there is eventually a complete elimination of the ONL. Even at this stage critical electron microscopic examination reveals the presence of discrete, isolated photoreceptor cell perikarya along the outer aspect of the neural retina (Figure 9). These cells are still characteristic by the typical perikaryal morphology of the rod or cone types. An axonemal structure consisting of a long cilium surrounded by plasma membrane is present at the receptor end of the cell and a number of membranous vesicles are still located in the vicinity of the cilium. A typical inner segment is not readily demarcated but the base of the cilium and the perikaryal cytoplasm adjoining the cilium are reminiscent of the paraboloid and the myeloid regions of the inner segments of normal photoreceptor cells as the accumulated presence of mitochondria and Golgi cisternae implies (Figure 10). Within the terminals of such photoreceptor cells, which are often somewhat atypically aligned due to cell displacement, essential elements of a photoreceptor synapse are regularly observed.

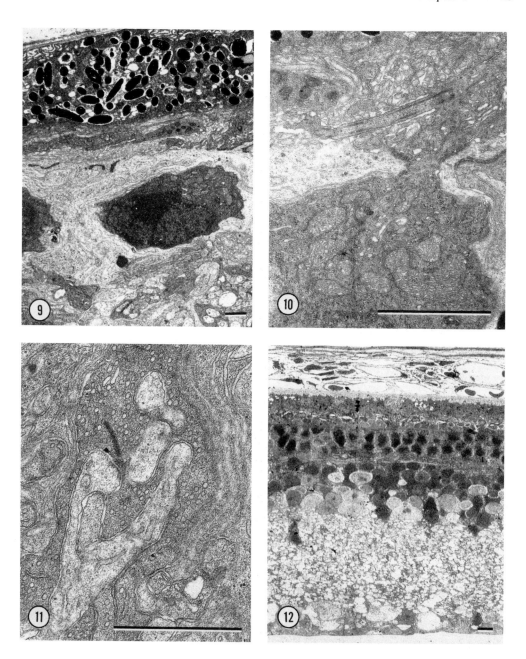

Figure 9. Electron micrograph of outer retina from a 15 month old homozygous <u>rds</u> mutant pigmented mouse; most photoreceptor cells have degenerated but a few isolated cells are still present. Bar=1μm.

Figure 10. The receptor end of a photoreceptor cell in the 15 month old pigmented <u>rds/rds</u> mouse shown in Figure 9. Bar=1μm.

Figure 11. Synaptic structures in a spherule type receptor terminal in the outer plexiform layer of the same retina. Bar=1μm.

Figure 12. Retina from a 3 year old heterozygous <u>rds</u> mutant mouse; note 2-3 rows of photoreceptor cells are still present. Bar=10μm.

While many of these (Figure 11) consist of a single synaptic ribbon, flanked laterally by endings of horizontal cell processes, and medially by bipolar cell dendrites, some of these terminals also show presence of synapses with multiple ribbons and enlarged profiles of such processes. This growth of the synaptic structures within the surviving rod cells have been previously described in detail and has been interpreted as resulting from functional compensation following partial deafferentiation caused by loss of photoreceptor cells.[3,31] Pedicles of cones containing multiple synapses are also observed.

In the retina of heterozygous mutant mice the photoreceptor cells do not degenerate completely. Two or three rows of outer nuclei are still present even in the oldest of the animals examined (Figure 12). The receptor ends of these cells still contain whorls of ROS membranes. These are slightly reduced in length but are otherwise comparable to those of the younger animals. The photoreceptor terminals also contain synaptic structures resembling those of the rods and cones of younger heterozygotes. Therefore it can be concluded on the basis of morphological findings that the primary phenotypic effect of the rds gene is on the structure of the ROS disc membranes. The effect is not immediately lethal and for so long as the photoreceptor cells survive in the retina of the homozygous and heterozygous mutant mice, the cellular phenotypes, as altered by the dose dependent expression of the rds gene, remain stable.

VI. SUMMARY AND CONCLUSIONS

In the developing photoreceptor cells, both opsin and S-antigen are initially localized over the perikarya and no difference between the normal and mutant retinas is detected. With the emergence and growth of the inner and outer segments, opsin is increasingly localized over the Golgi cisternae, ciliary plasma membrane and finally over the disc membranes of the rods, while the membranes over the rest of the cell become free from opsin. In this time-period of development of the homozygous mutant mice retina the plasma membrane over the ciliary protrusion becomes immunoreactive for both proteins. Although ROS discs remain absent, the emerging membrane bound vesicles show immunoreactivity for both proteins, but the plasma membranes over the perikarya and the receptor terminals continue to show immunoreactivity for both proteins as well. In the heterozygotes cellular localization of both opsin and S-antigen are comparable to normal even though ROS discs are grossly abnormal in form. Although there is some decline in the level of immunoreactivity in the retina of relatively older mutant mice, the cellular localization of both opsin and S-antigen in the photoreceptor cells remains unaltered throughout the survival period of these cells.

Immunoassay of opsin and S-antigen in the retinal extracts of normal and mutant mice at different ages have shown an initial rise accompanying the postnatal development of the retina; the peak levels are reached around the age of 4 weeks in all three genotypes, but the S-antigen level is much less affected by the mutation than the opsin level. Thereafter a slow decline in the levels of both of these proteins is recorded with age. This decline in the photoreceptor specific protein closely parallels the rate of photoreceptor cell loss.

Thus on the basis of immunohistochemical observations and immunoassay it can be concluded that the photoreceptor cells in the rds mutant retina continue to synthesize key molecular components necessary for photosensory function.

Ultrastructural observations on the photoreceptor cells at different ages, particularly in the very old animals at an advanced stage of the disease, have confirmed that the receptor elements, though characteristically altered in the homozygous and heterozygous mutants, are retained. The synaptic contacts of the cells are also maintained and, in some instances even enlarged. Thus on the basis of ultrastructure, immunohistochemistry and immunoassay it can be concluded that the altered phenotypic trait is structurally stable. In other words, the photoreceptor cells in the rds mutant mice during the long period that intervenes between the initial and primary effect of the gene and ultimate cell death, retain their functional potential.

We propose, that this aspect has an important clinical perspective. An essential starting point in the development of a therapeutic approach in confronting the clinical problem of Retinitis Pigmentosa will have to aim at identifying the factors that prolong the life of the photoreceptor cells. As an animal model, the rds mice with a long but variable survival period of the photoreceptor cells in the homozygous and heterozygous individuals, appear to be a very promising test material for experimental animal studies addressing this aspect.

Acknowledgement. Authors' thanks are due to R. K. Hawkins, Mrs. E. D. Kuhlmann for expert technical assistance, Ellen Voigt for management of the mouse colony and René Jansen for the graphic work. The study was supported by Grant EY 06841 (SS) and EY 01244 (GA) from the National Eye Institute, Bethesda, Md., RP Foundation Fighting Blindness and the Swedish Natural Science Research Council Grant 4644300 (TvV).

VII. REFERENCES

1. Van Nie, R., Iványi, D. and Démant, P., A new H-2 linked mutation, rds causing retinal degeneration in the mouse, Tissue Antigens, 12, 106, 1978.
2. Sanyal, S. and Jansen H. G., Absence of receptor outer segments in the retina of rds mutant mice, Neurosci. Letters, 21, 23, 1981.
3. Jansen, H. G., Sanyal, S., Development and degeneration of retina in rds mutant mice: Electron microscopy, J. Comp. Neurol., 224, 71, 1984.
4. Sanyal, S., De Ruiter, A. and Hawkins, R. K., Development and degeneration of retina in rds mutant mice: Light microscopy, J. Comp. Neurol., 194, 193, 1980.
5. Hawkins, R. K., Jansen, H. G. and Sanyal, S., Development and degeneration of retina in rds mutant mice: Photoreceptor abnormalities in the heterozygotes, Exp. Eye Res. 41, 701, 1985.
6. Sanyal, S., Cellular site of expression and genetic interaction of the rd and the rds loci in the retina of the mouse, Degenerative Retinal Disorders: Clinical and Laboratory Investigations, Hollyfield, J. G., Anderson, R. E. and LaVail, M. M., Eds., Alan Liss, Inc., New York, 1987, 175.
7. Sanyal, S. and Zeilmaker, G. H., Development and degeneration of

retina in <u>rds</u> mutant mice: light and electron microscopic observations in experimental chimaeras, <u>Exp. Eye Res.</u>, 39, 231, 1984.

8. Sanyal, S., Dees, C. and Zeilmaker, G. H., Development and degeneration of retina in <u>rds</u> mutant mice: observations in chimaeras of heterozygous mutant and normal genotype, <u>J. Embryol. exp. Morph.</u>, 98, 111, 1986.

9. Travis, G. H., Brennan, M. B., Danielson, P. E., Kozak, C. A. and Sutcliffe, J. G., Identification of a photoreceptor specific mRNA encoded by the gene responsible for retinal degeneration slow (<u>rds</u>), <u>Nature</u>, 338, 70, 1989.

10. Connel, G. J. and Molday, R. S., Molecular cloning, primary structure and orientation of the vertebrate photoreceptor cell protein peripherin in the rod outer segment disk membrane, <u>Biochemistry</u>, 29, 4691, 1990.

11. Pfister, C., Chabre, M., Plouet, J., Tuyen, V. V., De Kozak, Y., Faure, J. P. and Kuehn, H., Retinal S antigen identified as the 48K protein regulating light dependent phosphodiesterase in rods, <u>Science</u>, 228, 891, 1985.

12. Broekhuyse, R. M., Tolhuizen, E. F. J., Janssen, A. P. M. and Winkens, H. J., Light induced shift and binding of S-antigen in retinal rods, <u>Curr. Eye Res.</u>, 4, 613, 1985.

13. Wilden, U., Hall, S. W. and Kühn, H., Phosphodiesterase activation by photoexcited rhodopsin is quenced when rhodopsin is phosphorylated and binds the intrinsic 48-kDa protein of rod outer segments, <u>Proc. Natl. Acad. Sci. USA</u>, 83, 1174, 1986.

14. Van Veen, T., Cantera, R., Narfstrom, K., Nilsson, S. E., Sanyal, S., Wiggert, B. and Chader, G. J., <u>Degenerative Retinal Disorders: Clinical and Laboratory Investigations</u>, Hollyfield, J. G., Anderson, R. E. and LaVail, M. M., Eds., Alan Liss, Inc., New York, 1989, 275.

15. Jansen, H. G., Aguirre, G. D., Van Veen, T. and Sanyal, S., Development and degeneration of retina in <u>rds</u> mutant mice: Ultraimmunohistochemical localization of S-antigen, <u>Curr. Eye Res.</u>, 9, 903, 1990.

16. Jansen, H. G., Sanyal, S., De Grip, W. J. and Schalken, J. J., Development and degeneration of retina in <u>rds</u> mutant mice: Ultraimmunohistochemical localization of opsin, <u>Exp. Eye Res.</u>, 44, 347, 1987.

17. Usukura, J. and Bok, D., Opsin localization and glycosylation in the developing Balb/c and <u>rds</u> mouse retina, <u>Degenerative Retinal Disorders: Clinical and Laboratory Investigations</u>, Hollyfield, J. G., Anderson, R. E. and LaVail, M. M., Eds., Alan Liss, Inc., New York, 1987, 195.

18. Nir, I. and Papermaster, D. S., Immunocytochemical localization of opsin in the inner segment and ciliary plasma membrane of photoreceptors in retina of <u>rds</u> mutant mice, <u>Invest. Ophthalmol. Vis. Sci.</u>, 27, 836, 1986.

19. Cohen, A. I., Some cytological and initial biochemical observations on photoreceptors in retinas of <u>rds</u> mice, <u>Invest. Ophthalmol. Vis. Sci.</u>, 24, 832, 1983.

20. LaVail, M. M., Kinetics of rod outer segment renewal in the developing mouse retina, <u>J. Cell Biol.</u>, 58, 650, 1973.

21. Sanyal, S. and Hawkins, R. K., Development and degeneration of

retina in <u>rds</u> mutant mice: altered disc shedding pattern in the albino heterozygotes and its relation to light exposure, <u>Vision Res.</u>, 28, 1171, 1988.

22. Sanyal, S. and Hawkins, R. K., Development and degeneration of retina in <u>rds</u> mutant mice: altered disc shedding pattern in the heterozygotes and its relation to ocular pigmentation, <u>Curr. Eye Res.</u>, 8, 1093, 1989.

23. Reuter, J. H. and Sanyal, S., Development and degeneration of reina in <u>rds</u> mutant mice: the electroretinogram, <u>Neurosci.Lett.</u>, 48, 231, 1984.

24. Sanyal, S. and Hawkins, R. K., Development and degeneration of retina in <u>rds</u> mutant mice: Effects of pigmentation, constant light and light deprivation on the rate of degeneration, <u>Vision Res.</u>, 26, 1177, 1986.

25. Carter-Dawson, L. D., LaVail, M. M. and Sidman, R. L., Differential effect of the <u>rd</u> mutation on rods and cones in the mouse retina, <u>Invest. Ophthalmol. Visual Sci.</u>, 17, 489, 1978.

26. Schalken, J. J., Janssen, J. J. M., De Grip, W. J., Hawkins, R. K. and Sanyal, S., Immunoassay of rod visual pigment (opsin) in the eyes of <u>rds</u> mutant mice lacking receptor outer segments, <u>Biochem. Biophys. Acta</u>, 839, 122, 1985.

27. Schalken, J. J., Janssen, J. J. M., Sanyal, S., Hawkins, R. K. and De Grip, W. J., Development and degeneration of retina in <u>rds</u> mutant mice: immunassay of the rod visual pigment rhodopsin, <u>Biochem. Biophys. Acta</u>, 1033, 103, 1990.

28. Nir, I., Agarwal, N. and Papermaster, D. S., Opsin gene expression during early and late phases of retinal degeneration in <u>rds</u> mice, <u>Exp. Eye Res.</u>, 51, 257, 1990.

29. Broekhuyse, R. M. and Kuhlmann, E. D., Assay of S-antigen immunoreactivity in mammalian retinas in relation to age, ocular dimension and retinal degeneration, <u>Jpn. J. Ophthalmol.</u>, 33, 243, 1989.

30. Shinohara, T., Donoso, L., Tsuda, M., Yamaki, K. and Singh, V. K., S-antigen: structure, function and experimental autoimmune uveitis (EAU), <u>Progr. Ret. Res.</u> 8, 51, 1988.

31. Sanyal, S. and Jansen, H. G., A comparative survey of synaptic changes in the rod photoreceptor terminals of <u>rd</u>, <u>rds</u> and double homozygous mutant mice, <u>Inherited and environmentally induced retinal degenerations</u>, LaVail, M. M., Hollyfield, J. G. and Anderson, R. E., Eds., Alan Liss, Inc., New York, 1989, 233.

RETINAL DEGENERATION IN VITRO: COMPARISON OF POSTNATAL RETINAL
DEVELOPMENT OF NORMAL, rd AND rds MUTANT MICE IN ORGAN CULTURE

A.R.Caffé and S.Sanyal

Department of Anatomy, Erasmus University Rotterdam, Faculty of
Medicine, P.O.Box 1738, 3000 DR Rotterdam, Netherlands.

I. INTRODUCTION

Earlier attempts to simulate retinal degeneration in vitro have
reported limited success[1,2] and Sidman observed that the rate of
degeneration i.e., photoreceptor cell loss was, to a certain degree,
dependent on optimal development of the retina, more particularly the
receptor elements.[3] Recently we have described an organ culture
technique whereby the whole neural retina of the neonatal mouse can be
grown in vitro for 3 to 4 weeks.[4] In this system, the retinal explant
from genetically normal mouse develops a histotypic pattern comparable
to the in vivo counterpart. Perikaryal differentiation of rods and
cones was regularly obtained and electron microscopic observations
further revealed that receptor outer segments (ROS) containing profuse
disc membranes were also developed in explants containing retinal
pigment epithelium (RPE). Elements of synaptic contacts were also
regularly observed in the cultured retinas at the end of 3-4 weeks.
Although the ROS were reduced in length and irregular in form, and the
synaptic structures, formed in vitro, were also somewhat retarded in
comparison to those of mature retina, the essential components of the
photoreceptor cells were clearly recognized to have differentiated.
This partial success in obtaining some degree of photoreceptor
differentiation in vitro prompted us to apply the technique to the
analysis of mice bearing mutations causing retinal degeneration.
    In human Retinitis Pigmentosa (RP) visual cells selectively
degenerate due to mutant genes (see review).[5] Inquiries into how
genetic lesions lead to visual cell death have made experiments with
animal models having similar defects essential. The rd (retinal
degeneration)[6] and rds (retinal degeneration slow)[7] mice show an
inherited retinal degeneration reminiscent of human RP. In the rd
mouse the affected photoreceptor cells show rudimentary outer segments
in the first postnatal week.[8,9] However, further development is
arrested and is followed by rapid visual cell death leading to one row
of cone nuclei within 3 weeks.[10] In the homozygous rds mouse the outer
segments are never formed[11,12] and the photoreceptor cells degenerate
slowly over a period of about one year.[13]
    In this chapter we describe the first observations on the
genotypic differentiation of retina from the homozygous mutant rd and
rds mice in organ culture. This will be compared with similarly
cultured retinas from the genetically normal mouse. The purpose is to
evaluate and discuss the suitability of the in vitro system to study
the factors affecting the pathogenesis in the diseased retina.

II. MATERIALS AND METHODS

Pigmented C3H<u>rd</u>[+] mice, a subline of C3HfHeA<u>rd</u> strain, in which the <u>rd</u> gene has been substituted by the normal allele[9] were used as the source of normal retina. Two congenic lines of mice, C3H<u>rd</u>/<u>rd</u> and C3H<u>rds</u>/<u>rds</u> provided the two mutant retinas. All animals used in this study were obtained from sib matings. Maintenance and use of animals were undertaken in strict accordance with ethical standards guided by the Experiments on Animals Act of the Netherlands.

A. CULTURE TECHNIQUE

Newborn mice, between 36 and 48 hours after birth were used in all experiments and were found to be the most satisfactory in terms of separation of the neural retina with the RPE from the rest of the ocular tissues. Animals were quickly decapitated with a pair of scissors and the heads were dipped in 70% ethanol and transferred to a laminar flow cabinet in the culture room where all subsequent handling were performed in sterile conditions. The eyes were immediately removed and placed in a petridish containing culture medium at room temperature. The culture medium R 16 was prepared[14] from basal medium (GIBCO) as described earlier.[4]

A brief enzyme treatment of the eyeball at this stage facilitated isolation of the intact neural retina with the attached RPE. For this purpose, the eyeballs were incubated in 1.2% proteinase K (BDH) dissolved in the culture medium, without added serum, for 10-15 minutes at 37° C. After enzyme treatment the eyes were washed twice in culture medium with 10% fetal calf serum and transferred back to medium without added serum. Next, using a dissecting microscope, an incision was made in the eyeball behind the limbus and extended around the eye with iridectomy scissors. The cornea-iris complex, lens and the vitreous body were removed, and the retina with RPE attached was separated from the eyecup. The tissue was placed flat on a carrier membrane device with the vitreal surface facing upwards. Low water extractable nitrocellulose filters (HATF 04700, pore size 0.45 μm were purchased from Millipore. Pieces of approximately 10 mm square were prepared and soldered on a coarse-meshed polyamide gauze grid of 2 cm square. The carrier devices were sterilized by exposure to ethylene oxide gas.
The carrier device with explant attached was placed in a 6-well culture dish with 1.3-1.6 ml of culture medium, containing 10% fetal calf serum. The amount of culture medium was so applied as to reach to the upper surface of the explant. The culture dish was placed on a rocking apparatus in the incubator (Figure 1). The rocking system was mildly tilted once in every 30 seconds. There was no light in the incubator. Organ cultures were incubated at 37°C in a humidified 5% CO_2, 95% air atmosphere for one to 4 weeks. The culture medium was replaced three times a week.

B. HISTOLOGICAL PROCEDURE

After scheduled culture period, the tissues, still attached to the carrier device, were fixed in either 4% paraformaldehyde or 2% glutaraldehyde in 0.1 M Cacodylate buffer pH 7.2 for 2 to 3 hours. The membrane filter with fixed explant was then detached from the supporting grid. The filter, attached with the tissue facilitated the histological processing and avoided tissue damage. Subsequently the tissue was dehydrated in graded ethanol and embedded in paraffin. Sections were stained with haematoxylin. Explants were routinely examined after 7, 11, 14, 21 and 28 days in culture. Data from 74, 62 and 39 normal, <u>rd</u> and <u>rds</u> explants, respectively, were collected for the present report. At least 6 explants of each age were included.

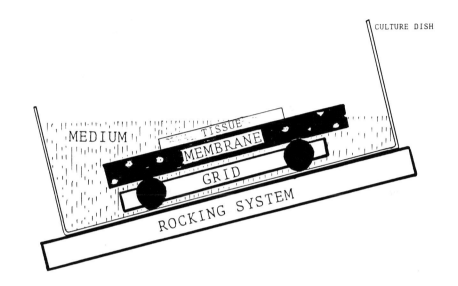

Figure 1. A cross sectionional diagram of the organ culture set up used for growing whole neonatal mouse retina. The retina adhered to the membrane filter along the scleral surface of the retinal pigment epithelium. Culture medium reached upto the vitreal side of the tissue. The intermittent movement of the rocking system facilitated metabolic exchange at the various interfaces.

III. RESULTS

The retinal materials, used for culture, were in all cases obtained from neonatal mice, between 36 and 48 hours after birth. The enzyme treatment of younger tissue caused patchy attachment of the RPE to the neural retina, and longer enzyme incubations led to tissue damage. The best type of explant was that of neural retina with RPE attached, since it had been shown that presence of RPE was essential for the development of ROS. Retina with RPE and mesenchymal tissue gave increased variability in tissue lamination. Therefore, neural retina with RPE attached was adopted as the standard starting material for cultivation <u>in</u> <u>vitro</u>. The explants attached firmly to the membrane; irregularities in carrier membrane or infolding of the explant sometimes resulted in distortion of the laminar organization of the retina. The use of excess culture medium also appear to cause increased

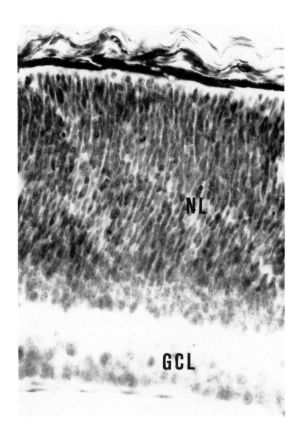

Figure 2. Section of the retina from a newborn mouse at the beginning of the culture period. Note that the retina consists of one neuroblast layer (NL) and a presumptive ganglion cell layer (GCL) at this stage of development. RPE, retinal pigment epithelium.

cell death and distortion of the explant.

At the time of explantation the neonatal retinas of normal, rd and rds mutant mice appeared morphologically similar (Figure 2) and consisted of a thick layer of neuroblast cells and a well demarcated multiple cell layer of presumptive ganglion cells. The course of development in the first week in vitro was the same for all types of tissue. In all explants examined the neuroblast layer developed into distinct inner and outer nuclear layers with intervening plexiform layers. A number of pycnotic nuclei, normal to this developmental stage, were observed in the outer and inner nuclear layer. After 7 to 8 days in culture all explants had an outer nuclear layer of comparable thickness (Figure 3) which was similar to their in vivo counterparts. In the center of the explants the thickness of the tissue was often slightly thinner than that of the retina in vivo but the difference was not really large. However, all the explants progressively became thinner at their margins. In all explants some degree of folding or waviness could be detected and a few small rosette like arrangements were also formed. But these were localized to small regions of the explants and did not disturb the normal lamination or thickness of the retina.

A. IN VITRO HISTOGENESIS OF NORMAL RETINA

After 11 days in vitro the photoreceptor layer of the genetically normal retina had increased in width. This thickness of the outer nuclear layer (ONL) did not change to any appreciable degree during the entire culture period for up to 4 weeks. The rod and cone nuclei could be easily distinguished. Furthermore, at 14 days in vitro (Figure 4a), developing receptor elements could be observed as a distinct layer

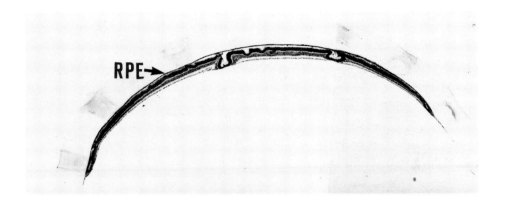

Figure 3. Section of neural retina with retinal pigment epithelium (RPE) of normal mouse after 11 days in culture. Note the distinct inner and outer nuclear layers and the plexiform layers. Some waving and rosette formation characteristic of most explants can be observed.

over the outer limiting membrane. These receptor elements elongated with further development of the tissue during the culture period (Figure 4b). However, they never attained the length of photoreceptor outer segments of comparable age in vivo. In general, normal explants could be cultured for 4 weeks without significant loss of retinal cells or distortion of gross tissue morphology.

B. IN VITRO HISTOGENESIS OF RD RETINA

Retina from the homozygous rd mutant mouse developed inner and outer nuclear layers by 7 to 8 days in vitro as in the normal mice. By 11 days an increased number of pycnotic nuclei was observed in the ONL. The degenerative changes in the rd retina proceeded further with the extension of the culture period. At 14 days, the outer nuclear layer was reduced to about 4 rows. This reduction of the photoreceptor cell nuclei occured over the whole explant (Figure 5a), but a moderate degree of variability in thickness of nuclear layer was observed between the different parts of an explant and also between the explants. At 21 or 28 days in vitro only a single row of dispersed photoreceptor cell nuclei were encountered in the rd retina (Figure 5b). At light microscopical level, the neuronal and glial cells comprising the inner retina appeared to be normal and comparable with that of its in vivo counterpart.

C. IN VITRO HISTOGENESIS OF RDS RETINA

At 11 days in vitro the retina from the homozygous rds mice developed a normal histotypic morphology. The ONL comprised of many rows of visual cell nuclei. Rod and cone perikarya could be distinguished and no sign of abnormal photoreceptor cell degeneration was encountered at 14 days in culture (Figure 6a). At 3 and 4 weeks (Figure 6b) in culture, the outer nuclear layer of the rds retina still

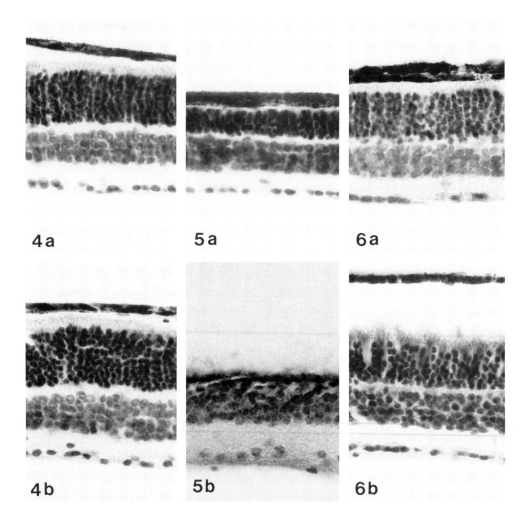

4a   5a   6a

4b   5b   6b

Figure 4-6. Photomicrographs of sections from organ cultured retina from normal, rd and rds mutant mice after (a) 14 days and after (b) 28 days in vitro.

Figure 4. Retina from the normal mouse.

Figure 5. Retina from the rd mutant mouse. Note reduction in the thickness of the ONL after 14 days (a); after 4 weeks (b) a single row of outer nuclei is present.

Figure 6. Retina from the rds mutant mouse. The ONL is seen to be only marginally reduced after 28 days (b).

had a healthy appearance. However, some degree of variability in the thickness of the ONL was present between the explants. In most cases the ONL appeared to be of normal thickness, while in some cases the layer was slightly reduced. A reduced receptor layer, could still be observed in the older cultures.

IV. DISCUSSION

The foregoing results demonstrate that the organ culture technique described here supports large scale cultivation of neonatal mouse retina that permits histotypic differentiation of normal and mutant genotypes for relatively long term. The postnatal development of retina from mice of the three different genotypes observed _in vitro_ can be divided in two distinct phases. The first phase involves the histogenesis of the retinal layers, including the differentiation of the photoreceptor cell layer. In very general terms and as observed at the light microscopical level, the explants from the normal and the two mutant retinas show signs of developmental progress as _in vivo_ until about 10-11 days _in vitro._ Electron microscopic observations on the cultured normal retina at this stage have revealed consistent presence of ROS discs and synaptic structures.[10] Immunohistochemical studies in progress[15] have succeeded in localizing photoreceptor specific proteins such as opsin, intercellular retinol binding protein and S-antigen; glial specific glial fibrillary acidic protein (GFAP) as well as transmitter substances such as GABA in different compartments of the cultured retina. Although some deviations from the normal pattern have been identified these observations have provided evidence for tissue specific differentiation of the retinal cells _in vitro_.

The second phase of the postnatal development _in vitro_ has registered differential survival of the photoreceptor cells in the normal and the two different mutant retinas. The main intention of this study is to examine this phase of retinal development _in vitro_ and examine the suitability of the methodological approach in realizing an _in vitro_ system for the analysis of gene expression on retina. In the normal retinal explant, the cell population in the different layers remain essentially intact over the culture period. In a number of recent studies specific factors mediating through cellular interactions such as between RPE and photoreceptor cells,[16] glial[17] and ganglion cells[18] have been recognized or anticipated as necessary for prolonged cell survival. Similarly, survival crisis encountered in sustaining normal photoreceptor cells from neonatal mouse retina in dispersed cell culture has been attributed to failure or breakdown in the working of such factors.[19,20] Thus the organ culture technique used for the cultivation of neural retina together with the attached RPE appears to fulfill at least the minimum essential requirements for the sustained growth, development and survival of the mouse retina.

In the rd/rd retina _in vitro,_ the beginning of photoreceptor cell death, marked by the appearance of pycnotic nuclei, at 11 days and rapid progress of the disease process, marked by the reduction of the ONL, appear to be very similar to the degeneration pattern observed _in vivo,_[8,9] the rest of the retinal layers remaining largely intact. Therefore, under the conditions of the organ culture, the expression of the rd gene can be evaluated to be as effective as _in vivo_. In the rds/rds retina on the other hand, despite the early effect of the gene observed in the altered phenotype of the photoreceptor cells, actual photoreceptor cell death is very slow, and is even slower in the pigmented C3H mice[21] used in this study. The marginal reduction of the ONL and preservation of the retinal layers in the rds/rds retina at the end of 4 weeks in vitro also appear to parallel the histogenetic changes in vivo. Therefore, the differential survival of the photo-receptor cells in the rd, rds mutant, and normal retinal explants results from true phenotypic expressions of their genotypic dif-ferences.

Recently the primary molecular defects in the rd and rds disorders have been identified. In the rd retina, changes in the beta subunit of the enzyme phosphodiesterase[22] is the underlying defect leading to excess accumulation of cyclic GMP and eventual cell death.[23] In the rds retina, an insertion within the sequence of the gene[24] results in malfunction of peripherin, a key protein essential for the assembly of ROS discs.[25,26] In both of these disorders, the immediate cause of cell death is not known. In other words, it is yet to be learned how the primary molecular defects affect the metabolic pathways of the photoreceptor cells and produce their lethal effect. The large scale cultivation of normal and mutant retinas allowing reasonably normal and comparable to in vivo development makes the tissue accessible to direct experimentation and adds a new dimension to the usefulness of these mutants as models for RP.

V. SUMMARY

An organ culture technique has been developed which supports the histogenesis of retina from newborn mouse over the postnatal period. In this technique the whole neural retina with the RPE attached is separated from the eye by partial enzyme digestion and microdissection and cultivated in toto on a flat membrane filter support. In a comparative study retinas from genetically normal, rd and rds mutant homozygous mice have been grown for periods up to four weeks and their histogenetic state has been examined at regular intervals. During the early phase, development of the different layers in the retina of the three different genotypes is similar and the tissue appears normal. At the end of the 4 weeks, the normal retina still remained intact and largely comparable to the in vivo retina except for a reduced receptor and outer plexiform layer. In the rd/rd retina a selective loss of photoreceptor cells, starting from around 11 days in vitro resulted in rapid reduction of the ONL to a single row at 3-4 weeks as in vivo. In the rds/rds retina reduction of the ONL, during the same period in vitro, was only marginal. The other retinal layers remained intact, healthy and similar in all the three types of explants. Therefore the in vitro system developed here can be considered as capable of providing necessary support for the differentiation of the essential components of the photoreceptor cells to the point that symptoms of genetically caused pathogenesis are easily defined and follow a time course that is comparable to the disease process in vivo. Thus organ culture of mammalian retina as a model system offers a unique opportu-nity to undertake direct experimental studies on factors controlling gene expression and eventually photoreceptor cell survival.

Ackowledgements. Authors' thanks are due to Richard Hawkins and Ellen Voigt for technical assistance and maintance of the mouse colony. This work was supported by Grant EY 06841 from the National Eye Institute, Bethesda, Md.

REFERENCES

1. Lucas, D. R., Inherited retinal dystrophy in the mouse: its appearance in eyes and retinae cultured <u>in</u> <u>vitro</u>, <u>J. Embryol. Exp. Morph.</u>, 6, 589, 1958.

2. Sidman, R. L., Tissue culture studies of inherited retinal dystrophy, <u>Dis. Nerv. System.</u> 22, 14, 1961.

3. Sidman, R. L., Organ culture analysis of inherited retinal degeneration in rodents, <u>Natl. Cancer Inst. Monogr.,</u> 11, 227, 1963.

4. Caffé, A.R., Visser, H., Jansen, H. G., and Sanyal, S., Histotypic differentiation of neonatal mouse retina in organ culture, <u>Curr. Eye Res.,</u> 8, 1083, 1989.

5. Bird, A. C., Clinical investigations of Retinitis Pigmentosa, <u>Degenerative Retinal Disorders: Clinical and Laboratory Investigations,</u> Hollyfield, J. G., Anderson, R. E. and LaVail, M. M., Eds., Alan Liss, Inc., New York, 1987, 3.

6. Sidman, R.I., and Green, M.C., Retinal degeneration in the mouse; Location of the <u>rd</u> locus in linkage group XVIII, <u>J. Hered.,</u> 56, 23, 1965.

7. Van Nie, R., Ivanyi, D., and Demant, P., A new H-2 linked mutation, <u>rds</u> causing retinal degeneration in the mouse, <u>Tiss. Antigens,</u> 12, 106, 1978.

8. Caley, D. W., Johnson, C. and Liebelt, R. A., The postnatal development of the retina in the normal and rodless CBA mouse: a light and electron microscopic study, <u>Am. J. Anat.,</u> 133, 179, 1972.

9. Sanyal, S., and Bal, A.K., Comparative light and electron microscopic study of retinal histogenesis in normal and <u>rd</u> mutant mice. <u>z. Anat. EntwGesch.,</u> 142, 219, 1973.

10. Carter-Dawson, L. D., LaVail, M. M. and Sidman, R. L., Differential effect of the <u>rd</u> mutation on rods and cones in the mouse retina, <u>Invest. Ophthalmol. Vis. Sci.,</u> 17, 489, 1978.

11. Sanyal, S., and Jansen, H. G., Absence of receptor outer segments in the retina of the <u>rds</u> mutant mice, <u>Neurosci. Lett.,</u> 21, 23, 1981.

12. Jansen, H. G. and Sanyal, S., Development and degeneration of retina in <u>rds</u> mutant mice: Electron microscopy, <u>J. Comp. Neurol.,</u> 224, 71, 1984.

13. Sanyal, S., De Ruiter, A., and Hawkins, R.K., Development and degeneration of retina in <u>rds</u> mutant mice: Light microscopy, <u>J. Comp. Neurol.,</u> 194, 193, 1980.

14. Romijn, H. J., De Jong, B. M. and Ruyter, J. M., A procedure for culturing rat neocortex explants in a serum-free nutrient medium, <u>J. Neurosci. Methods,</u> 23, 75, 1988.

15. Caffé, A. R., Sanyal, S., Chader, G. J. and Van Veen, T., unpublished data, 1990.

16. Spoerri, P.I., Ulshafer, R.J., Ludwig, H.C., Allen, C.B. and Kelley, K.C., Photoreceptor cell development *in vitro*: influence of pigment epithelium conditioned medium on outer segment differentiation, *Eur. J. Cell Biol.*, 46, 362, 1988.

17. Burke, J.M., Growth in retinal glial cells in vitro is affected differentially by two types of cell contact-mediated interactions, *Exp. Cell Res.*, 180, 13, 1989.

18. Lehwalder, D., Jeffrey, P.L. and Unsicker, K., Survival of purified embryonic chick retinal ganglion cells in the presence of neurotrophic factors, *J. Neurosci. Res.*, 24, 329, 1989.

19. Politi, L. E. and Adler, R., Selective failure of long term survival of isolated photoreceptors from both homozygous and heterozygous *rd* (retinal degeneration) mice, *Exp. Eye Res.*, 47, 269, 1988.

20. Adler, R. and Politi, L., Expression of a "survival crisis" by normal and *rd/rd* mouse photoreceptor cells *in vitro*, in *Inherited and Environmentally Induced Retinal Degeneration*, Hollyfield, J.G., Anderson, R.E., and LaVail, M.M., Eds., Alan R. Liss, New York, 1989, 169.

21. Sanyal, S. and Hawkins, R. K., Development and degeneration of retina in *rds* mutant mice: effects of light on the rate of degeneration in albino and pigmented homozygous and heterozygous mutant and normal mice, *Vision Res.*, 26, 1177, 1986.

22. Bowes, C., Tiansen, L., Danciger, M., Baxter L. C., Applebury, M. L. and Farber, D. B., Retinal degeneration in the *rd* mouse is caused by a defect in the ß subunit of rod cGMP-phosphodiesterase, *Nature*, 347, 677, 1990.

23. Farber, D. B. and Lolley, R. N., Cyclic guanosine monophosphate: Elevation in degenerating photoreceptor cells of the C3H mouse retina, *Science*, 186, 449, 1974.

24. Travis, G.H., Brennen, M.B., Danielson, P.E., Kozak, C.A., and Sutcliffe, J.G., Identification of a photoreceptor-specific mRNA encoded by the gene responsible for retinal degeneration slow (RDS), *Nature*, 338, 70, 1989.

25. Connell, G., Boscom, R., McInnes, R. and Molday, R. S., Photoreceptor cell peripherin is the defective protein responsible for retinal degeneration slow (rds), *Invest. Ophthalmol. Vis. Sci.*, 31, (Suppl.) 309, 1990.

26. Connel, G. J. and Molday, R. S., Molecular cloning, primary structure and orientation of the vertebrate photoreceptor cell protein peripherin in the rod outer segment disc membrane, *Biochemistry*, 29, 4691, 1990.

CONGENITAL NIGHT BLINDNESS AND PARTIAL DAY BLINDNESS IN THE BRIARD DOG

Sven Erik G. Nilsson[a], Anders Wrigstad[a] and Kristina Narfström[a,b]

[a]Department of Ophthalmology, University of Linköping, S-581 85 Linköping, Sweden and [b]Department of Surgery and Medicine, Faculty of Veterinary Medicine, Swedish University of Agricultural Sciences, S-750 07 Uppsala, Sweden

I.   INTRODUCTION

Human congenital stationary night blindness (CSNB) is found in two main types, the Schubert-Bornschein type[1] and the Riggs type.[2] The former type may be subdivided into a complete and an incomplete type.[3] The Schubert-Bornschein type shows a normal a-wave an absent or very reduced b-wave in the electroretinogram (ERG) (a "negative" ERG).[1] In such a case, the rhodopsin concentration and rate of regeneration after bleaching (fundus reflectometry) were found to be normal.[4] Therefore, this type has been considered to be a neural (synaptic) transmission defect.[4,5] In the Riggs type, the ERG a- and b-waves are generally both very reduced.[2] Sometimes only a minimal photopic response can be elicited. Also in such a case, both the concentration and rate of regeneration after bleaching of rhodopsin were found to be normal.[4] On this basis, the Riggs type has been thought to be a transduction defect.[4,5] In light microscopy, retinal and pigment epithelial (PE) histology was found to be normal in cases of CSNB.[6]

The Appaloosa horse model of hereditary night blindness showed an ERG, where only the a-wave could be recorded (similar to the Schubert-Bornschein type).[7] The retina was ultrastructurally normal. Transmission densitometry of the isolated retina showed an ample supply of rhodopsin.[5] The night blind Pearl mouse also showed normal photoreceptor outer and inner segments and normal rhodopsin content, but a reduced number of melanosomes and basal membrane infoldings in the PE, as well as changes in the PE basal lamina and in the photoreceptor synapses. The retinal ganglion cell axon responses were reduced.[8]

A strain of Briard dogs with congenital night blindness (CNB) and normal or nearly normal day vision was observed in Sweden (Narfström). Inheritance is still uncertain, but will be clarified after more matings. Initial AC ERG recordings demonstrated that the a- and b-waves were barely recordable or non-recordable (similar to Riggs type).[9] The 30 Hz flicker ERG was reduced but present, indicating that cones were better preserved than rods.

An American strain of Briard dogs was presented at ARVO 1989.[10] These dogs showed a plasma concentration of arachidonic acid which was doubled, as well as elevated levels of cholesterol and other lipids (LDL). Lipid inclusions were found in the PE, and the photoreceptors were damaged.

We were able to investigate further the offspring of a brother and a sister of the original CNB Briard dogs. This second generation of dogs showed an aggravation of the disease, however, since in addition to night blindness they also showed markedly to severely reduced day vision. Thus, the results presented here refer to dogs with night blindness and more or less reduced day vision. The ultrastructural and ERG findings were presented in a preliminary form at ARVO 1990.[11] So far, it seems that the disease is stationary, but we cannot be certain until the dogs have been followed for a longer period of time.

II. MATERIAL AND METHODS

A. DOGS

The eyes of 10 affected Briard puppies, 6 weeks to 1 year old, all belonging to the same litter, and 3 normal controls: 1 Border Collie, 1 Hamilton Harrier and 1 German Shepherd, 2 -13 years old, were studied ultrastructurally. Direct current (DC) electroretinography was performed on 5 affected Briard puppies, 7-12 months old, all belonging to the same litter as those mentioned above, and 3 normal controls: 2 Briards, 2-4 years old, and 1 Beagle, 1 year old.

B. CLINICAL EXAMINATIONS

The clinical examination included testing of direct and indirect pupillary light reflexes, ability to manage an obstacle course, ability to see falling cotton balls or hand movements in dim and bright light, as well as ophthalmoscopy, slit-lamp biomicroscopy and fundus photography.

C. ELECTRON MICROSCOPY

Within 2 min of sacrifice (an overdose of sodium thiopentone intravenously), the right eye was enucleated and hemisected at the ora serrata. The posterior eye-cup was fixed by immersion for 1-3 weeks in cold (4°C) solution of 2% glutaraldehyde in 0.1 M sodium cacodylate buffer (pH 7.2). After post-fixation in 1% osmium tetroxide in Veronal acetate buffer, pieces, about 3 x 5 mm, were cut under a dissecting microscope from three locations within the tapetal area (the posterior pole - temporally to the optic disc, the midperiphery and the periphery) as well as from the peripheral non-tapetal area. The pieces were dehydrated in acetone and embedded in Vestopal W. Ultrathin sections were cut and stained with uranyl acetate and lead citrate and examined in a JEOL 2000 EX or a JEOL 100 SX electron microscope. This investigation, as well as the ERG studies, conformed to the ARVO Resolution on the Use of Animals in Research.

D. DC ELECTRORETINOGRAPHY

The dogs were anaesthetised using intravenous sodium thiopentone and intubated. The pupils were fully dilated with 0.5% atropine and 10% phenylephrine. Dark adaptation time was 30 min. A computerised DC ERG system, including suction contact lenses, matched calomel half-cell electrodes and low-drift DC amplifiers, was employed, as described in detail earlier.[12] Ten sec white light stimuli, provided through fibre optics, were used. The stimulus intensity - amplitude relationship was investigated, using intensities ranging from slightly below the normal b-wave threshold (set at 20 μV) to 5 log rel. units above this threshold, changes being made in 0.5 log rel. unit steps. Furthermore, responses to a 30 Hz flickering (photopic) light as well as responses to single flashes of bright white light were recorded after 10 min of light adaptation.

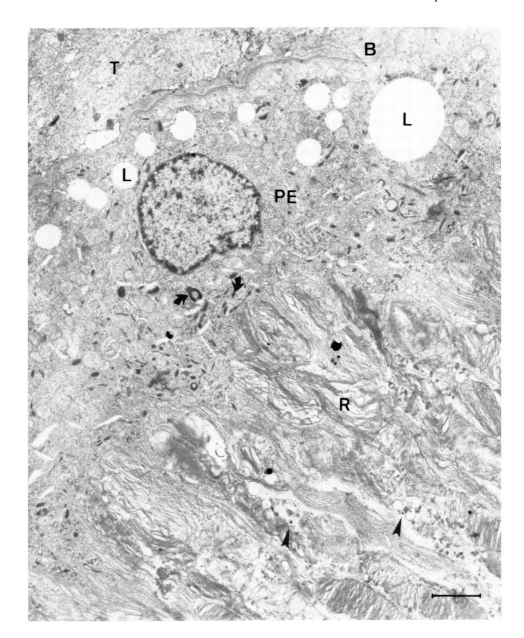

Figure 1. Parts of tapetum (T), pigment epithelium (PE) and rod outer segments (R) from the central tapetal area of an affected dog. Large, electron-lucent (L) and small, electron-dense (arrows) inclusions are seen in the pigment epithelium. The tapetum is fairly structureless. Most rod outer segments show disoriented and disrupted disc membranes. Small, electron-dense granules are present between and probably also within the damaged rod outer segments (arrowheads). B: Bruch's membrane. Bar: 2μ.

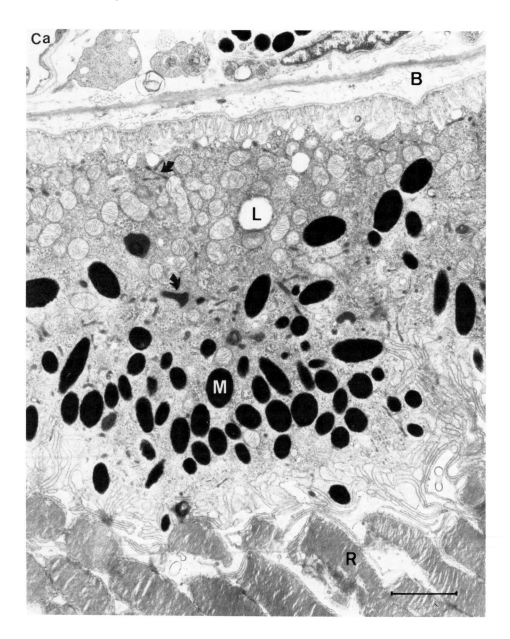

Figure 2. Pigment epithelium from the peripheral, extratapetal area of an affected dog. Large (L) and small (arrows) inclusions are seen, as well as abundant melanin granules (M). In this area, the rod outer segments (R) are unchanged. B: Bruch's membrane. Ca: capillary. Bar: 2μ.

III. RESULTS

A. CLINICAL FINDINGS

All affected dogs were nyctalopic (night blind). Some of them appeared nearly day blind as well, whereas others could see hand movements and falling white cotton balls in strong illumination. Direct and indirect pupillary light reflexes were present in all animals. The external structures of the eyes as well as the fundus seemed normal. The control dogs had normal vision.

B. ULTRASTRUCTURE

1. Pigment Epithelium, Bruch's Membrane, Tapetum

Two major changes were found in the PE of the affected dogs. The most striking one was the presence of large spherical, electron-lucent ("empty") inclusions in the central, tapetal area (Figure 1) as well as in the peripheral, non-tapetal area (Figure 2). Some of these were clearly membrane-bound, whereas in many cases a membrane could not be resolved. These inclusions seemed to be somewhat higher in number in the central than in the peripheral regions, and the distribution was patchy. In addition, a large number of smaller, electron-dense inclusions, sometimes round but more often elongated and slightly curved, were seen in both the central and peripheral areas (Figures 1 and 2). These inclusions were membrane-bound. Such structures were sometimes seen also in controls, but in smaller numbers. Other cell organelles, such as mitochondria, the Golgi apparatus, both types of endoplasmic reticulum and phagosomes, as well as the basal infoldings, seemed normal (Figures 1 and 2).

Bruch's membrane was sometimes normal-appearing in the affected dogs, but often thickened and including electron-dense material in much larger amounts than found in control animals (Figure 3). In certain places, the tapetum, consisting mainly of distinct and very regularly layered fibrils, showed bundles of more irregular and larger diameter tubular structures, sometimes even containing an amorphous material (Figure 1). Such structures, which could be seen also in the non-tapetal area, seemed to be more common in affected than in control dogs.

2. Photoreceptors, Inner Retina

In the affected dogs, the rod outer segments were damaged over large areas in the form of disoriented and disorganised disc membranes, sometimes vesiculated (Figures 1 and 4). In certain places, small membrane-bound, electron-dense granules were seen in PE processes between the photoreceptor outer segments and occasionally even within the damaged rod outer segments (Figure 1). Areas with normal rod outer segments could be seen in many places (Figure 2), i.e. the disease was patchy, at least at this stage. The number of PE inclusions and the rod damage did not always parallel each other. It seemed that rod changes occurred more frequently in the central, tapetal area than in the peripheral, non-tapetal area. The rod inner segments appeared mainly normal. Microtubules were seen. Most cone outer and inner segments appeared normal (Figure 4). The photoreceptor synapses were not analysed in detail yet, but no alterations were seen. No definite changes were found in the inner retina so far.

C. DC ELECTRORETINOGRAPHY

1. The a- and b-waves, Flicker Responses

The a- and b-waves of the dark adapted ERG from a normal dog in response to a stimulus intensity 5 log rel. units above b-wave threshold are demonstrated in Figure 5. Under the same conditions, there were no or extremely small and delayed responses from

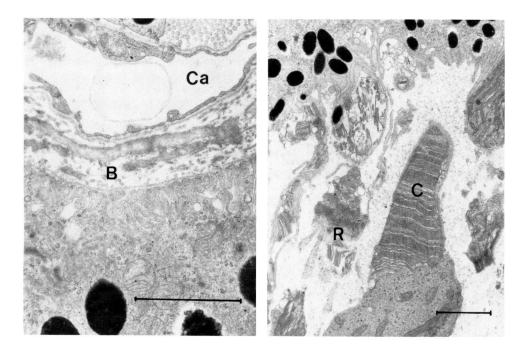

Figure 3. (Left.) Bruch's membrane (B) in an affected dog shows accumulation of electron-dense material. Ca: capillary. Bar: 2μ.

Figure 4. (Right.) A normal cone (C) among damaged rod outer segments (R) in an affected dog. Bar: 2μ.

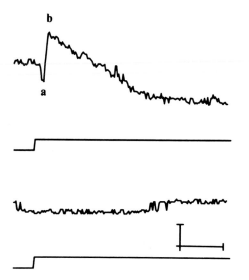

Figure 5. Top tracing: a- and b-waves of the dark adapted ERG in a normal Briard dog in response to a 10 sec white light stimulus, 5 log rel. units above the normal b-wave threshold. Bottom tracing: a recording under the same conditions from an affected dog. No definite response can be seen. Amplitude and time calibrations: 100 μV and 100 msec, respectively.

the affected dogs (Figure 5). Thus, rod function was very severely impaired. Thirty Hz flicker responses were present in all dogs, but reduced by about 50-70%, showing that cones were preserved better than rods.

2. Slower Responses

DC recordings to demonstrate the slower c-wave in a normal control dog are found in Figure 6. The c-wave is very small in the dog, sometimes approaching the base-line. In the affected dogs, the responses were quite different (Figure 7). No a-, b- or c-waves were seen. At lower intensities, there were no responses at all. From about 3 log rel. units above the normal b-wave threshold, a slow negative potential appeared. Both the latency and the peak time were very long, about 5-7 sec and about 12-15 sec, respectively. With increasing stimulus intensity, the latency as well as the peak time became shorter and shorter and the amplitude larger and larger. At the highest intensity, 5 log rel. units above the normal b-wave threshold, the peak time was 1-2 sec. The maximum amplitude recorded was 2,400 μV. At the highest intensities, the return of the potential was often fairly steep in the early phase, but thereafter much slower.

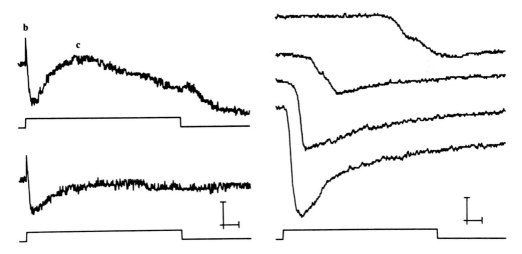

Figure 6. (Left.) DC ERG recordings from a normal, dark adapted control dog, showing the b-wave and the slow and small c-wave in response to 10 sec light stimuli, 3 log rel. units (top tracing) and 5 log rel. units (bottom tracing), respectively, above b-wave threshold. Amplitude and time calibrations: 100 μV and 1 sec.

Figure 7. (Right.) DC ERG recordings from an affected dog (dark adapted) in response to 10 sec stimuli, from top to bottom 3.0, 3.5, 4.0 and 5.0 log rel. units, respectively, above the normal b-wave threshold. No a-, b- or c-waves are seen. Instead, a slow negative response is present, increasing in amplitude and decreasing in latency and peak time with increasing stimulus intensities. Amplitude and time calibrations: 500 μV and 1 sec.

IV. DISCUSSION

It is interesting to note from a genetic point of view that the offspring of two dogs (sister and brother) with night blindness but normal or nearly normal day vision became severely affected also regarding day vision. This means that not only rod function but also cone function was impaired. These dogs are still rather young, and it is too early to make a definite statement whether the disease is stationary or not.

Whereas the Appaloosa horse model showed normal retinal histology,[7] and the Pearl mouse model normal photoreceptor outer and inner segments,[8] our model demonstrated disorganised rod outer segment disc membranes. Such disorganisation was observed already at the age of 5 weeks, but the changes have not been quantified yet in a longitudinal direction. The question is whether the outer segment damage may be secondary to the PE changes.

The rhodopsin concentration has not been measured yet in our dogs, but some photoreceptor proteins (opsin, transducin-a, S-antigen and IRBP) have been investigated immunohistochemically in collaboration with T. van Veen (to be published) and found to be normal. In human CSNB, rhodopsin concentration was found to be normal,[4] while the Pearl mouse showed a normal content of rhodopsin,[8] and the Appaloosa horse had an ample supply of rhodopsin.[6] When in spite of this, there is no ERG a-wave, an outer segment transduction defect is suspected.[4,5] If there is an a-wave but no b-wave, a synaptic transmission defect seems likely.[4,5] The Pearl mouse model was found to have ultrastructural changes associated with the synaptic lamellae.[8] We have not seen such changes in the affected dogs, although our analysis has not been completed yet. Microtubules are involved in axonal transport of a variety of cytoplasmic components, including synaptic vesicles, neurotransmitters and their precursors.[5] It has been suggested that defective microtubules, impairing axonal transport and synaptic transmission, may be one of several possible explanations of hereditary night blindness.[5,13] The rods of our affected Briard dogs do not lack microtubules. A quantitative comparison with normal controls will be performed.

The large, translucent PE inclusions observed in our affected dogs appear to be similar to the lipid inclusions described for the American strain of Briard dogs.[10] These latter dogs were found to have twice the normal plasma concentration of arachidonic acid, as well as hypercholesterolemia and elevated levels also of other lipids. On this basis, one could speculate whether lipid changes may be primary in the disease, interfering first with the PE function and secondarily with the photoreceptors. The large inclusions were observed in our dogs already at the age of 5 weeks, but again, a quantitative, longitudinal analysis has not been performed yet. The plasma lipids of our dogs are now under investigation. The small electron-dense inclusions found in much larger numbers in the PE of our affected dogs than in normal controls may be related to the large ones. They could possibly be precursors. Since they are membrane-bound, often elongated and slightly curved, they are reminiscent of structures derived from the Golgi apparatus, where their content may be accumulated. The electron-dense, membrane-bound granules observed in PE processes between the photoreceptor outer segments in certain areas, and occasionally even within rod outer segments, showed some similarity to the electron-dense inclusions in the PE and may be of the same origin. If so, they may be harmful to the photoreceptors.

The changes in Bruch's membrane may reflect either deposits originating from the disease process or primary changes in Bruch's membrane, impairing transport mechanisms. The deviant structures in the tapetum and at the corresponding level in the non-tapetal area may represent degenerative changes, but this is still unclear.

All the changes described were found in a patchy organisation. It seemed that healthy areas were less frequent in central than in peripheral regions, but this has to be quantified more precisely. Strangely enough, changes in the PE and in the photoreceptor outer segments did not always parallel each other in severity.

The absence of distinct scotopic ERG a- and b-waves reflects the very severely impaired rod function. However, since immunocytochemistry showed normal opsin, and since the ultrastructural rod outer segment damage was not extensive enough to account for the absence of a- and b-waves, it seems that the generation of the a- and b-waves is blocked or markedly delayed by other mechanisms. The PE inclusions and the scattered granules observed in the photoreceptor layer may imply an accumulation of a substance which is toxic to photoreceptor structure and function. A second possibility is that the PE is unable to eliminate a toxic substance from the photoreceptor. Finally, the PE may fail in supplying the photoreceptors with a substance needed by these cells or instead eliminate too much of such a substance from the photoreceptors. The PE changes found in the Pearl mouse are proposed to be involved in the mechanism behind its night blindness.[8] The proposal is strongly supported by the fact that the reduced ganglion cell axon responses were restored after the neuroretina was isolated from the PE and superfused.[8]

Cone structure and function were preserved better than rod structure and function, as seen both in the electron micrographs and in the flicker responses. On the other hand, cone function was markedly impaired in the puppies in comparison with that of their parents. This implies a functional defect not showing ultrastructurally, possibly related to the PE inclusions also regarding cone function.

Since AC ERG recordings in the Riggs type of CSNB as well as in our dogs show no or extremely reduced scotopic responses, we were very surprised to find a prominent slow, negative potential in DC recordings. The threshold of this potential was about 2-3 log rel. units above the normal b-wave threshold, and at such an intensity it appeared very late, 5-7 sec after the start of the stimulus. The response seems to show that some kind of transduction is taking place after all, although very delayed. We do not know yet what constitutes the hindrance (although the PE changes may be suspected as primary) or whether the cascade is involved. So far, only part of the cascade has been studied in the Briard dogs, i.e. transducin-a was normal immunohistochemically. It is very interesting to find in the data published on human CSNB that a case of Schubert-Bornschein CSNB showed a long and deep negative potential, replacing the c-wave.[14]

What may be the explanation of the slow, negative potential? The c-wave of the ERG is the sum of a positive potential (PI), generated in the PE in response to the decrease in potassium ion concentration occurring in the extracellular space surrounding the photoreceptors upon light stimulation,[15-17] and a negative potential (slow PIII), generated in the Müller cells, in response to the same potassium change.[18-21] At high light intensities, the negative potential in the dogs resembles to a large extent the slow PIII. For slow PIII to be generated, some kind of transduction would have to take place, sufficient to change the potassium concentration. This potential is clearly demonstrated after injuring the PE with $NaIO_3$ and thereby abolishing the c-wave of the ERG.[22,23] Such an explanation would agree with a damaged PE, e.g. through the inclusions demonstrated ultrastructurally in the Briard dogs. The fact that the PE in cases of human CSNB was found to be histologically normal[6] does not exclude ultrastructural changes. Furthermore, the fact that the EOG light peak may be normal (but often reduced) in human CSNB,[9,14,24,25] does not necessarily speak against a PE defect, since the light peak and the c-wave are generated in the PE through different mechanisms.[26] On the other hand, the mechanism behind human CSNB may differ from that in the dog.

A second and perhaps even more plausible explanation would be that the negative potential represents a delayed photoreceptor potential or a combination of a photoreceptor potential and slow PIII. The dog has a small c-wave but a deep trough after the b-wave. This trough, which resembles the initial phase of the negative potential in the affected dogs, represents the photoreceptor potential (fast PIII).[27] If transduction is obstructed in some way, it may take much longer to set up a photoreceptor potential. The first part of the slow negative potential would then reflect the photoreceptor potential (fast PIII), followed by slow PIII in response to the photoreceptor-induced change in extracellular potassium. As proposed above, the damaged PE would not be able to respond (properly) to the potassium change. According to this hypothesis, we have a delayed photoreceptor potential.

It is known that arachidonic acid may activate potassium channels in cardiac cells[28] and smooth muscle cells[29] as well as increase voltage-dependent potassium currents in neurons.[30] Furthermore, arachidonic acid inactivates chloride channels in certain epithelia.[31,32] It cannot be excluded that such interference occurs also in the retina and RPE. If so, the large increase in arachidonic acid plasma concentration found in the night blind American Briard dogs[10] may possibly have some relation to the electrophysiological changes and the visual disturbances observed in our dogs.

Why do we not see a delayed b-wave from the inner retina? The explanation may be that these dogs suffer from 2 defects, a slowed down transduction and, in addition, a defective transmission of a kind similar to the Schubert-Bornschein type of CSNB and the Appaloosa horse model. It seems that intraretinal recordings from affected dogs would be very valuable in elucidating further the origin of the slow negative response.

V. ACKNOWLEDGEMENTS

These investigations were supported by the Swedish Medical Research Council (Project No. 12X-734), the Crown Princess Margaretas Foundation for the Visually Handicapped, the U.S. National Retinitis Pigmentosa Foundation, and by the Research Foundation of Synfrämjandet. We are indebted to Miss Barbro Swenson for excellent technical assistance.

REFERENCES

1.   Schubert, G., and Bornschein, H., Beitrag zur Analyse des menschlichen Elektroretinogramms, *Ophthalmologica,* 123, 396, 1952.
2.   Riggs, L.A., Electroretinography in cases of night blindness, *Am. J. Ophthalmol.,* 38, 70, 1954.
3.   Miyake, Y., Yagasaki, K., Horiguchi, M., Kawase, Y., and Kanda, T., Congenital stationary night blindness with negative electroretinogram. A new classification, *Arch. Ophthalmol.,* 104, 1013, 1986.
4.   Carr, R.E., Ripps, H., Siegel, I.M., and Weale, R.A., Rhodopsin and the electrical activity of the retina in congenital night blindness, *Invest. Ophthalmol.,* 5, 497, 1966.
5.   Ripps, H., Night blindness revisited: from man to molecules. Proctor lecture, *Invest. Ophthalmol. Vis. Sci.,* 23, 588, 1982.
6.   Babel, J., Constatations histologiques dans l'amaurose infantile de Leber et dans diverses formes d'héméralopie, *Ophthalmologica,* 145, 399, 1963.

7. Witzel, D.A., Smith, E.L., Wilson, R.D., and Aguirre, G.D., Congenital stationary night blindness: an animal model, *Invest. Ophthalmol. Vis. Sci.*, 17, 788, 1978.

8. Pinto, L.H., Williams, M.A., Suzuki, H., Mangini, N.J., Balkema, G.W., Jr., and Vanable, J.W., Jr., A hypothesis for the mechanism for subnormal retinal sensitivity in the Pearl mouse model for human congenital night blindness, in *Retinal Degeneration: Experimental and Clinical Studies*, LaVail, M.M., Hollyfield, J.G., and Anderson, R.E., Eds., Alan R. Liss, Inc., New York, 1985, 257.

9. Narfström, K., Wrigstad, A., and Nilsson, S.E.G., The Briard dog: a new animal model of congenital stationary night blindness, *Brit. J. Ophthalmol.*, 73, 750, 1989.

10. Riis, R.C., and Siakotos, A.B., Inherited lipid retinopathy within a dog breed, *Invest. Ophthalmol. Vis. Sci.*, 30, ARVO Suppl., 308, 1989.

11. Narfström, K., Wrigstad, A., and Nilsson, S.E., Congenital night blindness in the Briard dog, *Invest. Ophthalmol. Vis. Sci*, **31**, ARVO Suppl., 545, 1990.

12. Nilsson, S.E.G., and Andersson, B.E., Corneal D.C. recordings of slow ocular potential changes such as the ERG c-wave and the light peak in clinical work. Equipment and examples of results, *Docum. Ophthalmol.*, 68, 313, 1988.

13. Ripps, H., Mehaffey, L., III, Siegel, I.M., and Niemeyer, G., Vincristine-induced changes in the retina of the isolated arterially-perfused cat eye, *Exp. Eye Res.*, 48, 771, 1989.

14. Heilig, P., Thaler, A., and Bornschein, H., Slow potentials of ERG in hemeralopia congenita, Xth ISCERG Sympos., Los Angeles, 1972, *Docum. Ophthalmol. Proc. Ser.*, W. Junk B.V. Publishers, The Hague, The Netherlands, 1973, 219.

15. Steinberg, R.H., Schmidt, R., and Brown, K.T., Intracellular responses to light from cat pigment epithelium: origin of the electroretinogram c-wave, *Nature (Lond.)*, 227, 728, 1970.

16. Oakley, B., II, and Green, D.G., Correlation of light-induced changes in retinal extracellular potassium concentration with c-wave of the electroretinogram, *J. Neurophysiol.*, 39, 1117, 1976.

17. Oakley, B.,II, Steinberg, R.H., Miller, S.S., and Nilsson, S.E.G., The in vitro frog pigment epithelial cell hyperpolarization in response to light, *Invest. Ophthalmol. Vis. Sci.*, 16, 771, 1977.

18. Witkovsky, P., Dudek, F.E., and Ripps, H., Slow PIII component of the carp electroretinogram, *J. Gen. Physiol.*, 65, 119, 1975.

19. Oakley, B., II, Potassium and the photoreceptor-dependent pigment epithelial hyperpolarization, *J. Gen. Physiol.*, 70, 405, 1977.

20. Welinder, E., Textorius, O., and Nilsson, S.E.G., Effects of intravitreally injected DL-a-aminoadipic acid on the c-wave of the D.C.-recorded electroretinogram in albino rabbits, *Invest. Ophthalmol. Vis. Sci.*, 23, 240, 1982.

21. Karwoski, C.J., and Proenza, L.M., Relationship between Müller cell responses, a local transretinal potential, and potassium flux, *J. Neurophysiol.*, 40, 244, 1977.

22. Noell, W.K., *Studies on the electrophysiology and the metabolism of the retina*, US Air Force, SAM Project 21-1201-0004, Randolph Field, Texas, 1953.

23. Nilsson, S.E.G., Knave, B., and Persson, H.E., Changes in ultrastructure and function of the sheep pigment epithelium and retina induced by sodium iodate. II: Early effects, *Acta Ophthalmol.*, 55, 1007, 1977.

24. Carr, R.E., and Siegel, I.M., *Visual Electrodiagnostic Testing; a practical guide for the clinician*, Williams and Wilkins, Baltimore, London, 1982.

25. Takahashi, Y., Onoe, S., Asamizu, N., Mori, T., Yoshimura, Y. and Tazawa, Y., Incomplete congenital stationary night blindness: Electroretinogram c-wave and electrooculogram light rise, *Docum. Ophthalmol.*, 70, 67, 1988.

26. Linsenmeier, R.A., and Steinberg, R.M., Origin and sensitivity of the light peak in the intact cat eye, *J. Physiol. (Lond.)*, 331, 653, 1982.

27. Frishman, L.J., and Steinberg, R.H., Intraretinal analysis of the light-adapted ERG of the cat, *Invest. Ophthalmol. Vis. Sci.*, 30, ARVO Suppl., 63, 1989.
28. Kim, D., and Clapham, D.E., Potassium channels in cardiac cells activated by arachidonic acid and phospholipids, *Science*, 244, 1174, 1989.
29. Ordway, R.W., Walsh, Jr., J.V., and Singer, J.J., Arachidonic acid and other fatty acids directly activate potassium channels in smooth muscle cells, *Science*, 244, 1176, 1989.
30. Schweitzer, P., Madamba, S. and Siggins, G.R., Arachidonic acid metabolites as mediators of somatostatin-induced increase of neuronal M-current, *Nature*, 346, 464, 1990.
31. Hwang, T.C., Guggino, S.E. and Guggino, W.B., Arachidonic acid block of epithelial Cl⁻ channels in tracheal airway cells, *Biophys. J.* 57, 88a, 1990.
32. Anderson, M.P. and Welsh, M.J., Fatty acids inhibit apical membrane chloride channels in airway epithelia, *Proc. Natl. Acad. Sci. USA*, (In press.)

HEREDITARY ROD CONE DEGENERATION IN THE ABYSSINIAN CAT:

MORPHOLOGICAL AND IMMUNOCYTOCHEMICAL ASPECTS

Kristina Narfström,[a,b] Sven Erik Nilsson,[b] Barbara Wiggert,[d] Geetha Kutty,[d], Gerald J. Chader[d] and Theo van Veen[c]

[a]Department of Medicine and Surgery, Faculty of Veterinary Medicine, Swedish University of Agriculutral Sciences, Uppsala, Sweden,
[b]Department of Ophthalmology, University of Linköping, Linköping, Sweden,
[c]Laboratory of Molecular Neuroanatomy, Department of Zoology, University of Lund, Sweden and
[d]Laboratory of Retinal Cell and Molecular Biology, National Eye Institute, Bethesda, Maryland, USA.

I. INTRODUCTION

The Abyssinian cat has been shown to be affected by a recessively inherited retinal degenerative disease that shares many similarities with human retinitis pigmentosa (RP).[1] The disease is relatively late in onset with ophthalmoscopical lesions first observed in young adulthood (1.5-2 years). After these, slowly progressive changes begin, resulting in generalized retinal atrophy by the time the cats are middle-aged or older.[2] Electrophysiological and morphologic studies have demonstrated that the disease primarily affects the rod visual cells but that there is a successive involvement also of the cone system.[3,4]

Developmental studies using electroretinography (ERG) showed that a group of affected cats, homozygous for the gene defect could be differentiated from a similar group of normal cats by the age of 8-12 weeks.[5] Even though the retinas of affected cats were still normal appearing at this early age by ophthalmoscopy, significantly reduced maximum amplitudes of the dark adapted b-wave were found when affected animals were compared to controls. Electron microscopic studies performed on groups of affected and normal cats during the time of retinal development and maturation demonstrate that alterations are observed already at the age 5 weeks in kittens that are homozygous for the genetic defect.[6] At this age, the rod and cone outer segment lamellar discs appear adult-like in the normal cat as to disc orientation.[7] In the affected kitten, however, at the age of 5 weeks, many of the outer segments are still "immature" in appearance with the majority of lamellar discs still being disoriented.

Degenerative changes are first observed in affected kittens at the age of 5 months.[6] Disintegration of discs with vacuolization and clumping of disc material is then seen and there is some formation of debris in the subretinal space. Then a successive drop out, primarily of immature rods, is observed followed by a slow, progressive degeneration of rods that appear to have developed and matured normally. Cones are normal at this young age; and it is not until 2-3 years of age that degenerative changes are observed also in cone photoreceptors.

The present report concerns laboratory studies that have been performed in mixed and pure-bred cats, homozygous for the genetic defect which causes the rod-cone degeneration. Results of light- and electron microscopic studies of retinas from affected pure- and mixed-bred cats will be described as well as immunocytochemical and immunochemical investigations mainly of photoreceptor-related proteins from retinas of affected animals.

II. MATERIALS AND METHODS

ANIMALS
The cats used in this study were bred and maintained by the first author in a closed animal facility at the Faculty of Veterinary Medicine, Swedish University of Agricultural Sciences, Uppsala. Different types of controled matings were initiated. Pure-bred Abyssinian cats with the defect as well as mixed-bred cats that were heterozygous for the defect were used in order to produce affected and non-affected, pure-breed and mixed breed cats. The animals were housed in spacious cages or rooms with timer-controlled, cyclic fluroescent lights (12 hr on, 12 hr off). Commercial cat food was fed twice daily; water was allowed **ad libitum**. Ophthalmoscopic examinations were performed at monthly intervals using indirect ophthalmoscopy (Fison indirect ophthalmoscope, Keeler, England) and biomicroscopy (Kowa SL2, Japan), following the induction of mydriasis with 1% tropicamide. This investigation conformed to the ARVO Resolution on the Use of Animals in Research.

MORPHOLOGY
Thirteen cats, homozygous for the defect, were used ranging from 12 weeks to 7 years of age. One of the affected (homozygous) cats was a 2-year old mixed-breed cat. As controls, 10 non-related domestic short-haired cats or cats, heterozygous for the defect, were used, aged 12 weeks to 2 years. Enucleations were performed in ordinary room light, 6-9 hr after light onset, in animals under general anesthesia, using sodium thiopentone intravenously or intraperitoneally. The right eye was hemisected at the ora serrata and the posterior eye-cup was fixed by immersion in a cold solution of 2% glutaraldehyde (pH 7.2) in 0.1 M sodium cacodylate buffer from 1-3 hrs. The eye-cup was then cut into 3 x 5 mm pieces before or after post-fixation in 1% osmium tetroxide in Veronal acetate buffer. Pieces from three locations (area centralis region, peripheral tapetal and peripheral non-tapetal retina) were dehydrated and embedded in epoxy resin (Epon 812). For light-microscopy 1 µm sections were cut and stained with toluidine blue and examined and photographed using a Zeiss Photomicroscope. Ultrathin sections were stained with uranyl acetate and lead citrate and examined in a JEOL 2000EX electron microscope.

IMMUNOCYTOCHEMISTRY
The left eye from affected pure-breed animals described above were used for the immunocytochemical investigations. For controls, 3 cats from 12 weeks to 2 years of age were used. The eye was hemisected and the posterior eye-cup immersed for 12 hours in 4% formaldehyde in 0.1 N phosphate buffer (pH 7.2). It was subsequently washed and transferred to 25% sucrose solution in Tyrode buffer. Sections were serially cut in a cryostat set to 10 µm section thickness. Phosphate-buffered saline (PBS) containing 0.25% bovine serum albumin (BSA) and 0.25% Triton-X-100 was used to dilute the antisera. The sections were incubated with rabbit anti-bovine TD-α (1:1000-1:3000) (a kind gift from Dr. A. Spiegel, NIH), rabbit anti-bovine S-antigen (48-K protein) (1:1000-1:3000) (a kind gift from Dr. I. Gery, NIH), sheep antibovine opsin (1:10 000) (a kind

gift from Dr. D.S. Papermaster), and monoclonal chicken anti-cone (1:400) (a kind gift of Dr. V. Lemmon) for 12 hours at room temperature. Goat anti-bovine IRBP was used at a dilution of 1:1500. Secondary antibodies were swine anti-rabbit IgG, rabbit anti-goat IgG, and rabbit anti-mouse IgG. Because of the strong cross reactions between antibodies raised in sheep with goat-IgG, this system could also be used for identifying the localization of the opsin immunoreactivity. Incubation with rabbit or goat peroxidase anti-peroxidase complex (1:50 for 30 min) was performed as the last step in the immunoreactions. The slides were rinsed with PBS containing 0.25% Triton-X-200 between each step. The immunoreactions were visualized by using 3,3'-diaminobenzidine tetrahydrochloride 0.03% and 0.0013% H_2O_2 in TRIS-HCI buffer (Ph 7.6) for 5-15 min. The sections were dehydrated and mounted. The controls were: 1. sections processed without the primary antibody, 2. sections treated without the reagents needed for the color development and 3. sections treated with primary antiserum preabsorbed with the proteins investigated.

IMMUNOCHEMISTRY
Quantitation of IRBP in the samples relative to purified IRBP standards was accomplished by slot-blot analysis as previously described.[8] Affected cats at well-defined specific stages of the disease[2] were used as well as control normal cats of mixed breed. Protein concentrations in the supernatant samples were determined using the method of Bradford.[9]

III. RESULTS

MORPHOLOGY
Since a detailed study of the electronmicroscopic findings in the disease in Abyssinian cats has been previously reported,[6] mainly the results of serial sections at the light-microscopic (LM) level will be given for pure-breed and mixed-breed affected cats. Results from electron microscopic studies of the affected, mixed breed cat will be reported.

Using light-microscopy, degenerative changes were first observed at 5 months of age in the outer retina of Abyssinian cats, homozygous for the disease. At this age, a slight reduction in the number of photoreceptor nuclei was seen, mainly in the mid-peripheral and peripheral retina. Macrophages could be observed in the subretinal space from this early age and onwards. Between the age of 5 months and 1.5 years, the retinal degenerative changes were extremely slow. Afterwards degenerative changes became more severe, affecting the retina in a more widespread manner. Then, a significant reduction of the outer nuclear layer was observed both centrally and peripherally with an obvious reduction in length of photoreceptor outer and inner segments. No differences were found when superior, inferior, nasal and temporal quadrants were compared as to degenerative changes in photoreceptor cells. Degenerative lesions were patchy, however, in all quadrants. The mid-periphery was always more severely affected than the central and peripheral areas although, after the age of 2 years the retinal changes were even more variable than previously with marked patchiness. Thus, there could be areas with a slightly reduced outer nuclear layer and normal appearing outer and inner segments and quite nearby a transitional area with only one or two rows of photoreceptor nuclei next to an area where photoreceptors were lacking. It appeared as if the degenerative changes progressed even more rapidly after the age of 2-3 years. The degenerative changes were then not only observed in rods but also in cones (Figure 1). The earliest alterations observed by electron microscopy in cones were, just as in rods, disorientation and disorganization of outer segment lamellar discs. With further progression of disease, in 3

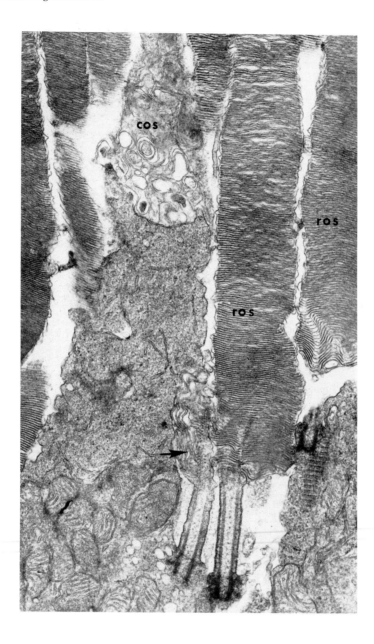

Fig. 1. Parts of rod and cone outer and inner segments from the retina of a 2-year-old mixed-breed cat. There is disorganization of a rod outer segment (ros) (arrow) next to completely normal appearing ones. Note also the disorganization and some early degenerative changes in the cone outer segment (cos). (×6,500.)

year-old cats and older, there was a generalized marked reduction of outer nuclear layer with areas where most outer and inner segments of rods and cones were lost. Most severe lesions were, as found at earlier ages, found in the mid-periphery while a central streak appeared to be spared late in the disease process. After the age of 4 years, only remnants of photoreceptor cells could be observed, most often centrally, near the disc and in some cases also in the far periphery. In these late stages of disease, a difference was seen between the tapetal and non-tapetal pigment epithelial cells. Usually the non-tapetal pigment epithelial cells were larger than normally, bulging outward into the subretinal space. At the end stage, usually in 4-year-old cats, there was a generalized thinning of the retina, to about 2/3 of its normal thickness, with a marked gliosis. Sometimes pigment-laden cells were seen in the outer and inner retina as well.

By light- and electron microscopy, the retinal lesions of the mixed-breed affected cat were similar to those found in the pure-breed Abyssinian cats at a comparable stage of disease.

IMMUNOCYTOCHEMISTRY

The intensity, distribution and cellular compartmentation of the immunoreaction (IR) using anti-opsin, anti-S-antigen and anti-cone antibodies were identical to those of the control retinae up to the age of 2 years in affected cats. Opsin-immunoreactivity was present mainly in the outer segments. S-antigen-IR was found in all areas of the photoreceptor cell (Figure 2A,B). More intense staining was found, however, in the outer segments than in the synaptic area and lower in the cell somata and in the inner segments. Anti-cone immunoreactivity clearly labeled cone outer segments (Figure 2C,D). For the α-subunit of transducin, (TD-α), the intracellular distribution of immunolabel differed slightly between control and affected retinae. In affected 2-year-old cats, the reaction product was located in the photoreceptor outer and inner segments but little immunoreactivity was present in the terminals. This was in contrast with the control retinae, where a considerable amount of reaction product was located in the terminals of the photoreceptor cells (Figure 3A,B). The distribution for IRBP showed only slight differences between affected and controls in young animals (Figure not shown). After the age of 1,5 years, however, the IRBP-IR was significantly reduced. Therefore specific quantitation of IRBP was performed (see immunochemistry, below).

In 2-3 year old animals with more advanced disease, distinct immunoreacitivity for S-antigen opsin and TD-α was observed. For opsin and TD-α, however, there appeared to be a dramatic shift in IR from the outer segments, which were severely shortened or lost, to the entire photoreceptor cell somata (Figure 3C,D). For IRBP the immunoreactivity was completely absent in the peripheral retina while only a weak reaction was detectable centrally. Using anti-cone antibodies some staining was observed in the central retina and sporadically also in the far periphery. At this moderately advanced stage of disease, the immunocytochemical studies clearly demonstrated the patchiness of the degenerative lesions (Fig. 3D).

At the end stage of the disease, the number of immunoreactive elements in the outer nuclear layer is low and consists almost exclusively of morphologically severely altered cells. Centrally, there are patches of cells that show co-localization of S-Ag, opsin and TD-α IR. In the peripheral retina the cells were mainly s-antigen-positive. IRBP was not present in any retinal areas. Also, there was no IR using anti-cone antibodies.

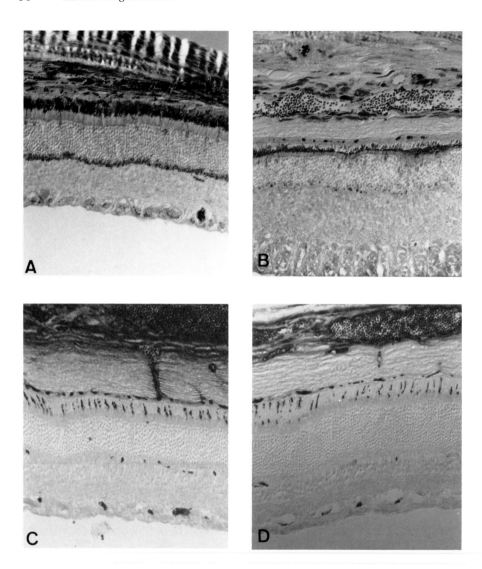

Fig. 2. A: S-antigen-IR of normal retina. The immunoreactivity is found in the entire photoreceptor cell with the highest intensity in outer segments and synaptic area. B: Moderately advanced stage of disease in a 3-year-old cat. Note the short and degenerating outer and inner segments as well as the reduced outer nuclear layer. S-antigen-IR is, however, distributed as in the control. C: Anti-cone-IR in a normal retina. D: Anti-cone-IR in an affected 1.5-year-old cat with early disease. The IR in the affected is similar to that found in normal retina. Note also the slightly reduced outer nuclear layer in the affected retina (D).

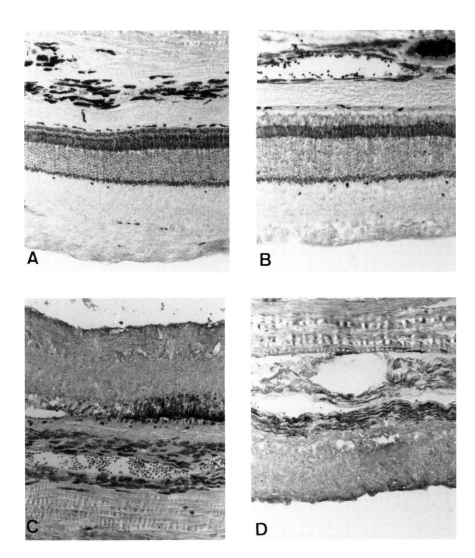

Fig. 3. A: α-Transducin-IR of normal cat. B: α-Transducin-IR of 1.5-year-old affected animal. IR in A and B is located in photoreceptor outer and inner segments and in their terminals. **D**: Midperipheral tapetal area of an affected retina in a 3-year-old cat. Note the loss of photoreceptor cells and of IR. **C**: Central area of the same animal as in **D**. Note patchiness of the disease and the shift or IR from the outer and inner segments to the entire cell somata.

IMMUNOCHEMISTRY

Slot-blot assays demonstrated significantly lower levels of IRBP when affected retinae were compared to those of controls.[10] In adult cats, control levels of IRBP ranged from 650 to 1000 ng IRBP/mg of total protein. At stage 2 and stage 3 of the disease, the level was reduced to approximately 400 ng/mg. In a 3-year-old affected cat, for example (stage 3), the IRBP concentration was 391 ng/mg protein. A preliminary finding is that even 4-6 week-old kittens, homozygous for the defect, shows much reduced IRBP levels (data not shown). This is particularly significant since abnormalities in the retinae are minimal at this early age.

IV. DISCUSSION

Through selected breeding, the gene for rod-cone degeneration in the Abyssinian cat has now been transferred to mixed breed cats. The morphological characteristics of the disease in these cats appear similar to what now and previously has been described for pure-bred Abyssinian cats. This study emphasizes the fact that photoreceptor cell death in this disease advances from the mid-periphery to the central regions of the retina. The development of this retinal degenerative disease thus resembles that of RP in man.[11,12] The similarity is marked at late stages, when the outer nuclear layer in the midperiphery is depleted of photoreceptor cells while the central and peripheral areas retain some patches of cell remnants. The latter is visualized as patches of severely-altered cells with distinctive patterns of photoreceptor-specific immunoreactivity.

In the Abyssinian cat rod-cone degenerative disease, it is clear that there is normal production of rod and cone disc membranes in the young retina. However, there appears to be abberation in the ordering of disc membranes into neat stacks in specific rod outer segments already at an early age. This "immaturity" is also seen in normal cats up to postnatal age 5 weeks.[6] In the affected retina, however, this disorganization of lamellar discs persists in some of the rod outer segments and it appears as if it is primarily these immature-like rod outer segments that degenerate first. Degenerative changes are not seen by light-microscopy, however, until 5 months postnatally. Macrophages are then observed in the subretinal space and there is a slight reduction of the outer nuclear layer, indicative of photoreceptor cell death. The degenerative lesions progress rather slowly at this time. It is not until after 1-2 years of age, that there is a generalized effect on photoreceptor cells. Abberations are then also seen in cones. Early structural changes observed in cone outer segments in affected cats are similar to those found in rods, i.e. disorganization of lamellae and subsequently, disintegration and more generalized degeneration.

Although the cause of the disease is yet unknown, reduced levels of important photoreceptor proteins or abnormalities in intracellular transport and/or release of specific substances could lead to photoreceptor cell death. Immunocytochemistry was therefore performed in order to investigate the cellular distribution of known photoreceptor markers such as opsin.[13] α-subunit of transducin,[14,15,16] S-antigen (48K protein),[17,18,19] IRBP[20,21] and cone pigments. All of these proteins showed normal-appearing IR early in the disease process. For example anti-cone IR is identical in normal and affected retinas of young adult animals demonstrating that cones do not drop-out until there are severe degenerative changes in the outer retina. There is, however, a reduction in the immunoreacitivty of IRBP at a stage of disease when photoreceptors are still rather intact. We recently have found that the levels are reduced already in very young kittens (manuscript in preparation), a finding which could play a role in this rod-cone degenerative disease. It is well known that IRBP is an important carrier of retinoids[22] which are extremely toxic to the photoreceptors,[23] if not "buffered". A reduction of IRBP levels in the subretinal space could cause extensive damage to the sensitive photoreceptor membranes. Further studies should clarify if the reduced concentration of IRBP is a primary defect in this disease or if it is a secondary event.

V. ACKNOWLEDGEMENTS

These studies were supported by the Swedish Medical Research Council (Project No. 12X-734), the Crown Princess Margaretas Foundation for the Visually Handicapped, the U.S. Retinitis Pigmentosa Foundation, the Research Foundation of Synfrämjandet, and the Swedish Natural Science Research Council (NFR 4644-110). The authors are indebted to Drs. I. Gery, A. Spiegel, D.S. Papermaster and V. Lemmon for their generous gift of antibodies and to Carina Rasmussen and Christl Dahlin for skilful laboratory assistance.

REFERENCES

1. Narfström, K., Hereditary progressive retinal atrophy in the Abyssinian cat, *J. Hered.*, 74, 273, 1989.
2. Narfström, K., Progressive retinal atrophy in the Abyssinian cat: Clinical characteristics, *Invest. Ophthalmol. Vis. Sci.*, 26, 193, 1985.
3. Narfström, K., Nilsson, S.E.G. and Andersson, B.E., Progressive retinal atrophy in the Abyssinian cat. Studies of the DC-recorded electroretinogram and the standing potential of the eye. *Br. J. Ophthalmol.*, 69, 618, 1985.
4. Narfström, K. and Nilsson, S.E.G., Progressive retinal atrophy in the Abyssinian cat: Electron microscopy, *Invest. Ophthalmol. Vis. Sci.*, 27, 1569, 1986.
5. Narfström, K., Wilén, M. and Andersson, B.E., Hereditary retinal degeneration in the Abyssinian cat: Developmental studies using clinical electroretinography, *Doc. Ophthalmol.*, 69, 111, 1988.
6. Narfström, K. and Nilsson, S.E.G., Morphological findings during retinal development and maturation in hereditary rod-cone degeneration in Abyssinian cats, *Exp. Eye Res.*, 49, 611, 1989.
7. Morrison, J.D., Morphogenesis of photoreceptor outer segments in the developing kitten retina, *J. Anat.*, 136, 521, 1983.
8. van Veen, T., Ekström, P., Wiggert, B., Lee, L., Hirose, Y., Sanyal, S. and Chader, G., A developmental study of interphotoreceptor retinoid-binding protein (IRBP) in the homozygous or heterozygous rd and rds mutant mouse retina, *Exp. Eye Res.*, 47, 291, 1988.
9. Bradford, M., A rapid and sensitive method for the quantitation of microgram quantities of protein using the principle of protein dye binding, *Anal. Biochem.*, 72, 248, 1976.
10. Narfström, K., Nilsson, S.E.G., Wiggert, B., Lee, I., Chader, J. and van Veen, T., Reduced IRBP level, a possible cause for retinal degeneration in the Abyssinian cat, *Cell and Tissue Res.*, 247, 631, 1989.
11. Krill, A.E., Retinitis Pigmentosa: A review, *Sight Sav. Rev.*, 42, 21, 1972.
12. Gartner, S. and Henkind, P., Pathology of Retinitis Pigmentosa, *Ophthalmology*, 89, 1425, 1982.
13. Jan, L.Y. and Revel, J.P., Ultrastructural localization of rhodopsin in the vertebrate retina, *J. Cell Biol.*, 62, 257, 1974.

14. van Veen, T., Ostholm, T., Gierchik, P., Spiegel, A., Somers, R., Korf, H. and Klein, D.C., α-Transducin immunoreactivity in retinae and sensory pineal organs of adult vertebrates, *Proc. Natl. Acad. Sci.*, USA, 83, 912, 1986.
15. Lerea, C., Somers, D., Hurley, J., Klock, I. and Bunt-Milam, A., Identification of specific transducin-α subunits in retinal rod and cone photoreceptors, *Science*, 234, 77, 1986.
16. Grunwald, G.B., Gierchik, P., Nirenberg, M. and Spiegel, A., Detection of α-transducin in retinal rods but not cones, *Science*, 231, 856, 1986.
17. Broekhuyse, R.M. and Winkins, H.J., Photoreceptor cell-specific localization of S-antigen in retina, *Curr. Eye Res.*, 4, 703, 1985.
18 Korf, H.W., Möller, M., Gery, I., Zigler, J.S. and Klein, D.C., Immunocytochemical demonstration of retinal S-antigen in the pineal organ of four mammalian species, *Cell Tissue Res.*, 239, 81, 1985.
19. van Veen, Th., Elofsson, R., Hartwig, H.-G., Gery, I., Mochizuki, M., Cena, V. and Klein, D.C., Retinal S-antigen: Immunocytochemical and immunochemical studies on distribution in animal photoreceptors and pineal organs, *Exp. Biol.*, 45, 15, 1986.
20. Wiggert, B., Lee, L., Rodriques, M., Hess, H., Redmond, T. and Chader, G., Immunochemical distribution of interphotoreceptor retinoid-binding protein in selected species, *Invest. Ophthalmol. Vis. Sci.*, 27, 1041, 1986.
21. van Veen, Th., Ekström, P., Wiggert, B., Lee, L., Hirose, Y., Sanyal, S. and Chader, G., A developmental study of interphotoreceptor retinoid-binding protein (IRBP) in the homozygous or heterozygous rd and rds mutant mouse retina, *Exp. Eye Res..*, 47, 291, 1988.
22. Okajima, T.-I., Pepperberg, D.R., Ripps, H., Wiggert, B. and Chader, G., Interphotoreceptor retinoid-binding protein promotes rhodopsin regeneration in toad photoreceptors, *Proc. Natl. Acad,.Sci.*, USA, 87, 6907, 1990.
23. Meeks, R.G., Zaharevitz, D. and Chen, F., Membrane effects of retinoids: possible correlation with toxicity, *Arch. Biochem. Biophys.*, 207, 141, 1981.

INHERITED AND ENVIRONMENTALLY INDUCED
RETINAL DEGENERATIONS IN *Drosophila*

William S. Stark, J. Scott Christianson, Linnette Maier, and De-Mao Chen
Division of Biological Sciences, Lefevre Hall,
University of Missouri, Columbia, MO 65211

I. INTRODUCTION

The present era of research involving *Drosophila* mutants to analyse the visual system was initiated with early publications from Pak's laboratory[e.g.1] "Nonphototactic mutants in a study of vision in *Drosophila*" and from Benzer's laboratory[e.g.2] "Genetic dissection of the *Drosophila* nervous system..." This latter publication introduced two genes, originally named the receptor degeneration I and II cistrons, now *rdgA* and *rdgB* respectively.[3] These genes have since been the subject of scores of studies [references[4, 5]].

The purpose of this chapter is to critically evaluate issues in the use of *Drosophila* as an animal model of retinal degeneration. Exactly what is meant by retinal degeneration? The importance of this issue is exemplified by the suggestion[3] that one mutant, namely *ora* [= *o*uter *r*habdomeres *a*bsent] had specific nonformation of the visual organelles [rhabdomeres, the fly equivalent of the vertebrate outer segments] while it was later shown that the rhabdomeres form then diminish [degenerate?] without cell death.[6, 7] What are the forms of retinal degeneration and how do these compare with vertebrate models? It is now recognized that, in addition to "degeneration" mutants, there are other degeneration syndromes caused by [1] pharmacological manipulations relevant to cell signalling;[8,9] [2] "transduction" mutants;[5,10-13] and [3] light stimuli in white-eyed [otherwise non-mutant] flies [the *Drosophila* equivalent of the vertebrate albino] such as [i] intense ultraviolet [UV] and blue light,[14,15] [ii] prolonged exposure to cyclic room light,[16] and [iii] exposure to constant room light.[12] Finally we discuss what the recent progress tells us about the mechanisms of normal photoreceptor function and the pathogenesis when that function is disrupted.

II. RESULTS AND DISCUSSION

A. LIGHT INDUCED DEGENERATION IN *rdgB* AND OTHER MUTANTS
When Harris and Stark[17] extensively analysed retinal degeneration in *Drosophila*

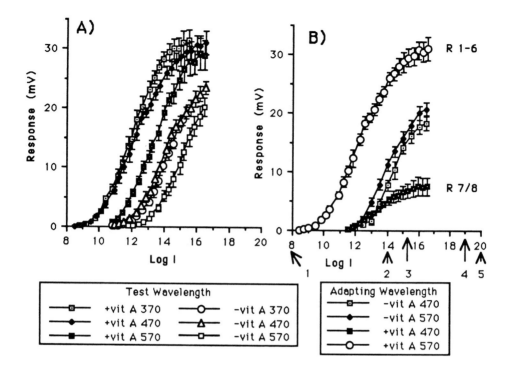

FIGURE 1. Intensity - response data for the ERG receptor component of white-eyed *Drosophila* [averaged from 4 - 8 eyes per curve with standard errors shown] helps to understand many of the findings discussed.

Graph A shows functions from dark adapted eyes for test wavelengths of 370 nm [near UV], 470 nm [blue] and 570 nm [yellow] for carotenoid replete [+vit A] and deprived [-vit A] flies. Note that the responsivity is surprisingly high, with maxima around 30 mV; this helps to explain the usefulness of ERG analyses applied to *Drosophila*. Sensitivity is highest in the blue and UV; deprivation decreases sensitivity throughout the spectrum but preferentially in the UV.[18]

Graph B shows the responses to a 470 nm test wavelength after adaptation with 570 nm [which nearly maximizes rhodopsin] vs. 470 [which favors metarhodopsin] in carotenoid replete [+vit A] vs. deprived [-vit A] flies. Note that, in replete flies, 570 nm adaptation maintains an ERG dominated by R1-6 as labeled while 470 nm adaptation inactivates R1-6 via a PDA [see text] leaving a diminished ERG generated by R7/8 as labeled. There is no PDA in carotenoid deprived flies.

In Graph B, the arrows on the abscissa help to put these intensities into perspective. Arrow # 1 marks a threshold at which approximately 1 quantum is being absorbed per rhabdomere per second.[18] Arrow # 2 very approximately [with the proviso that comparisons of white vs. monochromatic intensities are very difficult] indicates a photopic intensity of white room light from a desk lamp [perhaps 100 lux]. Arrow #3 marks an intensity which, if it were blue and delivered for 1 sec, would convert about half of the rhodopsin to metarhodopsin and induce a maximal PDA.[19] Arrow #4 is the threshold for UV induced intense light damage if delivered for 1 sec[14] and the intensity for nearly complete conversion of the rhodopsin - metarhodopsin visual pigment to M' [see text].[15] Finally, Arrow #5 marks the corresponding blue damage threshold[14] and blue induced visual pigment alteration.[15]

mutants, *rdgB* was considered to be more interesting than *rdgA* in that *rdgB*'s degeneration was light induced. Electrophysiological recording during the response to the light which initiated the demise [enough blue to maximally convert the 480 nm absorbing rhodopsin to its 570 nm absorbing stable metarhodopsin] showed that one specific subset of receptors in the compound eye, namely R1-6, was unable to maintain its poststimulus depolarization [PDA = prolonged depolarizing afterpotential, see Fig. 1]. Many factors which should inhibit the effectiveness of stimulation inhibited degeneration. These factors included dark rearing, lower temperature, eye color pigments, carotenoid deprivation [since deprivation decreases visual pigment], and the *ora* mutant [which eliminates visual pigment, see below]. The *norpA* [*no* receptor *potential*, see below] mutants also blocked degeneration. The most exciting suggestion was the finding that an allele specific suppressor of degeneration in *rdgB* was an allele of *norpA* which did not block the receptor potential. This suggested, on the basis of genetic evidence [in an era when molecular biology was in its infancy], that the gene products of these two genes interact directly in the process of phototransduction.

The *rdgB* gene has been frustratingly difficult to characterize biochemically or to clone. Thus, at the present time, the most thorough investigation of the degeneration mechanism is the pharmacological work of Minke and coworkers.[e.g.8] They suggest that a phosphoprotein phosphatase is deficient in the mutant.[9] This is consistent with the finding that structural degeneration is first witnessed in the receptor cell terminals.[5] However, the molecular biology is progressing rapidly, and a more direct answer to the cause of *rdgB*'s degeneration will probably be available in the near future.

Meanwhile, there has been substantial progress on other *rdg* genes in *Drosophila*. An example is *rdgA*, whose degeneration is independent of light.[17] Different alleles of *rdgA* differ in their severity and receptor specificity;[20-22] an extreme allele, namely *BS12* is very degenerate upon pupal emergence but does not suffer the ravages of time as much as another allele, *PC47*, suggesting that *BS12* has even lost the competence for further degeneration.[21] *rdgA* was shown to be deficient in the activity of diacylglycerol kinase,[23] responsible for the conversion of the putative cellular signalling molecule and product of phospholipase C, namely diacylglycerol, into phosphatidic acid. Also another gene, namely *rdgC*, was identified, and mutants were shown to have light induced retinal degeneration.[24] This mutant's degeneration depends on substantial rhodopsin activation in R1-6 but is curiously independent of phospholipase C in that *norpA* does not block the degeneration. This, as well as other mutants will continue to be of significant value in determining the mechanisms of visual excitation and of maintenance of the photoreceptor cells.

B. THE OPSIN GENE IN *Drosophila* AND HUMAN

The *ninaE* gene was cloned and shown to code for the opsin [Rh1] specific to the R1-6 subset of receptors in the compound eye.[25,26] *NinaE* is the *E* gene whose mutants suffer from *n*either *i*nactivation *n*or *a*fterpotential. The afterpotential is a "locking-in" of R1-6's depolarization [PDA, see above] caused by maximal conversion of its rhodopsin to metarhodopsin;[27,28] such maximal conversion inactivates R1-6.[28,29] It turns out[6,30] that one of the first[3,31] and best characterized[7,32] visual mutants, namely *ora* [see I. INTRODUCTION], is a strong allele of *ninaE*. The designation *outer rhabdomeres absent* is actually an overstatement in that *ora* actually begins its adult life with small rhabdomeres;[6,7] the microvilli of *ora* are devoid of the P-face particles that are normally interpreted as opsin molecules in freeze fracture electron microscopy.[32,33] As mentioned in the introduction, the suggestion[3] that *ora* had nonformation of the rhabdomeres is now more accurately stated: rhabdomeres form then diminish, making the boundary of distinction concerning the diagnosis of "degeneration" subtle indeed. An extreme example of this situation is provided by the example of *ey-2*.[34] This is a mutant with an adult *eyeless* phenotype; an examination of the larval eye imaginal disk, the pre-metamorphosis eye primordium, shows extensive cell death, once again suggesting degeneration rather than nonformation.

Recent research has left us with a fascinating parallel since several genetic lines of human autosomal dominant retinitis pigmentosa[35-37] turn out to be rod rhodopsin missense mutations. It seems odd, at first glance, that a defect in a protein as fundamental as rhodopsin, which comprises 90% of the outer segment protein, would cause a disorder taking years to fully express itself. However, in the autosomal dominant case, a heterozygous normal rhodopsin allele can compensate for the defective allele. In the human disorder, the mechanism of degeneration is not clear yet. It will be important to eventually determine whether the mutant rhodopsin is actually functional and / or forms a "toxic" product.

In the example of the *ora* mutant of the fly, opsin is neither synthesized nor deployed and the rhabdomeres, small at first, "degenerate" [diminish, however, cell death does not occur[32]]. However, the rhabdomere decline is not associated with the appearance of normal autophagic bodies [multivesicular bodies = MVB's].[7] In flies, autophagy, rather than the vertebrate's phagolysosomal system involving the retinal pigment epithelium, recycles membrane, and the MVB is the fly equivalent of the vertebrate phagosome.[16] Unfortunately, the mechanism by which the absence of opsin leads to the demise of the organelle is not known; further, carotenoid deprivation, which also produces a similar opsin decrease, does not lead to such complete demise of the rhabdomeres [see next section].

C. CAROTENOID DEPRIVATION & REPLACEMENT IN *Drosophila* & RAT

In the 1970s, a most remarkable finding was made concerning carotenoid deprivation in the fly: P-face particles are greatly reduced[17,38] while the microvilli of the rhabdomere remain intact. Sensitivity as measured by the ERG[28,29,39] and visual pigment content, as measured using *in vitro* spectrophotometry[17] and *in vivo* microspectrophotometry[40,41] are also drastically reduced in *Drosophila*. Pertinent to retinal dystrophy, what was not known until recently was that rhabdomeres are substantially smaller when *Drosophila* are reared from egg to adult on carotenoid deprivation.[42]

Using carotenoid deficiency to decrease rhabdomeric opsin, unlike using *ora* [discussed above], does not lead to the total loss of the rhabdomere. In order to investigate this phenomenon further, we followed the electroretinographic [ERG] sensitivity of white-eyed deprived flies as a function of time. Sensitivity increases rapidly when deprived flies are given carotenoid "replacement therapy" by placing the deprived flies in a vial with nothing but carrot juice to drink. Surprisingly, in deprived flies maintained on the deprivational medium, sensitivity increases as a function of adult age after pupal emergence by 1.64 log units as of 3 days, then decreases again 2.47 log units by 11 days. Although we suspected that this decline might be associated with degeneration, we found that sensitivity rebounds by 3.98 log units in 1 day when 11-day deprived flies are given carrot juice. This means that, even after deprived flies' sensitivity has waxed and waned, visual receptors are still healthy.

We further investigated trophic effects of vitamin A on rhabdomere and opsin maintenance in visual receptors using microspectrophotometry as well as electron micrographic morphometry and immunocytochemistry. Rhabdomeres enlarge[41] and visual pigment increases[16,43] when adults are carotenoid-replaced using carrot juice. We used a monoclonal antibody to the rhodopsin [called Rh1] in R1-6 receptors in the compound eye to further quantify opsin recovery in such carotenoid replacement therapy. Density of immunogold, specific to R1-6 [vs. R7], increases between days 1 and 3 of replacement as visual pigment and rhabdomeres recover. In summary, sensitivity, visual pigment, opsin and the opsin-containing organelle recover in unison during carotenoid replacement therapy in carotenoid deprived *Drosophila*. At one day of replacement therapy, when opsin synthesis and deployment are high, opsin immunogold labeling is especially high in the rough endoplasmic reticulum of the retinula cells.[42] While this is consistent with the possibility that vitamin A may even regulate fly opsin gene expression at the mRNA level,[44] the situation in the invertebrate is far from resolved since R. White [personal communication] did not observe a decrease in opsin mRNA, assayed with a *ninaE* probe in the moth [*Manduca*].

In the fly, carotenoid deprivation and replacement is relatively straightforward; in the vertebrate this is not the case, which may explain the relative paucity of such data in higher animals. The long-standing dogma for the rat is that deprivation leads to degeneration.[45,46] The effects of vitamin A deprivation were recently reexplored in the rat with the surprising finding that vitamin A's control of opsin is strikingly different in the fly vs. rat.[47,48] Deprivation for 26 weeks decreases rhodopsin by over 85% as measured spectrophotometrically but it does not decrease opsin density as determined by P-face particle counts or quantification of EM immunogold labeling of an opsin antibody. However, the volume of the outer segments is reduced to 42%, and the amount of vitamin A remaining even after 26 weeks of deprivation is still sufficient to support the synthesis of the outer segment's opsin. Even though bleached opsin is regenerated to rhodopsin by chromophore supplied from the adjacent retinal pigment epithelial cells, there is evidence that the chromophore is added in the inner segment during synthesis.[49] It would be interesting to determine whether further deprivation does, in fact, lead to degeneration and if replacement would allow for the reestablishment of normal outer segments as it does for rhabdomeres in *Drosophila*.

D. OTHER REGULATORS OF SYNTHESIS AND DEPLOYMENT

In the vertebrate, rhodopsin is glycosylated, and tunicamycin, which blocks N-linked glycosylation at asparagine residues decreases opsin incorporation into the outer segment and eventually causes degeneration.[50,51] Tunicamycin experiments had also been done in the moth.[52] During pupal development tunicamycin caused a withdrawal of microvilli within a few hours after injection suggesting that it affects certain proteins which are necessary for rhabdomere maintenance; however it did not affect well developed adult microvilli. It was claimed in the fly that the rhodopsin is not glycosylated[53] which seems counterintuitive because of the prevalence of glycosylation among membrane proteins. However, this suggestion was verified and extended by the finding that the mature rhabdomeric opsin is not glycosylated while, during synthesis or deployment it is, and only at one of the two possible sites.[54,55]

We pursued this finding in *Drosophila* with tunicamycin injections much as White and Bennett did in the moth.[52] Carotenoid deprived white-eyed flies within 36 hrs after emergence were fixed to a microscope slide with nail polish. Each fly was then pressure injected [through a glass micropipette[12]] with a solution of 20 mg tunicamycin [B family from Sigma which is fairly specific] per ml of DMSO or a control saline solution. [We had attempted applying tunicamycin onto the eye with DMSO, a good solvent and potential carrier, without an effect; further, we tried to feed the drug but could not find a sublethal dose which had an effect.] The visual pigment was immediately measured using microspectrophotometry, and the flies were then carefully removed from the microscope slide. After removal, flies were carotenoid

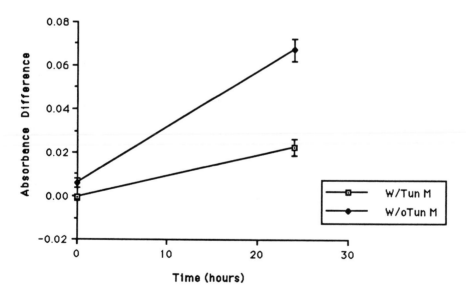

FIGURE 2. Carotenoid replacement therapy experiments on two groups of animals: those injected with tunicamycin have their recovery greatly diminished relative to those given a sham injection. N = 10 for each group with the standard error shown.

replaced by introduction to a vial with 2 ml of carrot juice applied to a kimwipe. At 24 hrs ± 30 min, flies were fixed on the microscope slide and their visual pigment was again measured. Within the 24 hr period, approximately 20% of the flies died due to the injection procedure, and these flies were not counted. The results for male white-eyed *Drosophila* are shown in Fig. 2 As expected, the visual pigment at the beginning of the experiment was virtually zero. Tunicamycin significantly decreased the recovery afforded by carotenoid replacement therapy relative to the "sham" injected controls. This finding is consistent with the data that opsin is glycosylated during cellular synthesis but not in the mature rhabdomeric form.[54,55]

Because *norpA* lacks phospholipase C [see below], the phospholipid and fatty acid composition of *Drosophila* heads is of interest.[56] Organic extracts of heads broken off after freezing in liquid nitrogen were separated by 2 or 3 solvent system HPTLC. Phospholipids were labeled by feeding flies with ^{32}P phosphate. Spots on TLC plates were counted. The profile of labeling after 24 hr of feeding was approximately as follows: phosphatidylethanolamine=PE - 47%, PE plasmalogen=PE_{pl} - 1.5%, phosphatidylcholine=PC - 24%, PC_r [an unknown, likely PC, but with different fatty acids] - 4%, phosphatidylinositol=PI - 12%, lysophospholipids LPE - 2.5%, LPC - 1.6%, LPI - 1.4%, poly-PI's PIP_2 - 0.2%, PIP - 0.2%, phosphatidic acid=PA - 0.4%, phosphatidylserine=PS - 1.6% and the cardiolipins CL_1 - 2.5% and CL_2 - 1.1%. A fraction of a percent of cerebroside is likely present. Relative to rat brain[57] the most notable differences were that, in *Drosophila* heads, PE is higher, PC is lower, PC_r is present and there is probably no sphingomyelin. Fatty acids of PS, PI, PE and PC were analysed by GC. Fatty acid composition differed for the above phospholipids: 14:0 - 2%, 16:0 - 9-34%, 16:1 - 2-10%, 18:0 - 8-25%, 18:1 - 22-33%, 18:2 - 18-28% 18:3 - 1-15%. Triglycerides comprise around 70% of head lipids and have high 14:0 and 14:1. Although docosahexaenoic acid [22:6] is high in vertebrate photoreceptors and nervous system,[58] *Drosophila* heads had none. We confirm and extend the earlier finding that PI lacks arachidonic acid [20:4].[59]

There are no fatty acids longer than 18 carbons in fly heads, but neither are there any in the food. Using several different media which differed in fatty acid composition, it was shown that the fatty acid composition of the heads could be readily manipulated. Thus, we decided to supplement the fly food with menhaden oil, a rich source of long chain fatty acids. We found that the ultrastructure of the photoreceptors of the fish oil supplemented flies was normal and that there was a small but significant increase in the electrophysiological sensitivity, especially in the UV. While these ERG findings should be considered as preliminary, they open the possibility of important trophic influences of dietary fatty acids.

E. THE *norpA* [*no receptor potential*] MUTANT

The mechanism of signal transduction has long been of interest. For photoreceptors, it has long been suspected that transduction defects can lead to retinal dystrophies. In vertebrate vision, a unique G protein mechanism in which cGMP phosphodiesterase [PDE] is inhibited is well established, and the recent evidence that the *rd* [*r*etinal *d*egeneration] gene[60] in mice codes for cGMP's PDE β subunit[61] adds credence to the transduction - integrity link.

In *Drosophila* vision, one of the oldest[1] and best studied[5,12,13,22] mutants, *norpA* [*no r*eceptor *p*otential] has a transduction defect involving a much more commonly used means of signal transduction, namely G protein mediated activation of phospholipase C [PLC]: mutants lack activity of a PLC[62] which acts on PIP_2 as well as PI,[63] and the gene, now cloned, proves to be a PLC gene.[64] [In the strictest sense, PLC is a PDE,[65] so these mechanisms may not be so far removed from each other after all.] Visual pigment is normal in newly emerged *norpA* flies.[11-13,66,67] In *norpA*, there is a demise of the rhabdomeres and an accumulation of membranous material called "zippers," and these phenomena are the subject of recent reports.[5,12,13] Interestingly, there are vertebrate models in which receptors apparently have rhodopsin, but the transduction is deficient; the parallel between *norpA* and congenital stationary night blindness in the human has already been discussed.[13] The newly hatched *rd* chicken has rhodopsin but no receptor potential; however an abnormal cone visual pigment protein is the current explanation of the chicken's "*norpA*"-like phenotype.[68]

Curiously, in a white-eyed strain of the *norpA* mutant, microspectrophotometry [MSP], electron microscopy [EM] and electroretinography [ERG] revealed that light mediates receptor demise in *norpA* even though *norpA* lacks phototransduction.[11, 12] Visual pigment and the rhabdomere which houses it decrease with increasing age in *norpA* but not in *w* with rearing on a 12 hr light / 12 hr dark cycle. At warm room temperature [about 28°C] in *norpA;cn bw* and *w* reared in constant light, visual pigment decreases, rhabdomeres diminish and cells die. This finding, incidentally, introduces an entirely new form of retinal degeneration in *Drosophila* in that white-eyed otherwise nonmutant flies show a retinal demise when placed in a constant light [L / L] regimen for about 10 days. Importantly, dark rearing blocked visual pigment loss in *norpA;cn bw*;[12] the M-potential, an ERG reflection of visual pigment level,[18,20,67,69,70] corroborated this finding.[12]

It seemed amazing to us that the rhabdomere demise should be light-dependent in a mutant which did not have a response to light. We explained the result by suggesting that light initiated the need for "housekeeping" or receptor maintenance, but that depolarization [or at least the transduction steps leading to depolarization] was necessary to put proper photoreceptor maintenance into effect. The ease with which additional manipulations can be applied in *Drosophila* is exemplified by our further experiments [Fig. 3]. We found that decreasing the rhodopsin activation by carotenoid deprivation blocked the rhabdomere demise in the constant light condition in white-eyed otherwise wild-type flies and in the light / dark cycle as well as in the constant light condition in white-eyed *norpA* flies. Of course the rhabdomeres were smaller to begin with [i.e. in constant darkness] in flies which had been reared without carotenoids in the diet [see above, C. CAROTENOID DEPRIVATION ...]. Further, we found that decreasing the photic stimulation by making the flies red-eyed afforded the same protections [with the caveat that different but equally strong alleles of *norpA* were used: *norpA*[P24] in the white-eyed strain and *norpA*[EE5] in the red eyed strain].

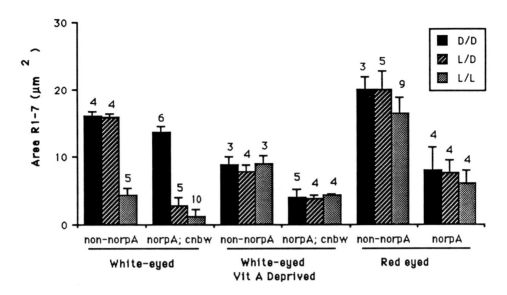

FIGURE 3. The cross sectional area of 10-day post-eclosion white-eyed non-*norpA* vs. *norpA* rhabdomeres with rearing on normal medium vs. on carotenoid [vit A] deprivation; also compared are flies which are red-eyed. N = the number of ommatidia with the standard deviation between ommatidia shown; one animal for each bar except *norpA;cnbw* L/L, vit A deprived *norpA;cnbw* D/D and wild-type [non-*norpA*, red-eyed] L / L where two animals each were pooled. These experiments go beyond those reported earlier[12] by establishing the protective effects of red eye color pigments and carotenoid deprivation.

Both *ora* and *norpA* have a rhabdomere demise. However, *norpA* has MVB's while *ora* does not. We decided to further analyse the resource of electron micrographs available from the Fig. 3 experiment for MVB counts to answer the question as to the interaction of lighting conditions, caroteniod rearing conditions, and genotype with respect to *norpA*. We were initially hesitant about this for the following reason: we have been regularly plagued with what seemed like bad fixation [we called it "ghosty cytoplasm"] in the deprived flies. We now think there is a reason, namely that there is less structure there. The most important finding in this analysis is so qualitative in this regard that we do not hesitate to present it: carotenoid deprivation brings the MVB count to zero, virtually; we say "virtually" because, if we look hard enough in the EM, we can find a few MVB's, though these micrographs turned up none.

F. ENVIRONMENTALLY INDUCED RETINAL DEGENERATION

Environmental manipulations have been used to accelerate or prevent retinal degeneration in mutants. For instance, the results on *norpA* show that light and visual pigment level play a role in the rhabdomere's demise. Further, in *rdgB*, decreases in temperature, visual pigment [via carotenoid deprivation as well as combination with *ora*] and light [by genetically replacing white eyes with wild-type red eyes] all inhibit degeneration.[17] What is less well appreciated is that degeneration can occur in "normal" flies as a result of environmental, as opposed to genetic, manipulations. By "normal," we mean *w* [flies made white-eyed with white or other eye color mutations]. White-eyed flies have been used for decades to eliminate the spectrally selective effects of the red eye color pigments on the basis of a substantial body of information suggesting that it is only the screening function of these pigments which is deficient.

One of the most dramatic examples of light induced degeneration in white-eyed otherwise wild-type *Drosophila* is the effect of intense UV and blue stimulation. These effects were first noted as a consequence of using the intense light sources of the incident illuminator of a fluorescence microscope to study photopigments microspectrofluorometrically.[15,18,71,72] The threshold for UV-induced damage is about 10^{19} quanta/cm^2 [quantum flux multiplied by time], while for blue it is about 10^{20} [Fig. 1].[14] These thresholds are precisely the thresholds needed for conversion of the visual pigment to an intense light photoproduct termed M' to differentiate it from M [the normal metarhodopsin photoproduct of rhodopsin, induced by about 3 orders of magnitude lower illumination, Fig. 1]. This line of work, together with the finding that carotenoid deprivation protects against degeneration, suggests that it is overstimulation of the photopigment system itself which induces retinal degeneration. There is an amazing parallel with the results on aphakic rhesus monkeys[73] in the absolute thresholds of UV and blue damage as well as in the greater efficiency of UV light for inducing damage.

The fact that intense UV and blue stimulation caused retinal degeneration came as no surprise. More recently, it was shown that constant light rearing for 10 days, at warm room temperature, caused a dramatic receptor demise in white-eyed otherwise wild-type *Drosophila*.[12] It was our impression that the *norpA* mutant actually protected somewhat against this degeneration. Also, a scattering of visual receptor cells are lost when flies are reared for 3 weeks on a light / dark cycle of ordinary white room light.[16]

III. CONCLUSIONS AND FUTURE DIRECTIONS

Knowledge is an expanding sphere of light in a universe of darkness: as knowledge increases, so does its contact with the unknown. As pessimistic as this view sounds, it is the *sine qua non* of scientific progress in that each round of answers gives rise to the next, more probing, questions. So it has been through two decades in the application of interdisciplinary cell biological approaches to study *Drosophila* as an animal model of retinal degeneration. Some aspects of *Drosophila's* visual system are uniquely different from that of the vertebrate, such as the nonbleaching metarhodopsin and the PDA. From a basic science standpoint, it is through studying the differences as well as the similarities of organisms that we can gain our fullest level of understanding. But as molecular biology is increasingly applied to the vertebrate as it has been to *Drosophila*, a new unity in the family tree of life paves the way for a new optimism; new homologies such as the rhodopsin - G protein receptor family tree are constantly being elaborated. And, as *Drosophila* remains at the forefront of molecular technology[e.g.74], it remains likely that *Drosophila* will continue to answer questions about the mechanisms underlying one of our most precious gifts, our eyesight.

ACKNOWLEDGEMENTS

This work has been supported mainly by NSF and NIH, most recently by NIH grant EY07192 and NSF grant BNS 88 11062. We thank Randall J. Sapp who was the electron microscopy technician, Kent Studer who assisted with the tunicamycin experiments and Jenny Jackson and Sandra Straughn for technical assistance.

REFERENCES

1. **Pak, W. L., Grossfield, J., and Arnold, K.**, Mutants of the visual pathway of *Drosophila melanogaster*, *Nature (Lond.)*, 222, 518, 1970.

2. **Hotta, Y. and Benzer, S.**, Genetic dissection of the *Drosophila* nervous system by means of mosaics, *Proc. Nat. Acad. Sci. (USA)*, 67, 1156, 1970.

3. **Harris, W. A., Stark, W. S., and Walker, J. A.**, Genetic dissection of the photoreceptor system in the compound eye of *Drosophila melanogaster*, *J. Physiol. (Lond.)*, 256, 415, 1976.

4. **Stark, W. S., Chen, D.-M., Johnson, M. A., and Frayer, K. L.**, The *rdgB* gene in *Drosophila*: Retinal degeneration in different mutant alleles and inhibition of degeneration by *norpA*, *J. Insect Physiol.*, 29, 123, 1983.

5. **Stark, W. S. and Sapp, R. J.**, Retinal degeneration and photoreceptor maintenance in *Drosophila*: *rdgB* and its interaction with other mutants, in *Inherited and Environmentally Induced Retinal Degenerations*, LaVail, M. M., Anderson, R. E., and Hollyfield, J. G., Eds., Liss, New York, 1989, 467.

6. **O'Tousa, J. E., Leonard, D. S., and Pak, W. L.**, Morphological defects in *ora^{JK84}* photoreceptors caused by mutation in R1-6 opsin gene in *Drosophila*, *J. Neurogenet.*, 6, 41, 1989.

7. **Stark, W. S. and Sapp, R. J.**, Ultrastructure of the retina of *Drosophila melanogaster*: the mutant *ora* (outer rhabdomeres absent) and its inhibition of degeneration in *rdgB* (retinal degeneration-B), *J. Neurogenet.*, 4, 227, 1987.

8. **Rubenstein, C. T., Bar-Nachum, S., Selinger, Z., and Minke, B.**, Chemically induced retinal degeneration in the *rdgB* (retinal degeneration B) mutant of *Drosophila*, *Vis. Neurosci.*, 2, 541, 1989.

9. **Minke, B., Rubenstein, C. T., Sahly, I., Bar-Nachum, S., Timberg, R., and Selinger, Z.**, Phorbol ester induces photoreceptor-specific degeneration in a *Drosophila* mutant, *Proc. Nat. Acad. Sci. (USA)*, 87, 113, 1990.

10. **Meyertholen, E. P., Stein, P. J., Williams, M. A., and Ostroy, S. E.**, Studies of the *Drosophila norpA* phototransduction mutant, *J. Comp. Physiol.*, 161, 793, 1987.

11. **Ostroy, S. E.**, Characteristics of *Drosophila* rhodopsin in wild-type and *norpA* vision transduction mutants, *J. Gen. Physiol.*, 72, 717, 1978.

12. **Zinkl, G., Maier, L., Studer, K., Sapp, R., Chen, D.-M., and Stark, W. S.**, Microphotometric, ultrastructural and electrophysiological analyses of light dependent processes on visual receptors in white-eyed wild-type and *norpA* (no receptor potential) mutant *Drosophila.*, *Vis. Neurosc.*, in press, 1990.

13. **Stark, W. S., Sapp, R. J., and Carlson, S. D.**, Photoreceptor maintenance and degeneration in the *norpA* (no receptor potential-A) mutant of *Drosophila melanogaster*, *J. Neurogenet.*, 5, 49, 1989.

14. **Stark, W. S. and Carlson, S. D.**, Blue and ultraviolet light induced damage to the *Drosophila* retina: ultrastructure., *Curr. Eye Res.*, 3, 1441, 1984.

15. **Stark, W. S., Walker, K. D., and Eidel, J. M.**, Ultraviolet and blue light induced damage to the *Drosophila* retina: microspectrophotometry and electrophysiology, *Curr. Eye Res.*, 4, 1059, 1985.

16. **Stark, W. S., Sapp, R. J., and Schilly, D.**, Rhabdomere turnover and rhodopsin cycle: maintenance of retinula cells in *Drosophila melanogaster*, *J. Neurocytol.*, 17, 499, 1988.

17. **Harris, W. A., Ready, D. F., Lipson, E. D., Hudspeth, A. J., and Stark, W. S.**, Vitamin A deprivation and *Drosophila* photopigments, *Nature (Lond.)*, 266, 648, 1977.

18. **Stark, W. S., Ivanyshyn, A. M., and Greenberg, R. M.**, Sensitivity and photopigments of R1-6, a two-peaked photoreceptor, in *Drosophila*, *Calliphora* and *Musca*, *J. Comp. Physiol.*, 121, 289, 1977.

19. **Stark, W. S., Frayer, K. L., and Johnson, M. A.**, Photopigment and receptor properties in *Drosophila* compound eye and ocellar receptors, *Biophys. Struct. Mechanism*, 5, 197, 1979.

20. **Harris, W. A. and Stark, W. S.**, Hereditary retinal degeneration in *Drosophila melanogaster*: a mutant defect associated with the phototransduction process, *J. Gen. Physiol.*, 69, 261, 1977.

21. **Stark, W. S. and Carlson, S. D.**, Retinal degeneration in *rdgA* mutants of *Drosophila melanogaster* meigen (Diptera: Drosophilidae), *Int. J. Insect Morphol. & Embryol.*, 14, 343, 1985.

22. **Stark, W. S., Sapp, R. J., and Carlson, S. D.**, Ultrastructure of the ocellar visual system in normal and mutant *Drosophila melanogaster*, *J. Neurogenet.*, 5, 127, 1989.

23. **Inoue, H., Yoshioka, T., and Hotta, Y.**, Diacylglycerol kinase defect in a *Drosophila* retinal degeneration mutant *rdgA*, *J. Biol. Chem.*, 264, 5996, 1989.

24. **Steele, F. and O'Tousa, J. E.**, Rhodopsin activation causes retinal degeneration in *Drosophila rdgC* mutant, *Neuron*, 4, 888, 1990.

25. **O'Tousa, J. E., Baehr, W., Martin, R. L., Hirsh, J., Pak, W. L., and Applebury, M. L.**, The *Drosophila ninaE* gene encodes an opsin, *Cell*, 40, 839, 1985.

26. **Zuker, C. S., Cowman, A. F., and Rubin, G. M.**, Isolation and structure of a rhodopsin gene from D. melanogaster, *Cell*, 40, 851, 1985.

27. **Stark, W. S.**, Spectral selectivity of visual response alterations mediated by interconversions of native and intermediate photopigments in *Drosophila*, *J. Comp. Physiol.*, 96, 343, 1975.

28. **Stark, W. S. and Zitzmann, W. G.**, Isolation of adaptation mechanisms and photopigment spectra by vitamin A deprivation in *Drosophila*, *J. Comp. Physiol.*, 105, 15, 1976.

29. **Stark, W. S., Ivanyshyn, A. M., and Hu, K. G.**, Spectral sensitivities and photopigments in adaptation of fly visual receptors, *Naturwissen.*, 63, 513, 1976.

30. **Scavarda, N. J., O'Tousa, J., and Pak, W. L.**, *Drosophila* locus with gene-dosage effects on rhodopsin, *Proc. Nat. Acad. Sci. (USA)*, 80, 4441, 1983.

31. **Koenig, J. H. and Merriam. J. R**, Autosomal ERG mutants, *Dros. Inform. Serv.*, 52, 50, 1977.

32. **Stark, W. S. and Carlson, S. D.**, Ultrastructure of the compound eye and first optic neuropile of the photoreceptor mutant *ora^{JK84}* of *Drosophila*, *Cell Tiss. Res.*, 233, 305, 1983.

33. **Schinz, R. H., Lo, M. V. C., Larrivee, D. C., and Pak, W. L.**, Freeze-fracture study of the *Drosophila* photoreceptor membrane: Mutations affecting membrane particle density, *J. Cell Biol.*, 93, 961, 1982.

34. **Eissenberg, J. C., and Ryerse, J. S.**, *ey-2*: a recessive eyeless mutation on the second chromosome of *Drosophila melanogaster, Dros. Inform. Serv.*, in press, 1991.

35. **Dryja, T. P., McGee, T. L., Reichel, E., B., H. L., Cowley, G. S., Yandell, D. W., Sandberg, M. A., and Berson, E. L.**, A point mutation of the opsin gene in one form of retinitis pigmentosa, *Nature (Lond.)*, 343, 364, 1990.

36. **Humphries, P., Farrar, J., Kenna, P., Bradley, D., Humphries, M., Sharp, E., Lawlor, M., and McWilliam, P.**, Studies on the molecular genetics of autosomal dominant retinitis pigmentosa, presented at Int. Symp. Retinal Degen., Stockholm, July 24-27, 1990.

37. **Olsson, J. E.**, Missence mutations within the rhodopsin gene in patients with autosomal dominant retinitis pigmentosa, presented at Int. Symp. Retinal Degen., Stockholm, July 24-27, 1990.

38. **Boschek, C. B. and Hamdorf, K.**, Rhodopsin particles in the photoreceptor membrane of an insect, *Z. Naturforsch.*, 31C, 763, 1976.

39. **Stark, W. S., Schilly, D., Christianson, J. S., Bone, R. A., and Landrum, J. T.**, Photoreceptor-specific efficiencies of β-carotene, zeaxanthin and lutein for photopigment formation deduced from receptor mutant *Drosophila melanogaster, J. Comp. Physiol.*, 166, 429, 1990.

40. **Stark, W. S., and Johnson, M. A.**, Microspectrophotometry of *Drosophila* visual pigments: Determinations of conversion efficiency in R1-6 receptors, *J. Comp. Physiol.*, 140, 275, 1980.

41. **Sapp, R. J., Christianson, J. S., Maier, L., Studer, K., and Stark, W. S.**, Carotenoid replacement therapy in *Drosophila* : recovery of membrane, opsin and rhodopsin., *Exp. Eye Res.*, in press, 1990.

42. **Sapp, R. J., Stark, W. S., Christianson, J. S., Maier, L., and Studer, K.**, Immunocytochemistry & morphometry of carotenoid replacement in *Drosophila, Invest. Ophthal. Vis. Sci. Suppl.*, 31, 77, 1990.

43. **Stark, W. S., Hartman, C. R., Sapp, R. J., Carlson, S. D., Claude, P., and Bhattacharyya, A.**, Vitamin A replacement therapy in *Drosophila, Dros. Inf. Serv.*, 1987, 136, 1987.

44. **Schwemer, J. and Spengler, F.**, Opsin mRNA level in fly photoreceptors is modulated by 11-*cis* retinoid, presented at Int. Symp. Signal Transduc. Photorecep. Cells, Julich, 41, Aug. 8-11, 1990.

45. **Dowling, J. E. and Wald, G.**, Vitamin A deficiency and night blindness, *Proc. Natl. Acad. Sci. USA*, 44, 648, 1958.

46. **Dowling, J. E. and Wald, G.**, The biological activity of vitamin A acid, *Proc. Nat. Acad. Sci. (USA)*, 46, 587, 1960.

47. **Katz, M. L., Stark, W. S., White, R. H., Gao, C. L., and Kutryb, M.**, Influence of dietary vitamin A on opsin density in the photoreceptor outer segment disc membranes., *Invest. Ophthalmol. Vis. Sci. Suppl.*, 31, 77, 1990.

48. **Katz, M. L., Gao, C. L., Kutryb, M., Norberg, M., White, R. H., and Stark, W. S.**, Maintenance of opsin density in photoreceptor outer segments of retinoid-deprived rats, *Invest. Ophthalmol. Vis. Sci.*, submitted, 1991.

49. **St. Jules, R. S., Wallingford, J. C., Smith, S. B., and O'Brien, P. J.**, Addition of the chromophore to rat rhodopsin is an early post-translational event, *Exp. Eye Res.*, 48, 653, 1989.

50. **Fliesler, S. J. and Basinger, S. F.**, Tunicamycin blocks the incorporation of opsin into retinal rod outer segment membranes, *Proc. Natl. Acad. Sci. USA*, 82, 1116, 1985.

51. **Fliesler, S. J., Rapp, L. M., and Hollyfield, J. G.**, Photoreceptor-specific degeneration caused by tunicamycin, *Nature (Lond.)*, 311, 575, 1984.

52. **White, R. H. and Bennett, R. R.**, Effects of rhodopsin defiency and tunicamycin on ultrastructure of insect photoreceptors, *Invest. Ophthalmol. Vis. Sci. Suppl.*, 28, 343, 1987.

53. **deCouet, H. G. and Tanimura, T.**, Monoclonal antibodies provide evidence that rhodopsin in the outer rhabdomeres of *Drosophila melanogaster* is not glycosylated, *Euro. J. Cell Biol.*, 44, 50, 1987.

54. **Paulsen, R., Bentrop, J., Plangger, A., and Huber, A.**, Post-translational modification of dipteran opsin: phosphorylation and glycosylation, presented at Int. Symp. Signal Transduc. Photorecep. Cells, Julich, 26, Aug. 8-11,1990.

55. **Huber, A. and Paulsen, R.**, The glycosylation state of *Calliphora* R1-6 opsin during biogenesis of photoreceptor membranes, presented at Int. Symp. Signal Transduc. Photorecep. Cells, Julich, 36, Aug. 8-11, 1990.

56. **Stark, W. S., Lin, T. N., Brackhahn, D., and Sun, G. Y.**, Genetic dissection of lipids in *Drosophila* heads by using eye mutants, presented at Molec. Neurobiol. *Drosophila*. Cold Spring Harbor, 45, Oct. 4-8, 1989.

57. **Sun, G. Y. and Lin, T. N.**, Time course for labelling of brain membrane phosphoinositides and other phospholipids after intracerebral injection of ^{32}P-ATP: Evaluation by an improved HPTLC procedure, *Life Sci.*, 44, 489, 1989.

58. **Bazan, N. G.**, Lipid-derived metabolites as possible retina messengers: Arachidonic acid, leukotrienes, docosanoids, and platelet activating factor, in *Extracellular and Intracellular Messengers in the Vertebrate Retina*, Eds., Alan R. Liss, Inc., New York, 1989, 269.

59. **Yoshioka, T., Inoue, H., Kasama, T., Seyama, Y., Nakashima, J., Nozawa, Y., and Hotta, Y.**, Evidence that arachidonic acid is deficient in phosphatidylinositol of *Drosophila* heads, *J. Biochem.*, 98, 657, 1985.

60. **Bowes, C., Danciger, M., Kozak, C. A., and Farber, D. B.**, Isolation of a candidate cDNA for the gene causing retinal degeneration in the *rd* mouse, *Proc. Nat. Acad. Sci. (USA)*, 86, 9722, 1989.

61. **Bowes, C., Li, T., Danciger, M., Applebury, M. L., and Farber, D. B.**, The rd gene codes for the beta-subunit of cGMP-phosphodiesterase, presented at Int. Symp. Retinal Degen., Stockholm, July 24-27, 1990.

62. **Yoshioka, T., Inoue, H., and Hotta, Y.**, Absence of phosphotidylinositol phosphodiesterase in the head of a *Drosophila* visual mutant, norpA (no receptor potential A), *J. Biochem.*, 97, 1251, 1985.

63. **Inoue, H., Yoshioka, T., and Hotta, Y.**, Membrane-associated phospholipase C of *Drosophila* retina, *J. Biochem.*, 103, 91, 1988.

64. **Bloomquist, B. T., Shortridge, R. D., Schnewly, S., Perdew, M., Montell, C., Steller, H., Rubin, G., and Pak, W. L.**, Isolation of a putative phospholipase C gene of *Drosophila*, *norpA*, and its role in phototransduction, *Cell*, 54, 723, 1988.

65. **Berridge, M. J.**, The molecular basis of communication within the cell, *Sci. Am. (Nov.)*, 253, 142, 1985.

66. **Ostroy, S. E., Wilson, M., and Pak, W. L.**, *Drosophila* rhodopsin: photochemistry, extraction and differences in the *norpA*^{P12} phototransduction mutant, *Biochem. Biophys. Res. Comm.*, 59, 960, 1974.

67. **Pak, W. L. and Lidington, K. L.**, Fast electrical potential from a long-lived, long-wavelength pho-

toproduct of fly visual pigment, *J. Gen. Physiol.*, 63, 740, 1974.

68. **Ulschafer, R. J., Clausnitzer, E. L., Sherry, D. M., Szel, A., and Rohlich, P.**, Innunocytochemical identification of outer segment proteins in the *rd* chicken, *Exp. Eye Res.*, 51, 209-216, 1990.

69. **Minke, B. and Kirschfeld, K.**, Fast electrical potentials arising from activation of metarhodopsin in the fly, *J. Gen. Physiol.*, 75, 381, 1980.

70. **Stephenson, R. S. and Pak, W. L.**, Heterogenic components of a fast electrical potential in *Drosophila* compound eye and their relation to visual pigment photoconversion, *J. Gen. Physiol.*, 75, 353, 1980.

71. **Stark, W. S., Stavenga, D. G., and Kruizinga, B.**, Fly photoreceptor fluorescence is related to UV sensitivity, *Nature (Lond.)*, 280, 581, 1979.

72. **Miller, G. V., Itoku, K. A., Fleischer, A. B., and Stark, W. S.**, Studies of fluorescence in *Drosophila* compound eyes: changes induced by intense light and vitamin A deprivation, *J. Comp. Physiol.*, 154, 297, 1984.

73. **Ham, W. T., Mueller, H. A., Ruffolo, J. J. J., Guerry, D. I., and Guerry, R. K.**, Action spectrum for retinal injury from near ultraviolet radiation in the aphakic monkey, *Am. J. Ophthalmol.*, 93, 199, 1982.

74. **Palazzolo, M. J., Hyde, D. R., Raghaven, K. V., Mecklenburg, K., Benzer, S., and Meyerowitz, E.**, Use of a new strategy to isolate and characterize 436 *Drosophila* cDNA clones corresponding to RNAs detected in adult heads but not in early embryos, *Neuron*, 3, 527, 1989.

SECTION II

SYSTEMIC, LOCAL, AND ENVIRONMENTAL FACTORS
AFFECTING PHOTORECEPTORS

It has long been known that environmental factors such as light and oxygen play important roles in retinal degeneration. Systemic diseases such as diabetes and hypertension may also lead to destruction of the retina. However, little is known about the role of systemic factors in retinal diseases, and only recently have local retinal factors been identified that promote survival of photoreceptors.

The first four papers in this section relate to the role of local factors in the retina in regulating the differentiation and even survival of photoreceptor cells. One describes the development of photoreceptor cells in culture, while two others discuss the role of basic fibroblast growth factor in photoreceptor cell survival. The last considers the role of glial cells in the retina.

The next four papers deal with the role of docosahexaenoic acid (22:6n-3) in photoreceptors. One paper describes the effects of 22:6n-3 deficiency on function of primate retinas, and another discusses delivery of 22:6n-3 to the retina. Two others discuss the role of n-3 polyunsaturated fatty acids in inherited retinal degenerations in humans and animals.

Environmental factors affecting photoreceptor integrity are discussed in two papers. One deals with the role of UVA in retinal degeneration and the other with protection from light damage by natural and synthetic antioxidants.

Accumulation of high levels of normal cellular metabolites may lead to retinal degeneration. Two chapters deal with this topic: one discusses cyclic GMP in the retina and the other the fluorophores in the retinal pigment epithelium.

The interphotoreceptor matrix has received considerable attention in recent years because of the importance of the retina-pigment epithelium relationship. Three subjects covered in this area are the role of rod outer segment carbohydrates on recognition and phagocytosis by the pigment epithelium, proteoglycans in the interphotoreceptor matrix, and light-induced changes in the interphotoreceptor matrix.

MOLECULAR FACTORS REGULATING THE SURVIVAL AND DIFFERENTIATION OF PHOTORECEPTOR CELLS

Ruben Adler and A. Tyl Hewitt
The Wilmer Eye Institute
The Johns Hopkins University
School of Medicine
Baltimore, Maryland

I. INTRODUCTION: THE "TROPHIC" CONCEPT

The concept that the survival and differentiation of neuronal cells are regulated by "trophic factors" has as its basis the correlation between developmental neuronal death and the association of neurons with their postsynaptic targets[1]. In short, only those neurons which are successful in interacting with their targets will survive. Trophic factors can be perceived as regulatory molecules which provide the environment needed to mobilize a cell's metabolic machinery (e.g. enzymes and nutrients) resulting in long term cell survival. In this regard, trophic factors are similar to hormones. However, while hormones are delivered by a vascular route, trophic factors are produced in the immediate neighborhood of their site of action (i.e. "locally" derived). Because of the often complex local cellular environment in which these factors would be expected to have an effect, cell culture has played a pivotal role in their investigation. Obviously, it is necessary to separate the neurons of interest from possible sources of trophic support in order to investigate their trophic requirements *in vitro*, before verifying the effects of trophic agents *in vivo*.

In spite of the discovery of NGF (nerve growth factor) several decades ago,[2,3] the field of trophic factor research did not gain universal recognition until recently when such culture systems became available. Since then there has been a change in the general perception of these factors by the scientific community resulting from the cloning of both NGF and its receptor, by the discovery, purification and cloning of other trophic factors, such as BDNF (brain-derived neuronotrophic factor),[4] and CNTF (ciliary neuron trophic factor),[5] and by observations that several recognized growth factors, including EGF and FGF, were also active on cells of the nervous system.[6-9] The observation that several of the degenerating neuronal groups in Alzheimer's disease require NGF for their survival has brought into focus the possible application of neuronotrophic factors as therapeutic agents.[10,11]

As mentioned above, the identification of trophic factors requires the availability of adequate *in vitro* bioassays consisting of isolated neuronal populations which eventually die off in culture. The development of cell cultures for isolated photoreceptor cells has opened the possibility of investigating their trophic requirements. In this paper, we will describe the characteristics of the cells in these cultures and discuss our studies on the influence of several classes of molecules on their survival and expression of differentiated properties.

II. THE CULTURE SYSTEM

In this system, embryonic chick retina are dissociated and plated at low density on polyornithine-coated tissue culture dishes.[12,13] Under these conditions, neurons develop in the absence of glial, epithelial, or endothelial cells. From detailed analyses of these cultures,[12,14–19] it can be concluded that many of the differentiated properties expressed by the photoreceptors are acquired by the cells early in their development, and can be expressed without physical contact with other cells (Figure 1). This concept derives from the finding that retinal precursor cells, removed from their microenvironment <u>before</u> they begin to differentiate and then allowed to grow *in vitro* in the absence of intercellular contacts, express a complex phenotype which includes not only the synthesis of cell-specific molecules, such as opsin, but also a complex pattern of morphological organization which includes structural and molecular polarity (Table 1). In addition, these cells express photo-

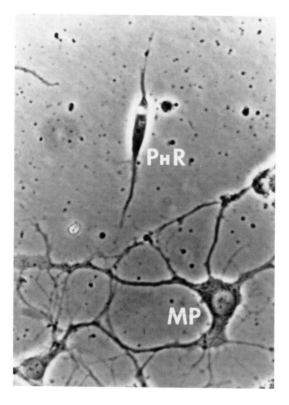

Figure 1. Phase contrast photomicrograph of a 5-day-old culture generated from 8-day-old embryonic chick neural retina. Both multipolar neurons (MP) and photoreceptors (PhR), with their characteristic lipid droplet, are identifiable. See Table 1 for additional characteristics of photoreceptors in these cultures. [Reprinted from reference 22, with permission].

TABLE 1
Properties of Cultured Photoreceptors

Compartmentalized Organization

Short neurite
Cell body
Inner segment
Short outer segment

Asymmetry and Polarization

Morphological
Biochemical (e.g. Na$^+$,K$^+$ ATPase, opsin)

Molecular Specialization

Opsin
Peanut agglutinin receptors
Specific uptake mechanisms

mechanical movements when grown in a light cycle,[20] demonstrating that their differentiation is functional as well as molecular and structural. The identity of the molecular signals which determine photoreceptor cells early in development is not known, but their identification is an area of intense interest. It is our hypothesis that the photoreceptor phenotype represents the "default" developmental pathway for retinal precursor cells in the absence of positional signals normally available during cell migration.[19] The recent observation that isolated retinal precursor cells undergoing terminal mitosis *in vitro* differentiate predominantly as photoreceptors may serve as a bioassay in these investigations.[21]

III. PHOTORECEPTOR SURVIVAL-PROMOTING ACTIVITY

Our observations have indicted that the cells survive and differentiate normally through the first 4 or 5 days in culture. However, the photoreceptors die in large numbers between *in vitro* days 7 and 10. This phenomenon has been used as a bioassay for the investigation of photoreceptor survival-promoting agents. The logical candidates as sources for these activities are the postsynaptic cells to which photoreceptors are connected, the glial cells of Müller, and the retinal pigment epithelium. The interphotoreceptor matrix (IPM), which is bordered by the latter two cell types and by photoreceptors, was thought to be a reasonable starting material for these investigations. Initial studies, using IPM preparations derived from either adult chicken or bovine eyes by gentle rinsing of retinas with saline,

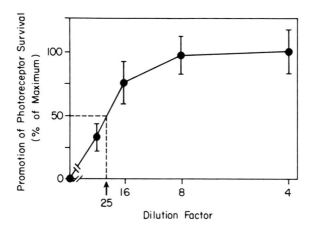

Figure 2. A dilution series of crude IPM preparations indicates that the promotion of photoreceptor survival is concentration-dependent and saturable. Using a dilution series, a trophic unit (TU) can be defined as the amount of activity in 1 ml of medium supporting survival at 50% of the maximal level. The number of TU/ml in this preparation is read directly from the plot as being 25 TU/ml (i.e. 1 TU was achieved with a 25-fold dilution). [Reprinted from reference 22, with permission].

indicated the presence of an activity that promoted photoreceptor survival in a concentration-dependent manner (Figure 2). Interestingly, other types of neurons present in the same cultures failed to show any responses indicating the specificity of the effect. The activity does not appear to stimulate differentiation of photo-receptors since cell counts during the culture period indicate that the number of photoreceptors increased in parallel in IPM-treated and control cultures to a maximum reached after 3-4 days *in vitro*. What appears to be affected is the onset and/or the rate of photoreceptor degeneration during the second half of the culture period. Studies on the physical and chemical properties of the activity indicate that the activity is thermolabile and sensitive to pH <6.5 and >8. Its apparent sensitivity to freezing at -70°C can be overcome by initially freezing in liquid nitrogen. The well characterized IPM molecule, interphotoreceptor retinoid-binding protein (IRBP), had no effect in the bioassay. In addition, purified NGF, CNTF and FGF failed to mimic the activity of crude IPM preparations.[22]

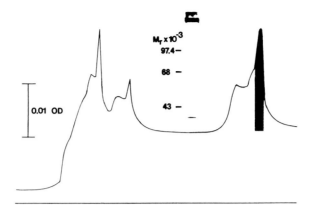

Figure 3. Chromatogram (absorbance at 280 nm) of a representative IPM preparation separated by chromatofocusing. This procedure develops a descending pH gradient with molecules eluting near their isoelectric point. The hatched peak represents the localization of the trophic activity which elutes at ~pH=5.5. When this material is subsequently chromatographed on a heparin-agarose column, the bound material, which contains the activity, produces the protein profile on SDS-gels as indicated in the inset.

Behavior on a variety of chromatographic supports have been investigated to develop a strategy for isolating the activity. The activity can be fractionated by gel filtration on Sephacryl S-200 (1.5 x 100 cm) from which it eludes in two peaks (M_r ~ 400 kDa and 33 kDa).[22] Our studies suggest that the activity readily aggregates to form high molecular weight complexes. The activity binds to heparin affinity columns, and is eluted at 0.5 M NaCl, which is lower than that required for other known growth factors, such as FGF. The combination of heparin affinity chromatography with hydrophobic interaction chromatography results in a 720-fold purification with a unit of biological activity (defined as a concentration necessary to obtain 50% of the maximum survival promoting activity) corresponding to 40 ng/ml.[22] While this activity is yet to be purified to homogeneity, recent studies combining chromatofocusing and heparin affinity chromatography showed substantial simplification of the protein profile (Figure 3). While these studies are promising, there are still many questions remaining regarding mechanism, cellular origin, etc. The production of antibodies is our current short term goal which will provide us with useful tool for answering these important questions.

IV. EFFECTS OF RETINOIDS ON OPSIN EXPRESSION
BY PHOTORECEPTORS *IN VITRO*

Retinoids are a family of molecules which are known to be related to photoreceptor well-being and function in at least two different ways. In addition to the well known role of 11-cis retinal in visual transduction, it has been observed that rats deprived of vitamin A suffer first from night blindness and eventually from photoreceptor degeneration.[23-26] The mechanism underlying the "trophic" effects of vitamin A remains unknown. These latter observations and the finding that retinoic acid has been shown to regulate the differentiation of a variety of cell types[27-30] has led us to investigate the effects of various retinoids on isolated photoreceptor cells *in vitro*. In both embryonic chick and newborn mouse retinal cultures, the inclusion of retinoids into the culture medium results in a pronounced increase in the concentration of opsin immunoreactive materials measured with a slot blot assay as well as in the number of opsin-positive photoreceptor cells.[31] The increase in cellular opsin-immunoreactivity was accompanied in many photoreceptor cells by the development of an enlarged outer segment-like process at the apical end of the cells. Similar effects were obtained regardless of whether 11-*cis* retinaldehyde, all-*trans* retinol or retinoic acid was used. The effects were concentration dependent, with a maximum response at concentrations (10^{-8}-10^{-7} M) which are considered "physiological" in the literature. Interestingly, the increase in opsin expression seems to be specific since neither IRBP levels, nor GABA and glutamate high affinity uptake activities appeared to be affected.[31] Similarly, the overall survival of photoreceptor cells in the cultures did not change in response to retinoid treatment. Although it is possible that the increase in opsin expression in cultured photoreceptor cells could be due to mechanisms other than increased gene expression, the well known function of retinoids, such as retinoic acid, in regulating gene expression suggests this as a likely mechanism.[32] Changes in the levels of opsin message in response to retinoic acid treatment is currently being investigated using probes for chick rod and cone visual pigment genes.

V. SUMMARY

Our *in vitro* studies and those *in vivo* and *in vitro* from other laboratories using a variety of systems seem to indicate that what is true for other PNS and CNS neurons is also true for photoreceptor cells: their survival and differentiation are regulated in a specific manner through the interaction of one or more molecular agents. Some of these factors are apparently "local" in nature and seem to fulfill the definition of a trophic factor, while others may act in a more systemic manner. In any event, it is reasonable to speculate that, as we learn more about these regulatory agents, photoreceptor degenerative disorders may represent a situation similar to that being discussed in connection with Alzheimer's disease and that these factors may represent possible therapeutic agents.

ACKNOWLEDGMENTS

The authors are most grateful to Ms. Doris Golembieski for her exceptional assistance in the preparation of this paper. This work was supported in part by USPHS NEI grants EY04859 (R.A.), EY05404 (R.A.) and EY06963 (A.T.H.).

REFERENCES

1. Adler, R., Trophic factors in neuronal development, in *Handbook of Human Growth and Developmental Biology*, Meisami, E. and Timiras, P., Eds., CRC Press, Inc., Boca Raton, 1988. 67.

2. Levi-Montalcini, R. S. and Angeletti, P. U., Nerve growth factor, *Physiol. Rev.* 48, 534, 1968.

3. Levi-Montalcini, R., The nerve growth factor 35 years later, *Science*, 237, 1154, 1987.

4. Barde, Y. A., Edgard, D. and Thoenen, H., New neuronotrophic factors, *Ann. Rev. Physiol.*, 45, 601, 1982.

5. Barbin, G., Manthorpe, M. and Varon, S., Purification of the chick eye ciliary neuronotrophic factor, *J. Neurochem.*, 43, 1468, 1984.

6. Walicke, P., Cowan, W. M., Ueno, N., Baird, A. and Guillemin, R., Fibroblast growth factor promotes survival of dissociated hippocampal neurons and enhances neurite extension, *Proc. Natl. Acad. Sci. U.S.A.* 83, 3012, 1986.

7. Morrison, R. S., Kornblum, H. I., Leslie, F. M. and Bradshaw, R. A., Trophic stimulation of cultured neurons from neonatal rat brain by epidermal growth factor, *Science*, 238, 72, 1987.

8. Morrison, R. S., Sharma, A., deVellis, J. and Bradshaw, R. A., Basic fibroblast growth factor supports the survival of cerebral cortical neurons in primary culture, *Proc. Natl. Acad. Sci. U.S.A.* 83, 7537, 1986.

9. Faktorovich, E. G., Steinberg, R. H., Yasumura, D., Matthes, M. T. and LaVail, M. M., Photoreceptor degeneration in inherited retinal dystrophy delayed by basic fibroblast growth factor, *Nature*, 347, 83, 1990.

10. Hefti, F. and Mash, D. C., Localization of nerve growth factor receptors in normal human brain and in Alzheimer's disease, *Neurobiol. Aging* 10, 75, 1989.

11. Hefti, F., Hartikka, J. and Knusel, B., Function of neuronotrophic factors in the adult and aging brain and their possible treatment of neurodegenerative diseases, *Neurobiol. Aging* 10, 515, 1989.

12. Adler, R., Lindsey, J. D. and Elsner, C. L., Expression of cone-like properties by chick embryo neural retina cells in glial-free monolayer cultures, *J. Cell Biol.*, 99, 1173, 1984.

13. Adler, R., Preparation, enrichment, and growth of purified cultures of neurons and photoreceptors from chick embryos and from normal and mutant mice, in *Methods in Neurosciences*, Vol. 2, *Cell Culture*, Conn, P. M., Ed., Academic Press, Inc. Orlando, 1990. 134.

14. Adler, R., Developmental predetermination of the structural and molecular polarization of photoreceptor cells, *Dev. Biol.*, 117, 520, 1986.

15. Adler, R., Nature and nurture in the differentiation of retinal photoreceptors and neurons, *Cell Differ.*, 20, 183, 1987.

16. Adler, R., The differentiation of retinal photoreceptors and neurons *in vitro*, in *Progress in Retinal Research*, Vol. 6, Osborne, N. and Chader, G., Eds., Pergamon Press, London, 1987. 1.

17. Madreperla, S. A. and Adler, R., Opposing microtubule- and actin-dependent forces in the development and maintenance of structural polarity in retinal photoreceptors, *Dev. Biol.* 131, 149, 1989.

18. Madreperla, S. A., Edidin, M. and Adler, R., Na^+,K^+-Adenosine triphosphatase polarity in retinal photoreceptors: A role for cytoskeletal attachments, *J. Cell Biol.* 109, 1483, 1989.

19. Adler, R. and Hatlee, M., Plasticity and differentiation of embryonic retinal cells after terminal mitosis, *Science*, 243, 391, 1989.

20. Stenkamp, D. and Adler, R., Photomechanical responses of isolated embryonic chick photoreceptors in cell culture, *Invest. Ophthalmol. Vis. Sci. (Suppl.)*, 31, 4, 1990.

21. Repka, A. and Adler, R., Differentiation of retinal precursor cells undergoing terminal mitosis *in vitro*, *Invest. Ophthalmol. Vis. Sci. (Suppl.)*, 31, 284, 1990.

22. Hewitt, A. T., Lindsey, J. D. Carbott, D. and Adler, R., Photoreceptor survival-promoting activity in interphotoreceptor matrix preparations: Characterization and partial purification, *Exp. Eye Res.*, 50, 79, 1990.

23. Wald, G., The biochemistry of vision, *Annu. Rev. Biochem.*, 22, 497, 1953.

24. Dowling, J. E., Chemistry of visual adaptation in the rat, *Nature (London)*, 188, 114, 1960.

25. Dowling, J. E. and Wald, G., The biological function of vitamin A acid, *Proc. Natl. Acad. Sci. U.S.A.*, 46, 587, 1960.

26. Dowling, J. E. and Gibbons, I. R., The effect of vitamin A deficiency on the fine structure of the retina, in *The Structure of the Eye*, Smelser, G. K., Ed., Academic Press, New York, 1961. 85.

27. Brockes, J. P., Retinoids, homeobox genes and limb morphogenesis, *Neuron*, 2, 1285, 1989.

28. Eichele, G., Retinoids and vertebrate limb pattern formation, *Trends Gen.*, 5, 246, 1989.

29. Giguere, V., Ong, E. S., Segui, P. and Evans, R. M., Identification of a receptor for the morphogen retinoic acid, *Nature*, 300, 624, 1989.

30. Maden, M., Ong, D. E. and Chytil, F., Retinoid-binding protein distribution in the developing mammalian nervous system, *Development*, 109, 75, 1990.

31. Adler, R. and Politi, L. E., Effects of 11-cis retinal and other retinoids on opsin expression by isolated mouse and chick photoreceptor cells in culture, *Invest. Ophthalmol. Vis. Sci. (Suppl.)*, 30, 157, 1989.

32. Stark, W. and Katz, M., Opsin gene expression: control by vitamin A in rat vs fly, *Soc. Neurosci. Abst.* 16, 1076, 1990.

FIBROBLAST GROWTH FACTOR AND PHOTORECEPTOR-RETINAL PIGMENTED EPITHELIUM CELL BIOLOGY

HICKS, D., MALECAZE, F., MASCARELLI, F., BUGRA, K. AND COURTOIS, Y.
UNITE DE GERONTOLOGIE
INSERM U 118
29, rue Wilhem - 75016 PARIS, FRANCE

1. GENERAL INTRODUCTION

In recent years, trophic factors have become widely implicated in regulating various aspects of central nervous system (CNS) development and function. Nerve growth factor (NGF) has been shown to be crucial for the survival of cholinergic CNS neurons[1], but in addition novel neurotrophic molecules have been identified properties have been demonstrated to influence neuronal metabolism. The first category includes such molecules as brain derived neurotrophic factor (BDNF)[2], whilst the second includes such well known substances as epidermal growth factor (EGF) and fibroblast growth factor (FGF)[3]. Particularly this latter family of low molecular weight polypeptides has emerged as a strong candidate for representing a true group of neurotrophic agents. The evidence for this activity is based mainly on demonstrations of FGF's stimulation of cell survival and neurite outgrowth in neuronal cell lines[4,5] and primary cultures[6-8]. They have also been shown to enhance neuronal survival <u>in vivo</u> following surgical ablation[9].

The retina, which develops as an outgrowth of the neural tube early in embryogenesis, is no exception to this rule. Trophic factors were isolated from this tissue many years ago[10], and subsequently shown to be identical to brain-derived FGF. Acidic FGF (aFGF), the form predominant in nervous tissue, was also subsequently purified from photoreceptor outer segments (OS), where its binding was shown to be cyclic nucleotide and phosphorylation dependent[11,12]. Autoradiographic localization of radiolabelled FGF binding in the retina reveals low affinity basement membrane[13] and high affinity cell surface[14] binding sites. aFGF has been shown to stimulate opsin levels in cultured retinal photoreceptors[15] and axon regeneration in cultured retinal ganglion cells[16]. Finally, and perhaps most dramatically, intraocular injection of FGF stimulates complete regeneration of the neural retina from the retinal pigmented epithelium (RPE)[17].

Given these data on the implication of FGF in retinal differentiation and function, its possible role in inherited retinal degenerations and other ocular pathologies becomes evident. aFGF has recently been implicated in epiretinal membrane formation subsequent to retinal surgery[18]. Importantly, chimaeric recombination[19] and tissue transplant[20] studies suggest the presence of a diffusible trophic factor secreted by normal RPE which can rescue photoreceptor cells from an otherwise progressive deterioration and death in animal models of retinal dystrophy. The possibility that this molecule is FGF is raised by the facts that RPE cells synthesize FGF[21], and that intraocular injections of FGF into rats suffering from retinal dystrophy (the RCS rat) similarly rescue photoreceptor cells destined to die[22].

We chose to examine two aspects of the involvement of FGF in photoreceptor and RPE cell biology :
1) FGF effects on normal and dystrophic rat and mouse photoreceptors in vitro
2) FGF effects on and synthesis by normal and RCS rat RPE in vitro.

2. FGF AS A TROPHIC FACTOR FOR PHOTORECEPTOR CELLS

A. THE RCS RAT

The neural retina of newborn normal sighted (Long-Evans black hooded or RCS-rdy+-p tan hooded) or dystrophic (RCS-rdy-p+ black hooded) rats is essentially composed of a thick neuroblastic zone containing undifferentiated neuroblasts overlying a primitive inner plexiform layer and ganglion cell layer. Immunolabelling of such retina with anti-opsin antibodies reveal that a few positively labelled cells, corresponding to differentiating photoreceptors, are already present at the scleral surface. In both normal and RCS rats the number of positively stained cells and intensity of labelling increase over the first postnatal week[23], so that by 7-8 days after birth the emerging outer segments (OS), inner segments (IS) and photoreceptor cell bodies (outer nuclear layer = ONL) are all heavily labelled by anti-opsin antibodies (Figures 1a-d). Whereas normal retinas maintain this general aspect of labelling into maturity, with the OS, IS and ONL all brightly labelled (Figure 1e, f), the RCS retina begins to degenerate after about three weeks, and eventually the photoreceptor layer is reduced to a zone of opsin immunoreactive debris (Figure 1g, h).

Newborn rat retinas were isolated, cut into small fragments, digested and seeded as cell suspensions as previously described[15]. When seeded onto substrates such as laminin and maintained in serum supplemented media, cell attachment and process outgrowth occur rapidly (Figures 2a, b). Retinal glial cells proliferate rapidly to form a confluent carpet by about 5 days in vitro, upon which the retinal neurons form a network of cell bodies and processes (Figure 2f). Culture morphology retains this aspect for 8-14 days, depending on the substrate, initial seeding density or number of media changes, after which the glial monolayer begins to disintegrate and cell death follows within a few days (Figure 2e). This is true for both normal and RCS retinal cells. Addition of aFGF, basic FGF (bFGF), or EGF to such cultures induces an increase in glial cell proliferation, as observed by examination of living cultures (Figures 2c, d) and ^{3}H-thymidine uptake (Figure 3). NGF does not stimulate any mitogenic response. Thus FGF

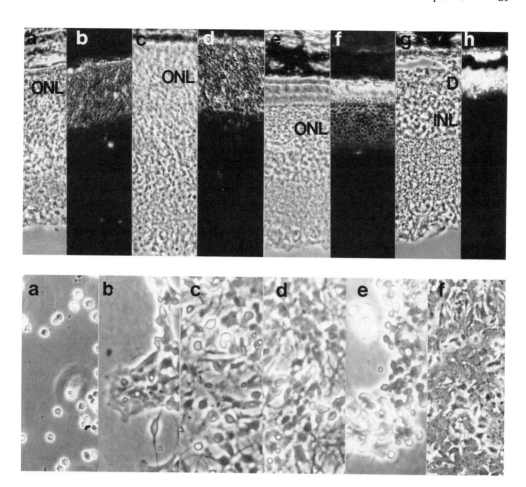

Figure 1 (top) : Light microscope immunocytochemistry of
normal and dystrophic retinas labelled with rho-4D2 anti-
opsin antibody. a) Phase contrast of normal 7 day postnatal
rat retina. b) Rho-4D2 binds to the ONL and emerging OS. c)
Phase contrast of dystrophic 7 day rat retina. d) Rho-4D2
labelling resembles the normal retina. e) Phase contrast of
30 day normal rat retina. f) Rho-4D2 binding is very
intense in the OS and ONL. g) Phase contrast of 90 day
dystrophic rat retina, showing reduced thickness due to
disappearance of the ONL. h) Rho-4D2 binding is restricted
to a band of membranous debris (D). Abbreviations as in
text. ×175.

Figure 2 (bottom) :Morphology of newborn normal retinal
cells in vitro. a) Newly seeded dissociated cells. b)
Untreated culture after 4 days in vitro : the glial cells
have spread out on the substrate. c) 4 day culture with 50
ng/ml aFGF : much more glial cell growth has occurred. d) 4
day culture with 20 ng/ml EGF : again glial cell
proliferation is much greater than in controls. e)
Untreated culture after 15 days in vitro : the glial cell
monolayer has begun to break up. f) At 7 days in vitro all
treatments resemble each other closely : untreated
(pictured here), FGF, EGF and NGF treated cultures are all
confluent with randomly dispersed neurons. Magnification :
a,f x 330 ; b-e ×390.

and EGF treated cultures reach confluency 24-48h before
untreated or NGF treated cultures. However, the appearance
of all cultures subsequent to attainment of confluency is
indistinguishable (Figure 2f). This is also true for normal
or RCS rat retinal cultures.

Plating of similar cells onto more complex substrates
such as extracellular matrix which contains molecules such
as laminin, collagen IV, entactin and proteoglycan, can
result in much longer survival times in vitro, even in the
absence of exogenous growth factors. We have maintained
such monolayer cultures from dystrophic RCS rats for 2
months, by which time all the photoreceptor cells have died
in vivo (Figures 4a, b).

Harvesting of such cells at different time points
within the culture period, followed by solubilization and
aliquoting in microtitre plates permits an analysis of
photoreceptor development by radioimmunoassay (RIA). Using
specific anti-opsin antibodies followed by ^{125}I goat anti-
mouse antibody, we have previously shown that whereas opsin
levels in untreated normal retinal cultures remained very
low, aFGF addition resulted in a 5-10 fold increase around
day 7, levels remaining high thereafter[15]. A similar
phenomenon is seen with bFGF (Figure 5a). Dystrophic RCS
rate retinal cultures also manifest this FGF-induced
increase, in fact opsin levels rising even higher than in
the normal retina (Figure (5b). As is also seen in cultures

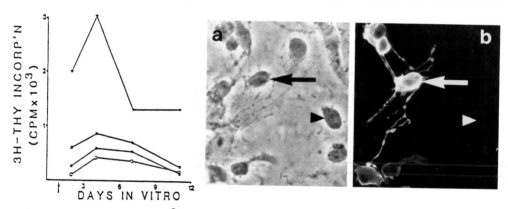

Figure 3 (left) : ^{3}H-thymidine incorporation into cultured
retinal cells with or without exogenous growth factors.
Cells were plated in serum-supplemented medium for 24h,
after which the medium was carefully replaced with defined
medium with or without growth factors. The incorporation of
[3]H-thymidine was measured in triplicate for each treatment
at different times in vitro. Open circles : untreated
cultures ; closed circles : 50 ng/ml aFGF added ; closed
squares : 10 ng/ml aFGF/ 10 μg/ml heparin added ; closed
triangles : 20 ng/ml EGF added.

Figure 4 (right) :Dystrophic retinal cells growing on
extracellular matrix after 83 days in vitro. a) Phase
contrast showing numerous birefringent neurons overling
glial cell monolayer. b) Rho-4D2 shows several brightly
labelled photoreceptors (arrow), whilst other neurons
(arrowhead) are completely unlabelled. ×880.

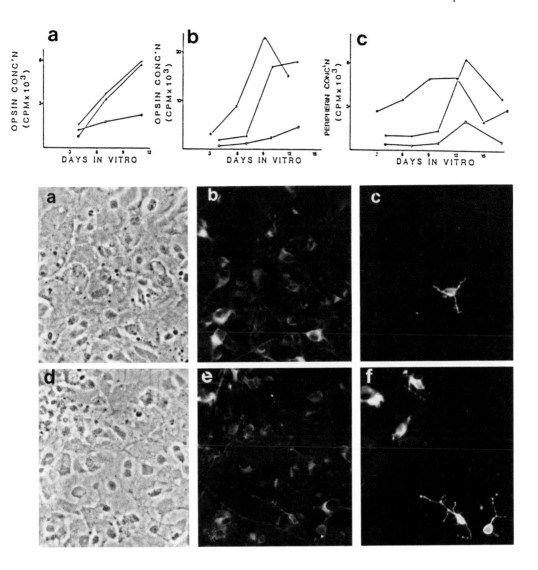

Figure 5 (top) :Solid phase radioimmunoassay of cultured normal and dystrophic retinal cells. Each point was calculated from duplicate wells of solubilized cultured cells incubated sequentially with the primary antibody (anti-opsin or anti-peripherin monoclonals) and goat anti-mouse IgG. a) Normal newborn retinal cells either without (open circles) or with 50 ng/ml aFGF (closed circles) or 1 ng/ml bFGF (closed triangles). Opsin levels are increased with FGF treatment. b) Dystrophic newborn retinal cell cultures in the absence (open circles) or presence of 50 ng/ml aFGF (closed circles) or 20 ng/ml aFGF/ 10 ng/ml heparin (closed squares). Large increases in opsin levels are noted in the treated cultures. c) Dystrophic newborn retinal cells cultured in the absence (open circles) or presence of 50 ng/ml aFGF (closed circles) or 20 ng/ml aFGF: 10 ng/ml heparin (closed squares). Large increases in the levels of peripherin are observed in the treated cultures.

Figure 6 (previous page, middle panel) : Newborn dystrophic RCS rat retinal cells after 7 days <u>in vitro</u> in the absence (a-c) or presence (d-f) of 10 ng/ml bFGF. Phase contrast images of untreated (a) and FGF treated (d) cultures are similar at this time, as are the number and distribution of total neurons immunoreactive for neuron specific enolase (b = untreated, e = FGF). However, FGF treated cultures exhibit many more opsin-immunoreactive photoreceptors (f) than the controls (c). Magnification ×615.

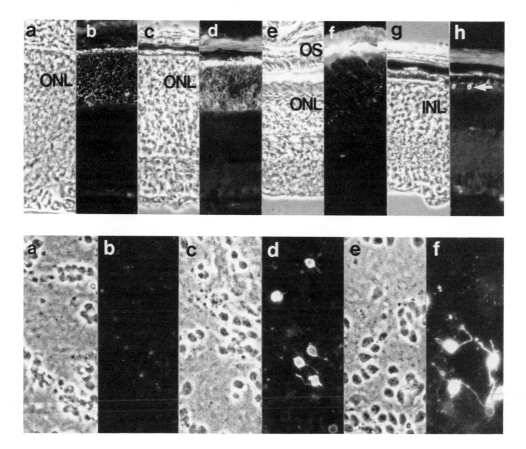

Figure 7 (top) : Opsin immunoreactivity in developing normal and <u>rd</u> mouse retina. At postnatal day 8, the retina is relatively mature in control (a) and <u>rd</u> (c) mice, and opsin-positive photoreceptor cell bodies fill the ONL (b and d respectively). Whereas the normal retina retains this pattern throughout life (e, f), 12 days later the ONL has almost entirely disappeared in the <u>rd</u> mutant (g), with rare opsin immunoreactive cells (arrow in h). ×260.

Figure 8 (bottom) : Newborn rd mouse retinal cells maintained for 10 days <u>in vitro</u> in the absence (a, b) or presence of 0.1 N acetic acid retinal extract (c, d) or purified native aFGF (10 ng/ml) and heparin (10 µg/ml). Opsin containing photoreceptors are only left in the treated cultures (d, f). ×390.

of normal retina, inclusion of heparin in the culture medium accelerates the rate at which RCS retinal cultures attain maximal levels of opsin expression (Figure 5b). In addition, levels of the photorecepor OS-specific protein peripherin[24] are also increased by aFGF in both normal and dystrophic retinal cultures (Figure 5c). Interestingly, the rise in peripherin concentration occurs with a lag of 2-3 days relative to opsin, reflecting the different temporal appearances of these two proteins in vivo.

Although we previously could not see any evidence of an increase in the number of opsin-expressing cells to account for this effect of FGF, recent refinement of the dissociation technique and use of double labelling immunocytochemistry has enabled us to demonstrate that indeed FGF stimulates a 3-8 fold increase in the number of retinal cells labelled by anti-opsin antibodies (manuscript submitted). This is also true for dystrophic retina (Figure 6a-f). Additionally, treatment of cultures with other growth factors known to exhibit neurotrophic properties, EGF[25] and NGF[1], does not have any effect on opsin expression. FGF effects are not through general enhancement of neuronal survival, as total numbers of neurons (as revealed by immunoreactivity for neuron specific enolase) do not change. Neither do the increases in opsin-expressing photoreceptor numbers correlate with glial cell numbers, which in fact vary little between untreated, FGF or EGF treated cultures at confluency.

B. THE rd MOUSE

Similar studies have been undertaken on the rd mouse, another animal model for retinal degenerations in which photoreceptor cell death occurs rapidly during the 3rd week of postnatal life. This time the lesion does not appear to be within the RPE[26], but has recently been mapped to the β sub-unit of cGMP phosphodiesterase[27].

Opsin immunocytochemistry of developing normal and rd in vivo retina, as for the RCS rat, shows the two to be initially similar and then a rapid disappearance of the ONL in the pathological mutant (Figures 7a-h). In vitro studies have previously demonstrated that under certain conditions both normal and mutant photoreceptor cells die rapidly after about 8 days[28]. In the present case, both normal and rd photoreceptor cells maintained in the absence of exogenous FGF also disappeared around day 10 in vitro (Figures 8a,b). However, cultures maintained with the addition of crude retinal FGF extracts (Figures 8c, d) or aFGF and heparin (Figures 8e, f) survived for several days longer. Due to the small amount of tissue obtained from newborn mouse eyes, quantitation by radioimmunoassay was not possible.

Although we cannot say whether these effects observed in vitro in both mice and rat retinas are direct or indirect, acting through the glial cell feeder layer by stimulating some other trophic factor or cell surface molecule, these data demonstrate that FGF is the first characterized molecule to modulate photoreceptor cell differentiation or survival. Taken together with the findings on the rescue of RCS rat photoreceptors by

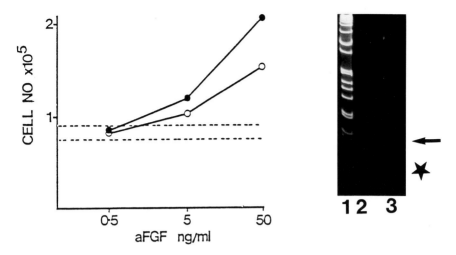

Figure 9 (left) : Proliferation of normal (closed circles) and dystrophic (open circles) RPE cells in response to aFGF addition. There is some variation in the half-maximal response between experiments on these primary cultured cells, but differences in normal and dystrophic ED_{50}'s (9 and 10 ng/ml respectively) were not statistically significant. Dashed lines = cell numbers in untreated wells of normal (upper) and RCS (lower) RPE.

Figure 10 (right) : aFGF mRNA transcripts in normal (lane 2) and dystrophic (lane 3) RPE revealed by polymerase chain reaction (PCR) analysis of confluent monolayers. The positions and intensities of the bands (arrow) are similar in both cases, after 24 cycles of amplification. Lane 1 : Molecular weight markers. Lower bands (star) : nitrate reductase standards.

intraocular injection of FGF[22], the evidence suggests photoreceptors are highly sensitive to and dependent on this trophic factor. The <u>in vitro</u> system we have developed should be very useful to analyse the cellular events triggered by FGF stimulation culminating in photoreceptor stimulation.

3. FGF SYNTHESIS BY AND PROLIFERATIVE STIMULATION OF RPE

The evidence existing demonstrating the RPE as the site of the primary lesion in RCS retinal dystrophy[19], the possible involvment of soluble factors in this condition[20], and the synthesis of bFGF by normal RPE[21], all led us to investigate the presence and action of FGF on normal and RCS RPE.

For the studies reported below, we used purified primary cultures of normal (RCS-rdy$^+$-p) and dystrophic (RCSrdy-p+) rat RPE cells, prepared by previously published methods[29].

A. PROLIFERATION OF RPE

Cells were seeded at densities of $8-30 \times 10^3$/well in 24 well plates, growth factors added on the first and third day of culture and cell numbers determined on the 5th day. aFGF was mitogenic for both normal and dystrophic RPE (Figure 9), the ED_{50} varying between 2-17 ng/ml for the two strains, with a mean ED_{50} of 11.5 and 9.7 ng/ml respectively for normal and RCS RPE. These values are in agreement with previously published activities on other cell types. Depending on the initial densities, both factors stimulated a 2-4 fold increase in cell numbers over the experimental period, and no significant differences were noted between normal or dystrophic.

B. FGF SYNTHESIS BY RPE

It has been reported that RPE contain bFGF mRNA but not aFGF mRNA[21]. Using a highly specific anti-aFGF polyclonal antibody, we have recently observed the presence of aFGF in pigmented cells within epiretinal membranes[18]. Furthermore, polymerase chain reaction (PCR) analysis using specific aFGF primers reveals that equal amounts of aFGF mRNA are present in primary cultures of normal and dystrophic RPE (Figure 10). Hence aFGF in addition to bFGF is expressed by these cells, and within dystrophic RPE. It is still possible that the molecule is released in an inactive form in the RCS rat. We are presently examining the presence of bFGF mRNA in normal and dystrophic RPE cells, and examining the activities present in conditioned media.

4. GENERAL DISCUSSION

The data presented in this chapter indicate that FGF is a vitally important molecule in the normal functioning of the retinal photoreceptor cell. FGF has been shown to have important effects on neuronal survival and development in other areas of the CNS [4-9], so it is perhaps not surprising to discover it has similar effects within the retina.

Possible in vivo sources of FGF for photoreceptors are the RPE, the retinal Muller cells, the photoreceptors themselves and circulating levels. The RPE synthesizes aFGF (present study) and bFGF[21], and presumably secretes FGF into the inter-photoreceptor matrix (IPM), which has been shown to contain substantial amounts of FGF[11]. Here it may bind to receptors on the photoreceptor cell, such as have been demonstrated at the level of the IS[14] or OS[12]. Muller cells are unlikely to be an important source of FGF as they do not appear to synthesize bFGF as examined by in situ hybridization[30], and contain only very low levels of aFGF mRNA as detected by PCR (data not shown). The photoreceptors synthesize aFGF, as do all retinal neurons[31], whereas it appears that only the photoreceptors are capable of synthesizing bFGF within the neural retina[30]. Finally, the retinal circulation sems to contain immunologically detectable bFGF during angiogenesis[32]. When one considers that RPE21, Muller cells[33] and photoreceptors[14] all contain high affinity surface receptors for FGF, the possibilities of autocrine and paracrine interactions are numerous. We still need to know more about the release of FGF's under physiological conditions into the IPM to be able to infer more accurately their role (s).

One should also consider the presence of co-factors and other molecules which may modulate growth factor action. The presence of retinal proteoglycans is well established[34] and RPE and Muller cells express ECM molecules such as proteoheparan sulfate and laminin[35] at their surfaces. Apart from their roles in cellular adhesion and cellular recognition, such molecules may also control FGF efficacy and accessibility to receptors.

Other trophic factors surely exist which are important in retinal metabolism. One partially characterized molecule stimulates photoreceptor survival in vitro[36] : this molecule bears certain resemblances to FGF, such as its affinity for heparin, but does not appear to be identical. It may thus represent another member of the heparin binding growth factor family.

Hence in conclusion, a large body of work now attests to the synthesis, presence and binding of FGF to the retina in vivo, and at least in certain in vitro conditions it markedly stimulates cellular differentiation and survival. The surprising potential of FGF as a therapeutic agent has also been revealed by its ability to prevent or delay photoreceptor cell death in genetically programmed dystrophies[22], although much more work on possible undesirable side-effects such as neovascularization[3] will have to be performed. We also recently demonstrated that RPE cells isolated from the RCS contain only 30% the number of FGF receptors found in normal congenic RPE cells (Malecaze et al, manuscript submitted), further extending the possibilities of FGF involvement in retinal pathologies. The next important step in research on FGF action in the outer retina will be the analysis of the transduction mechanisms within the cells and the cascade of molecular events leading to modification of gene expression

; we now possess the model systems, the probes and the techniques to tackle such questions.

5. REFERENCES

1. Korsching, S. The fate of nerve growth growth factor in the CNS. <u>Trends Neurosci</u>.. 9, 570, 1986
2. Barde, Y.A., Davies, A.M., Johnson, J.E., Lindsay, R.M. and Thoenen, H. Brain derived neurotrophic factor. <u>Prog. Brain Res</u>. 71, 185, 1987
3. Gospodarowicz, D., Neufeld, G. and Schweigerer, L. Molecular and biological characterization of fibroblast growth factor, an angiogenic factor which also controls the proliferation and differentiation of mesoderm and neuroectoderm-derived cells. <u>Cell Differ</u>. 19, 1, 1986
4. Neufeld, G., Gospodarowicz, D., Dodge, L. and Fujii, D.K. Heparin modulation of the neurotropic effects of acidic and basic fibroblast growth factors and nerve growth factor on PC 12 cells. <u>J. Cell PHysiol</u>. 131, 131, 1987
5. Rydel, R.E. and Greene, L.A. Acidic and basic fibroblast growth factor promote stable neurite outgrowth and neuronal differentiation in cultures of PC 12 cells. <u>J. Neurosci</u>. 7, 3639, 1987
6. Walicke, P.A., Cowan, W.M., Ueno, N., Baird, A. and Guillemin, R. Fibroblast growth factor promotes survival of dissociated hippocampal neurons and enhances neurite extension. <u>Proc. Natl. Acad. Sci</u>. USA. 83, 3012, 1986
7. Schubert, D., Ling, N. and Baird, A. Multiple influences of a heparin binding growth factor on neural development. <u>J. Cell Biol</u>. 104, 635, 1987
8. Hatten, M.E., Lynch, M., Rydel, R.E., Sanchez, J., Joseph-Silverstein, J., Moscatelli, D. and Rifkin, D.B. In vitro neurite extension by granule neurons is dependent upon astroglial derived fibroblast growth factor. <u>Dev. Biol</u>. 125, 280, 1988
9. Anderson, K.J., Dan, D., Lee, S. and Cofman, C.W. Basic fibroblast growth factor prevents death of lesioned cholinergic neurons in vivo. <u>Nature</u> 332, 360, 1988
10. Arruti, C. and Courtois, Y. Morphological changes and growth stimulation of bovine epithelial lens cells by a retinal extract in vitro. <u>Exp. Cell Res</u>. 117, 283, 1978
11. Plouet, J., Mascarelli, F., Loret, M.D., Faure, J-P. and Courtois, Y. Regulation of eye derived growth factor bindindgto membranes by light, ATP or GTP in photoreceptor outer segments. <u>EMBO J</u>. 7, 373 , 1988
12. Mascarelli, F., Raulais, D. and Courtois, Y. Fibroblast growth factor phosphorylation and receptors in rod outer segments. <u>EMBO J</u>. 8, 2265, 1989
13. Jeanny, J-C., Fayein, N.A., Moenner, M., Chevallier, B., Barritault, D. and Courtois, Y. Specific fixation of bovine brain and retinal acidic and basic fibroblast growth factors to mouse embryonic eye basement membranes. <u>Exp. Cell Res</u>. 171, 63, 1987
14. Fayein, N.A., Courtois, Y. and Jeanny, J-C. Ontogeny of basic fibroblast growth factor binding sites in mouse ocular tissues. <u>Exp. Cell Res</u>. 188, 75, 1990
15. Hicks, D. and Courtois, Y. Acidic fibroblast growth

factor stimulates opsin levels in retinal photoreceptor cells in vitro. FEBS Lett. 234, 475, 1988

16. Lipton, S.A., Wagner, J.A., Madison, R.D. and D'Amore, P.A. Acidic fibroblast growth factor enhances regeneration of processes by postnatal mammalian retinal ganglial cells in culture. Proc. Natl. Acad. Sci. USA. 85, 2388, 1988

17. Parks, C.A. and Hollenberg, M.J. Basic fibroblast growth factor induces retinal regeneration in vivo. Dev. Biol. 134, 201, 1988

18. Malecaze, F., Mathis, A., Arné, J-L., Raulais, D., Courtois, Y. and Hicks, D. Localization of acidic fibroblast growth factor in proliferative vitreoretinopathy membranes. Arch. Ophthalmol., submitted

19. Mullen, R.J. and La Vail, M.M Inherited retinal dystrophy : primary defect in pigment epithelial cells determined with experimental rat chimeras. Science 192, 799, 1976

20. Li, L. and Turner, J.E. Inherited retinal dystrophy in the RCS rat : prevention of photoreceptor degeneration by pigment epithelial cell transplantation.Exp. Eye Res. 47, 911, 1988

21. Schweigerer, L., Malerstein, B., Neufeld, G. and Gospodarowicz, D. Basic fibroblast growth factor is synthesized in cultured retinal pigment epithelial cells. Biochem. Biophys. Res. Commun. 143, 934, 1987

22. Faktorovich, E.G., Steinberg, R.H., Yasumura, D., Matthes, M.T and La Vail, M.M. Photoreceptor degeneration in inherited retinal dystrophy delayed by basic fibroblast growth factor. Nature 347, 83, 1990

23. Hicks, D. and Barnstable, C.J. Different rhodopsin monoclonal antibodies reveal different binding patterns on developing and adult retina. J. Histochem. Cytochem. 35, 1317, 1987

24. Molday, R.S., Hicks, D. and Molday, L.L. Peripherin : a rim-specific membrane protein of rod outer segment disks. Invest Ophthalmol. Vis. Sci. 28, 50, 1987

25. Morrison, R.S., Kornblum, H.I., Leslie, F.M and Bradshaw, R.A. Trophic stimulation of cultured neurons from neonatal rat brain by epidermal growth factor. Sci§ence 238, 72, 1987

26. La Vail, M.M and Muller, R.J. Role of the pigment epithelium in inherited retinal degeneration analyzed with experimental mouse chimeras. Exp. Eye Res. 23, 227, 1976

27. Bowes, C., Li, T., Dansiger, M., Baxter, L.C., Applebury, M.L and Farber, D.B. Retinal degeneration in the rd mouse is caused by a defect in the β-subunit of rod cGMP-phosphodiesterase. Nature 347, 677, 1990

28. Politi, L and Adler, R. Selective failure of long-term survival of isolated photoreceptors from both homozygous and heterozygous rd (retinal degeneration) mice. Exp. Eye Res. 47, 269, 1988

29. Edwards, R.B. Culture of rat retinal pigmented epithelium. In vitro 13, 301, 1977

30. Noji, S., Matsuo, T., Koyama, E., Yamaai, T., Nohno, T., Matsuo, N and Taneguchi, S. Expression pattern of acidic and basic fibroblast growth factor in adult rat eyes. Biochem. Biophys Res. Comm. 168, 343, 1990

31. Jacquemin E., Halley, C., Alterio, J., Laurent, M.,

Courtois, Y and Jeanny, J.C. Localization of acidic fibroblast growth factor (aFGF) mRNA in mouse and bovine retina by in situ hybridization. <u>Neurosci. Lett.</u> 116, 23, 1990

32. Hanneken, A., Lutty, G.A., McLeod, D.S., Robey, F., Harvey, A.K and Hjelmeland, L.M. Localization of basic fibroblast growth factor to the developing capillaries of the bovine retina. <u>J. Cell Physiol</u>. 138, 115, 1989

33. Mascarelli, F., Tassin, J and Courtois, Y. Effect of FGF's on adult bovine Muller cells : proliferation binding and internalization. <u>Growth Factors</u>, in press.

34. Hewitt, A.T.Extracellular matrix molecules : their importance in the structure and function of the retina. In : The retina : a model for cell biology, Adler and Farber, eds. Acad. Press, 1986, 169

35. Wakakura, M and Foulds, W.S. Laminin expressed by cultured Muller cells stimulates growth of retinal neurites. <u>Exp. Eye Res</u>. 48, 577, 1989

36. Hewitt, A.T., Lindsey, J.D., Carbott, D and Adler, R. Photoreceptor survival promoting activity in interphotoreceptor matrix preparations : characterization and partial purification. <u>Exp. Eye Res</u>. 50, 79, 1990

PHOTORECEPTOR RESCUE IN RETINAL DEGENERATIONS BY BASIC FIBROBLAST GROWTH FACTOR

Ella G. Faktorovich, Roy H. Steinberg, Douglas Yasumura,
Michael T. Matthes and Matthew M. LaVail

Departments of Anatomy, Physiology and Beckman Vision Center
University of California, San Francisco
San Francisco, CA 94143-0730, USA

I. INTRODUCTION

It is widely known that the normal functioning and viability of photoreceptors depends on multiple interactions with the retinal pigment epithelium (RPE).[1] This is readily apparent in the Royal College of Surgeons (RCS) rat, in which a genetic defect in the RPE results secondarily in the death of photoreceptor cells.[2] In experimental chimeras produced from RCS and normal rat embryos, where mutant and wild-type RPE cells had been intermingled, photoreceptors survived in those regions immediately adjacent to normal, wild-type RPE cells.[2] In addition, extension of the rescue effect beyond the boundaries of the wild-type RPE cells suggested a role for diffusible factors produced by the normal RPE cells.[2]

We were encouraged to search for such a putative diffusible factor(s) by two additional and more recent findings. First, in experiments where normal RPE cells were transplanted into the retinas of RCS rats before substantial PR cell death occurred, the normal RPE cells rescued photoreceptors from degenerating.[3,4] The rescue effect was found both adjacent to the transplanted RPE cells and beyond their boundaries, similar to the earlier observations in the experimental chimeras. Second, several recent studies demonstrated that the acidic and basic fibroblast growth factors (aFGF and bFGF, respectively) are present in the retina[5-9] and RPE,[10,11] and that rod outer segments have receptors for both FGFs.[8,9] These growth factors are widely known to act as mitogens and as differentiation-promoting agents in many systems; bFGF can induce retinal regeneration from the RPE;[12] and bFGF acts as a neurotrophic agent following axonal injury in several regions of the central nervous system.[13-15]

Could it be that either aFGF or bFGF is the diffusible factor responsible for photoreceptor rescue beyond the borders of the RPE cells in the experimental chimeras and transplantation experiments? To explore this question, we have studied the effect of these heparin-binding peptides on degenerating photoreceptor cells in two forms of retinal degeneration, inherited retinal dystrophy in the RCS rat and light damage in albino rats.

II. MATERIALS AND METHODS

The methods used in these studies are described in detail elsewhere.[16] Briefly, at selected ages, 1 μl of aFGF or bFGF dissolved in phosphate buffered saline (PBS) (500, 820 or 1150 ng/μl) was injected transsclerally into the subretinal (interphotoreceptor) space or into the vitreous of anesthetized rats. For buffer control experiments, 1 μl of PBS alone was injected in some animals, and in others the surgical control of a dry needle insertion was performed with no injection. Each of these was compared to uninjected animals.

The injections in RCS rats were made at postnatal day (P) 23 when photoreceptor cells had just begun to degenerate.[17] The eyes were taken 1 or 2 months later (P53 or P83) and prepared for histological analysis using either 1 μm thick plastic sections or 10 μm thick polyester wax serial sections.[16] Experiments with light damage were carried out in the same way on 2- to 4-month-old F344 or Sprague-Dawley rats obtained from Simonsen Laboratories and maintained in our cyclic light environment 7 or more days before intraocular injections. Injections were made 2 days before the rats were placed in a constant light environment (115-130 ft-c) produced by fluorescent bulbs as described elsewhere.[18] Eyes were taken after 1 week of light exposure. In some cases after constant light exposure, the animals were returned to cyclic light for 10 days before eye removal to allow for possible regeneration of photoreceptor inner and outer segments. All procedures involving the rats adhered to the ARVO Resolution on the Use of Animals in Research and the guidelines of the UCSF Committee on Animal Research.

III. RESULTS

A. INHERITED RETINAL DYSTROPHY

At the time of injection, the retinas of RCS rats at P23 showed a mostly normal structure, with only a few dying, pyknotic nuclei and an outer segment zone that had an accumulation of debris membranes at the apical surface of the RPE (Figure 1a). The debris accumulation results from the failure of the RPE to phagocytize outer segment membranes.[19,20] By P53, the uninjected RCS retinas had degenerated considerably. The ONL was reduced to only 1-2 rows of photoreceptor nuclei, no photoreceptor inner segments were present and the outer segment zone consisted only of debris membranes (Figure 1b). When bFGF was injected subretinally, however, the retina near the site of injection was remarkably well-preserved at P53, and in some instances, was indistinguishable from the RCS retina at P23 (Figure 1c).

The degree of photoreceptor rescue following bFGF injection was somewhat less at P83 than at P53, but the ONL still consisted of 5-7 rows of nuclei, and photoreceptor inner segments were still present. The area of photoreceptor rescue from a single subretinal injection, as judged by serial section analysis, often extended through most of the superior hemisphere of the eye where the injection was made. When the injection was made intravitreally, photoreceptor rescue was even more extensive and occurred throughout almost the entire retina.

The injection of aFGF did not produce an extensive area of photoreceptor rescue like that provided by bFGF, but rather, produced a small region of rescue that was restricted to the site of the injection. However, both the PBS and needle controls also produced a small area of rescue localized to the site of injection. In a small number of

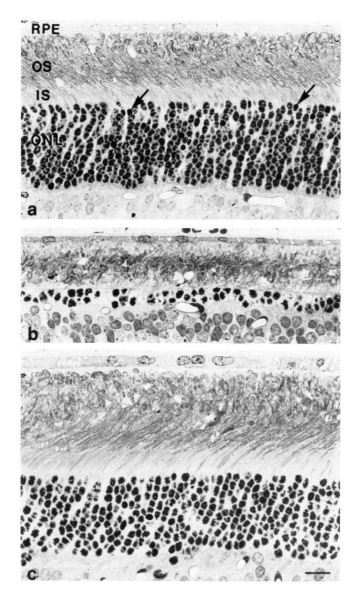

Figure 1. Plastic-embedded sections of RCS rat retinas. **a**, P23, at the age of injections. Photoreceptors have just begun to degenerate, and some nuclei are pyknotic (arrows). Photoreceptor inner segment (IS) and outer segments (OS) are present, and some outer segment debris membranes have accumulated at the apical surface of the RPE. **b**, P53, uninjected control retina. The ONL has degenerated to 1-2 rows of nuclei, and no discrete photoreceptor inner or outer segments are present. **c**, P53, adjacent to the site of subretinal bFGF injection in a region of maximal photoreceptor rescue. The retina appears almost unchanged from the time of injection, whereas the retina in the opposite hemisphere of the same eye was fully degenerated and indistinguishable from that in Figure b. Toluidine blue stain, scale bar, 16 μm. (From Faktorovich et al., 1990, with permission from Macmillan Magazines Ltd.)

animals in which either an epiretinal membrane formed or there was obvious intraocular bleeding at the time of injection, rosettes of photoreceptor cells were present and the area of rescue was extensive, generally about 75% of that seen with intravitreal injections of bFGF. The quantitative data describing these and other studies has been presented elsewhere.[16] It should also be noted that in all cases of intravitreal injection of bFGF, numerous invading macrophages were seen in the inner retinal layers and in the outer segment debris zone.

It should be emphasized that the bFGF-induced photoreceptor rescue observed in the RCS rat was not permanent. Preliminary observations of retinas taken 3 and 4 months after bFGF injection showed progressively fewer surviving photoreceptors. It is possible that serial bFGF injections could have further prolonged the rescue effect, and experiments to test this hypothesis are currently underway in our laboratory. In addition, despite photoreceptors surviving in bFGF-injected eyes for one to several months longer than in untreated RCS retinas, bFGF (as well as the aFGF, PBS and needle controls) did not actually reverse the genetically induced phagocytosis defect. The RPE showed no obvious phagosomes, even when the retinas were taken during the peak of outer segment disc shedding,[21] and outer segment debris characteristic of retinal dystrophy was present at the apical surface of the RPE in virtually all instances (e.g., Figure 1c).

B. LIGHT DAMAGE

To determine whether bFGF-induced photoreceptor rescue was effective only in inherited retinal dystrophy, we explored the effect of the peptide growth factor on a non-genetic form of retinal degeneration, light damage. As expected from previous light-damage studies,[22-24] after 1 week of constant light the ONL was reduced from the normal 8-10 rows of nuclei (Figure 2a) to about 2 rows (Figure 2b) in the most sensitive region of the retina in the superior hemisphere of the eye.[23] There was also a loss of most photoreceptor inner segments in this region (Figure 2b), and a loss of almost all outer segments throughout the retina.

When bFGF was injected intravitreally 2 days before light exposure, far less photoreceptor degeneration occurred (Figure 2c). In the most degenerated region of the retinas, the ONL still showed 4-5 (F344 strain) or 6-8 (Sprague-Dawley, Figure 2c) rows of nuclei, and many inner and outer segments remained (Figure 2c). When control rats and bFGF-treated rats were allowed to recover after the constant light exposure for 10 days in cyclic light, the bFGF-treated retinas showed much more extensive regeneration of inner and outer segments than did the control retinas. In addition, when a dry needle was inserted into the subretinal space 2 days before constant light exposure, a significant degree of protection from light damage was provided, at least in the superior hemisphere where the needle had been inserted.

IV. DISCUSSION

When it was discovered that bFGF retarded the pace of inherited retinal dystrophy in the RCS rat,[16] it was suggested that bFGF may play a neurotrophic role in normal photoreceptor RPE cell interactions. Indeed, the suggestion is attractive based on the observations that bFGF is synthesized by the RPE[10,11] and rod outer segments have bFGF receptors,[9] although it has yet to be shown how bFGF is released from cells. It was also pointed out that the accumulation of debris membranes or an abnormal accumulation of

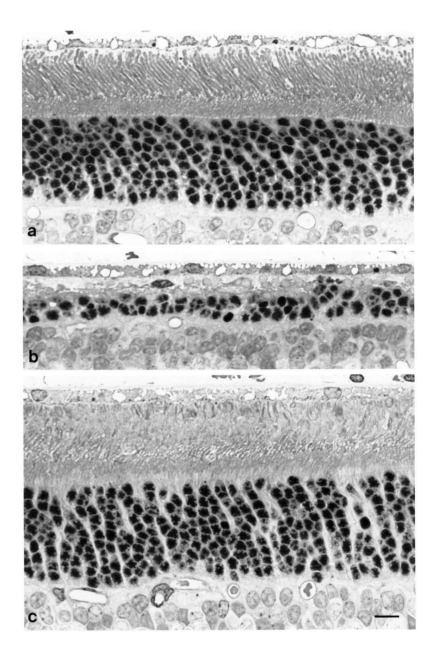

Figure 2. Plastic-embedded sections of 3-month-old Sprague-Dawley albino rats. **a**, Normal retina from a rat reared in cyclic light. **b**, Retina from an uninjected rat exposed to constant light for 7 days. The ONL is reduced to about 2 rows of nuclei, and no normal appearing photoreceptor inner or outer segments are present. **c**, Retina from a rat that received an intravitreal injection of bFGF 2 days before a 7-day constant light exposure. The ONL is 6-8 rows in thickness, and some discrete photoreceptor inner and outer segments are present, although many outer segments are disorganized. Toluidine blue stain, scale bar, 10 μm.

interphotoreceptor matrix in the RCS rat[25] may bind bFGF released from the RPE and prevent it from reaching the photoreceptor cells. Thus, it is possible that the exogenous bFGF provided by our injections in some way overcame a deficit in synthesis, release, uptake or abnormal binding of bFGF in the RCS rat.

Two important questions that still remain are the mechanism of bFGF rescue and the normal role of bFGF in the retina. Does the finding that bFGF protects photoreceptors from degenerating in both inherited retinal dystrophy and light damage provide any insight into these questions? Superficially, the mechanisms of light damage and inherited retinal dystrophy appear quite different. The defect in RPE phagocytosis of outer segment disc membranes in the RCS rat[19,20] is not seen in light damage, while oxidative mechanisms are thought to result in photoreceptor degeneration in light damage.[26-28] Since bFGF protects photoreceptors from degenerating in these two quite different disorders, bFGF may act as a non-specific survival promoting factor. This interpretation gains some strength from the finding that bFGF reduces or delays the degeneration of other classes of neurons, as well.[13-15] It is possible, however, that both retinal degenerative conditions interfere with a normal role of bFGF. For example, it has been observed that at all stages of light damage, an abnormal distribution of the interphotoreceptor matrix occurs,[29] similar to that seen in the RCS rat.[25] Thus, it is possible that light damage and inherited retinal dystrophy share at least one common cytopathologic feature that could explain the disruption of a putative normal movement of bFGF from the RPE to the photoreceptors in the two disorders. Hopefully, the effect of bFGF (or lack thereof) on other forms of retinal degeneration that do not have the same sort of IPM accumulation will clarify the cellular mechanism of bFGF rescue and the normal role of bFGF in the retina.

It is important to discuss the current status of bFGF as a possible therapeutic agent for inherited retinal degenerations. For several reasons, the growth factor should not be considered for therapeutic use at the present time. First, the rescue effect that we have observed is short-lived relative to the slowly progressing human retinal degenerations. Second, it is not yet known whether bFGF will have a comparable rescue effect on other forms of inherited retinal degeneration. Third, bFGF has widely known mitogenic and angiogenic effects that could possibly cause serious side effects. Fourth, the injection of bFGF apparently stimulates the influx of macrophages into the retina, and the consequences of these cells in the retina are unknown. Nevertheless, the action of bFGF on RCS photoreceptor cells marks the first time that the pace of an inherited retinal degeneration has been slowed significantly by pharmacological means. Thus, we are hopeful that the finding represents a first step in research toward a pharmacological therapeutic measure for some forms of retinal degeneration.

V.   ACKNOWLEDGEMENTS

We thank D. Gospodarowicz for helpful discussions and the gift of aFGF and bFGF, and N. Lawson and G. Riggs for technical and secretarial assistance. This work was supported in part by NIH Research Grants EY01919, EY06842, EY01429, Core Grant EY02162 and funds from the Retinitis Pigmentosa Foundation Fighting Blindness, Research to Prevent Blindness and That Man May See, Inc. Dr. LaVail is the recipient of a Research to Prevent Blindness Senior Scientific Investigators Award.

VI. REFERENCES

1. Steinberg, R. H., Research update: report from a workshop on cell biology of retinal detachment, *Exp. Eye Res.*, 43, 695, 1986.
2. Mullen, R. J. and LaVail, M. M., Inherited retinal dystrophy: primary defect in pigment epithelium determined with experimental rat chimeras, *Science*, 192, 799, 1976.
3. Li, L. and Turner, J. E., Inherited retinal dystrophy in the RCS rat: prevention of photoreceptor degeneration by pigment epithelial cell transplantation, *Exp. Eye Res.*, 47, 911, 1988.
4. Lopez, R., Gouras, P., Kjeldbye, H., Sullivan, B., Reppucci, V., Britis, M., Wapner, F. and Goluboff, E., Transplanted retinal pigment epithelium modifies the retinal degeneration in the RCS rat, *Invest. Ophthalmol. Vis. Sci.*, 30, 586, 1989.
5. D'Amore, P. A. and Klagsbrun, M., Endothelial cell mitogens derived from retina and hypothalamus: biochemical and biological similarities, *J. Cell Biol.*, 99, 1545, 1984.
6. Baird, A., Esch, F., Gospodarowicz, D. and Guillemin, R., Retina- and eye-derived endothelial cell growth factors: partial molecular characterization and identity with acidic and basic fibroblast growth factors, *Biochem.*, 24, 7855, 1985.
7. Mascarelli, F., Raulais, D., Counis, M. F. and Courtois, Y., Characterization of acidic and basic fibroblast growth factors in brain, retina and vitreous chick embryo, *Biochem. Biophys. Res. Comm.*, 146, 478, 1987.
8. Plouët, J., Mascarelli, F., Loret, M. D., Faure, J. P. and Courtois, Y., Regulation of eye derived growth factor binding to membranes by light, ATP or GTP in photoreceptor outer segments, *EMBO J.*, 7, 373, 1988.
9. Plouët, J., Molecular interaction of fibroblast growth factor, light-activated rhodopsin and s-antigen, in *Molecular Biology of the Eye: Genes, Vision and Ocular Disease*, Piatigorsky, J., Toshimichi, S. and Zelenka, P. S., Eds., Alan R. Liss, Inc., New York, 1988, 83.
10. Schweigerer, L., Malerstein, B., Neufeld, G. and Gospodarowicz, D., Basic fibroblast growth factor is synthesized in cultured retinal pigment epithelial cells, *Biochem. Biophys. Res. Comm.*, 143, 934, 1987.
11. Sternfeld, M. D., Robertson, J. E., Shipley, G. D., Tsai, J. and Rosenbaum, J. T., Cultured human retinal pigment epithelial cells express basic fibroblast growth factor and its receptor, *Curr. Eye Res.*, 8, 1029, 1989.
12. Park, C. M. and Hollenberg, M. J., Basic fibroblast growth factor induces retinal regeneration *in vivo*, *Dev. Biol.*, 134, 201, 1989.
13. Sievers, J., Hausmann, B., Unsicker, K. and Berry, M., Fibroblast growth factors promote the survival of adult rat retinal ganglion cells after transection of the optic nerve, *Neurosci. Lett.*, 76, 157, 1987.
14. Anderson, K. J., Dam, D., Lee, S. and Cotman, C. W., Basic fibroblast growth factor prevents death of lesioned cholinergic neurons *in vivo*, *Nature*, 332, 360, 1988.
15. Otto, D., Frotscher, M. and Unsicker, K., Basic fibroblast growth factor and nerve growth factor administered in gel foam rescue medial septal neurons after fimbria fornix transection, *J. Neurosci. Res.*, 22, 83, 1989.
16. Faktorovich, E. G., Steinberg, R. H., Yasumura, D., Matthes, M. T. and LaVail, M. M., Photoreceptor degeneration in inherited retinal dystrophy delayed by basic fibroblast growth factor, *Nature*, 347, 83, 1990.
17. LaVail, M. M. and Battelle, B. A., Influence of eye pigmentation and light deprivation on inherited retinal dystrophy in the rat, *Exp. Eye Res.*, 21, 167, 1975.

18. LaVail, M. M., Gorrin, G. M., Repaci, M. A., Thomas, L. A. and Ginsberg, H. M., Genetic regulation of light damage to photoreceptors, *Invest. Ophthalmol. Vis. Sci.*, 28, 1043, 1987.
19. Bok, D. and Hall, M. O., The role of the pigment epithelium in the etiology of inherited retinal dystrophy in the rat, *J. Cell Biol.*, 49, 664, 1971.
20. LaVail, M. M., Sidman, R. L. and O'Neil, D. A., Photoreceptor-pigment epithelial cell relationships in rats with inherited retinal degeneration. Radioautographic and electron microscope evidence for a dual source of extra lamellar material, *J. Cell Biol.*, 53, 185, 1972.
21. LaVail, M. M., Rod outer segment disc shedding in rat retina: relationship to cyclic lighting, *Science*, 194, 1071, 1976.
22. Noell, W. K., Walker, V. S., Kang, B. S. and Berman, S., Retinal damage by light in rats, *Invest. Ophthalmol.*, 5, 450, 1966.
23. Rapp, L. M. and Williams, T. P., A parametric study of retinal light damage in albino and pigmented rats, in *The Effects of Constant Light on Visual Processes*, Williams, T. P. and Baker, B. N., Eds., Plenum Press, New York, 1980, 135.
24. LaVail, M. M., Gorrin, G. M., Repaci, M. A. and Yasumura, D., Light-induced retinal degeneration in albino mice and rats: strain and species differences., in *Degenerative Retinal Disorders: Clinical and Laboratory Investigations*, Hollyfield, J. G., Anderson, R. E. and LaVail, M. M., Eds., Alan R. Liss, Inc., New York, 1987, 439.
25. LaVail, M. M., Pinto, L. H. and Yasumura, D., The interphotoreceptor matrix in rats with inherited retinal dystrophy, *Invest. Ophthalmol. Vis. Sci.*, 21, 658, 1981.
26. Noell, W. K., Possible mechanisms of photoreceptor damage by light in mammalian eyes, *Vision Res.*, 20, 1163, 1980.
27. Anderson, R. E., Rapp, L. M. and Wiegand, R. D., Lipid peroxidation and retinal degeneration, *Curr. Eye Res.*, 3, 223, 1984.
28. Wiegand, R. D., Jose, J. G., Rapp, L. M. and Anderson, R. E., Free radicals and damage to ocular tissues, in *Free Radicals in Molecular Biology, Aging, and Disease*, Armstrong, D., Sohal, R. S., Cutler, R. G. and Slater, T. F., Eds., Raven Press, New York, 1984, 317.
29. Uehara, F., Yasumura, D. and LaVail, M. M., unpublished observations, 1990.

REACTIVE GLIOSIS IN RETINAL DEGENERATIONS

Vijay Sarthy,
Departments of Ophthalmology and Cell, Molecular and Structural Biology, Northwestern University Medical School, Chicago, IL 60611

I. INTRODUCTION

The vertebrate central nervous system (CNS) is remarkable for its morphological complexity and functional sophistication. Hence, it is rather surprising that such a highly evolved system lacks efficient repair mechanisms for neuronal regeneration and functional recovery following trauma. This limited regenerative capacity of the mammalian CNS might be due to a number of reasons: (i) the inability to reinitiate critical steps that occur during normal development such as expression of trophic and guidance molecules; (ii) the presence of active 'inhibitory' molecules in the adult tissue; and (iii) the formation of glial scars by nonneuronal cells which in turn might form physical barriers (1).

An important feature of glial cells is their response to nerve injury. This reaction of glial cells -reactive gliosis- involves hypertrophy and proliferation of glial cells at the site of injury (1). It has been presumed that activated glia perform phagocytic functions and are additionally involved in restoring breaches in the blood-brain barrier by formation of scar tissue. Gliosis is also seen in subependymal and subpial regions with aging (1). Studies of reactive glia have immediate, direct and fundamental relevance to human retinal diseases since varying degrees of gliosis are manifested in many of these disorders.

II. RETINAL GLIA

The vertebrate retina contains three types of glial cells—Müller cells, astrocytes, and microglia, with Müller cells constituting the major cell type (2). The morphology and fine structure of Müller cells have been described at both light and electron microscopic levels in a number of vertebrates (for complete list, see ref. 3). The Muller cell body is located in the inner nuclear layer and its processes span the retina extending from the outer limiting membrane to the inner limiting membrane. The astrocytes which are less numerous are located in the ganglion cell layer and send their processes into both ganglion cell and nerve fiber layers (4). Retinal microglia which are probably specialized macrophages are distributed across the entire retina and are usually found close to the retinal vasculature (4).

Müller cells appear to perform a multitude of functions in the retina. Since their plasma membrane is highly permeable to K^+, these cells have been suggested to be involved in two important processes in the retina—generation of the b-wave of the electroretinogram and K^+ spatial buffering. Müller cells have also been implicated in neurotransmitter metabolism, glycogen storage, pH regulation, vitamin A cycle, and neuronal migration in developing retina (5).

Recent investigations show that astrocytes and Muller cells are derived from separate lineages. Retroviral and dye marking studies reveal that retinal neurons and Muller cells arise from a common progenitor (6-9). Developmental studies of astrocytes, and tissue culture studies of retina and optic nerve strongly suggest that retinal astrocytes are not formed in the retina but actually migrate from the optic nerve (10-12).

In response to retinal injury or degeneration, both astrocytes and Muller cells appear to undergo reactive gliosis. In addition, gliosis by Muller cells is also observed with retinal aging (Sarthy, unpublished data). Although the functional significance of gliotic response is poorly understood, some of the cytological changes observed in glia have important consequences. For example, in atrophic macular lesions characterized by the loss of RPE and photoreceptors, reactive Müller cells adhere to the denuded Bruch's membrane, and may help to maintain the outer blood-retina barrier (13,14).

III. EPIRETINAL GLIA

Epiretinal membranes consist of sheets of cells embedded in a network of extracellular matrix and arise as a complication in several ocular disorders (15). Such membrane formation occurs on both inner and outer surfaces of the retina as well as on the posterior hyaloid. Epiretinal membranes have been identified in proliferative diabetic retinopathy, retinal detachment, macular pucker, sickle cell disease, retinitis pigmentosa and following many types of ocular surgery (15). The pathogenesis involves an initial inflammatory reaction followed by migration, proliferation and synthesis of extracellular matrix molecules.

Several cell types have been found in epiretinal membranes based on light, electron microscopic and immunocytochemical studies (for complete list, see ref. 16,17). These comprise retinal pigment epithelial cells, fibrous astrocytes, fibroblasts, macrophages and Muller cells. Many questions need to be addressed before we can understand, and possibly interfere with membrane formation. What triggers the cells to migrate? What mitogens induce proliferation? Which cells produce the matrix molecules?

IV. BIOCHEMICAL MARKERS FOR REACTIVE GLIOSIS

A characteristic feature of Muller cells and astrocytes is the occurrence of 9 nm filaments in their cytoplasm (18). These intermediate filaments (IFs) sorround the nucleus and send parallel bundles into the cell processes. In reactive glial cells, there is a substantial increase in the filament content (1). In the mammalian nervous system, the major components of the glial filaments have been identified as Vimentin and Glial Fibrillary Acidic Protein (GFAP), two closely related proteins that belong to the intermediate filament protein family (19, 20). The availability of highly specific, polyclonal and monoclonal antibodies has made it possible to localize these proteins to known cell types by immunocytochemistry. However, the cellular function of these proteins remains unknown (20).

Vimentin is a ~ 53KDa protein that occurs mainly in cells of mesenchymal origin. The protein has also been found in undifferentiated cells in tissues, and usually reappears when cells are grown *in vitro* (20). In neural tissue, astrocytes, radial glial cells and Bergmann glial cells contain vimentin during development and in adult tissue (19, 21).

In the vertebrate retina, vimentin has been found in both astrocytes and Muller cells although its presence in astrocytes has been questioned (4). Moreover, an increase in vimentin level in Muller cells has been reported in detached cat retina (22). Unfortunately, vimentin appears not be a cell type-specific marker for Muller cells because horizontal cells have also been found to express vimentin (23).

Glial fibrillary acidic protein (GFAP) is a ~50 KDa protein that is normally found in large amounts in mature astrocytes (24). It is a major component of glial filaments and is generally accepted as a cell type-specific marker for astrocytes. However, GFAP has also been observed in tanycytes, ependymal cells and Schwann cells during regeneration (24). GFAP has been widely used as a marker for following development of astrocytes both *in vivo* and in vitro. In addition, GFAP antibodies have employed in studies of PNS to CNS grafts, intraocular transplants and intracerebral/intracerebellar transplants (25).

In normal adult brain, GFAP is detectable by immunohistochemical techniques in fibrous but not protoplasmic astrocytes. In response to a stab wound, however, both cell types stain intensely for GFAP. Furthermore, this pattern of staining is maintained for periods of up to two months (26). A parallel increase in GFAP levels has also been noted in cases of reactive gliosis (24). The response of glia to injury appears also to depend on the age of the animal. Gliosis and GFAP immunostaining are much less pronounced in immature brain compared to the adult. In addition, the spread of GFAP reactivity away from a lesion is age dependent with reactivity being well confined to regions neighboring the lesion in immature animals. In adults, GFAP reactivity may spread across the entire hemisphere (for complete list of refs., see ref. 25). This observation suggests that diffusible factors may be involved in induction of gliosis in adult CNS.

In the normal retina, GFAP is present at low levels or is not detectable at all in Müller cells depending on the species examined (for complete list of refs., see ref. 27). In contrast, loss of retinal integrity as a result of injury, detachment or photoreceptor degeneration results in the appearance of intense GFAP-immunoreactivity in Müller cells (27). Recently, the mechanism of GFAP expression has been investigated in the mouse retina with photoreceptor degeneration (27). Using a combination of Western blot analysis, steady state mRNA level comparison, nuclear 'run-on' assay and *in situ* hybridization it was shown that transcription of the GFAP gene was activated in Muller cells in retinas with photoreceptor degeneration. These observations indicate that disruption of normal neuron-glia interactions as a result of photoreceptor degeneration results in activation of the GFAP gene in Müller cells (27). Although these experiments demonstrate that GFAP expression is regulated mainly at the level of transcription, the molecular mechanisms responsible for changes in transcriptional activity remain to be elucidated. These alterations could involve modifications such as methylation at the gene level, changes in chromatin organization or both.

Expression of other glial cell-specific proteins has also been examined in retinal degeneration and detachment. The results obtained, however, appear to differ among the animal models examined. While glutamine synthetase and carbonic anhydrase levels are not measurably altered in retinas with photoreceptor degeneration, a sharp decline in the enzyme content has been reported in the case of detached retina (22). Similarly, immunostaining for cellular retinaldhyde binding protein (CRALBP), a specific marker for Muller cells, appears not be affected in RCS rats while the protein is barely detectable in detached cat retina after several weeks (22). Whether these discrepancies are due to the differences in species used or are the result of differences in the gliotic mechanisms operating in retinal detachment and degeneration remains currently unclear.

Finally, other proteins have also been advanced as putative markers for reactive gliosis. These include laminin, 37 KDa protein and M1 antigen (28, 29); however, their usefulness as markers for Muller cells is unknown.

V. GLIAL CELL PROLIFERATION

An important feature of gliosis is the proliferation of glial cells around the site of injury. The mechanisms that regulate glial cell proliferation in the normal tissue and the factors that trigger cell proliferation are subjects of current research interest. A scheme for gliotic response was put forward by Del Rio-Hortega and Penfield (30) according to which glial response to brain injury begins with an initial period of phagocytic activity by microglia followed by hypertrophy and amitotic division of astrocytes. Subsequently, the astrocytes arrange radially around the wound to form a sorrounding connective tissue zone. Finally, the tissue contracts resulting in sealing off of the affected area. Although this proposal provided a useful description of glial response, it also provoked several controversial questions such as (i) Is reactive gliosis an intrinsic property of glia or does it require external signals that come from break down of the blood-brain barrier? (ii) Do both microglia and astrocytes perform phagocytic activity or only microglia carry out this function? (iii) Do astrocytes undergo proliferation or only exhibit amitotic division? (iv) Do the glial scars serve as physical barriers and prevent axonal growth through the region?

Although a large number of studies have been carried out to address these questions, the results obtained have been less than conclusive (25, 31). To summarize, it appears that the extent to which intrinsic and extrinsic glial cells proliferate depends on the severity and type of trauma. While microglial cells account for the majority of dividing cells in highly inflammatory wounds, astrocytes make up a large fraction of proliferating cells in other situations. The oligodendrocytes appear to be the least responsive to injury. Furthermore, kainic acid lesion experiments show that reactive gliosis can occur even when there is no breaching of the blood-brain barrier. The question as to whether both fibrous and protoplasmic astrocytes can undergo gliosis and proliferation has also been examined. Immunocytochemical studies using multiple markers suggests that the majority of reactive astrocytes are of the type I (protoplasmic) class (32).

The capacity of glial cells to proliferate *in vitro* has been extensively investigated (25). In general. it appears that it is possible to obtain primary cultures of glial cells from embryonic and early postnatal CNS tissue. In contrast, it has been rather difficult to prepare glial cell cultures from the adult tissue. One reason for this difference could be that since the majority of glial cells are present as undifferentiated precursors in the developing tissue, the cells retain their capacity to proliferate *in vitro*. Such capacity ceases or is diminished, however, in postmitotic glial cells in adults.

In this regard, it is of interest that glial cell cultures can be obtained from adult CNS including the retina after induction of reactive gliosis (for detaills, see ref. 25). It is possible that at the site of injury, glia have undergone dedifferentiation and reentered the mitotic cycle. Alternatively, these cells could be derived from proliferation of glial precursors in cultures. In either case, an understanding of the molecular mechanisms that induce mitotic activity in glial cells in the adult tissues would be of considerable interest. Recently, a soluble molecule which appears to inhibit mitogenic activity in adult brain has been reported. Brain injury was found to result in an increase in Epidermal growth factor (EFG) receptor levels on astrocytes (33). Intracerebral injection of anti EGF resulted in the appearance of reactive astrocytes. The data suggest the existence of an astrocyte mitogen inhibitor that is immunologically related to the EGF receptor.

In the retina, glial cell proliferation has been noted in a variety of pathological conditions such as proliferative vitreoretinopathy, macular pucker, proliferative diabetic retinopathy and idiopathic preretinal macular gliosis (15, 34). It is presumed that the dividing glia are usally fibrous astrocytes. In massive retinal gliosis, however, Muller cell proliferation has been proposed (35). RPE and glial cell proliferation has also been described in the detached cat retina.(36). Recent studies with glial cell cultures suggest that Muller cells may have phagocytic functions in the retina (37).

VI. GLIAL CELL MIGRATION

Migration of glial cells from retina into ectopic locations is an important event in determining the sites of epiretinal membrane formation and probably the severity of glial reaction. This migration has to occur across limiting membranes and probably involves chemotactic movement of cells. The chemotactic responses of glial cells to purified growth factors such as Platelet derived growth factor (PDGF) and Fibroblast growth factor (FGF) have been studied in cell cultures (summarized in ref. 34).

Similar studies have also been carried out with cultures of retinal glial cells (34). In order to facilitate such investigations, monolayer cultures of retinal glia have been obtained by several experimental approaches. Burke and Foster (38) used explants of rabbit retina and recovered cells that grew out of the tissue. These cultures were used to demonstrate that rabbit retinal glia are not responsive to PDGF (39). Roberge et al. (40) employed conditioned medium from concavalin A-stimulated spleen cell cultures. Sarthy (41) used a separate strategy which is based on the ability of reactive glia to proliferate *in vitro*. He used rat retinas with photoreceptor degeneration resulting from either constant light damage or RCS mutation to obtain monolayer cultures that contained ~ 90% Muller cells. More recently, Hicks and Courtois (42) produced cultures of Muller cells from rat retina using a protocol developed for culturing retinal pigment epithelial cells. These cultures will be important in testing the effects of growth factors on migratory and proliferative behavior of retinal glia.

VII. GROWTH FACTORS AND INHIBITORS

The biological effects of a large number of known growth factors have been examined on glial cells from the CNS (34,43,44). In addition, astrocytes have been shown to synthesize neuronotrophic factors such as bFGF, S100b, Nexin, insulin-like growth factors (IGF-I and II) and apolipoprotein E (43). PDGF, a mediator of wound healing, has been shown to be a potent mitogen for both mesodermal cells and glia (43). Besides EGF, glial cells also respond to other growth factors such as aFGF, bFGF, Glial Maturation Factor, Glial Growth Factor and Astroglial Growth Factor (34). In addition, interleukin-1 and related cytokines produce by microglial cells are mitogenic for glial cells (34). In summary, CNS glial cells respond to a wide variety of mitogens derived from macrophages, platelets and plasma.

The influence of known growth factors on retinal glial cells has also been examined by several investigators (34,43). While rabbit glial cells were found to be unresponsive to PDGF, rat retinal glia cells showed considerable mitotic activity (34,39). It appears that bFGF is the most effective mitogen for retinal cells (34, 44). Recent studies in RCS rats show that bFGF can retard degeneration of photoreceptors. The mechanisms involved in this phenomenon are, however, unknown (45) It is possible that exogenous FGF acts directly on photoreceptors or RPE cells; alternatively, it could act on either Muller cells or macrophages which in turn produce other 'factors' that mediate rescue. In addition, vitreous injection experiments suggest that macrophages produce molecules that are highly mitogenic (45). Isolation and characterization of the mitogens present in these preparations remains a challenging task.

In addition to neuronotrophic factors, the CNS may also contain molecules that prevent regeneration. Recent evidence suggests that certain endogenous inhibitor molecules produced by CNS myelin suppress sprouting and regeneration of neurons (47). Moreover, antibodies specific to these proteins promote axonal outgrowth *in vivo*. It is possible that such molecules are also present in the adult mammalian retina and retinal regeneration is inhibited by them.

VIII. RELEVANCE TO REGENERATION AND TRANSPLANTATION

Although the response of glial cells to injury has been studied in great detail, it is far from clear whether the inability for neuronal regeneration in the mammalian CNS is due to some intrinsic property of neurons or is the result of indirect intervention by nonneuronal cells. While glial scar formation in highly inflammatory CNS wounds could block regeneration, it appears that in majority of cases where the injury is milder, neuronotrophic factors or inhibitory molecules might play a more important role. In retinal degenerations, gliotic reaction of Muller cells might have a similar effect.

At present, there is considerable interest in the use of transplants to rescue photoreceptor degeneration in animal models of retinal dystrophy.(e.g. see related articles in this book) Both RPE cells and photoreceptor cell preparations have been used for this purpose. Although RPE replacement is useful in cases where the defect has been localized to RPE, in other situations, photoreceptor transplantation would be a natural choice. Here, it is important to know whether the transplanted cells will attach to the outer limiting membrane. Since outer limiting membrane changes occur in reactive gliosis, the question as to whether the altered membrane can mediate normal photoreceptor-Muller cell interactions remains an important one. Cell culture studies of photoreceptors and reactive Muller cells should be useful in addressing this issue.

IX. ACKNOWLEDGEMENTS

During the preparation of this review, the author was supported by NIH grants, EY-03523 and EY-03664 and an unrestricted grant from the Research To Prevent Blindness Foundation, Inc. I wish to thank Dr. Richard O'Grady for his helpful comments.

X. REFERENCES

1. Duffy, P.E., Astrocytes: Normal, Reactive, and Neoplastic. Raven Press, New York, 1983, 1.
2. Ogden, T. The glia of the retina, in Retina, Vol.1, Ryan, S.J., C.V. Mosby Co., St. Louis, 53, 1989.
3. Gaur, V.P., Eldred, W. and Sarthy, P.V. , Distribution of Muller cells in the turtle retina: an immunocytochemical study. J. Neurocytol. 17, 683, 1988.
4. Schnitzer, J. , Astrocytes in mammalian retina. Prog. Retina Res. 7, 209, 1988.
5. Ripps, H. and Witkovsky, P., Neuron-glia interaction in the brain and retina. Prog. Retina Res. 4, 181, 1985.
6. Turner, D.L. and Cepko, C.L. , A common progenitor for neurons and glia persists in rat retina late in development. Nature, 238, 131, 1987.
7. Turner, D.L., Snyder, E.Y. and Cepko, C.L. Lineage-independent determination of cell type in the embryonic mouse retina. Neuron. 4, 833, 1990.
8. Wetts, R., and Fraser, S.E., Multipotent precursors can give rise to all major cell types of the frog retina. Science. 239, 1142, 1988.
9. Holt, C.E., Bertsch, T.W., Ellis, H.M. and Harris, W.A., Cellular determination in the Xenopus retina is independent of lineage and birthdate. Neuron, 1, 15, 1988.
10. Watanabe, T. and Raff, M.C. , Retinal astrocytes are immigrants from the optic nerve. Nature, 332, 834, 1988.
11. Stone, J. and Dreher, Z., Relationship between astrocytes, ganglion cells and vasculature of the retina. J. Comp. Neurol. 255, 35, 1987.
12. Ling, T. and Stone, J. The development of astrocytes in the cat retina: evidence of migration from the optic nerve. Dev. Brain Res. 44, 73, 1988
13. Weiter, J. and Fine, B.S., A histologic study of regional choroidal dystrophy. Am. J. Ophthlmol. 83, 741, 1977
14. Eagle, RC., Jr., Lucier, A.C., Bernardino, V.B., and Yanoff, M. Retinal pigment epithelial abnormalities in fundus flavimaculatus. Ophthalmol. 87, 1189, 1980.
15. McDonald, H.R. and Schatz, H. Introduction to epiretinal membranes, in Retina, Vol. 2, Ryan, S.J. Ed. C.V. Mosby Co., St. Louis, 789, 1989.
16. Weller, M., Hemann, K. and Wiedemann, P., Immunochemical analysis of periretinal membranes. Review and outlook., in Developments in Ophthalmology, Straub, W., Ed., S. Karger, Basel, 54, 1989.
17. Guerin, C.J., Wolfshagen, R.W., Eifrig, D.E. and Anderson, D.H., Immunocytochemical identification of Muller's glia as a component of human epiretinal membranes. Invest. Ophthalmol. Vis. Sci. 31, 1483, 1990.

18. Uga, S. and Smelser, G.K., Comparative study of the fine structure of retinal Muller cells in various vertebrates. Invest. Ophthalmol. 12, 434, 1973

19. Kalnins, V.L., Subrahmanyan, L. and Opas, M. The cytoskeleton, in Astrocytes, Vol. 3, Federoff, S. and Vernadakis, A., Eds., Academic Press, Inc. Orlando, FL., 27, 1986.

20. Lazarides, E, Intermediate filaments: A chemically heterogeneous, developmentally regulated class of proteins. Ann. Rev. Biochem. 51, 219, 1982.

21. Wilkin, G.P. and Levi, G., Cerebellar astrocytes. in Astrocytes, Vol. 3, Federoff, S. and Vernadakis, A., Eds., Academic Press, Inc. Orlando, FL., 245, 1986.

22. Lewis, G.P., Erickson, P.A., Guerin, C.J., Anderson, D.H. and Fisher, S.K., Changes in the expression of specific Muller cell proteins during long term retinal detachment. Exp. Eye Res. 48, 93, 1989.

23. Drager, U.C. Coexistence of neurofilaments and vimentin in a neurone of adult mouse retina. Nature. 303, 169, 1983.

24. Dahl, D., Bjorklund, H. and Bignami, A. Immunological markers in astrocytes. in Astrocytes, Vol. 3, Federoff, S. and Vernadakis, A., Eds., Academic Press, Inc. Orlando, FL. 1, 1986.

25. Lindsay, R.M. Reactive gliosis. in Astrocytes, Vol. 3, Federoff, S. and Vernadakis, A., Eds., Academic Press, Inc. Orlando, FL. 231, 1986.

26. Bignami, A. and Dahl, D. The astroglial response to stabbing. Immunofluorescence studies with antibodies to astrocyte-specific protein (GFA) in mammalian and submammalian vertebrates. Neuropathol. Appl. Neurobiol. 2, 99, 1976.

27. Sarthy, P.V. and Fu, M. Transcriptional activation of an intermediate filament protein gene in mice with retinal dystrophy. DNA, 8, 437, 1989.

28. Politis, M.J., Pellegrino, R.G., Oaklanders, A.L. and Ritchie, J.M. Reactive glial protein synthesis and early appearance of saxitoxin binding in degenerating rat optic nerve. Brain Res, 273, 392, 1983.

29. Schachner, M. Glial antigens and the expression of neuroglial phenotypes. Trends Neurosci. 5, 225, 1982.

30 Del Rio-Hortega, P. and Penfield, W. Cerebral cicatrix. The reaction of neuroglia and microglia to brain wounds. Bull. John's Hopkins Hosp. 41, 278, 1927.

31. Korr, H. Proliferation and cell cycle parameters of astrocytes. in Astrocytes, Vol. 3, Federoff, S. and Vernadakis, A., Eds., Academic Press, Inc. Orlando, FL. 77, 1986.

32. Miller, R.H., Abney, E.R., David, S., Ffrench-Constant, C., Lindsay, R.M., Patel, R., Stone, J. and Raff, M.C. Is reactive gliosis a property of a distinct population of astrocytes? J. Neurosci. 6, 22, 1986.

33. Nieto-Sampedro, M. Astrocyte mitogen inhibitor related to epidermal growth factor receptor. Science 240, 1784, 1988.

34. Hjelmeland, L.M. and Harvey, A.K. Gliosis of the mammalian retina: Migration and proliferation of retinal glia. Prog. Ret. Res. 7, 259, 1988.

35. Nork, T.M., Ghobrial, M.W., Peyman, G.A. and Tso, M.O.M. Massive retinal gliosis, A reactive proliferation of Muller cells. Arch. Ophthalmol. 104, 1383, 1986.

36. Fisher, S.K., Anderson, D.H., Erickson, P.A., Guerin, C.J. and Lewis, G.P. The response of Muller cells in experimental retinal detachment and reattachment. in Proc. 9th Int. Soc. Eye Res. Congress, 76, 1990.

37. Mano, T. and Puro, D.G. Phagocytosis by human retinal glial cells in culture. Invest. Ophthalmol. Vis. Sci. 31, 1047, 1990.

38. Burke, J.M. and Foster, S.J., Culture of adult rabbit retinal glial cells: methods and cellular origin of explant outgrowth. Curr. Eye Res. 3, 1169, 1984.

39. Burke, J.M. Cultured retinal glial cells are insensitive to platelet derived growth factor. Exp. Eye Res. 35, 663, 1982.

40. Roberge, F.G., Caspi, R.R., Chan, C.C., Kuwabara, T. and Nussenblatt, R,B, Long-term culture of Muller cells from adult rats in the presence of activated lymphocytes/monocytes products. Curr. Eye Res. 4, 975, 1985.

41. Sarthy, P.V. Establishment of Muller cell cultures from adult rat retina. Brain Res. 337, 138, 1985.

42. Hicks, D. and Courtois, Y. The growth and behavior of rat retinal Muller cells *in vitro*. 1. An improved method for isolation and culture. Exp. Eye Res. 51, 119, 1990.

43. Walicke, P.A. Novel neurotrophic factors, receptors and oncogenes. Ann Rev. Neurosci. 12, 103, 1989.

44. Folkman, J. and Klagsburn, M. Angiogenic factors. Science. 235, 442, 1987.

45. Faktorovich, E.G., Steinberg, R.H., Yasumura, D., Matthes, M.T. and LaVail, M.M. Photoreceptor degeneration in inherited retinal dystrophy delayed by basic fibroblast growth factor. Nature, 347, 83, 1990.

46. Burke, J.M. and Foster, S.J. Injured vitreous stimulates DNA synthesis in retinal pigment epithelium in culture and within the vitreous. Graefes Arch. Clin. Exp. Ophthalmol. 218, 153, 1982.

47. Caroni, P. and Schwab, M.E. Antibody against myelin associated inhibitor of neurite outgrowth neutralizes nonpermissive substrate properties of CNS white matter. Neuron. 1, 85, 1988.

DIETARY OMEGA-3 FATTY ACIDS: EFFECTS ON RETINAL LIPID COMPOSITION AND FUNCTION IN PRIMATES

Martha Neuringer, William E. Connor, Don S. Lin, Gregory J. Anderson
and Louise Barstad
Oregon Health Sciences University and Oregon Regional Primate Research Center

I. INTRODUCTION

Docosahexaenoic acid (DHA, 22:6ω3*) is a major fatty acid in the excitable, fluid, and metabolically active membranes of the retina and nervous system, including synaptic and photoreceptor outer segment membranes.[1-4] With six double bonds, DHA is the most polyunsaturated fatty acid commonly found in biological tissue, a characteristic which affects the biophysical and functional properties of the membranes in which it is a structural component.[4,5] Because animal tissues cannot synthesize de novo either DHA or its precursor, α-linolenic acid (18:3ω3), these fatty acids must be obtained from dietary sources. Many plant foods contain α-linolenic acid, and most animals possess enzyme systems to form longer-chain ω3 fatty acids, including DHA and EPA (eicosapentaenoic acid, 20:5ω3), by carbon chain elongation and insertion of additional double bonds.

DHA is present at uniquely high levels in the phospholipids of photoreceptor outer segment disk membranes. It is most concentrated in the ethanolamine and serine glycerophospholipids, where it can account for up to 50% of the total fatty acid content.[2,3] In the sn-2 position of these phospholipids, the percentage of DHA reaches 75-100%.[6-9] Their sn-1 position in most tissues is occupied by saturated or monounsaturated fatty acids such as palmitic (16:0), stearic (18:0) and oleic (18:1), but in disk membranes this position also contains a substantial proportion of DHA.[6-9]

The high content of DHA in the retina and brain is maintained within individual animals and across vertebrate species despite wide variations in dietary fatty acid intakes, and is lowered substantially only by dietary manipulation during development.[10-13] A key factor is the dietary ratio of α-linolenic acid to linoleic acid (18:2ω6), the precursor for essential fatty acids of the ω6 family. This ratio appears to be more important than the absolute amount of ω3 fatty acids in determining degree of depletion,[14] presumably due to competitive inhibition between the two fatty acid families for desaturating enzymes. For this reason, diets containing natural fats in which the ω6/ω3 ratio is very high, such as safflower or sunflower oils, are most effective in producing ω3 fatty acid depletion.[12,15] When developing animals are fed such diets, ω3 fatty acids are replaced by ω6 fatty acids in their tissue phospholipids. DHA is quantitatively replaced by longer-chain ω6 fatty acids, especially 22:5ω6,[12-15] so that the total content of 22-carbon polyunsaturated fatty acids is generally maintained. Despite the seemingly subtle nature of this alteration in lipid composition, it is associated with changes in retinal function and vision.

The pioneering studies of Benolken, Wheeler and Anderson[16,17] were the first to demonstrate that specific dietary depletion of ω3 fatty acids leads to abnormalities in the electroretinogram (ERG). Deficient rats had diminished amplitudes of the ERG A-wave and, to a lesser degree, the B-wave, a result which has since been replicated in other

---

*Fatty acid nomenclature: first number indicates length of carbon chain; second number, following colon, specifies number of double bonds; third number, after ω (or omega- or n-) gives number of carbons between first double bond and methyl terminal group.

laboratories.[18-20] In other studies, deficient rats performed poorly in visually-cued learning tasks, but it is difficult to know if these results were due to impairments in retinal function or deficits in learning or performance.[12,20-22]

We have examined the effects of dietary deprivation of ω3 fatty acids in a nonhuman primate species, the rhesus monkey. We have demonstrated that dietary deprivation during prenatal and postnatal development leads to depletion of ω3 fatty acids from the phospholipids of the retina and brain.[23] These biochemical changes are accompanied by functional changes in deficient monkeys including subnormal development of visual acuity,[24] abnormalities in the electroretinogram,[23] and changes in nonvisual functions including fluid intake.[25]

II. METHODS

A. ANIMALS AND DIETS

This study was conducted in accordance with the ARVO Resolution on the Use of Animals in Research and the NIH Guide for the Care and Use of Laboratory Animals.

Rhesus mothers and their infants were fed safflower oil diets containing very low levels of ω3 fatty acids ($\leq 0.3\%$ of total fatty acids as 18:3ω3) and a very high ratio of ω6 to ω3 fatty acids (~250). They were compared to control monkeys fed diets containing soybean oil, which is relatively rich in 18:3ω3 (8% of total fatty acids) and provided an ω6/ω3 ratio of 7.[23,24] Adult females received these semipurified diets for a minimum of two months before mating and throughout pregnancy, and their infants were fed similar diets, in liquid form, from the day of birth.

In five deficient monkeys, beginning at ages from 10 to 24 months, the reversibility of the deficiency was tested by repletion with high levels of dietary fish oil (12% of diet by weight + 3% safflower oil to provide adequate linoleic acid). The repletion diet provided 9% of total fatty acids as DHA and 13% as EPA. In these animals, longitudinal monitoring of changes in neural tissue fatty acid composition was made possible by 15-25 mg biopsies of prefrontal cerebral cortex gray matter, obtained via craniotomy under general anesthesia. The biopsies produced pinpoint cortical lesions which had no discernable effect on the animals' behavior. Biopsies were obtained at 2-8 week intervals (4 biopsies per animal) from 1-28 weeks after fish oil feeding began.[26]

B. BIOCHEMICAL ANALYSES OF TISSUE PHOSPHOLIPIDS

1. Fatty Acid Composition

Lipids of the retina and cerebral cortex were extracted by standard procedures. Phospholipids were isolated by thin-layer chromatography (TLC), and individual phospholipid classes (ethanolamine, choline, serine and inositol glycerophospholipids) were then separated by further TLC.[23] The fatty acids of each phospholipid class were transmethylated with boron trifluoride in methanol[27] and the methyl esters analyzed by capillary gas-liquid chromatography,[28] using a two-column instrument equipped with hydrogen flame ionization detectors (Perkin-Elmer Model Sigma 3B) and 30 meter SP 2330 fused silica capillary columns. A Hewlett-Packard HP 85 computer, connected directly to the integrators, was used to identify each fatty acid. A mixture of fatty acid standards was run daily.

2. Phospholipid Molecular Species

To characterize changes in fatty acid composition in more detail, we determined the molecular species composition of ethanolamine glycerophospholipids (EGP) in the cerebral cortex of monkeys fed control and deficient diets and in deficient monkeys repleted with fish oil.[29] Each phospholipid molecule is made up of a glycerol backbone connecting two fatty acid chains and a phosphate-linked head group (ethanolamine in the case of EGP). Analysis of molecular species defines the pairs of fatty acids present in phospholipid molecules and the position (*sn*-1 or *sn*-2) of each fatty acid. We initially focused on EGP because they are the most abundant highly polyunsaturated class of phospholipids in retina and brain. Molecular species were analyzed based on the method of Blank et al.,[30] as modified by us.[29] Briefly, phospholipid classes were separated by TLC, and the EGP were hydrolyzed by phospholipase C. Diradylglycerobenzoates were then prepared and separated into the diacyl, alkenylacyl (plasmalogen) and alkylacyl subclasses by TLC on silica gel G with benzene/hexane/ethyl ether (50:45:4 by volume). Molecular species were eluted from a 3.9 x 30 cm Nova-pak HPLC column with acetonitrile/isopropanol at 1 ml/min[30] and peaks identified by retention time and gas chromatographic analysis of the fractions.[28]

C. ELECTRORETINOGRAPHY

Full-field electroretinograms were recorded at ages from 3-4 months to 2 years. Pupils were maximally dilated with 1% cyclopentolate plus 10% phenylephrine, and the animals were then anesthetized with intravenous thiamylal sodium. Recordings were obtained with bipolar corneal contact lens electrodes. The signal was amplified at a gain of 10,000, passband 1-1000 Hz for cone responses and at gain 5000, passband 0.3-1000 Hz for rod responses. The stimuli were 10 μsec flashes (1.75 cd/m²-sec) produced by a Grass PS-22 photostimulator and diffused within a spherical dome.

Cone-dominated responses were isolated using 31.25 Hz flicker or flashes at 2 Hz superimposed on an 80 cd/m² adapting background. Rod-dominated ERGs were elicited at 20-second intervals after at least 30 minutes of dark adaptation. Signal averaging of 100 cone responses or 4-10 rod responses was accomplished with an Apple II+ computer and custom software. The averaged responses were analyzed to determine amplitudes of the A-wave (the major cornea-negative component generated by the photoreceptors) and B-wave (the later major cornea-positive component) and implicit times (latencies to the peak of the B-wave). In addition, repetitive stimulation was used to test the recovery (relative refractory period) of dark-adapted responses. Trains of flashes (1.75 cd/m²-sec, sufficient luminance to produce maximal B-wave amplitudes) were presented at intervals from 1 to 20 seconds. For shorter intervals, the relative A-wave and B-wave amplitudes were calculated as a percent of the maximal amplitudes obtained at 20-second intervals.

III. RESULTS

A. BIOCHEMICAL ANALYSES OF TISSUE PHOSPHOLIPIDS

1. Fatty Acid Composition

Dietary deprivation of ω3 fatty acids resulted in abnormally low levels of DHA in all retinal phospholipids, including ethanolomine glycerophospholipids (EGP) (Figure 1).[23] Deprivation of pregnant females reduced retinal DHA in their newborn infants to 50% of control levels by the time of birth; when deprivation continued postnatally, levels fell to 20% by 2 years of age. As in previous studies of ω3 fatty acid deprivation, reductions in DHA were almost quantitatively matched by increases in 22:5ω6, the most unsaturated fatty acid of the ω6 series. This fatty acid is normally present at very low levels, but its synthesis increases dramatically when ω3 series precursors are unavailable, so that the overall degree of polyunsaturation is nearly maintained. These changes in fatty acid composition were closely mirrored in cerebral cortex gray matter (Figure 1). DHA levels in this tissue are not as high as in the retina, but showed similar changes in response to dietary deprivation. Thus, the composition of the more abundant and accessible cerebral cortex can provide a reliable index of retinal fatty acid levels.

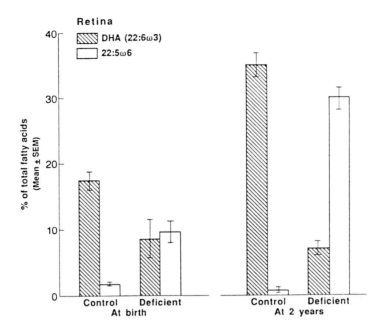

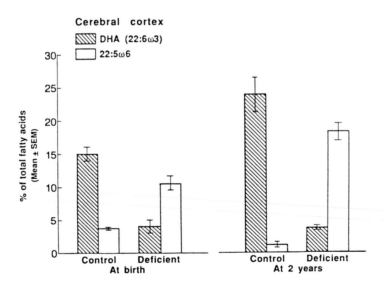

Figure 1. Levels of DHA (22:6ω3) and 22:5ω6 (weight % of total fatty acids) in the ethanolamine gycerophospholipids of the retina (top) and prefrontal cerebral cortex gray matter (bottom) of control and ω3 fatty acid-deficient rhesus monkeys near the time of birth and at 2 years of age. In both tissues, reduced DHA levels in the deficient group were matched by compensatory increases in the levels of 22:5ω6.

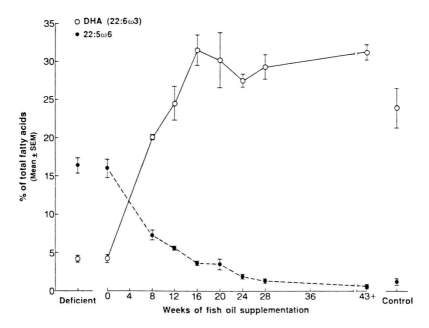

Figure 2. Levels of DHA (22:6ω3) and 22:5ω6 (weight % of total fatty acids) in the ethanolamine glycerophospholipids of prefrontal cerebral gray matter in ω3 fatty acid-deficient rhesus monkeys before and after repletion with dietary fish oil. Values for 2-year-old control and deficient monkeys are shown for comparison.

The reversibility of the effects of ω3 fatty acid deficiency was tested beginning at ages from 10 to 24 months by feeding a diet high in fish oil, a rich source of DHA and EPA. Although it was not possible to monitor longitudinal changes in fatty acid composition in the retina, we were able to examine serial biopsies of prefrontal cortical gray matter in order to determine the time course of these changes. Changes in fatty acid composition occurred rapidly (Figure 2). In EGP, levels of DHA increased to control levels within 12 weeks and plateaued at levels approximately 30% above those seen in controls, while levels of 22:5ω6 declined more slowly.[26] Levels of DHA in the EGP of the retina, determined after 10 months or more of supplementation, also increased above control levels by 25% (Figure 3). However, the fish oil diet also produced an abnormal increase in the levels of EPA (20:5ω3), another ω3 fatty acid which is abundant in fish oil but is normally absent or very low in tissues. EPA increased from 0 to 3.1% of total fatty acids in the frontal cerebral cortex and from 0.3% to 7.0% in the retina. Meanwhile, levels of longer-chain ω6 fatty acids, including 22:5ω6 and 20:4ω6 (arachidonic acid), fell below control levels after fish oil feeding.

2. Phospholipid Molecular Species

In the EGP of rhesus monkey cerebral cortex gray matter, three DHA-containing molecular species were present: 16:0-22:6ω3, 18:0-22:6ω3 and 18:1-22:6ω3 (given as *sn*-1:*sn*-2). In deficient monkeys, as expected from the overall fatty acid composition, these three species were much reduced in all EGP subclasses (diacyl, alkenylacyl, and alkylacyl), and there were compensatory increases in the corresponding three species containing 22:5ω6.[29] However, these changes were not evenly distributed, because 22:5ω6 did not pair with the three possible *sn*-1 fatty acids in the same pattern as DHA.

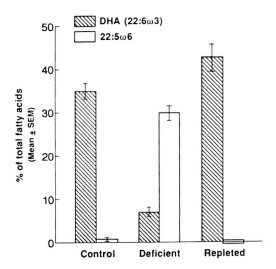

Figure 3. Levels of DHA (22:6ω3) and 22:5ω6 (weight % of total fatty acids) in the retinal ethanolamine glycerophospholipids of 2-year-old control and ω3 fatty acid-deficient rhesus monkeys and in deficient monkeys after repletion with dietary fish oil.

In particular, it did not pair with 18:1 to the same extent. Over all three subclasses, the proportion of DHA paired with 18:1 in the deficient animals (19%) was significantly higher than the proportion of 22:5ω6 paired with 18:1 (6%), and was also higher than in control animals (12.5%) (Figure 4). That is, there was a relative sparing of the 18:1-22:6ω3 species in the deficient group. In the control animals, of the small amount of 22:5ω6 which was present, we detected none paired with 18:1. Another unexpected result was that the species 16:0-18:1, normally present in all EGP subclasses at a level of 3-5%, was completely absent from the diacyl and alkyacyl subclasses in deficient monkeys. Thus, ω3 fatty acid deficiency did not produce a simple replacement of ω3 fatty acids with ω6 fatty acids, but rather involved a more complex remodeling of membrane phospholipids. Such changes are likely to have important consequences for membrane function.[31] The selective sparing of 18:1-22:6ω3 is intriguing, and could be part of a mechanism to maintain fluidity or other biophysical properties of the membrane despite the loss of DHA. Preliminary results indicate an even more dramatic retention of this species in the retina of deficient monkeys; indeed, despite an 80% decrease in total DHA in retinal EGP, the weight percent of 18:1-22:6ω3 was maintained at or above control levels in both the diacyl and alkylacyl subclasses.

In the cerebral cortex of deficient monkeys repleted with fish oil, the proportion of total EGP species containing DHA increased as expected, and in most cases the individual species exceeded control levels.[29] The proportion of 22:6ω3 paired with 18:1 fell to 14.6%, not significantly different from the control value (Figure 4). In addition, 18:0-20:5ω3 increased from zero to 2.5% in diacyl, 2.7% in alkylacyl and 4.5% in alkenylacyl EGP. In contrast, species containing 22:5ω6 and 20:4ω6 (arachidonic acid) decreased below control levels, in agreement with the overall fatty acid composition data. However, species containing 20:4ω6 showed a differential response similar to that found for DHA in deficient animals: 18:1-20:4ω6 actually increased in both the alkylacyl and alkenylacyl subclasses. This increase contributed to a statistically significant rise in the proportion of total species containing 18:1 in the *sn*-1 position.

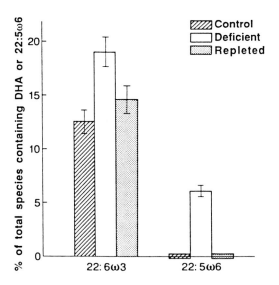

Figure 4. Percent of 22:6ω3-containing molecular species which had 18:1 in the *sn*-1 position [18:1-22:6ω3 / (16:0-22:6ω3 + 18:0-22:6ω3 + 18:1-22:6ω3)] and corresponding values for species containing 22:5ω6, averaged across the three subclasses of ethanolamine glycerophospholipids of the prefrontal cerebral cortex in control and ω3 fatty acid-deficient rhesus monkeys and in deficient monkeys repleted with dietary fish oil.

B. ELECTRORETINOGRAPHY

At 3-4 months, deficient monkeys had significantly reduced amplitudes of the cone and rod A-waves (Figure 5). Similar effects have been reported in ω3 fatty acid-deficient rats.[16-20] However, amplitudes decreased with age in control monkeys more than in the deficient group, so that no group differences were found at later ages. Bourre et al.[20] recently reported a similar disappearance of the amplitude effect with age in deficient rats. B-wave amplitudes were not significantly affected at any age in deficient monkeys.

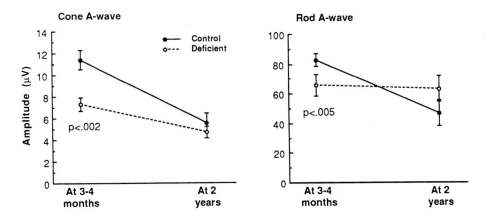

Figure 5. A-wave amplitudes of the cone- and rod-dominated ERG in control and ω3 fatty acid-deficient rhesus monkeys at 3-4 months and 2 years of age. Cone-dominated ERGs were elicited by flashes on an adapting background.

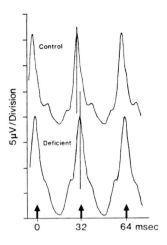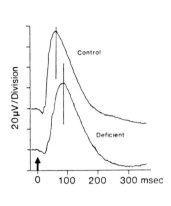

Figure 6.   Representative ERG waveforms in 2-year-old control and ω3 fatty acid-deficient rhesus monkeys, illustrating prolonged implicit times (latencies to the B-wave peak) in the deficient group.   Left: Cone-dominated ERG evoked by 31.25 Hz flicker (32 msec interval between flashes). Right: Rod-dominated ERG elicited by moderate intensity flash. Arrows indicate time of flash; vertical lines are drawn through the peaks to facilitate comparison.

Deficient monkeys also showed changes in the timing and recovery (relative refractory period) of the ERG.   Cone- and rod-dominated B-wave implicit times were significantly prolonged in older deficient monkeys (Figure 6). The recovery of dark-adapted A- and B-wave amplitudes after a saturating flash also was significantly impaired,[23] as best represented by the relative amplitudes of responses at short inter-flash intervals, compared to maximal responses obtained with 20-second intervals (Figure 7). This effect was present by 3-4 months and increased in magnitude with age, so that it was correlated with the degree of retinal DHA depletion. It is related to the rapid phase of dark adaptation and does not involve regeneration of visual pigment, as flash intensities were too low for significant rhodopsin bleaching. Thus, ω3 fatty acid deficiency produced a slowing of processes involved in generation and regeneration of a full ERG response.

In the repletion study, ERGs recorded after 12, 24 and 36 weeks of supplementation showed no improvement in the abnormal implicit times or recovery functions induced by the deficiency, suggesting that these effects may not be reversible after 10 months of age. This absence of recovery may have been due to the failure of fish oil feeding to restore a completely normal retinal fatty acid composition, the new compositional abnormalities induced by the fish oil diet, or a lasting effect of early deficiency on retinal development.

IV. DISCUSSION

During prenatal development, the human fetus is supplied with a rich supply of DHA by the placenta, richer than that found in the maternal circulation.[32,33] After birth, infants appear to be limited in their capacity to synthesize DHA from α-linolenic acid, as elongation and desaturation occur too slowly to keep pace with the high demand imposed by rapid growth. Animal studies have shown that pre-formed dietary DHA or EPA are more efficient sources for DHA incorporation into developing neural tissue than α-linolenic acid.[34,35] Human milk, in addition to supplying α-linolenic acid, contains

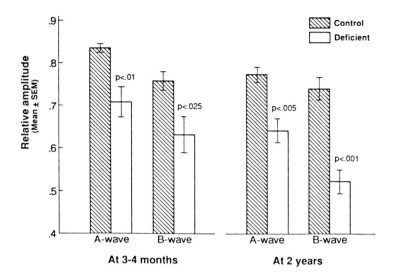

Figure 7. The effect of repetitive stimulation at 3.2-second intervals on the amplitude of the dark-adapted ERG A-wave and B-wave. Relative amplitude represents amplitude at 3.2-second inter-flash intervals as a fraction of the maximal amplitude obtained at 20-second intervals.

DHA in sufficient amounts to account for its rapid accumulation in developing neural tissue.[36] Synthetic infant formulas, on the other hand, contain widely varying levels of α-linolenic acid and none contain DHA or EPA. Human infants fed these formulas show a postnatal drop in erythrocyte membrane DHA compared to infants receiving human milk, even when the formula contains a relatively rich source of α-linolenic acid.[37-40] Supplementation with small amounts of fish oil produces erythrocyte DHA levels comparable to those in breast-fed infants.[41,42]

Two recent studies in human infants provide evidence, in agreement with results in rats and monkeys, that dietary ω3 fatty acids are necessary for optimal visual development. Very low birth weight infants fed a formula based on corn and coconut oils, relatively low in α-linolenic acid, had lower maximum amplitudes and higher thresholds for the rod ERG B-wave at 36 weeks post-conception than those fed either human milk or a fish oil-supplemented formula.[42] Infants fed a formula containing soybean oil, higher in α-linolenic acid but without DHA or EPA, had intermediate values for these ERG parameters, suggesting that the pre-formed longer-chain ω3 fatty acids may provide an advantage over α-linolenic acid alone. In another study, infants fed fish oil-supplemented formula had better visual acuity at 48 weeks of age than those fed standard formulas, and acuity was significantly correlated with erythrocyte DHA levels.[43]

Low plasma levels of DHA have been found in several families with retinitis pigmentosa, including ones with X-linked[44] and autosomal dominant[44,45] forms and Usher's syndrome.[46] However, the changes have not shown a consistent pattern, and the relationship of these findings to the disease process is unclear. The differences in some cases have been specific to DHA,[44,45] whereas others have involved decreases in both DHA and in arachidonic acid (20:4ω6),[44,46] suggesting a general defect in essential fatty acid metabolism. One recent study found significant increases, rather than decreases, in plasma DHA in affected members of a large family with the autosomal dominant form.[47] Among animal models of inherited retinal degenerations, the *rd* mouse shows alterations in photoreceptor fatty acid composition by postnatal day 5, before degenerative changes begin,[48] and the progressive rod-cone degeneration of miniature poodles is accompanied by low plasma DHA levels.[49] However, loss of DHA by itself does not lead to retinal degeneration: dietary deficiency of ω3 fatty acids fails to induce significant morphological abnormalities, despite more dramatic DHA depletion from plasma and from the retina.[16,50] But it is possible that plasma fatty acid changes associated with retinal degenerations may be markers for some abnormality in lipid metabolism which affects the integrity of retinal membranes. Candidates for such an abnormality include a deficiency of desaturase enzymes, a lack of fatty acid carriers or binding proteins, an unusual vulnerability to lipid oxidation or peroxidation, or a defect in phospholipid acylation or deacylation.

DHA's functional role in photoreceptor and neural membranes is poorly understood. The fatty acid composition and molecular species distribution of membrane phospholipids have been shown to modulate the activities of a number of membrane-associated receptors, enzymes, and transport systems.[5,31,51-53] The phospholipids immediately surrounding some membrane proteins appear to be selectively enriched with DHA,[53] and may create a microenvironment which facilitates mobility and changes in shape. Studies of synthetic phospholipid membranes have demonstrated that a DHA content of 50%, as in normal outer segment disks, is necessary for maximal photochemical activity of rhodopsin.[54] It has been proposed that DHA-rich phospholipids create a membrane with optimal thickness, or that they are best able to accommodate light-induced conformational changes in rhodopsin and the resulting expansion of the disk membrane.[55,56] Thus, DHA-rich phospholipids appear to provide an optimal lipid environment for the initial photochemical events in vision, and in synaptic membranes they may similarly facilitate neurotransmission. In addition, high DHA levels may provide a pool of precursor for functionally important lipoxygenase products, either directly or via retroconversion to EPA.[57] However, the high content of DHA can also be a biological liability; it may contribute to the instability of outer segment membranes by increasing their permeability and vulnerability to lipid peroxidation, and therefore may enhance their susceptibility to osmotic or peroxidative damage.[58,59]

Animal studies have demonstrated the importance of ω3 fatty acids for development of vision and retinal function, and some of these findings now have been confirmed by studies in human infants. However, ω3 fatty acid deficiency does not provide a straightforward model for retinal degenerative diseases, and we do not yet understand the mechanisms by which the deficiency induces functional changes in the retina.

V. ACKNOWLEDGEMENTS

This research was supported by NIH grants DK-29930 and RR-00163 and a grant from the National Retinitis Pigmentosa Foundation. This is publication number 1770 of the Oregon Regional Primate Research Center.

VI. REFERENCES

1. Cotman, C., Blank, M.L., Moehl, A., and Snyder, F., Lipid composition of synaptic plasma membranes isolated from rat brain by zonal ultracentrifugation, *Biochemistry* 8: 4606, 1969.
2. Anderson, R.E., Benolken, R.M., Dudley, P.A., Landis, D.J., and Wheeler, T.G., Polyunsaturated fatty acids of photoreceptor membranes, *Exp. Eye Res.* 18: 205, 1974.
3. Stone, W.L., Farnsworth, C.C., and Dratz, E.A., A reinvestigation of the fatty acid content of bovine, rat and frog retinal rod outer segments, *Exp. Eye Res.* 28: 387, 1979.

4. Fliesler, S.J., and Anderson, R.E., Chemistry and metabolism of lipids in the vertebrate retina, *Prog. Lipid Res.* 22: 79, 1983.

5. Stubbs, C.D., and Smith, A.D., The modification of mammalian membrane polyunsaturated fatty acid composition in relation to membrane fluidity and function, *Biochim. Biophys. Acta* 779: 89, 1984.

6. Anderson, R.E., and Sperling, L., Lipids of ocular tissues. VII. Positional distribution of the fatty acids in the phospholipids of bovine retina rod outer segments, *Arch. Biochem. Biophys.* 144: 673, 1971.

7. Wiegand, R.D., and Anderson, R.E., Phospholipid molecular species of frog rod outer segment membranes, *Exp. Eye Res.* 37:159, 1983.

8. Aveldaño, M.I., and Bazan, N.G., Molecular species of phosphatidylcholine, -ethanolamine, -serine, and -inositol in microsomal and photoreceptor membranes of bovine retina, *J. Lipid Res.* 24: 620, 1983.

9. Choe, H.-G., and Anderson, R.E., Unique molecular species composition of glycerolipids of frog rod outer segments, *Exp. Eye Res.* 51:159, 1990.

10. Crawford, M.A., and Sinclair, A.J., Nutritional influences in the evolution of the mammalian brain, in *Lipids, Malnutrition and the Developing Brain,* Ciba Foundation Symposium, Elsevier, Amsterdam, 1972, p. 267.

11. Neuringer, M., Anderson, G.J., and Connor, W.E., The essentiality of n-3 fatty acids for the development and function of the retina and brain, *Ann. Rev. Nutr.* 8: 517, 1988.

12. Lamptey, M.S., and Walker, B.L., A possible essential role for dietary linolenic acid in the development of the young rat, *J. Nutr.* 106: 86, 1976.

13. Tinoco, J., Babcock, R., Hincenbergs, I., Medwadowski, B., and Miljanich, P., Linolenic acid deficiency: Changes in fatty acid patterns in female and male rats raised on a linolenic acid-deficient diet for two generations, *Lipids* 13: 6, 1978.

14. Mohrhauer, H., and Holman, R.T., Alteration of the fatty acid composition of brain lipids by varying levels of dietary essential fatty acids, *J.Neurochem.* 10: 523,1963.

15. Galli, C., Trzeciak, H.I., and Paoletti, R., Effects of dietary fatty acids on the fatty acid composition of brain ethanolamine phosphoglyceride: Reciprocal replacement of n-6 and n-3 polyunsaturated fatty acids, *Biochim. Biophys. Acta* 248: 449, 1971.

16. Benolken, R.M., Anderson, R.E., and Wheeler, T.G., Membrane fatty acids associated with the electrical response in visual excitation, *Science* 182: 1253, 1973.

17. Wheeler, T.G., Benolken, R.M., and Anderson, R.E., Visual membranes: Specificity of fatty acid precursors for the electrical response to illumination, *Science* 188: 1312, 1975.

18. Nouvelot, A., Dedonder, E., Dewailly, P., and Bourre, J.M., Influence des n-3 exogènes sur la composition en acides gras polyinsaturés de la rétine, aspects structural et physiologique, *Cahier Nutr. Diet.* 20: 123, 1985.

19. Watanabe, I., Kato, M., Aonuma, H., Hasimoto, A., Naito, Y., Moriuchi, A., and Okuyama, H., Effect of dietary alpha-linolenate/linoleate balance on the lipid composition and electroretinographic responses in rats, *Adv. Biosciences* 62: 563, 1987.

20. Bourre, J.M., Francois, M., Youyou, A., Dumont, O., Piciotti, M., Pascal, G. and Durand, G., The effects of dietary α-linolenic acid on the composition of nerve membranes, enzymatic activity, amplitude of electrophysiological parameters, resistance to poisons and performance of learning tasks in rats, *J. Nutr.* 119: 1880,1989.

21. Yamamoto, N., Saitoh, M., Moriuchi, A., Nomura, M., and Okuyama, H., Effects of dietary α-linolenate/linoleate balance on brain lipid composition and learning ability of rats, *J. Lipid Res.* 28: 144, 1987.

22. Yamamoto, N., Hashimoto, A., Takemoto, Y., Okuyama, H., Nomura, M., Kitajima, R., Togashi, T., and Tamai, Y., Effects of the dietary alpha-linolenate/linoleate balance on brain lipid compositions and learning ability of rats. II. Discrimination process, extinction process and glycolipid compositions, *J. Lipid Res.* 29: 1013, 1988.

23. Neuringer, M., Connor, W.E., Lin, D.S., Barstad, L., and Luck, S., Biochemical and functional effects of prenatal and postnatal omega-3 fatty acid deficiency on retina and brain in rhesus monkeys, *Proc. Natl. Acad. Sci.* 83: 4021, 1986.

24. Neuringer, M., Connor, W.E., Van Petten, C., and Barstad, L., Dietary omega-3 fatty acid deficiency and visual loss in infant rhesus monkeys, *J. Clin. Invest.* 73: 272, 1984.

25. Reisbick, S., Neuringer, M., Connor, W.E., and Hasnain, R., Polydipsia in rhesus monkeys deficient in omega-3 fatty acids, *Physiol. Behav.* 47: 315, 1990.

26. Connor, W.E., Neuringer, M., and Lin, D.S., Dietary effects upon brain fatty acid composition: The reversibility of n-3 fatty acid deficiency and turnover of docosahexaenoic acid in the brain, erythrocytes and plasma of rhesus monkeys, *J. Lipid Res.* 31: 237, 1990.

27. Morrison, W.R., and Smith, L.M., Preparation of fatty acid methyl esters and dimethylacetals from lipids with boron trifluoride-methanol, *J. Lipid Res.* 5: 600, 1964.

28. Anderson, G.J., Connor, W.E., Corliss, J.D., and Lin, D.S., Rapid modulation of n-3 docosahexaenoic acid levels in the brain and retina of the newly hatched chick, *J. Lipid Res.* 30: 433, 1989.

29. Lin, D.S., Connor, W.E., Anderson, G.J., and Neuringer, M., The effects of dietary n-3 fatty acids on the phospholipid molecular species of monkey brain, *J. Neurochem.* 55: 1200, 1990.

30. Blank, M.L., Robinson, M., Fitzgerald, V., and Snyder, F., Novel quantitative method for determination of molecular species of phospholipids and diglycerides, *J. Chromatogr.* 298: 473, 1984.

31. Lynch, D.V., and Thompson, G.A., Retailored lipid molecular species: A tactical mechanism for modulating membrane properties, *Tr. Biochem. Sci.* 9: 442, 1984.

32. Crawford, M.A., Hassam, A.G., and Williams, G., Essential fatty acids and fetal brain growth, *Lancet* 1: 452, 1976.

33. Ruyle, M., Connor, W.E., Anderson, G.J., and Lowensohn, R.I., Placental transfer of essential fatty acids in humans: Venous-arterial difference for docosahexaenoic acid in fetal umbilical erythrocytes, *Proc. Natl. Acad. Sci.* 87: 7902, 1990.

34. Sinclair, A.J., Incorporation of radioactive polyunsaturated fatty acids into liver and brain of developing rat, *Lipids* 10: 175, 1975.

35. Anderson, G.J., Connor, W.E., and Corliss, J., Docosahexaenoic acid is the preferred dietary n-3 fatty acid for the development of the brain and retina, *Pediat. Res.* 27: 89, 1990.

36. Clandinin, M.T., Chappell, J.E., and Heim, T., Do low weight infants require nutrition with chain elongation-desaturation products of essential fatty acids? *Prog. Lipid Res.* 20: 901, 1981.

37. Crawford, M.A., Hassam, A.G., and Hall, B.M., Metabolism of essential fatty acids in the human fetus and neonate, *Nutr. Metab.* 21: 187, 1977.

38. Sanders, T.A.B., and Naismith, D.J., A comparison of the influence of breast feeding and bottle feeding on the fatty acid composition of erythrocytes, *Br. J. Nutr.* 4: 619, 1979.

39. Carlson, S.E., Carver, J.D., and House, S.G., Docosahexaenoic acid status of preterm infants at birth and following feeding with human milk or formula, *Am. J. Clin. Nutr.* 44: 798, 1986.

40. Pita, M.L., Fernandez, M.R., DeLucchi, C., Medina, A., Martinez-Valverde, A., Uauy, R., and Gil, A., Changes in the fatty acid pattern of red blood cell phospholipids induced by type of fat, dietary nucleotides and postnatal age in preterm infants, *J. Pediatr. Gastroenterol. Nutr.* 7: 740, 1988.

41. Carlson, S.E., Rhodes, P.G., Rao, V.S., and Goldgar, D.E., Effect of fish oil supplementation on the n-3 fatty acid content of red blood cell membranes in preterm infants, *Pediat. Res.* 21: 507, 1987.

42. Uauy, R.D, Birch, D.G., Birch, E.E., Tyson, J.E., and Hoffman, D.R., Effect of dietary omega-3 fatty acids on retinal function of very-low-birth-weight neonates, *Pediat. Res.* 28: 485, 1990.

43. Carlson, S. E., Cooke, R., Werkman, S., and Peeples, J., Docosahexaenoate (DHA) and eicosapentaenoate (EPA) supplementation of preterm (PT) infants: Effects on phospholipid DHA and visual acuity, *FASEB J.* 3: A1056 (abstract), 1989.

44. Converse, C.A., Hammer, H.M., Packard, C.J., and Shepherd, J., Plasma lipid abnormalities in retinitis pigmentosa and related conditions, *Trans. Ophthalmol. Soc. U.K.* 103: 508, 1983.

45. Anderson, R.E., Maude, M.B., Lewis, R.A., Newsome, D.A., and Fishman, G.A., Abnormal plasma levels of polyunsaturated fatty acid in autosomal dominant retinitis pigmentosa, *Exp. Eye Res.* 44: 155, 1987.

46. Bazan, N.G., Scott, B.L., Reddy, T.S., and Pelias, M.Z., Decreased content of docosahexaenoate and arachidonate in plasma phospholipids in Usher's syndrome, *Biochem. Biophys. Res. Commun.* 141: 600, 1986.

47. Newsome, D.A., Anderson, R.E., May, J.G., McKay, T.A., and Maude, M., Clinical and serum lipid findings in a large family with autosomal dominant retinitis pigmentosa, *Ophthalmology* 95: 1691, 1988.

48. Scott, B.L., Racz, E., Lolley, R.N., and Bazan, N.G., Developing rod photoreceptors from normal and mutant *rd* mouse retinas: Altered fatty acid composition early in development of the mutant, *J. Neurosci. Res.* 20: 202, 1988.

49. Anderson, R.E., Maude, M.B., Alvarez, R.A., Acland, G.M., Narfström, K., Nilsson, S.E.G., Wetzel, M., O'Brien, P., and Aguirre, G.D., Plasma lipid abnormalities in dogs, cats and humans with an inherited retinal degeneration, this volume.

50. Feeney-Burns, L., Neuringer, M., and Connor, W.E., unpublished data.

51. Brenner, R.R., Effect of unsaturated acids on membrane structure and enzyme kinetics, *Prog. Lipid Res.* 23: 69, 1984.

52. Spector, A.A., and Yorek, M.A., Membrane lipid composition and cellular function, *J. Lipid Res.* 26: 1015, 1985.

53. Salem, N., Kim, H.-Y., and Yergey, J.A., Docosahexaenoic acid: Membrane function and metabolism, in *Health Effects of Polyunsaturated Fatty Acids in Seafoods*, Simopoulos, A.P., Ed., Academic Press, New York, 1986, p. 263.

54. Weidmann, T.S., Pates, R.D., Beach, J.M., Salmon, A., and Brown, M.F., Lipid-protein interactions mediate the photochemical function of rhodopsin, *Biochemistry* 27: 6469, 1988.

55. Dratz, E.A., and Deese, A.J., The role of docosahexaenoic acid (22:6n-3) in biological membranes: Examples from photoreceptors and model membrane bilayers, in *Health Effects of Polyunsaturated Fatty Acids in Seafoods*, Simopoulos, A.P., Ed., Academic Press, New York, 1986, p. 319.

56. Dratz, E.A., Ryba, N., Watts, A., and Deese, A.J., Studies of the essential role of docosahexaenoic acid (DHA), 22:6ω3, in visual excitation, *Invest. Ophthalmol. Vis. Sci.* 28 (Suppl.3): 96 (abstract), 1987.

57. Bazan, N.G., The metabolism of omega-3 polyunsaturated fatty acids in the eye: The possible role of docosahexaenoic acid and docosanoids in retinal physiology and ocular pathology, *Prog. Clin. Biol. Res.* 312: 95, 1989.

58. Anderson, R.E., Rapp, L.M., and Wiegand, R.D., Lipid peroxidation and retinal degeneration, *Curr. Eye Res.* 3: 223, 1984.

59. Organisciak, D.T., Wang, H.-M., and Noell, W.K., Aspects of the ascorbate protective mechanism in retinal light damage of rats with normal and reduced ROS docosahexaenoic acid, in *Degenerative Retinal Disorders: Clinical and Laboratory Investigations*, Hollyfield, J.G., Anderson, R.E., and LaVail, M.M., Eds., Alan R. Liss, 1987, p. 455.

PLASMA LIPID ABNORMALITIES IN *prcd*-AFFECTED MINIATURE POODLES AND ABYSSINIAN CATS

Robert E. Anderson[1], Maureen B. Maude[1], Richard A. Alvarez[1],
Sven Erik G. Nilsson[2], Kristina Narfström[2,3], Gregory M. Acland[4],
and Gustavo Aguirre[4]

[1]Cullen Eye Institute, Baylor College of Medicine, Houston TX;
[2]Department of Ophthalmology, University of Linköping,
Linköping, Sweden; [3]Department of Medicine & Surgery,
Faculty of Veterinary Medicine, Swedish University of
Agricultural Sciences, Uppsala, Sweden; and
[4]Department of Clinical Studies, School of Veterinary
Medicine, University of Pennsylvania, Philadelphia PA

Retinitis pigmentosa (RP) is the name given to a number of inherited retinal degenerations whose clinical presentations are similar but not identical.[1] Usually, the first symptom is night blindness, followed by loss of peripheral vision. With time, there is a slow, progressive degeneration of retinal membranes that ultimately leads to death of photoreceptor cells and loss of visual function. The usual clinical picture of an elderly RP patient is that of an otherwise healthy person with very limited or no visual function.

With few exceptions, there are no extraocular manifestations of RP. Nevertheless, researchers have long sought systemic markers of inherited retinal degenerations in humans and animals, mostly to no avail. However, several years ago Converse and her colleagues[2,3] reported abnormalities in plasma lipids among several Scottish families with RP. This included hyperlipidemia in some patients, evidenced by elevated cholesterol and low density lipoprotein levels, and hypolipidemia in others. Jahn and co-workers[4] surveyed 250 unrelated RP patients in Germany and found an increase in total serum cholesterol in autosomal dominant RP, autosomal recessive RP, and isolated RP. The increase in dominant RP was due to elevations of both LDL and HDL, while only HDL was elevated in recessive and isolated RP. This group also examined the apoprotein E (apoE) phenotypes in 139 unrelated Germans with RP and found a ten-fold elevation in apo E_2E_2 phenotypes (10% vs. 1%).[5] Significant elevations were also found in phenotypes apo E_2/E_3 and apo E_3/E_4. Converse et al.[6] found normal apo E_2/E_2 in their Scottish population, but an eleven-fold elevation in apo E_4/E_4.

Abnormalities in plasma fatty acids have also been reported in human RP. Converse et al.[7] reported low plasma 22:6ω3 in some, but not all, of the X-linked and autosomal dominant RP families that they examined. Bazan et al.[8] found that patients with Usher's syndrome had significant reductions in the level of 22:6ω3 in plasma phospholipids compared to controls. Anderson et al.[9] reported lower plasma 22:6ω3 levels in autosomal dominant RP, but found no differences in X-linked or simplex RP. However, examination of two families with autosomal dominant RP showed no differences in plasma levels of 22:6ω3 between affected and controls.[10,11] Reduced plasma levels of 22:6ω3 and 20:4ω6 in one of three families with autosomal dominant RP was reported by Voaden et al.[12]

Taken together, these results suggest a systemic abnormality in polyunsaturated fatty acid metabolism in humans with retinitis pigmentosa. However, the differences between families and the metabolic heterogeneity of humans made any search for a metabolic defect in lipid metabolism an extremely difficult task in humans. Therefore, we turned our attention to two animal strains with inherited retinal degenerations that closely resemble autosomal recessive RP.

The miniature poodle[13,14] and the Abyssinian cat[15,16] with progressive rod-cone degeneration are among the best animal models of human retinitis pigmentosa. In both animals, the retina develops normally at first. In the Abyssinian cat, minor signs of outer segment degeneration are observed already at the age of 35 days. Degeneration, which occurs more markedly in the midperiphery and the periphery, proceeds slowly, however, and blindness does not occur until the age of 5-6 years. In the miniature poodle, degeneration is first noted in late adolescence and begins with changes in the peripheral retina that slowly progress centrally until all photoreceptor cells are destroyed. The metabolic basis for the degeneration is not known in either animal. There is no disturbance in cyclic nucleotide metabolism in affected poodles[17] or cats.[18] In the retina, the only known metabolic difference between affected and control poodles is the renewal rate of integral proteins of rod outer segments, which in affected dogs is one-half that of controls.[19]

We have examined the plasma lipids of affected and control miniature poodles,[20-22] Abyssinian cats,[23] and Irish setters.[22] Affected poodles and cats have lower levels of 22:6ω3 than controls. However, there were no differences in the Irish setter, in which a defect in cyclic GMP metabolism has been shown.[17] Our studies of lipid metabolism in these diverse strains are summarized in this chapter.

I. EXPERIMENTAL DESIGN

The miniature poodles and Irish setters we examined were from a colony that was maintained in a controlled animal care facility in Pennsylvania. All dogs were born and raised in this facility and fed Purina lab chow and Kal-Kan dog foods obtained from commercial sources. All Abyssinian cats were born, raised, and maintained in a controlled animal care facility in Sweden. They were fed commercial diets supplemented with an occasional piece of fish.

Blood was collected from fasting animals and blood elements were removed by centrifugation. Frozen plasma was mailed on dry ice to Houston for lipid analysis. After thawing, a known volume of plasma was extracted and the lipids made to a known volume in chloroform. An aliquot was removed for determination of lipid phosphorus and another aliquot was placed on a thin layer plate, which was developed in a neutral lipid solvent system. The phospholipids remaining at the origin were scraped into a glass tube and methyl esters prepared. An internal standard of 17:0 and 21:0 was added, and methyl esters were quantitated by capillary gas-liquid chromatography. These are standard procedures that have been previously described.[24]

Affected and control animals were compared using analysis of covariance (ANCOVA) with the animal's age (in months) serving as covariant. A total of 109 observations were made on 57 different miniature poodles, with blood being drawn on three different occasions (June, 1987; August, 1987; and July, 1988). A total of 28 observations were made on 28 Irish setters, with blood being drawn once. A total of 41 observations were made on 34 Abyssinian cats, with blood being drawn on two separate occassions (March, 1988 and September, 1988).

TABLE 1

Plasma Fatty Acids in Affected and Control Miniature Poodles,
Irish Setters, and Abyssinian Cats

Animal	Animal Status	Lipid Measure	Lipid Value	P-Value
Miniature Poodle	Affected	$22:6\omega3$	45.3 ± 5.0	< 0.01
	Control	(nmol/ml)	61.8 ± 5.4	
	Affected	$22:5\omega3/$	1.7 ± 0.1	< 0.001
	Control	$22:6\omega3$	1.1 ± 0.1	
Irish Setter	Affected	$22:6\omega3$	55.9 ± 7.1	NS
	Control	(nmol/ml)	55.1 ± 7.4	
	Affected	$22:5\omega3/$	1.8 ± 0.1	NS
	Control	$22:6\omega3$	1.8 ± 0.1	
Abyssinian Cat	Affected	$22:6\omega3$	95 ± 14	< 0.005
	Control	(nmol/ml)	174 ± 19	
	Affected	$22:5\omega3/$	0.25 ± 0.01	< 0.001
	Control	$22:6\omega3$	0.12 ± 0.02	

II. RESULTS

Table 1 contains the results of analysis of 22:6ω3 and 22:5ω3/22:6ω3 in plasma phospholipids of affected and control miniature poodles, Irish setters, and Abyssinian cats. Affected poodles and cats had lower plasma levels of 22:6ω3 than controls. The values for the poodles are the averages of the results from the three different times that blood was drawn, and the differences are significant at the 0.01 level. When each time point was considered separately, the differences between affected and control values were also significant. The ratios of 22:5ω3/22:6ω3 were significantly elevated in affected poodles and cats, compared to controls. No differences were seen in plasma levels of 22:6ω3 or in the 22:5ω3/22:6ω3 ratio between affected and control Irish setters. Thus, in the animal with defective cyclic GMP metabolism,[17] there is no evidence of a defect in 22:6ω3 metabolism.

III. DISCUSSION

The retinas of all animals, both vertebrates and invertebrates, have high levels of long chain ω3 polyunsaturated fatty acids (PUFA).[25] High levels of ω3 PUFAs are also found in brain[26] and reproductive tissues.[27] The major PUFAs of most other tissues are of the ω6 family, the most prominent two members being 18:2ω6 and 20:4ω6. Arachidonic acid (20:4ω6) is the precursor of most of the prostaglandins, thromboxanes, and leukotrienes. Omega-3 and ω6 PUFAs are essential fatty acids, since neither family of fatty acids can be synthesized *de novo* by animals. Long chain PUFAs of both families can be synthesized by animals from short chain precursors (18:2ω6 and 18:3ω3) through a series of elongation and desaturation reactions, depicted in Figure 1. The enzymes for these reactions are tightly bound to microsomes and none has been characterized at the molecular level.

The major fatty acid found in vertebrate rod outer segments is 22:6ω3.[25] This fatty acid must be obtained from the diet or synthesized from the appropriate precursor through the pathway shown in Figure 1. Plants are sources of 18:3ω3, while animals, especially those of marine origin, are sources of C-20 and C-22 ω3 PUFA's.

The final step in the synthesis of 22:6ω3 and 22:5ω6 is the desaturation reaction catalyzed by the enzyme Δ-4 desaturase. Our plasma fatty acid analyses in the miniature poodle[20-22] and Abyssinian cat[23] suggest these animals are deficient in this enzyme. This would account for the low levels of 22:6ω3 and the elevated ratio of 22:5ω3/22:6ω3. This conclusion is strengthened by two recent studies in the miniature poodle.

In the first,[28] five affected and five control miniature poodles were given daily oral supplements of linseed oil (enriched in 18:3ω3). Blood was drawn at predetermined times before, during, and after supplementation, and plasma phospholipid fatty acids were analyzed. In *prcd*-affected animals, the 22:5ω3/22:6ω3 ratio was significantly increased relative to controls during supplementation. The ratio

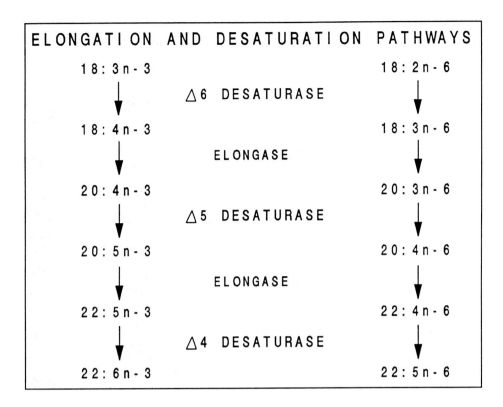

ELONGATION AND DESATURATION PATHWAYS

18:3n-3 → 18:4n-3 → 20:4n-3 → 20:5n-3 → 22:5n-3 → 22:6n-3

18:2n-6 → 18:3n-6 → 20:3n-6 → 20:4n-6 → 22:4n-6 → 22:5n-6

Δ6 DESATURASE

ELONGASE

Δ5 DESATURASE

ELONGASE

Δ4 DESATURASE

Figure 1. Pathways for elongation and desaturation of short-chain polyunsaturated fatty acids. The two families of fatty acids are identified by the position of the first double bond from the methyl terminus, designated either as $\omega 3$ and $\omega 6$ or n-3 and n-6.

declined once supplementation ceased, but remained significantly elevated above control values for up to ten days.

In the second study,[29] liver microsomes from three affected and three unaffected animals were incubated with ^{3}H-20:5ω3, which is first elongated to 22:5ω3 and then desaturated to 22:6ω3 (see Figure 1). The results showed no difference in specific activities in 22:5ω3 between groups, but a large difference in specific activity of 22:6ω3 (1.10 ± 0.16 Ci/mg/hr for affected vs 3.55 ± 0.46 for unaffected). This decrease in Δ-4 desaturase activity would result in the lowered plasma 22:6ω3 found in affected animals. One consequence of this would be lower levels of this important fatty acid being available to the photoreceptors.

Why is 22:6ω3 important to the retina? Docosahexaenoate is the major fatty acid of rod outer segments. Although it or its precursors must be obtained from the diet, dietary deprivation of ω3 fatty acids does not lead to dramatic alterations in the 22:6ω3 content in ROS. The retina (and the brain) have mechanisms to conserve ω3

PUFA's during ω3 deficiency.[30-32] Docosahexaenoate appears to be essential to some retinal function that is measurable by electroretinography. Slight alterations in 22:6ω3 in the rat retina brought about by dietary deprivation lead to reduction in amplitudes of the a- and b-waves of the electroretinogram.[33-36] Changes in visual acuity and the ERG have been reported in rhesus monkeys deprived of 22:6ω3 from birth.[37-39] Recently, Uauy et al.[40] reported premature human infants fed semi-synthetic diets depleted of 22:6ω3 had a delayed development of the electro-retinogram which could be corrected when the infants were placed on ω3 fatty acid-containing diets. In contrast, the ERG changes in the rhesus monkey (b-wave) could not be corrected by dietary supplementation of 22:6ω3.[39]

Does dietary deprivation of PUFAs lead to a retinal degeneration? In none of the studies on dietary deprivation of ω3 and/or ω6 fatty acids was there any report of retinal changes. Thus, it appears that, at least in the animal models tested, dietary deprivation of essential PUFAs does not lead to retinal degeneration. However, there are several points that must be considered before we can accept this conclusion. First, the degeneration observed in the *prcd*-affected miniature poodle, the Abyssinian cat, and humans with retinitis pigmentosa is a slow process that takes place over a long period of time. The lower plasma levels of 22:6ω3 in affected humans and animals may take an entire lifetime to proceed to total blindness. Long term morphological studies required to explore this possibility have not been done in animals deprived of dietary ω3 polyunsaturated fatty acids. Second, the low levels of plasma 22:6ω3 may not reflect the state of 22:6ω3 in the retina. We do not know the extent of uptake of 22:6ω3 into the pigment epithelium and its subsequent transfer into the retina. We presume from dietary studies[41] that the RPE selectively removes C-22 polyunsaturated fatty acids from the plasma. This conclusion is based on the absence of any C-18 and C-20 PUFA's (other than a small amount of arachidonic acid, 20:4ω6) in ROS phospholipids. Finally, there is a fundamental difference in the metabolism of PUFAs in essential fatty acid deprivation and Δ4-desaturase deficiency. In the deprivation studies, 22:6ω3 is replaced molecule-for-molecule by 22:5ω6.[31,32,41,42] In those animals that received ω6 supplements, large amounts of 22:6ω3 were replaced by 22:5ω6. Those animals receiving neither ω3 nor ω6 fatty acids retained their high ROS levels of 22:6ω3, but also incorporated enough 22:5ω6 to replace the small amounts of 22:6ω3 that were lost. Thus, the total C-22 PUFA levels did not change in the deprivation studies. In Δ4-desaturase deficiency, however, neither 22:6ω3 nor 22:5ω6 (see Figure 1) are synthesized. Therefore, the levels of both of these fatty acids would be reduced in the ROS, if there were no dietary source of these two acids. Thus, it is misleading and inappropriate to draw conclusions about the role of 22:6ω3 on retinal degenerations by comparing animals deficient in ω3 and/or ω6 PUFA with those that have a Δ4-desaturase deficiency. These are uniquely different conditions.

Are there conditions under which the level of 22:6ω3 can be reduced in the ROS without an increase in 22:5ω6? Penn and Anderson[43,44] showed that albino rats adapted to bright cyclic light (800 lux, 12L:12D) had a significant reduction in the level of 22:6ω3 compared to albino rats raised in dim cyclic light (5 and 300 lux, 12L:12D). The 22:6ω3 levels in the ROS of the bright-reared group was one-third that of the dim group (16% vs. 56%). They attributed this change to "adaptation" of the retinas to bright cyclic light. It was later demonstrated that the reduction of $22:6\omega3$ was achieved through a decreased synthesis of phospholipids containing $22:6\omega3$, rather than an increased turnover of $22:6\omega3$ containing phospholipids in the ROS.[45] Unlike what happens in $\omega3$ and $\omega6$ deprivation, in these adaptation experiments, there was no compensatory increase in $22:5\omega6$ to replace the $22:6\omega3$ that was reduced in the bright light animals. Thus, these retinas were responding in a manner consistent with that of a $\Delta4$-desaturase abnormality.

Did the rat retinas that adapted to bright cyclic light show any evidence of retinal degeneration? Yes. There were three morphological differences between rats raised in 5 lux and 800 lux cyclic light.[44,45] In the bright group, the ROS were much shorter, the ROS disks were disorganized, and there was a significant loss of photoreceptor cell nuclei. Penn and Anderson[44] made the point that the morphological appearance of these retinas did not indicate that the cells were dying, since every cell was affected and few pyknotic nuclei were observed. To the contrary, they emphasized that this state of disarray of the ROS was a chronic condition brought about by the adaptation of the cell to bright cyclic light.

How do these adaptation experiments in rats relate to our studies on dogs, cats, and humans with inherited retinal degenerations? The retinas of affected poodles[13,14] and cats,[15,16] like the retinas of the rats discussed above, show disorganization of the disks in their rod outer segments. Since the disease in these animals takes years to progress to the total loss of photoreceptors, this disorganization of disks must be considered a chronic condition, and not due to photoreceptor cell death. In fact, affected dogs generate an electroretinographic response and renew their ROS long after degenerative changes are evident. Furthermore, there are biochemical similarities between these two conditions. The ROS of the bright light-adapted rats have reduced levels of $22:6\omega3$ (without an increase in $22:5\omega6$), which would be expected in the animals deficient in $\Delta4$-desaturase activity. However, we do not know in either condition if low levels of $22:6\omega3$ are actually responsible for the disorganization of the ROS. Also, there is no reason *a priori* to assume that disorganized disks lead to photoreceptor cell death.

IV. WORKING HYPOTHESIS

Our working hypothesis is that miniature poodles, Abyssinian cats, and (perhaps) humans with an inherited retinal degeneration have a defective $\Delta4$-desaturase that leads to a reduction in the amount of $22:6\omega3$ available to the retina, and that prolonged deficiency of $22:6\omega3$ leads to a retinal degeneration. Support for this hypothesis in derived from the following studies:

1. Plasma levels of $22:6\omega3$ are reduced in miniature poodles,[20-22] Abyssinian cats,[23] and some humans with inherited retinal degenerations.[7-12]

2. Delta-4 desaturase activities are lower in livers of affected poodles compared to controls.[29]

3. Dietary supplementation of linseed oil containing 18:3ω3 to poodles results in a significant elevation of 22:5ω3/22:6ω3 in affected dogs compared to controls.[28]

V. PREDICTIONS OF THE HYPOTHESIS

If the hypothesis is correct, then several predictions follow:

1. The ROS of affected animals with evidence of retinal degeneration should have lower levels of 22:6ω3 than controls.

2. There may be a subset of humans with retinitis pigmentosa that have a deficiency of Δ4-desaturase activity.

3. Supplementation of diets of affected poodles and cats with 22:6ω3 may prevent their retinal degeneration. If Δ4-desaturase deficiency is found in humans with RP, supplementation may also prove beneficial.

ACKNOWLEDGEMENTS

This work was supported by NIH grants EY00871, EY04149, EY01244, EY06855, and EY02520, and grants from the Retinitis Pigmentosa Foundation Fighting Blindness, the Retina Research Foundation, The CERF, Inc.-PRA Research Fund, The Frances V. R. Seebe Trust, Research to Prevent Blindness, Inc., The Swedish Medical Research Council (Project No. 12X-734), and The Crown Princess Margareta's Foundation for the Visually Handicapped. Dr. Anderson is the recipient of a Senior Scientific Investigator Award from Research to Prevent Blindness, Inc. We are grateful to Dr. David Francis for assistance with the statistical analyses. We would also like to thank Mrs. Susan Nitroy and the staff of The Retinal Disease Studies facility at the University of Pennsylvania.

REFERENCES

1. Bird, A. C., Clinical investigation of retinitis pigmentosa, in *Progress in Clinical and Biological Research, Vol. 247, Degenerative Retinal Disorders: Clinical and Laboratory Investigations*, Hollyfield, J.G., Anderson, R.E., and LaVail, M.M., Eds., Alan R. Liss, Inc., New York, 1987. 3.

2. Converse, C. A., Hammer, H. M., Packard, C. J., and Shepherd, J., Plasma lipid abnormalities in retinitis pigmentosa and related conditions, *Trans. Ophthalmol. Soc. U. K.*, 103, 508, 1983.

3. Converse, C. A., McLachlan, T., Hammer, H. M., Packard, C. J., and Shepherd, J., Hyperlipidemia in retinitis pigmentosa, in *Retinal Degeneration: Experimental and Clinical Studies*, LaVail, M. M., Hollyfield, J. G., and Anderson, R. E., Eds., Alan R. Liss, Inc., New York, 1985. 63.

4. Jahn, C. E., Leiss, O., v. Bergmann, K., and Schäfer K., Serum lipoprotein concentrations in patients with retinitis pigmentosa, in *Advances in the Biosciences*, Vol. 62, *Research in Retinitis Pigmentosa*, Zrenner, E., Krastel, H., and Goebel, H. H., Eds., Pergamon Journals Ltd., Oxford, 1987. 571.

5. Jahn, C. E., Oette, K., Esser, A., v. Bergmann, K., and Leiß, O., Increased prevalence of apolipoprotein E2 in retinitis pigmentosa, in *Advances in the Biosciences*, Vol. 62, *Research in Retinitis Pigmentosa*, Zrenner, E., Krastel, H., and Goebel, H. H., Eds., Pergamon Journals Ltd., Oxford, 1987. 575.

6. Converse, C. A., Huq, L., McLachlan, T., Bow, A. C., and Alvarez, E., Apolipoprotein E isotypes in retinitis pigmentosa, *Invest. Ophthalmol. Vis. Sci.* (Suppl.), 29, 169, 1988.

7. Converse, C. A., McLachlan, T., Bow, A. C., Packard, C. J., and Shepherd, J., Lipid metabolism in retinitis pigmentosa, in *Progress in Clinical and Biological Research, Vol. 247, Degenerative Retinal Disorders: Clinical and Laboratory Investigations*, Hollyfield, J. G., Anderson, R. E., and LaVail, M. M., Eds., Alan R. Liss, Inc., New York, 1987. 93.

8. Bazan, N. G., Scott, B. L., Reddy, T. S., and Pelias, M. Z., Decreased content of docosahexaenoate and arachidonate in plasma phospholipids in Usher's syndrome, *Biochem. Biophys. Res. Comm.*, 141, 600, 1986.

9. Anderson, R. E., Maude, M. B., Lewis, R. A., Newsome, D. A., and Fishman, G. A., Abnormal plasma levels of polyunsaturated fatty acid in autosomal dominant retinitis pigmentosa, *Exp. Eye Res.*, 44, 155, 1987.

10. Newsome, D. A., Anderson, R. E., May, J. G., McKay, T. A., and Maude, M. B., Clinical and serum lipid findings in a large family with autosomal dominant retinitis pigmentosa, *Ophthalmology*, 95, 1691, 1988.

11. Dehning, D. O. and Garcia, C. A., Lipid abnormalities in autosomal dominant retinitis pigmentosa, *Invest. Ophthalmol. Vis. Sci.* (Suppl.), 28, 346, 1987.

12. Voaden, M. J., Polkinghorne, P. J., Belin, J., and Smith, A. D., Studies on blood from patients with dominantly inherited retinitis pigmentosa, in *Progress in Clinical and Biological Research, Vol.247, Inherited and Environmentally Induced Retinal Degenerations*, LaVail, M. M., Anderson, R. E., and Hollyfield, J. G., Eds., Alan R. Liss, Inc., New York, 1989. 57.

13. Aguirre, G., Alligood, J., O'Brien, P., and Buyukmihci, N. Pathogenesis of progressive rod-cone degeneration in miniature poodles. *Invest. Ophthalmol. Vis. Sci.* 23, 610, 1982.

14. Aguirre, G., Stramm, L., and O'Brien, P., Diseases of the photoreceptor cells - pigment epithelium complex: Influence of spatial, pigmentation and retinal factors, in *Retinal Degeneration: Experimental and Clinical Studies,* LaVail, M. M., Hollyfield, J. G., and Anderson, R. E., Eds., Alan R. Liss, Inc., New York, 1985. 401.

15. Narfström, K., and Nilsson, S. E., Progressive retinal atrophy in the Abyssinian cat: Electron microscopy, *Invest. Ophthalmol. Vis. Sci.*, 27, 1569, 1986.

16. Narfström, K., and Nilsson, S. E., Morphological findings during retinal development and maturation in hereditary rod-cone degeneration in Abyssinian cats, *Exp. Eye Res.*, 49, 611, 1989.

17. Aguirre, G. A., Farber, D., Lolley, R., Fletcher, R. T., and Chader, G. J., Rod-cone dysplasia in Irish setters: A defect in cyclic GMP metabolism in visual cells, *Science*, 201, 1133, 1978.

18. Narfstrom, K. and Nilsson, S. E. G., Hereditary rod-cone degeneration in a strain of Abyssinian cats, in *Progress in Clinical and Biological Research, Vol. 247, Degenerative Retinal Disorders: Clinical and Laboratory Investigations*, Hollyfield, J. G., Anderson, R. E., and LaVail, M. M., Eds., Alan R. Liss, Inc., New York, 349. 1987.

19. Aguirre, A. A. and O'Brien, P. J., Morphological and biochemical studies of canine progressive rod-cone degenerations, *Invest. Ophthalmol. Vis. Sci.* 27, 635, 1986.

20. Anderson, R. E., Maude, M. B., Alvarez, R. A., Acland, G. M., and Aguirre, G. D., Plasma levels of docosahexaenoic acid in miniature poodles with an inherited retinal degeneration, *Invest. Ophthalmol. Vis. Sci.* (Suppl.), 29, 169, 1988.

21. Wetzel, M. G., Fahlman, C., Maude, M. B., Alvarez, R. A., O'Brien, P. J., Acland, G. M., Aguirre, G. D., and Anderson, R. E., Fatty acid metabolism in normal miniature poodles and those affected with progressive rod-cone degeneration (*prcd*), in *Progress in Clinical and Biological Research, Vol. 314, Inherited and Environmentally Induced Retinal Degenerations*, LaVail, M. M., Hollyfield, J. G., and Anderson, R. E., Eds., Alan R. Liss, Inc., New York, 1989. 427.

22. Anderson, R. E., Maude, M. B., Alvarez, R. A., Acland, G. M., and Aguirre, G., Plasma lipid abnormalities in the miniature poodle with progressive rod-cone degeneration. *Exp. Eye. Res.*, 1990, in press.

23. Anderson, R. E., Maude, M. B., Nilsson, S. E. G., and Narfström, K., Plasma lipid abnormalities in the Abyssinian cat with a hereditary rod-cone degeneration. *Exp. Eye Res.*, 1991, submitted for publication.

24. Wiegand, R. D., and Anderson, R. E., Determination of molecular species of rod outer segment phospholipids, in *Methods in Enzymology, Vol. 81, Visual Pigments and Purple Membranes*, Packer, L., Ed., Academic Press, New York, 1982. 296.

25. Fliesler, S. J., and Anderson, R. E., Chemistry and metabolism of lipids in the vertebrate retina, in *Progress in Lipid Research*, Vol. 22, Holman, R. T., Ed., Pergamon Press, London, 1983. 79.

26. O'Brien, J. S. and Sampson, E. L., Fatty acid and aldehyde composition of the major brain lipids in normal gray matter, white matter, and myelin, *J. Lipid Res.*, 4, 357, 1965.

27. Neill, A. R. and Masters, C. J., Metabolism of fatty acids by ovine-spermatozoa, *J. Reprod. Fert.*, 34, 279, 1973.

28. Anderson, R. E., Maude, M. B., Acland, G. M., and Aguirre, G. A., Abnormal delta-4 desaturase in the *prcd* poodle, *Invest. Ophthalmol. Vis. Sci.* (Suppl.), 32, 1991.

29. Alvarez, R. A., Aguirre, G., and Anderson, R. E., A defective liver delta-4 desaturase in the *prcd* poodle may be responsible for its progressive retinal degeneration, *Invest. Ophthalmol. Vis. Sci.* (Suppl.), 32, 1991.

30. Futterman S., Downer J. L., and Hendrickson A., Effect of essential fatty acid deficiency on the fatty acid composition, morphology, and electroretinographic response of the retina, *Invest. Ophthalmol.*, 10, 151, 1971.

31. Anderson R. E. and Maude M. B., Lipids of ocular tissues: VIII. The effects of essential fatty acid deficiency on the phospholipids of the photoreceptor membranes of rat retina, *Arch. Biochem. Biophys.*, 151, 270, 1972.

32. Tinoco J., Dietary requirements and function of α-linolenic acid in animals, in *Progress in Lipid Research, Vol. 21*, Holman R. T., Ed., Pergamon Press, London, 1982. 1.

33. Benolken, R. M., Anderson, R. E., and Wheeler, T. G., Membrane fatty acids associated with the electrical response in visual excitation, *Science*, 182, 1253, 1973.

34. Wheeler, T. G., Benolken, R. M., and Anderson, R. E., Visual membranes: Specificity of fatty acid precursors for the electrical response to illumination, *Science*, 188, 1312, 1975.

35. Watanabe, I., Kato, M., Aonuma, H., Hashimoto, A., Naito, Y., Moriuchi, A., and Okuyama, H., Effect of dietary alpha-linolenate/linoleate balance on the lipid composition and electroretinographic responses in rats, in *Advances in the Biosciences, Vol. 62, Research in Retinitis Pigmentosa*, Zrenner, E., Krastel, H., and Goebel, H. H., Eds., Pergamon Journals Ltd., Oxford, 1987. 563.

36. Bourre, J-M., Francios, M., Youyou, A., Dumont, O., Piciotti, M., Pascal, G., and Durand, G., The effects of dietary α-linolenic acid on the composition of nerve membranes, enzymatic activity, amplitude of electrophysiological parameters, resistance to poisons and performance of learning tasks in rats, *J. Nutr.*, 119, 1880, 1989.

37. Neuringer, M., Connor, W. E., v. Petten, C., and Barstad, L., Dietary omega-3 fatty acid deficiency and visual loss in infant rhesus monkey, *J. Clin. Invest.* 73, 272, 1984.

38. Neuringer, M., Connor, W. E., Lin, D. S., Barstad, L., and Luck, S., Biochemical and functional effects of prenatal and postnatal omega-3 fatty acid deficiency on retina and brain in rhesus monkey, *Proc. Natl. Acad. Sci. USA*, 83, 4021, 1986.

39. Neuringer, M. and Connor, W. E., Omega-3 fatty acids in the retina, in *Dietary Omega-3 and Omega-6 Fatty Acids*, Galli, C., and Simopoulos, A. P., Eds., Plenum Press, New York, 1989. 177.

40. Uauy, R. D., Birch, D. G., Birch, E. E., Tyson, J. E., and Hoffman, D. R., Effect of dietary omega-3 fatty acids on retinal function of very-low-birth-weight neonates, *Pediatr. Res.*, 28, 485, 1990.

41. Anderson, R. E., Koutz, C. A., Stinson, A. M., and Wiegand, R. D., Effect of dietary fatty acids on 22-carbon polyunsaturates in rat rod outer segments, *Invest. Ophthalmol. Vis. Sci.* (Suppl.), 30, 286, 1989.

42. Connor W. E., Neuringer M., and Lin D. S., Dietary effects on brain fatty acid composition; the reversibility of n-3 fatty acid deficiency and turnover of

docosahexaenoic acid in the brain, erythrocytes and plasma of rhesus monkeys, *J. Lipid Res.*, 31, 237, 1990.

43. Penn, J. S., and Anderson, R. E., Effect of light history on rod outer segment membrane composition in the rat, *Exp. Eye Res.* 44, 767, 1987.

44. Penn, J. S., Naash, M. I., and Anderson, R. E., Effect of light history on retinal antioxidants and light damage susceptibility in the rat, *Exp. Eye Res.*, 44, 779, 1987.

45. Penn, J. S., Wiegand, R. D., Thum, L. A., and Anderson, R. E., Light environment affects the metabolism of docosahexaenoate-containing molecular species of glycerophospholipids in rat rod outer segments, *Invest. Ophthalmol. Vis. Sci.* (Suppl.), 31, 471, 1990.

SYNTHESIS OF N-3 POLYUNSATURATED FATTY ACIDS IN RETINITIS PIGMENTOSA

Carolyn A. Converse, Avril J. McColl, Tracey McLachlan,
Aileen G. Pollacchi, Donal Brosnahan,[*] Harold M. Hammer[*]
and Gawn G. McIlwaine[*]

Department of Pharmacy, University of Strathclyde, and
[*]Tennent Institute of Ophthalmology, Western Infirmary,
Glasgow, Scotland, U.K.

I. INTRODUCTION

Retinitis pigmentosa, a family of hereditary degenerative diseases of the retina, is often accompanied by disorders in lipid metabolism.[1-4] In particular, we have described low levels of a polyunsaturated fatty acid, docosahexaenoic acid (DHA; C22:6, n-3), in the plasma of patients affected with the X-linked form of the disease.[1,3,5] These findings have been confirmed in an American study, and in addition low DHA levels have been reported in autosomal dominant retinitis pigmentosa, in Usher syndrome and in a canine retinal degeneration resembling human retinitis pigmentosa.[6-9]

Docosahexaenoic acid is an essential fatty acid which is either obtained in the diet, primarily from fish oils, or synthesized from α-linolenic acid (ALA; C18:3, n-3) by the following pathway:

18:3,n-3 -> 18:4,n-3 -> 20:4,n-3 -> 20:5,n-3 -> 22:5,n-3 -> 22:6,n-3

Here 'n-3' refers to the position of the terminal double bond. This n-3 pathway is entirely distinct from the n-6 pathway, shown below, and there is no interconversion between n-3 and n-6 fatty acids.

18:2,n-6 -> 18:3,n-6 -> 20:3,n-6 -> 20:4,n-6 ->22:4,n-6 -> 22:5,n-6

DHA is the most abundant fatty acid in photoreceptor rod outer segments,[10,11] and it seems to be necessary for vision, as animals deprived of n-3 fatty acids in their diet show decreased visual function, for instance as measured by electroretinography.[12-15] Thus it is possible that retinitis pigmentosa patients with low levels of DHA in the blood may be supplying insufficient quantities of this fatty acid to the retina, and this may contribute to the etiology of the disease.

The aim of the present study was to find out whether retinitis pigmentosa patients with low plasma levels of DHA are able to make this polyunsaturated fatty acid from ALA, or they have a defect in the n-3 biosynthetic pathway.

II. MATERIALS AND METHODS

A. SUBJECTS

The families studied were for the most part obtained from the patient records for the retinitis pigmentosa clinic at the Tennent Institute of Ophthalmology. Type of retinitis pigmentosa (*i.e.*, mode of inheritance) was ascertained from family histories backed up by clinical examination of affected and unaffected members whenever practicable. Twelve-hour fasted blood samples were obtained in potassium-EDTA tubes, and the plasma prepared the same day and stored at -20°C until analysis.

B. FATTY ACID ANALYSIS

Total fatty acids were extracted with chloroform:methanol (2:1), saponified with methanolic NaOH then methylated using BF₃ in 14% methanol.[16] Packed column gas chromatographic analysis was used to compare new families with families previously analysed by this method (10% Silar 10C on 100/200 Gas Chrom Q, with temperature program 200°C for 4 min. then 5°C/min. to 235°C where it was held for 4 min.).[3] Results were expressed as weight-percentage of the total fatty acids recovered, and differences between affected and unaffected members of the same family analysed by the Mann-Whitney test.[17]

Capillary gas chromatography was used to analyse plasma fatty acids in the ALA feeding study (see below), as this gives better resolution of the intermediates in the n-3 pathway. A 25m BP20 column, internal diameter 0.32μ, film thickness 0.15μ was used, with temperature program 200°C for 5 min, then increased by 3°C min⁻¹ to 230°C, and held at 230°C for 20 min. Samples were analysed in triplicate and compared to known standards (PUFA-2, Supelco). Results were expressed as weight-percentage of total fatty acids recovered.

C. α-LINOLENIC ACID FEEDING STUDY

Initially, two female controls were used in a pilot study. Three 12-hour-fasting plasma samples over a 2-week period were analysed to determine basal levels of polyunsaturated fatty acids. Each subject then consumed 20g of uncooked edible linseed ("Linusit Gold", Fink GMBH, Herrenberg, FRG) per day for six weeks; this is equivalent to about 5g per day of ALA, or about ten times the normal dietary intake. Fasting blood samples were taken weekly for fatty acid analysis. Samples were also taken every 2-3 weeks for analysis of cholesterol, triglyceride, and lipoprotein levels.

Three affected and three unaffected members of the G family (X-linked) and and one affected and one unaffected person from the T family (autosomal dominant) were put on a similar regimen to that described above, except only two basal level blood samples were taken, separated by one week, before beginning 6 weeks of linseed consumption.

To analyse the data, fatty acid measurements (as weight-percentage) for each group were averaged at each time point. The average amount of each fatty acid was plotted against time, and the slope and y-intercept calculated by linear regression analysis; correlation co-efficients were also calculated. The rate of increase of each fatty acid with time was then calculated as the slope divided by the y-intercept.

III. RESULTS

A. FATTY ACID PROFILES OF FAMILIES

Three families, H, W, and T, have been analysed by packed-column gas chromatography, to add to the five families analysed previously.[3] The results for all eight families are presented in Table 1.

TABLE 1

Plasma Fatty Acids, Comparing Affected
to Unaffected People within Families

	X-linked							Autosomal Dominant
Family	G	Gl	H	Ra	S	W	Y	T
Affected (A)	4	4	3	4	2	2	3	15
Unaffected (U)	11	9	6	11	6	9	6	13
Fatty Acids:								
16:0	NS[a]	NS	NS	NS	NS	NS	NS	NS
16:1	NS	NS	U>A[c]	NS	NS	NS	NS	U>A[c]
18:0	NS	NS	NS	NS	NS	NS	NS	NS
18:1	NS	NS	U>A[c]	NS	NS	A>U[c]	NS	NS
18:2	NS	NS	NS	NS	NS	NS	NS	NS
20:4	NS	U>A[c]	NS	A>U[c]	NS	NS	U>A[c]	U>A[d]
22:6	U>A[c]	U>A[b]	NS	NS	U>A[b]	NS	U>A[c]	U>A[c]

[a]NS: not significantly different (Mann-Whitney test)
U>A: Unaffected significantly > Affected
A>U: Affected significantly > Unaffected
[b]$p<0.10$,   [c]$p<0.05$,   [d]$p<0.025$.

B. α-LINOLENIC ACID FEEDING STUDY

The average percentage increases in plasma levels of each fatty acid are shown in Figure 1. Although 12 fatty acids from 16:0 to 22:6 in length were measured, only those from 18:3, n-3 and above are relevant to the feeding study and are presented in Figure 1; the ratio of 22:6 to 16:0 is also presented. In this system, it was possible to distinguish 18:3, n-6 from 18:3, n-3, and these were measured separately. In Figure 1, "20:3" and "20:4" are n-6 and "20:5", "22:5" and "22:6" are n-3. Thus the most important fatty acids in the analysis, those involved in the n-3 pathway, are 18:3,n-3, 20:5, 22:5 and 22:6.

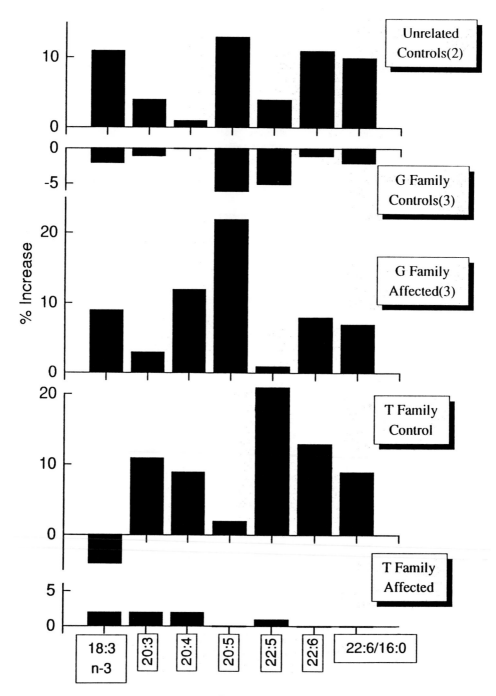

FIGURE 1.   Percentage Increase in Plasma Fatty Acid Content
             after Six Weeks' Ingestion of Linseed (20g day^{-1}).

(Controls: Unaffected. Numbers in parentheses: numbers in each group.)

IV. DISCUSSION

The results in Table 1 show that four of the seven X-linked families have a tendency towards low levels of 22:6 and sometimes 20:4 in affected members of each family, compared to unaffected members. In two of these families, the decrease in 22:6 is only statistically significant if p<0.10 is taken as the boundary for significance. However, in such a small sample, even a probability of 0.10 indicates a trend, and this is particularly interesting when the low levels of 22:6 in the other families are taken into account. It is possible that if larger families had been available, it would have been possible to show low levels of 22:6 in all the families; alternatively, there may be two different types of retinitis pigmentosa represented in these families.

The T family, with autosomal dominant retinitis pigmentosa, shows a significant decrease in both 20:4 and 22:6 in affected members of the family. The relatively large size of this family makes statistical analysis more reliable. It is interesting that in another large autosomal dominant family it has been shown that there is no decrease in levels of 22:6.[18] It is possible that these two families have different sub-types of autosomal dominant retinitis pigmentosa.

The G and T families were chosen for the ALA feeding study as members of these families showed the greatest and most consistent tendency towards low levels of DHA - indeed, the G family has maintained this tendency over more than seven years.[5] Unfortunately it was difficult to enlist many members of the T family in the study, as they live at a distance from Glasgow.

As is seen in Figure 1, the pilot study on two unrelated controls appears to show that it is possible to demonstrate an increase in later fatty acids in the n-3 pathway, including DHA, when subjects are fed linseed at a rate of 20 g per day for six weeks. The assumption is made that the additional ALA is converted directly into additional DHA and its precursors. Thus it appears that we can demonstrate that the n-3 biosynthetic pathway is functioning in these subjects.

Based on this pilot study, it was decided that increases of at least 7% in fatty acid levels from week 0 to week 6 would be regarded as significant; indeed, all the plots of fatty acid level against time, for all the subjects, showed a correlation coefficient > 0.50 when the increase was $\geq$ 7%, indicating that despite some scatter in points, there was in each case a definite upward trend. This was not true for increases of < 7%.

Thus, in the pilot study, there are significant increases in 18:3,n-3, 20:5 and 22:6. The ratio of 22:6 to 16:0 also increases by 10%. In the affected members of the G family a similar pattern is seen, with significant increases in 18:3,n-3, 20:5, 22:6 and 22:6/16:0. There is also a 12% increase in 20:4, not seen with the unrelated controls. Thus it appears likely that the affected members of this X-linked family are still able to synthesize longer-chain polyunsaturated fatty acids from 18:3, n-3, if our analysis is correct.

One problem is the failure to demonstrate any increase in any of the measured polyunsaturated fatty acids in the unaffected members of the G family. This is puzzling, considering the definite increases seen in the two unrelated controls. The most obvious explanation is non-compliance or under-compliance. Alternatively, there could have been a failure adequately to chew the linseeds to release the ALA, or they could have been cooked, destroying some of the polyunsaturated fatty acids. These suppostions are supported by the lack of net increase in plasma concentrations of ALA (18:3,n-3). In fact, the curve is biphasic, with an initial increase then a decrease after three weeks. That is, there may have been insufficient ALA in the plasma to drive the biosynthesis of the later fatty acids in the pathway.

The data from the T family are more difficult to interpret, with only two subjects. Certainly, the unaffected subject does show an increase in 22:5, 22:6, and 22:6/16:0. He also shows an increase in 20:4 and 20:3, from the n-6 pathway. There is no net increase in ALA, but again, this is a biphasic curve, with an increase to 4 weeks, then a decrease. It is possible that this subject stopped taking the seeds at this point or changed his eating habits; in any case, if our interpretation is correct, he is capable of synthesizing long-chain n-3 fatty acids.

In contrast, the affected member of this family showed no increase in plasma ALA and no increase in any of the longer-chain polyunsaturated fatty acids. If we assume compliance, there may a problem with availability of the ALA or its transport into the gut. There may also be a defect in the biosynthetic pathway (comparing him to the unaffected member of this family). It is important not to place too much emphasis on these results, however, as only two people were involved.

One assumption which underlies these studies is that when the plasma concentration of ALA is increased substantially, the extra molecules are converted directly into longer-chain derivatives, so an increase in these derivatives is a measure of the biosynthetic activity of the pathway. Alternatively, it is possible to postulate that excess ALA either causes release of DHA (for instance) from stores into the plasma or its synthesis by some other pathway (e.g., from very-long-chain-length polyunsaturated fatty acids). To counter these arguments, it is necessary to use radioactive precursors and analyse for radioactive products farther along in the synthetic pathway. These studies are now in progess, using cultured cells derived from the patients.

In conclusion, the data seem to suggest that the n-3 pathway is not defective in retinitis pigmentosa patients in the G family, and another cause, perhaps in lipid-handling, must be sought for the low levels of plasma DHA in these patients. It is possible there is a defect in this pathway in the T family, but further studies are required in both families.

V. ACKNOWLEDGEMENTS

We are grateful to members of the G and T families for agreeing to participate in this study. We are also grateful to Drs. M.M. Macartney, J. Clayton and Prof. J. Shepherd for assistance in obtaining blood samples. This research was supported by the National Retinitis Pigmentosa Foundation, Inc., George Gund Foundation, and W.H. Ross Foundation (Scotland) for the Study of Prevention of Blindness.

VI. REFERENCES

1. Converse, C.A., Hammer, H.M., Packard, C.J. and Shepherd, J., Plasma lipid abnormalities in retinitis pigmentosa and related conditions. *Trans. Ophthalmol. Soc. U.K.* 105, 508, 1983.
2. Converse, C.A., McLachlan, T., Hammer, H.M., Packard, C.J. and Shepherd, J., Hyperlipidemia in retinitis pigmentosa, in *Retinal Degeneration: Experimental and Clinical Studies*, LaVail, M.M., Hollyfield, J.G. and Anderson, R.E., Eds., Alan M. Liss, Inc., New York, 1985, 63.
3. Converse, C.A., McLachlan, T., Bow, A.C., Packard, C.J. and Shepherd, J., Lipid metabolism in retinitis pigmentosa, in *Degenerative Retinal Disorders: Clinical and Laboratory Investigations*, Hollyfield, J.G., Anderson, R.E. and LaVail, M.M., Eds., Alan M. Liss, Inc., New York, 1987, 93.
4. Converse, C.A., Keegan, W.A., Huq, L., Series, J., Caslake, M., McLachlan, T., Packard, C.J. and Shepherd, J., Further epidemiological studies on lipid metabolism in retinitis pigmentosa, in *Inherited and Environmentally Induced Retinal Degenerations*, LaVail, M.M., Hollyfield, J.G. and Anderson, R.E., Eds., Alan M. Liss, Inc., New York, 1989, 39.
5. McLachlan, T., McColl, A.J., Collins, M.F., Converse, C.A., Packard, C.J. and Shepherd, J., A longitudinal study of plasma n-3 fatty acid levels in a family with x-linked retinitis pigmentosa, *Bioch. Soc. Transact.* 18, 905, 1990.
6. Anderson, R.E., Maude, M.B., Lewis, R.A., Newsome, D.A., and Fishman, G.A., Abnormal plasma levels of polyunsaturated fatty acids in autosomal dominant retinitis pigmentosa, *Exp. Eye Res.* 44, 155, 1987.
7. Bazan, N.G., Scott, B.L., Reddy, T.S., and Pelias, M.Z., Decreased content of docosahexaenoate and arachidonate in plasma phospholipids in Usher's syndrome. *Biochem. Biophys. Res. Commun.* 141, 600, 1986.
8. Schaefer, E.J., personal communication, 1989.
9. Anderson, R.E., Maude, M.B., Alvarez, R.A., Acland, G.M., and Aguirre, G.D., Plasma levels of docosahexaenoic acid in miniature poodles with an inherited retinal degeneration, *Invest. Ophthalmol. Vis. Sci.* 29(suppl), 169, 1988.
10. Anderson, R.E., Benolken, R.M., Dudley, P.A., Landis, D.J. and Wheeler, T.G., Polyunsaturated fatty acids of photoreceptor membranes. *Exp. Eye Res.* 18, 205, 1974.
11. Stone, W.L., Farnsworth, C.C., and Dratz, E.A., A reinvestigation of the fatty acid content of bovine, rat and frog retinal rod outer segments, *Exp. Eye Res.* 28, 387, 1979.

12. Hands, A.R., Sutherland, N.S. and Bartley, W., Visual acuity of essential fatty acid-deficient rats, *Biochem. J.* 94, 279, 1965.

13. Wheeler, T.G., Benolken, R.M., and Anderson, R.E., Visual membranes: specificity of fatty acid precursors for the electrical response to illumination, *Science,* 188, 1312, 1975.

14. Neuringer, M, Connor, W.E., Van Petten, C., and Barstad, L, Dietary omega-3 fatty acid deficiency and visual loss in infant rhesus monkeys, *J. Clin. Invest.* 73, 272, 1984.

15. Birch, D., Uauy, R., Birch, E. and Tyson, J., Dietary omega-3 fatty acids and full-field ERGs in very low birth weight neonates (VLBWN), *Invest. Ophthalmol. Vis. Sci.* 30(suppl), 318, 1989.

16. Morrison, W.R. and Smith, L.M., Preparation of fatty acid methyl esters and dimethylacetals from lipids with BF_3-methanol, *J. Lipid Res.* 5, 600, 1964.

17. Conover, W.J., *Practical Nonparametric Statistics,* John Wiley and Sons, New York, 1971.

18. Dehning, D.O. and Garcia, C.A., Lipid abnormalities in autosomal dominant retinitis pigmentosa, *Invest. Opthalmol. Vis. Sci.* 28(3:suppl), 346, 1987.

DOCOSAHEXAENOIC ACID AND PHOSPHOLIPID METABOLISM IN PHOTORECEPTOR CELLS AND IN RETINAL DEGENERATION

NICOLAS G. BAZAN
ELENA B. RODRIGUEZ de TURCO
WILLIAM C. GORDON

LSU Eye Center and Neuroscience Center
2020 Gravier Street, Suite B
New Orleans, LA 70112 USA

I. INTRODUCTION

The essential fatty acids linoleic acid (18:2n6) and linolenic acid (18:3n3) are precursors of two families of polyunsaturated fatty acids, the n6 and the n3 series. The major fatty acids generated from 18:2n6 and 18:3n3 are arachidonic acid (20:4n6) and docosahexaenoic acid (22:6n3), which are produced by sequential elongation and desaturation enzymatic steps. Both of these fatty acids are esterified mainly at the C_2 position of the glycerol moiety of biomembrane phospholipids, and are required for normal structure and function. Experimental evidence indicates that each one plays unique and well defined cellular roles. A major role of 20:4n6 is as precursor of a variety of oxygenated metabolites (eicosanoids) with second messenger functions. Moreover, it has been suggested that oxygenated metabolites, termed docosanoids, generated from 22:6n3 by the retina, have biological activity.[1] While 20:4n6 and 22:6n3 are widely distributed among all cell membranes of different tissues, only 22:6n3 is highly concentrated in cellular membranes of the central nervous system. Membranes of photoreceptor outer segment discs and synaptic terminals are built with phospholipids selectively enriched in 22:6n3.[2-5]

Supraenoic molecular species of phospholipids are found in the retina.[2,6-10] They were defined by their behavior on silver-impregnated thin-layer chromatographs as more highly unsaturated than hexaenoic and contain two 22:6n3 moieties per molecule.[6] Molecular species containing more than 22 carbons and 6 double bonds, and esterified at the C_1 position, are also found in very high concentration in the retina and in outer segments of photoreceptor cells.[8,9,11,12]

The physiological reason for the selective enrichment in lipids containing 22:6n3 in phospholipids of these membranes is not defined at present. It may be that 22:6n3 is involved in the modulation of membrane fluidity. However, membrane fluidity generated by lipids containing only two double bonds is not appreciably increased once three or more double bonds are present.[13]

Because of the six double bonds in 22:6n3, it would be expected that this fatty acid has a short tissue half-life, and is very readily oxidized. However, neural tissues retain 22:6n3 for long periods of time and protect this highly unsaturated fatty acid from oxidation. The advantage of utilizing 22:6n3 in these systems must significantly outweigh the problems that its presence poses to the cell, suggesting some remarkable and unique role.

Although other long-chain polyunsaturated fatty acids, such as 22:5n6, are generated as a compensatory mechanism in the retinas of monkeys deprived of dietary n3 fatty acids during early postnatal life,[14] impairments in brain and visual function[14-18] have been reported. This suggests an irreplaceable role of 22:6n3 in excitable membranes.

Our approach to understanding the role of 22:6n3 in photoreceptor cells is based upon the hypothesis that impairments in the sustained, selective delivery involving the liver and uptake of 22:6n3 may result in cellular dysfunction and retinal degeneration.[19] This can be of critical importance, especially in the perinatal period, when photoreceptor morphogenesis and synaptogenesis are most active.

We provide here an overview of the conversion of dietary 18:3n3 to 22:6n3, as well as possible mechanisms involved in the selective delivery of 22:6n3 to the CNS and its subsequent fate within photoreceptor cells, as they first retain, and then recycle, 22:6n3 to preserve its endogenous content, even during prolonged dietary deprivation of 18:3n3. We have also summarized our studies showing that, early in the development of photoreceptor cells from the *rd* mouse, there are alterations in both the content and the metabolism of docosahexaenoic acid.

II. THE CENTRAL ROLE OF THE LIVER IN THE HANDLING OF 18:3n3 AND SUSTAINED DELIVERY OF 22:6n3 TO RETINA AND BRAIN

During the early postnatal life of vertebrates, there is very active delivery of 22:6n3 to the retina and brain. At this time active differentiation of photoreceptors and synaptogenesis occur. Retinal and neural cells use 22:6n3 to synthesize phospholipids that, in turn, become membrane components. Dietary 18:3n3 is delivered in chylomicrons to the liver where it is activated, elongated, and desaturated to generate 22:6n3.[20] In newborn mouse pups, within 2 h after injection of radiolabeled 18:3n3, most retinal labeling was in 16:0 (48%) and other saturated and monoenoic fatty acids (32%), with only 20% found in 22:5n3. Since there was no detectable labeling of 22:6n3, the 18:3n3 taken up by retinal cells was mainly oxidized and reutilized for the synthesis of other fatty acids. It is also possible that some or most of the labeled fatty acids found in the retina under these conditions are coming from other organs, such as liver or intestinal epithelium. In the liver, 18:3n3 was found at the earliest time points to be esterified into triacylglycerols. Once conversion to 22:5n3 and 22:6n3 had occurred, more than 90% was recovered in phospholipids. Within 24-72 h a progressive decrease in 22:6n3 labeling in the whole liver was accompanied by an increase of 22:6n3 labeling in brain and retina. This suggests that the liver plays a central role in supplying the brain and retina with 22:6n3 only after its conversion from 18:3n3, and probably releases the final product as 22:6-containing lipoproteins. Accumulation of labeled 22:5n3 in the retina also suggests that the activity of the Δ-4 desaturase, which converts 22:5n3 to 22:6n3, is the rate-limiting step in the 22:6n3 biosynthetic pathway. Since the CNS and retinal cells rely on a liver-mediated supply of 22:6n3 for maintenance and synthesis of excitable membranes (e.g. the constant renewal of disc membranes in photoreceptor cells), it has been postulated that blood-borne signals sent by the CNS to the liver control this process.[20]

III. TRAFFICKING OF 22:6n3 FROM THE BLOOD THROUGH THE PIGMENT EPITHELIUM TO PHOTORECEPTOR CELLS: POSSIBLE Apo-E INVOLVEMENT IN 22:6 UPTAKE BY PHOTORECEPTOR CELLS

Nutrients required by photoreceptor cells are selectively taken up from the choriocapillaris by pigment epithelial cells. It is likely that 22:6n3 carried by plasma lipoproteins[20] follows this route.[21] Therefore, a highly selective receptor-mediated mechanism may operate to assure the efficient uptake of 22:6n3 by the pigment epithelial cells. Autoradiographic studies of frogs injected with [3]H-22:6n3 revealed that the fatty acid was actively transferred from the pigment epithelial cells through the interphotoreceptor matrix to the photoreceptors.[21] Some label also accumulated in the oil droplets of the pigment epithelial cells, implying that neutral lipids (e.g. triacylglycerols) may function as a reservoir, buffering the supply of 22:6n3 to the matrix so that a relatively constant flux exists toward the photoreceptors. Experiments in frogs, injected *in vivo* with [3]H-22:6n3,[21] and *in vitro* incubations of human, monkey,[22] and frog[23] retinas with the same fatty acid, showed that it was avidly and selectively taken up by photoreceptor cells. Therefore, free and/or esterified 22:6n3 released by the pigment epithelial cells needs a carrier to transfer it to the final target, the photoreceptor cell. The presence in the interphotoreceptor matrix of proteins (e.g. interphotoreceptor retinoid-binding protein, IRBP) that bind 22:6n3 and other fatty acids suggests that these proteins could be involved in the intercellular transport of these fatty acids.[24]

The involvement of apolipoprotein E (Apo-E) in the transport of 22:6-containing lipids to retinal cells through interaction with specific receptors has recently been evaluated.[25] Apo-E, synthesized and secreted by hepatic tissue as a constituent of plasma lipoproteins (e.g. VLDL and HDL), serves to increase the efficiency of LDL receptor-lipoprotein interactions, facilitating the subsequent delivery of cholesterol and other lipids transported through the plasma to various tissues.[26] Apo-E is also produced by extrahepatic tissues to facilitate and direct cholesterol (and phospholipid) movement among cells. The nervous system is second only to liver in Apo-E production.[27] Astrocytes and Müller cells of the retina synthesize and release Apo-E, suggesting that other cells (e.g. neurons and photoreceptors) could be targets for the lipids associated with these Apo-E molecules. It was recently demonstrated that during nervous tissue repair and regeneration Apo-E plays a crucial role in the transport of cholesterol required by these cells for membrane synthesis.[28]

Retinas from 10-day old mouse pups were used to study Apo-E binding.[25] At this stage of development, photoreceptor cells are actively synthesizing new outer segment disc membranes enriched in 22:6-phospholipids and cholesterol.[29] These retinas, therefore, depend upon an active and efficient delivery of both 22:6n3 and cholesterol molecules. Photoreceptor cells isolated from retinas previously incubated with ^{125}I-Apo-E/dimyristoyl phosphatidylcholine (DMPC) exhibited specific and saturable binding and internalization of the labeled precursor. Subsequent studies with [3]H-22:6-phospholipids assembled into the Apo-E/DMPC discs revealed that [3]H-22:6-phospholipids were delivered with high selectivity to the photoreceptor cells. Therefore the presence of this Apo-E receptor-mediated mechanism assures the efficient phospholipid and/or cholesterol delivery to photoreceptors for membrane biogenesis.

IV. EARLY AND LONG-TERM FATE OF [3]H-22:6n3 IN RETINAL CELLS: BIOCHEMICAL AND AUTORADIOGRAPHIC ANALYSIS

The metabolism and cellular distribution of [3]H-22:6 among retinal cells were studied using two experimental approaches: a) *in vitro* short-term incubations (up to 6 h) of frog, monkey, and human retinas, and b) *in vivo* studies in frogs monitoring the fate of systemically injected [3]H-22:6n3.

Short-term *in vitro* studies with isolated frog retinas revealed by autoradiography that tritium appeared in the neural retina, and reached a concentration plateau after only 1 h, while photoreceptors immediately began to take up label, and continued to accumulate 22:6-phospholipids throughout the 6 h of incubations.[23,30] Of all [3]H-22:6 label incorporated into retinal lipids, 92% was concentrated in the photoreceptors while 8% was dispersed throughout the neural retina. Biochemical data, therefore, reflect the fate of [3]H-22:6 predominantly within photoreceptors. Tri-

and diacylglycerols accounted for 7% of the label and phospholipids for 88%, with approximately equal distribution among species of phosphatidylinositol (PI), phosphatidylcholine (PC), and phosphatidylethanolamine (PE). Within 30 min, label was detected in the myoid region of photoreceptors (where phospholipid synthesis occurs), and migrated proximally toward the synaptic terminal and distally into the ellipsoid region, where it continued to accumulate throughout the incubations. Density measurements of photoreceptor ellipsoids showed that the accumulated label in 435-rods was more than 3 times that in the 502-rods. Interestingly, cone ellipsoids did not label in the frog. However, nearby cone oil droplets sequestered label avidly.

Similar *in vitro* autoradiographic studies with human retinal biopsy tissue and monkey retinas also indicated that the majority of the label accumulated within photoreceptors (58% and 79%, respectively), while the neural retina labeled uniformly, with increased label in the synaptic regions.[22] In both cases, 80% of the total phospholipid labeling was recovered in PC and PE. Of interest is the fact that in monkey retinas incubated for 1 h there was seen, as in poikilotherm retinas, an initial, high labeling of PI (20%) and phosphatidic acid (PA, 11%).

After 1 or 4 h of incubation, human outer segments had diffusely labeled throughout their lengths, but, unlike frog retina, inner segments of both rods and cones became well labeled. In over-exposed material, the ellipsoid regions of both cell types increased their label density equally, and photoreceptor synaptic terminals were labeled.

When frogs were injected *in vivo* with ^{3}H-22:6n3 the retina rapidly accumulated label.[21] Autoradiography showed that rod photoreceptor cells took up the majority of the label. Both inner and outer segments labeled diffusely over their entire lengths, while outer segments continued to accumulate additional label in the region of disc morphogenesis. This dense region of accumulation expanded apically until it reached the tip of the photoreceptor, filling the outer segment.

Parallel experiments using ^{3}H-leucine as a protein marker demonstrated that the leucine band and the leading edge of the dense 22:6n3 label migrated apically at the same rate, arriving at the tip of the rod cell in 28 days.[21] This suggests that some labeled 22:6-rich lipid species were associated with opsin. In fact, close association of PC- and PS-containing dipolyunsaturated species with rhodopsin isolated from bovine retinas has been reported.[31] Since no ^{3}H-22:6n3 was detected in lipid-free protein residue of retina, the association of 22:6-containing phospholipids and opsin therefore must be noncovalent.[21] Phagosomes appearing in the pigment epithelium after 28 days retained the dense ^{3}H-22:6n3 label. However, after degradation of phagosomes, label appeared to accumulate in the cytoplasm of the pigment epithelium only diffusely, while heavy label accumulated within the oil droplets of these cells. This suggests that 22:6-containing phospholipids are recycled, either directly or by way of the liver, back to the inner segments of the photoreceptors to be reutilized in membrane biogenesis.[32] The retina has the ability, through day 46, to retain the label in 22:6n3 molecules. Even at 67 days after [3]H-22:6n3 delivery, only very small amounts of tritium appeared in other fatty acids, both within the retina and the liver.[21]

It can be concluded from these autoradiographic and biochemical studies that the photoreceptor cells avidly take up and incorporate 22:6n3 into phospholipids. While much 22:6n3 becomes associated with synaptic regions, even more appears within photoreceptor inner segments. Phospholipids containing 22:6n3 are subsequently incorporated into newly formed disc membranes in a manner that strongly suggests an association with opsin and, therefore, an active role in the visual process. The preferential uptake of 22:6n3 by rod photoreceptors in frogs, and by both rod and cone primate photoreceptors,[21-23,30] implies an important and unique cell-specific function for 22:6n3 in the retina.

V. RETINAL DEGENERATIONS

The continual and efficient supply of 22:6n3 through the liver to the retina is essential for retinal function.[19] This fatty acid is synthesized in the liver from dietary 18:3n3,[20] secreted as 22:6-containing lipoproteins, selectively taken up by retinal pigment epithelial cells, and finally, associated with a carrier system that facilitates delivery of 22:6n3 to its ultimate target, the photoreceptor cells. Although the handling of 22:6n3 is a multi-step process, this mechanism functions efficiently to provide 22:6n3 for the maintenance and synthesis of new membranes in photoreceptor cells and synaptic terminals. Obviously, an impairment at any of the trafficking steps from 18:3n3 to 22:6n3 could result in a reduced delivery of 22:6n3 and compromise retinal structure and function. In fact, rats[18] and monkeys[14-17] deprived of dietary 18:3n3 developed abnormal electroretinograms and decreased visual acuity. In the primate model, fatty acid deprivation occurred during the perinatal period, when there are large requirements for 22:6n3 by the retina. The essential role that 22:6n3 plays in the functioning of photoreceptor membranes is also emphasized by the ability of the system to preserve this fatty acid, even after long periods of 18:3n3 deficiency.[3,33,34] During the daily shedding of rod outer segment tips, the 22:6n3 present in phagocytosed membranes[21] may be recycled from the retinal pigment epithelium back to the photoreceptor cell inner segments.[24,32] Finally, the retina can elongate and desaturate 18:2n6 to 22:5n6[17] so that retinal cells might partially overcome long periods of 18:3n3, and therefore 22:6n3, deprivation and depletion.

In patients with Usher's syndrome (an autosomal recessive disease, retinitis pigmentosa), a decreased content of 22:6n3 in plasma was observed.[35-37] This implies that perturbations of the 22:6n3 metabolic pathways outside the affected organ could arise as a consequence of the genetic defect, perhaps affecting a putative retina-to-liver signal evoking delivery of 22:6n3 by the liver.[20] Regardless of the cause, a decreased supply of 22:6n3 to the eye may contribute to retinal dysfunction and, perhaps, to photoreceptor cell degeneration, if the interruption is prolonged.

VI. REDUCED CONTENT OF POLYUNSATURATED FATTY ACID-CONTAINING PHOSPHOLIPIDS AND ALTERED 22:6n3 METABOLISM IN THE DEVELOPING *rd* MOUSE RETINA

Studies of membrane lipid metabolism in photoreceptor cells isolated from control and *rd* mice during early postnatal development showed the course of enrichment in 22:6n3 and allowed the exploration of possible early alterations in the mutant. The lipid content and fatty acid composition of whole retina during development showed a constant increase for both control and *rd* mice up to 10 days after birth.[38] Differences between the two groups became apparent within 10 to 15 days, when photoreceptor cell outer segments started to develop.[39] A further accumulation of lipids enriched in 22:6n3 was observed at this time in control but not in *rd* mice. Normal mice maintained their 22:6n3 content from day 10 through day 30, when photoreceptor maturation was completed. The increase in fatty acids other than 22:6n3 (e.g. 18:0 and 20:4n6) was shifted to a later time in the retinal development of the *rd* mouse. This increase, similar to the 10-15-day increase in controls, occurred in *rd* mice between 20 and 25 days.[38]

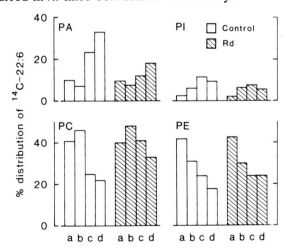

Figure 1   Percentage distribution of docosahexaenoic acid incorporated into retinal phospholipids *in vitro*. Values are the mean for 3-6 independent samples, which agree within 10%. Retinas were incubated with ^{14}C-22:6n3 (200 μM final concentration) for 5 min at 37 °C. Data were replotted from reference 38. Ages of pups: a, 3 days; b, 8-9 days; c, 14-15 days; d, 22-30 days.

In vitro incubation of retinas with [14]C-22:6n3 demonstrated a preferential labeling of PC and PE at 3 and 9 days (Figure 1). Within 10-14 days a shift toward PA-PI labeling concomitant with a decreased labeling of other phospholipids was observed. This implies that, at the time of outer segment development, stimulation of 22:6-PI synthesis occurs, likely through a *de novo* pathway. Recently, *in vitro* incubations of adult human, monkey, and frog retinas with [3]H-22:6n3 have shown high initial labeling of PI.[22,23] These observations suggest the involvement of 22:6-PI in specific retinal cell functions correlated during development with the formation of photoreceptor outer segments.

In retinas of *rd* mice, the shift toward PA-PI labeling at 15 days was less pronounced than in control mice, and the profile of lipid labeling remained similar to that seen at 8-9 days (Figure 1). While PC had the lowest endogenous content of 22:6n3 in the *rd* retina at 30 days, this phospholipid showed the highest labeling with [14]C-22:6n3 when it was offered to the tissue *in vitro*. In these experiments high concentrations (200 μM) of 22:6n3 were added to the incubation medium likely leading to free diffusion of the fatty acid through membranes, and preventing the

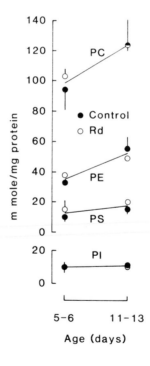

Figure 2   **Phospholipid content of photoreceptor cells dissociated from retinas of control and *rd* mice. Values are the average ± S.D. of at least 4 individual determinations. Data were replotted from reference 39.**

detection of differences in uptake by a carrier-mediated mechanism. However, the results suggest that *if* 22:6n3 can get into the photoreceptor cells, the enzymatic mechanisms involved in the conversion to 22:6-CoA, and subsequent esterification into phospholipids, are not impaired in *rd* mouse retinas.

Changes in the polyunsaturated fatty acid content of phospholipids became apparent in isolated photoreceptor cells from 5-6- and 11-13-day-old mouse pups, prior to and at the time when degeneration was histologically detected.[40] Control and *rd* mouse whole retinas showed no differences in the accumulation of phospholipids in photoreceptor cells between 5 and 11-13 days of age (Figure 2). However, fatty acid analysis showed a significant decrease in polyunsaturated fatty acids, which was compensated by an increase of saturated and monoenoic fatty acids in *rd* retinal phospholipids.[39] Phosphatidylethanolamine from retinas of 5-6-day-old *rd* mice showed a lower content of 20:3n6 and 22:5n6 (Figure 3). By 11-13 days, a proportionally higher content of 18:2n6 and a lower content of 20:3n6, 22:5n6, and 22:6n3 were observed. In PC, on the other hand, the n3 family was more affected, both at 5-6 days and 11-13 days after birth (Figure 4). The 22:6n3 content was decreased by 30% and 22:5n3 to undetectable levels.

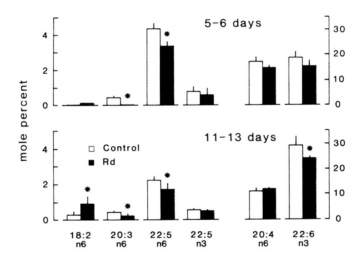

Figure 3   Polyunsaturated fatty acids of phosphatidylethanolamine in dissociated photoreceptor cells from retinas of control and *rd* mice. Values expressed as mole percent ± S.D. were recalculated from reference 39. Asterisk denotes differences from control values that are statistically significant (p < 0.05).

It is interesting that the elongation and desaturation products of 18:2n6 appear, in PC, to compensate, at least in part, for the dramatic reduction in 22:6n3 content. Lowered amounts of 22:6n3 in retinal lipids of *rd* mice are to be expected, since the 22:6-phospholipid-enriched rod outer segments fail to develop. However, alterations in the content of n6 fatty acids suggest that 22:6n3 availability, transport, and/or receptor-mediated uptake may also be impaired in *rd* mice. A higher uptake of 18:2n6 (accumulated in PE) and its conversion to 22:5n6 may be an inherent compensatory mechanism in retinal cells, which operates during times of dietary stress to maintain retinal function until additional n3 fatty acids can be obtained. This, coupled with high retention and recycling of existing 22:6n3 molecules, could represent the normal condition. The *rd* retina, on the other hand, may have a deficient delivery and/or uptake mechanism for 22:6n3 in photoreceptor cells. An inefficient mechanism of supply of phospholipids for photoreceptor membrane synthesis may result in damage to and degeneration of photoreceptors. These ideas are experimentally testable, and the impairments in the handling of 22:6n3 may play an important role in the pathogenesis of retinal degenerative disorders.

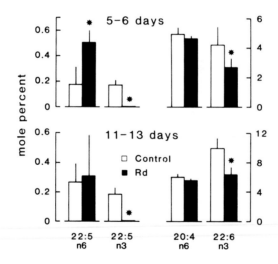

Figure 4 **Polyunsaturated fatty acids of phosphatidylcholine in dissociated photoreceptor cells from retinas of control and *rd* mice. Values expressed as mole percent ± S.D. were recalculated from reference 39. Asterisk denotes differences from control values that are statistically significant (p < 0.05).**

ACKNOWLEDGMENTS

This work was supported in part by United States Public Health Service Grant EY04428 from the National Eye Institute, National Institutes of Health, Bethesda, Maryland, and the support to the Ernest C. and Yvette C. Villere Chair for Retinal Degeneration at the Eye, Ear, Nose and Throat Hospital, New Orleans, Louisiana.

REFERENCES

1.   Bazan, N.G., Birkle, D.L., and Reddy, T.S., Docosahexaenoic acid (22:6,n3) is metabolized to lipoxygenase reaction products in the retina. *Biochem. Biophys. Res. Commun.* 125, 741, 1984.

2.   Aveldaño de Caldironi, M.I., and Bazan, N.G., Composition and biosynthesis of molecular species of retina phosphoglycerides. *Neurochem. Int.* 1, 381, 1980.

3.   Fliesler, S.J., and Anderson, R.E., Chemistry and metabolism of lipids in the vertebrate retina. *Prog. Lipid Res.* 22, 79, 1983.

4.   Wiegand, R.D., and Anderson, R.E., Phospholipid molecular species of frog rod outer segment membranes. *Exp. Eye Res.* 37, 159, 1983.

5.   Bazan, N.G., Reddy, T.S., Bazan, H.E.P., and Birkle, D.L., Metabolism of arachidonic and docosahexaenoic acids in the retina. *Prog. Lipid Res.*, 25, 595, 1986.

6.   Aveldaño de Caldironi, M.I., and Bazan, N.G., Acyl groups, molecular species, and labeling by ^{14}C-glycerol and ^{3}H-arachidonic acid of vertebrate retina glycerolipids. *Adv. Exp. Med. Biol.*, 83, 397, 1977.

7.   Miljanich, G.P., Sklar, L.A., White, D.L., and Dratz, E.A., Disaturated dipolyunsaturated phospholipids in the bovine retinal rod outer segment disk membrane. *Biochim. Biophys. Acta*, 55, 294, 1979.

8.   Aveldaño, M.I., and Bazan, N.G., Molecular species of phosphatidylcholine, -ethanolamine, -serine, and -inositol in microsomal and photoreceptor membranes of bovine retina. *J. Lipid Res.*, 24, 620, 1983.

9.   Aveldaño, M.I., Dipolyunsaturated species of retinal phospholipids and their fatty acids, in *Biomembranes and Nutrition*, Lèger, C.L., and Béreziat, G., Eds., Editions INSERM, Paris, 1989, 87.

10.   Louie, K., Wiegand, R.D., and Anderson, R.E., Docosahexaenoate-containing molecular species of glycerophospholipids from frog retinal rod outer segments show different rates of biosynthesis and turnover. *Biochemistry,* 27, 9014, 1988.

11.   Rotstein, N.P., and Aveldaño, M.I., Labeling of phosphatidylcholines of retina subcellular fractions by [1-^{14}C]eicosatetraenoate (20:4 (n-6)), docosapentaenoate (22:5 (n-3)), and docosahexaenoate (22:6 (n-3)). *Biochim. Biophys. Acta,* 921, 235, 1987.

12.   Aveldaño, M.I., A novel group of very long chain polyenoic fatty acids in dipolyunsaturated phosphatidylcholines from vertebrate retina. *J. Biol. Chem.,* 262, 1172, 1987.

13.   Dratz, E.A., and Deese, A.J., The role of docosahexaenoic acid (22:6 omega-3) in biological membranes: examples from photoreceptors and model membrane bilayers, in *Health Effects of Polyunsaturated Fatty Acids in Seafood,* Simopoulos, A.P., Kifer, R., and Martin, R.E., Eds., Academic Press, New York, 1986, 319.

14.   Neuringer, M., and Connor, W.E., n3 fatty acids in the brain and retina: evidence for their essentiality. *Nutrition Rev.,* 44, 285, 1986.

15.   Neuringer, M., Connor, W.E., Van Petten, C., and Barstad, L., Dietary omega-3 fatty acid deficiency and visual loss in infant rhesus monkeys. *J. Clin. Invest.,* 73, 272, 1984.

16.   Neuringer, M., Connor, W.E., Daigle, D., and Barstad L., Electroretinogram abnormalities in young infant rhesus monkeys deprived of omega-3 fatty acids during gestation and postnatal development or only postnatally. *Suppl. Invest. Ophthalmol. Vis. Sci.,* 29, 145, 1988.

17.   Neuringer, M., Connor, W.E., Lin, D.S., Barstad, L., and Luck, S., Biochemical and functional effects of prenatal and postnatal ω3 fatty acid deficiency on retina and brain in rhesus monkeys. *Proc. Nat. Acad. Sci. USA,* 83, 4021, 1986.

18.   Wheeler, T.G., Benolken, R.M., and Anderson, R.E., Visual membranes: specificity of fatty acid precursors for the electrical response to illumination. *Science,* 188, 1312, 1975.

19.　Bazan, N.G., Birkle, D.L., and Reddy, T.S., Biochemical and nutritional aspects of the metabolism of polyunsaturated fatty acids and phospholipids in experimental models of retinal degeneration, in *Retinal Degeneration: Experimental and Clinical Studies,* LaVail, M.M., Anderson, R.E., and Hollyfield, J., Eds., Alan R. Liss, Inc., 1985, 159.

20.　Scott, B.L., and Bazan, N.G., Membrane docosahexaenoate is supplied to the developing brain and retina by the liver. *Proc. Nat. Acad. Sci. USA*, 86, 2903, 1989.

21.　Gordon, W.C., and Bazan, N.G., Docosahexaenoic acid utilization during rod photoreceptor cell renewal. *J. Neurosci.*, 10, 2190, 1990.

22.　Rodriguez de Turco, E.B., Gordon, W.C., Peyman, G.A., and Bazan, N.G., Preferential uptake and metabolism of docosahexaenoic acid in membrane phospholipids from rod and cone photoreceptor cells of human and monkey retinas. *J. Neurosci. Res.*, 27, 522, 1990.

23.　Rodriguez de Turco, E.B., Gordon, W.C., and Bazan, N.G., Rapid and selective uptake, metabolism, and differential distribution of docosahexaenoic acid among rod and cone photoreceptor cells in the frog retina. Submitted.

24.　Bazan, N.G., Reddy, T.S., Redmond, T.M., Wiggert, B., and Chader, G.J., Endogenous fatty acids are covalently and noncovalently bound to interphotoreceptor retinoid-binding protein in the monkey retina. *J. Biol. Chem.*, 260, 13677, 1985.

25.　Bazan, N.G., and Cai, F., Internalization of apolipoprotein E (Apo-E) in rod photoreceptor cells by a low density lipoprotein receptor. *Suppl. Invest. Ophthalmol. Vis. Sci.*, 31, 471, 1990.

26.　Mahley, R.W., Innerarity, T.L., Rall, S.C., and Weisgraber, K.H., Plasma lipoproteins: Apolipoprotein structure and function. *J. Lipid Res.*, 25, 1277, 1984.

27.　Elshourbagy, N.A., Liao, W.S., Mahley, R.W., and Taylor, J.M., Apolipoprotein E mRNA is abundant in the brain and adrenals, as well as in the liver, and is present in other peripheral tissues of rats and marmosets. *Proc. Nat. Acad. Sci. USA,* 82, 203, 1985.

28.   Boyles, J.K., Zoellner, G.D., Anderson, L.J., Kosik, L.M., Pitas, R.E., Weisgraber, K.H., Hui, D.Y., Mahley, R.W., Gebicke-Haerter, P.J., Ignatius, M.J., and Shooter, E.M., A role for apolipoprotein E, apolipoprotein A-1, and low-density lipoprotein receptors, in cholesterol transport during regeneration and remyelination of the rat sciatic nerve. *J. Clin. Invest.*, 83, 1013, 1989.

29.   Boesze-Battaglia, K., Hennessey, T., and Albert, A., Cholesterol heterogeneity in bovine rod outer segment disk membranes. *J. Biol, Chem.*, 264, 8151, 1989.

30.   Gordon, W.C., and Bazan, N.G., Rhodopsin and some docosahexaenoyl (22:6-phospholipids are jointly displaced during rod outer segment renewal. *Suppl. Invest. Ophthalmol. Vis. Sci.*, 31, 284, 1990.

31.   Aveldaño, M.I., Phospholipid species containing long and very long polyenoic fatty acids remain with rhodopsin after hexane extraction of photoreceptor membranes. *Biochemistry*, 27, 1229, 1988.

32.   Bazan, N.G., Supply of n3 polyunsaturated fatty acids and their significance in the central nervous system, in *Nutrition and the Brain*, Vol. 8, Wurtman, R.J. and Wurtman, J.J., Eds., Raven Press, New York, 1990, 1.

33.   Tinoco, J., Dietary requirements and functions of α-linolenic acid in animals. *Prog. Lipid Res.*, 21, 1, 1982.

34.   Bazan, N.G., Reddy, T.S., Retina, in *Handbook of Neurochemistry*, Vol 8, Lajtha, A., Ed., Plenum Press, New York, 1985, 507.

35.   Anderson, R.E., Maude, M.B., Lewis, R.A., Newsome, D.A., and Fishman, G.A., Abnormal plasma levels of polyunsaturated fatty acid in autosomal dominant retinitis pigmentosa. *Exp. Eye Res.*, 44, 155, 1987.

36.   Bazan, N.G., Scott, B.L., Reddy, T.S., and Pelias, M.Z., Decreased content of docosahexaenoate and arachidonate in plasma phospholipids in Usher's syndrome. *Biochem. Biophys. Res. Commun.*, 141, 600, 1986.

37.   Converse, C.A., Hammer, H.M., Packard, C.J., and Shepherd, J., Plasma lipid abnormalities in retinitis pigmentosa and related conditions. *Trans. Ophthalmol. Soc. UK*, 103, 508, 1983.

38. Scott, B.L., Reddy, T.S., and Bazan, N.G., Docosahexaenoate metabolism and fatty-acid composition in developing retinas of normal and *rd* mutant mice. *Exp. Eye Res.*, 44, 101, 1987.

39. Scott, B.L., Racz, E., Lolley, R.N., and Bazan, N.G., Developing rod photoreceptors from normal and mutant *rd* mouse retinas: Altered fatty acid composition early in development of the mutant. *J. Neurosci. Res.*, 20, 202, 1988.

40. Blanks, J.C., Adinolfi, A.M., and Lolley, R.N., Photoreceptor degeneration and synaptogenesis in retinal-degenerative (*rd*) mice. *J. Comp. Neurol.*, 156, 95, 1974.

ABNORMALITIES IN cGMP PHOSPHODIESTERASE IN MICE HETEROZYGOUS FOR THE rd GENE

Mary J.Voaden, Ali A.Hussain and Nicholas J.Willmott.
Departments of Visual Science (MJV) and Clinical Ophthalmology,
Institute of Ophthalmology, London WC1H 9QS, UK.

I. CYCLIC GMP AND ITS PHOSPHODIESTERASE IN 'rd' MICE

The abnormal mouse gene, designated as rd, codes for the *beta* subunit of a rod-specific cyclic guanosine monophosphate phosphodiesterase (cGMP PDE) and leads to its malfunction.[1] Consequently, in mice homozygous for the gene (i.e. rd/rd), the normal PDE complex fails to form[2,3] and at least 90% of enzymic activity is lost[4-6] (cf.below). Diminished activity in the presence of a functional guanyl cyclase (GC) leads to the intracellular accumulation of cGMP and rod degeneration.[4] The effect is cell specific and is likely to relate to the fact that the excessive amount of free cGMP will maintain open, both in light and dark, a much higher than normal number of the cGMP-gated, cation channels, present in the rod outer segment (ROS) plasma membrane. In turn, this will lead to unremitting stimulation of the electrogenic Na^+/K^+ ATPase present in the inner limb of the cell,[7,8] and energy balance will be perturbed, potentially disrupting essential processes such as protein synthesis[9] and the visual cycle.

Retinal structure[10,11] and rhodopsin content,[12,13] are normal in adult, heterozygotic (+/rd) mice. However, there are abnormalities in metabolism and function that also arise from defects in cGMP PDE. Thus, the enzyme has a higher Km and, therefore, a lower affinity than normal for cGMP at its active centre[12] and a reduced capacity for cGMP binding at non-catalytic sites.[13] The net results are a reduced turnover rate for cGMP at concentrations below active site saturation (cf. Figure 1) and a 30-40% reduction in the overall endogenous concentration of the nucleotide in +/rd retinas as compared to normal.[12,14] The latter might arise because about 90% of ROS cGMP is bound, principally to non-catalytic binding sites on the PDE, and these determine the total.[7,15]

Although there have been no studies concerning non-catalytic cGMP binding to the rd/rd PDE, Farber and Lolley have reported the Km of the enzyme as normal.[5] Subsequently, however, Lolley, Lee and coworkers have found the purified enzyme to be inactive,[2,3,16] thereby implying that the activity determined in intact tissue was not of the rod PDE. Nevertheless, if current concepts of phototransduction are correct[7,8] (but compare Krapivinsky and coworkers[17]), complete dysfunction is unlikely as a scotopic PIII, albeit greatly reduced in amplitude and of prolonged latency, is present.[18]

Clearly, the rd/rd and +/rd PDE defects must be related and defining the relationship will tell us a great deal about the homozygous versus heterozygous expression of recessive genes. At the same time the more subtle defects in the +/rd retina are likely to provide information concerning normal phototransduction and adaptation, not only as regards the role(s) of non-catalytic binding of cGMP to PDE but also because the

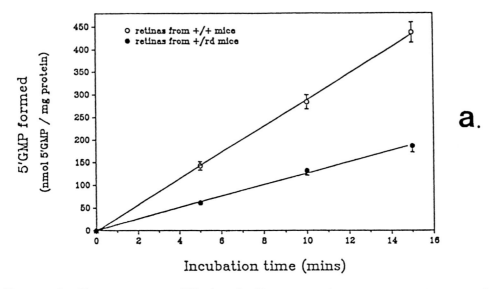

Figure 1. Photoreceptor cGMP phosphodiesterase in +/+ and +/rd retinal homogenates in light. Activity was determined at 37°C, as previously described[12], employing a substrate concentration of 500 µM [8-³H]-cGMP to delineate photoreceptor activity.[4] Points represent the mean of 4 estimations ± S.E.M.[12]

higher Km of the enzyme will lead to an increase in the concentration of <u>free</u> cGMP and, thus, a greater dark current,[7,8] and this, in turn, also perturbs function.

II. FUNCTION IN THE +/rd RETINA

It is predictable that a higher dark current will lead to an increase in the intracellular concentration of calcium in +/rd ROS.[7,8]

Reducing extracellular calcium to about 1.0 nM rapidly activates photoreceptor GC and, in dark-adapted retinas, leads to an increase in ROS cGMP.[19] Consistent with there being more calcium inside +/rd rods, the response of GC to a reduction in extracellular calcium is delayed but is speeded up if the calcium ionophore A23187 is included in the medium (Figure 2).[20]

Calcium via its actions on GC[21,22] and PDE[23,24] and/or rhodopsin kinase[7,25] potentially modulates rod sensitivity, response recovery and light adaptation.[7,8,22] Of these, +/rd retinas are already known to exhibit greater than normal sensitivity at low light intensity[20,26,27] and also delay in the termination of a photoresponse.[20,28] The former might arise from the combination of a greater dark current with a higher concentration of intracellular calcium since, in the presence of the latter, the activity of rhodopsin kinase may be inhibited or that of PDE increased, leading to a greater gain per photon absorbed by rhodopsin. Termination of fast PIII is aided by the reduction in intracellular calcium that normally follows closure of the cGMP-gated channels in the ROS plasma membrane, and the consequent stimulation of GC and, possibly,

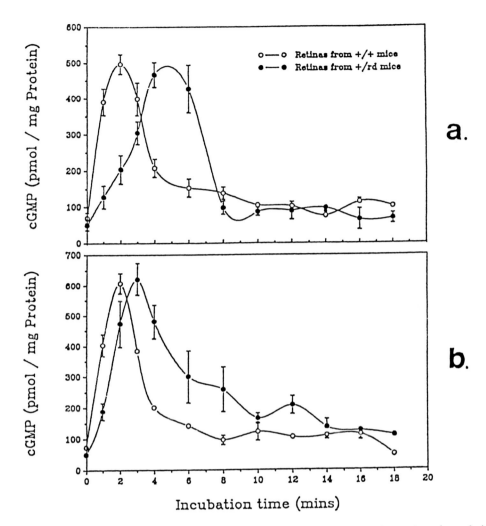

Figure 2. The concentration of cGMP in +/+ and +/rd retinas incubated in calcium depleted media. Dark-adapted retinas were incubated at 37°C, from zero time, in Eagle's MEM without calcium salts and supplemented (a) with 3.0 mM EGTA and (b) with 3.0 mM EGTA and 10.0 μM of the cation ionophore A23187. Cyclic GMP was assayed as described previously[12] and each point represents the mean of at least 4 estimations.[20] The response in +/rd retinas is of normal magnitude but is delayed. It is speeded up when A23187 is included in the medium.

rhodopsin kinase. Thus, if the resting level of calcium in +/rd retinas is higher than normal, termination of the response will be delayed. Equally, it is possible that the abnormality in cGMP binding is contributing to the delay by modifying interaction between the PDE and the mechanisms effecting its shutdown. The latter are incompletely understood. However, we have preliminary evidence suggesting that deactivation is normal.

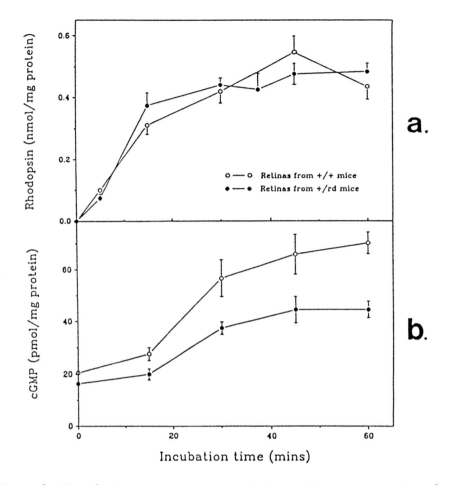

Figure 3. Visual pigment regeneration (a) and the concentration of cGMP (b) in retinas of +/+ and +/rd mice, incubated with 9- and 11-cis retinal. Mixed isomers of retinal (0.05 mg/ml), prepared by photoisomerization of the all-trans form, were encapsulated in phosphatidyl choline liposomes and applied to previously-bleached retinas at zero time as described previously.[13,29] Incubations were then continued in the dark at 37°C. Each point represents the mean ± S.E.M. of at least 5 estimations.[13]

The rod PDE is greatly activated by light[7,8] and the increased turnover persists in bleached tissue. Deactivation occurs in an isolated retina if visual pigment is regenerated with exogenously-applied 9- or 11-cis retinal.[29] We have found that the time course of the consequent increase in intracellular cGMP is the same in +/+ and +/rd retinas (Figure 3), suggesting that the underlying PDE deactivation is normal in the +/rd retina in spite of the differential in cGMP binding - shown in Figure 3 by the lower than normal concentration of cGMP in the +/rd rods throughout the study.[13]

The photoresponse time-to-peak is also increased in +/rd retinas.[28] We have confirmed this and have found that at -4.0 log units of stimulus light intensity, the normal +/+ PIII (as isolated with 10 mM sodium glutamate) peaks at 125 $\pm$ 7 msec (S.E.M., n=18) and the +/rd PIII at 150 $\pm$ 7 (n=15).[20] Several factors might contribute to the slower implicit time but if the rising phase is due to cGMP hydrolysis[7,8] rather than transducin binding to the cGMP-gated channels,[17] then reduced affinity of PDE for its substrate in +/rd ROS could underly the phenomenon.

It is likely that the +/rd retina will prove to be a highly informative 'model' not only for investigation of the determinants of the normal photoresponse waveform but also for several other aspects of phototransduction and adaptation.

REFERENCES
1. Bowes, C., Tiansen, L., Danciger, M., Baxter, L.C., Applebury, M.L. and Farber, D.B. Retinal degeneration in the rd mouse is caused by a defect in the β subunit of rod cGMP-phosphodiesterase, *Nature* 347, 677, 1990.
2. Lee, R.H., Lieberman, B.S., Hurwitz, R.L. and Lolley, R.N. Phosphodiesterase-probes show distinct defects in rd mice and Irish setter dog disorders, *Invest. Ophthalmol. Vis. Sci.* 26, 1569, 1985.
3. Lee, R.H., Navon, S.E., Brown, B.M., Fung, B.K.-K. and Lolley, R.N. Characterization of a phosphodiesterase-immunoreactive polypeptide from rod photoreceptors of developing rd mouse retinas, *Invest. Ophthalmol. Vis. Sci.* 29, 1021, 1988.
4. Farber, D.B. and Lolley, R.N. Enzymic basis for cGMP accumulation in degenerative photoreceptor cells of mouse retina, *J. Cyclic Nucleotide Res.* 2, 139, 1976.
5. Farber, D.B. and Lolley, R.N. Light-induced reduction in cyclic GMP of retinal photoreceptor cells *in vivo*: abnormalities in the degenerative diseases of RCS rats and rd mice, *J. Neurochem.* 28, 1089, 1977.
6. Fletcher, R.T., Sanyal, S., Krishna, G., Aguirre, G. and Chader, G.J. Genetic expression of cyclic GMP phosphodiesterase activity defines abnormal photoreceptor differentiation in neurological mutants of inherited retinal degeneration, *J. Neurochem.* 46, 1240, 1986.
7. Pugh, E.N. and Cobbs, W.H. Visual transduction in vertebrate rods and cones: a tale of two transmitters, calcium and cyclic GMP, *Vision Res.* 26, 1613, 1986.
8. Yau, K.-W. and Baylor, yclic GMP-activated conductance of retinal photoreceptor cells, *A. Rev. Neurosci.* 12, 289, 1989.
9. Ulshafer, R.J. and Hollyfield, J.G. Cyclic nucleotides alter protein synthesis in human and baboon retinas, in *The Structure of the Eye*, Hollyfield, J.G. Ed., Elsevier Biomedical, Amsterdam, 1982. 115.
10. Noell, W.K. Differentiation, metabolic organisation and viability of the visual cell, *Archs. Ophthalmol.* 60, 702, 1958.
11. Carter-Dawson, L., LaVail, M. and Sidman, R. Differential effect of the rd mutation on rods and cones in the mouse retina, *Invest. Ophthalmol. Vis. Sci.* 17, 489, 1978.
12. Doshi, M., Voaden, M.J. and Arden, G.B. Cyclic GMP in the retinas of normal mice and those heterozygous for early onset photoreceptor dystrophy, *Expl. Eye Res.* 41, 61, 1985.
13. Voaden, M.J. and Willmott, N.J. Evidence for reduced binding of cyclic GMP to cyclic GMP phosphodiesterase in photoreceptors of

mice heterozygous for the rd gene, *Current Eye Res.* 9, 643, 1990.

14. Ferrendelli, J.A. and Cohen, A.I. The effects of light and dark adaptation on the levels of cyclic nucleotides in retinas of mice heterozygous for a gene for photoreceptor retinal dystrophy, *Biochem. Biophys. Res. Commun.* 73, 421, 1976.

15. Yamazaki, A., Sen, I., Bitensky, M.W., Casnellie, J.E. and Greengard, P. Cyclic GMP-specific, high-affinity, non-catalytic binding sites on light-activated phosphodiesterase, *J. Biol. Chem.* 255, 11619, 1980.

16 Lolley, R.N., Navon, S.E., Fung, B.K.-K and Lee, R.H. Inherited disorders of rd mice and affected Irish setter dogs: evaluation of transducin and cGMP-phosphodiesterase, in *Degenerative Retinal Disorders: Clinical and Laboratory Investigations*, Hollyfield, J.G., Anderson, R.E. and LaVail, M.M., Eds., Alan R. Liss, New York, 1987. 269.

17. Krapivinsky, G.B., Filatov, G.N., Filatova, E.A., Lyubarsky, A.L. and Fesenko, E.E. Regulation of cGMP-dependent conductance in cytoplasmic membrane of rod outer segments by transducin, *FEBS Letters* 247, 435, 1989.

18. Noell, W.K. Aspects of experimental and hereditary retinal degeneration, in *Biochemistry of the Retina*, Graymore, C.N., Ed., Academic Press, New York, 1965. 51.

19. Cohen, A.I., Hall, A.I. and Ferrendelli, J.A. Calcium and cyclic nucleotide regulation in incubated mouse retinas, *J. Gen. Physiol.* 71, 595, 1978.

20. Hussain, A.A., Willmott, N.J., and Voaden, M.J. Cyclic GMP, calcium and photoreceptor sensitivity in mice heterozygous for the rod dystrophy gene designated 'rd', *Vision Res.* 1991, in press.

21. Lolley, R.N. and Racz, E. Calcium modulation of GMP synthesis in rat visual cells, *Vision Res.* 22, 1481, 1982.

22. Koch, W.-H. and Stryer, L. Highly cooperative feedback control of retinal rod guanylate cyclase by calcium ions, *Nature* 334, 64, 1988.

23. Robinson, P.R., Kawamura, S., Abramson, B. and Bownds, M.D. Control of the cyclic GMP phosphodiesterase of frog photoreceptor membranes, *J. Gen. Physiol.* 76, 631, 1980.

24. Detwiler, P.B. and Rispoli, G. Phototransduction in detached rod outer segments: calcium control of the cGMP economy, *Invest. Ophthalmol. Vis. Sci. (Suppl.)* 30, 162, 1989.

25. Wagner, R., Ryba, N. and Uhl, R. Calcium regulates the rate of rhodopsin disactivation and primary amplification step in visual transduction, *FEBS Letters* 242, 249, 1989.

26. Low, J.C. The corneal ERG of the heterozygous retinal degeneration mouse, *Von Graefe's Arch. Ophthal.* 225, 413, 1987.

27. Voaden, M.J., Willmott, N.J., Hussain, A.A. and Al-Mahdawi, S. Functional and biochemical abnormalities in the retinas of mice heterozygous for the rd gene, in *Inherited and Environmentally Induced Retinal Degenerations*, LaVail, M.M., Anderson, R.E. and Hollyfield, J.G., Eds., Alan R. Lork, 1989.183.

28. Arden, G.B. and Low, J.C. Altered kinetics of the photoresponse from retinas of mice heterozygous for the retinal degeneration gene, *J. Physiol.* 308, 80P,1980.

29. Huang, J.C., Voaden, M.J. and Marshall, J. Survival of structure and function in postmortem rat and human retinas: rhodopsin regeneration, cGMP and the ERG, *Current Eye Res.* 9, 151, 1990.

THE FLUOROPHORES OF THE RCS RAT RETINA AND IMPLICATIONS FOR RETINAL DEGENERATION

Graig E. Eldred

University of Missouri-Columbia
Department of Ophthalmology
Columbia, MO, 65212
U.S.A.

With advanced age, the retinal pigment epithelium (RPE) becomes packed with a large number of membrane-bound pigment granules (i.e., lipofuscin granules or age pigments).[1-2] The age-related accumulation of these granules has long been suspected to play some critical role in the etiology of age-related retinal dysfunctions.[3-6] A characteristic feature of these granules is that they emit a golden yellow autofluorescence when viewed under 366 nm illumination.[2] Many studies have been undertaken to try to identify the chemical composition of the granules,[7-9] but protein and lipid analyses reveal little as to why the granules accumulate, or as to what the nature of the fluorophores that give the granules their characteristic emission properties might be. When the fluorescent compounds are identified, a much better understanding of both the chemical mechanism(s) underlying lipofuscin granule accumulation, and the role that lipofuscin granules might play in age-related retinal dystrophies will be gained.

The goals of the present paper are: 1) to briefly describe how these fluorescent compounds are theorized to play a role in age-related macular degeneration (AMD), 2) to review the characteristics of the isolated human RPE lipofuscin fluorophores, 3) to demonstrate that several animal models have proven to be valuable in yielding potentially useful information on the mechanisms of formation of these fluorophores, 4) to present the spectral characteristics and tentative categorical identification of one of the most prominent fluorophores of the human RPE lipofuscin, and 5) to raise some new questions which have arisen as a result of these investigations.

I. WORKING HYPOTHESIS OF AGE-RELATED MACULAR DEGENERATION

AMD is one of the leading causes of blindness in the elderly.[10-11] Little is known of the cell biology of this disease. Correlations of disease occurrence with ocular pigmentation,[12] life and occupational histories of light exposure,[13-14] dietary zinc[15] and plasticizer[16] levels, etc., have led to a variety of ideas as to what factors might influence the onset of this disease. Of these hypotheses, the most widely accepted and investigated one is outlined briefly below. It is this hypothesis that serves as the basis for our interest in the fluorophores that accumulate with age in the RPE.

The microenvironment of the photoreceptor outer segments has three component features that could predispose the retina to potentially damaging chemical reactions: light, oxygen, and a rich supply of polyunsaturated fatty acids in the form of 22:6 n-3 (i.e., docosahexaenoic acid).[17] Under these conditions, a variety of photochemical and/or oxidative processes can stimulate free radical reactions within the photoreceptor outer segments which ultimately result in the formation of "damaged" or chemically modified molecular membrane components. Some of these components are thought to be rendered fluorescent as a result of this damage.[18]

As the tips of the photoreceptor outer segments are shed and phagocytosed by the RPE,[19] the normal components (lipids, proteins, vitamins, etc.) are enzymatically digested, removed and reprocessed. The modified molecules, however, are believed to be indigestable and over time start to accumulate within the lysosomal system of the RPE cells.[4] At the same time, other cellular components, including melanin, are turned over in the process of autophagy[2,20] and any similarly damaged components of these organelles enter the pool of residual indigestible materials within the lysosomal compartment. Over years of time, lysosomal residual bodies accumulate as lipofuscin and melanolipofuscin granules (age pigments), and come to fill the RPE cell.[21]

At some point, lipofuscin-packed cells are believed to attempt to relieve themselves of some of their excess intracellular burden by shedding dollops of cytoplasm basally in a process termed apoptosis.[22] The RPE-derived material cannot pass through Bruch's membrane so it starts to accumulate as local thickenings. The debris can serve as binding sites for other extraneous material and as loci for calcification. Eventually the debris deposits manifest themselves as wart-like humps called drusen. Drusen are one of the clinically recognizable hallmarks of age-related macular degeneration.[23,24]

The drusen and localized thickenings of Bruch's membrane are believed to impair nutrient and metabolite exchange between the retina and the choriocapillaris. As this starvation becomes acute, it is believed that a putative angiogenesis factor is produced by the retina which serves to promote new vessel growth,[25-26] especially in the areas of so-called "soft drusen".[27] This marks the onset of the potentially blinding neovascularization process. At this point clinical intervention is required to halt new vessel growth via laser ablation.[28]

The above is only a working hypothesis. Many of the specific details are currently being investigated in numerous laboratories. Our laboratory has been addressing questions related to the "damaged" molecules which accumulate in the RPE. What are they? How are they formed? Can they be removed or manipulated?

II. HUMAN RPE LIPOFUSCIN FLUOROPHORES

Human RPE lipofuscin granules can be isolated by discontinuous density sucrose gradient centrifugation.[29] Most, if not all, of the fluorescent components can be extracted by chloroform:methanol extraction procedures. We developed a solvent system for the separation of the fluorophores using thin-layer chromatography. A variety of autofluorescent molecules that range in fluorescence from green-emitting to orange-emitting have been isolated.[30] Two of the bands co-migrate with retinyl palmitate and free retinol standards,[31] and are therefore believed to represent unresolved retinyl esters and free vitamin A derivatives. The remaining fluorescent compounds remain unidentified.

As a starting point, our attention has focussed on one of the most prominent well-resolved orange-emitting fluorophores (i.e., from Fraction VIII).[30] In trying to identify this fluorophore, both animal studies and analytical studies have been pursued.

III. A SEARCH FOR ANIMAL MODELS FOR LIPOFUSCIN FLUOROPHORES

Working with Dr. Martin Katz, several animal models for autofluorescent pigment inclusions have been investigated, including vitamin E deficiency pigments,[32] Batten's disease pigments (the so-called ceroid lipofuscinosis pigments),[33] Best's disease pigment,[34] and in vitro lipid oxidation products.[35] None of these sources of fluorescent pigments proved comparable to the human RPE age pigment fluorophores based on the criteria of extractability, chromatographic mobilities, and fluorescence characteristics.

We next turned to the age pigments of Fisher rats and found that the fluorophoric composition of RPE lipofuscin from old rats was very comparable to that of human RPE lipofuscin.[36] Previous studies on Fisher rats had demonstrated that dietary vitamin A deficiency reduces RPE lipofuscin accumulation.[37-38] Repeating these experiments showed that dietary vitamin A deficiency also reduces the amounts of fluorophores in the RPE, specifically the orange-emitting pigment that we had chosen to study.[39]

It was also noticed by Katz and co-workers that the outer segment debris which accumulates over the RPE in RCS rats develops an autofluorescence which appears very similar to the age pigment fluorescence.[40] Extraction and chromatographic analysis of this fluorescence demonstrated that the pattern of fluorophores from the debris is very similar to the pattern obtained from age pigments, with the exception that one of the most prominent fluorophores is an orange-emitting fluorophore with a greater chromatographic mobility than the one we had chosen to study.[40] It appears that the RCS rat debris fluorophore may be a precursor to the age pigment fluorophore. Consistent with this interpretation is the fact that the RCS orange fluorophore is also reduced in dietary vitamin A deficiency.[41]

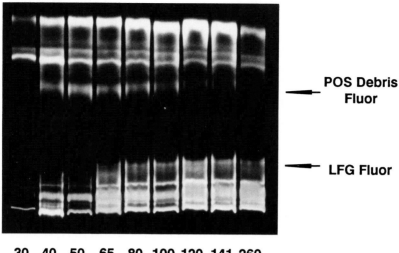

POS Debris
Fluor

LFG Fluor

30 40 50 65 80 100 120 141 260
Postnatal Age (days)

Figure 1. Fluorophores of the RCS rat retina/eyecup: age series. The orange-emitting fluorophore associated with the photoreceptor outer segment (POS) debris appears by postnatal day 40 and disappears in a time course paralleling the disappearance of the debris zone and degeneration of the retina. The age-related, lipofuscin fluorophore (LFG) begins to appear by postnatal day 65 and remains throughout the life of the animal.

Matthes and LaVail have expressed the opinion that the RCS debris zone fluorescence might actually be due to lipofuscin granule contamination.[42] To study this we ran an age series of rats and were able to demonstrate that the upper debris-related fluorophore was present only during the time that the outer debris zone is present and that it disappears as the debris zone disappears, and that the lower age-related, lipofuscin-derived fluorophore appears only with advanced age (Figure 1). A major advantage of using the RCS rat outer segment debris as a model for studying the factors that influence the formation of the fluorophores is the fact that the lipofuscin-like fluorescence evolves over less than two months time as opposed to nearly two years time for significant age pigment accumulation in normal rat eyes.

Both the vitamin A deficiency and the age series studies are consistent with the interpretation that the upper orange emitting fluorophore may serve as a precursor to the lower orange emitting fluorophore. Much remains to be done to prove that this is the case. To do so we will be purifying the fluorophores from the RCS rats and investigating several spectral properties. The specific features that we will be looking for will be based largely on our experience with the characterization of the human lipofuscin orange emitting fluorophore.

IV. CHEMICAL AND SPECTRAL ANALYSES OF THE HUMAN RPE LIPOFUSCIN ORANGE-EMITTING FLUOROPHORE

We have found that the human orange-emitting fluorophore displays the following characteristics:

1) In a battery of chromatographic spray reagent tests, the only chemicals that gave a positive reaction were antimony pentachloride and vanillin/sulfuric acid, both of which react with terpenoid compounds.[39]

2) UV/VIS absorbance spectra reveal three absorbance peaks at 285, 340, and 420 nm.[30] The long wavelength absorbance peaks are indicative of an extensive series of conjugated double bonds. The wide separation of the peaks may indicate that there are more than one such system in the molecule.

3) Corrected fluorescence excitation spectra reflect the absorbance spectra peaks and the emission spectrum displays peaks at 605, 633, and 672 nm,[30] which is consistent with the orange/red appearance of its fluorescent emission. Again, for a molecule to display such a long wavelength emission, there must be an extensive system of conjugated double bonds. Also, the large Stokes shift (i.e., the distance separating the absorbance and emission peaks) would indicate that a lot of the excitation energy is lost vibrationally before the molecule emits a photon to return to its ground state. This would be the case for a linear system of conjugated double bonds rather than a rigid fused ring system.

4) FTIR spectra reveal strong $C = C$ absorbance, a moderate $C = O$ absorbance, and possibly a weak OH absorbance.[39]

5) We have been unable to accumulate sufficient material for analysis by ^{1}H or ^{13}C nmr.

6) GC and direct probe mass spectroscopy proved disappointing in that the compound was nonvolatile and thermally labile so that a fragment occurred at every mass which makes structural interpretation very difficult. The low mass end of the spectrum did however display a fragmentation pattern typical of an unsaturated hydrocarbon.

7) More recent success has been obtained using a softer ionization techinique: fast atom bombardment. In the FAB spectrum discrete peaks are obtained which are more readily interpreted. While final details of this spectrum are being worked out, it appears that the molecule is a $4 + 2$ cyclodimer of a ketoretinal Schiff base and a ketoretinol. Similar retinoid dimers have previously been reported as natural products in whale liver oil,[43] and as photosensitized reaction products of synthetic aromatic retinoids.[44]

V. EFFECT OF DARK-REARING ON RCS DEBRIS FLUOROPHORES

To test whether the occurrence of the RCS rat orange-emitting fluorophore was dependent upon light exposure, rats were raised in total darkness, and all tissue handling was done under dim red illumination. After 66 days, it was found that the orange-emitting fluorophore was absent from dark-reared RCS rats but present in control light reared rats. Because it is known that the degeneration of the RCS rat retina is delayed in dark-reared rats,[45] the time of dark rearing was extended to 96 days. In these animals, some samples had no orange-emitting fluorophore, but one did have the fluorophore. Thus, it appears that the orange emitting fluorophore is capable of being generated in the absence of light, and may be more dependent on the state of degeneration of the retinal debris. These experiments bear repeating for clarification.

VI. NEW QUESTIONS ARISING

It now appears that vitamin A is a direct precursor to the human lipofuscin fluorophore. Therefore, evidence now exists that vitamin A esters and free vitamin A are present in the lipofuscin granule, and that modified vitamin A derivatives may also accumulate within the granules. This raises some new questions as to how RPE lipofuscin might affect the vitamin A cycle[19,46] with advanced age. It will be important to determine whether the granule is acting as an irreversible sink for these vitamin A compounds or whether it is acting as an exchangeable pool. If it is acting as a sink, is the vitamin A cycle being depleted of available vitamin A? If it is acting as an exchangeable pool, especially for the modified vitamin A derivatives, can these derivatives compete for binding sites in the metabolic and transport machinery that drives the vitamin A cycle, thereby deleteriously effecting vitamin A turnover in advanced age? Much work remains to be done to begin to approach the answers to these questions.

VII. ACKNOWLEDGEMENTS

Mass spectroscopic analyses have been performed in collaboration with Dr. Roger N. Hayes of the Midwest Center for Mass Spectroscopy, Department of Chemistry, University of Nebraska-Lincoln, Lincoln, Nebraska, U.S.A. 68588-0304. Supported by USPHS grant EY-06458 and by a grant from Research to Prevent Blindness, Inc.

VIII. REFERENCES

1.   Streeten, B. W., The sudanophilic granules of the human retinal pigment epithelium, Arch. Ophthalmol., 66, 391, 1961.

2. Feeney, L., Lipofuscin and melanin of human retinal pigment epithelium: Fluorescence, enzyme cytochemical and ultrastructural studies, Invest. Ophthalmol. Vis. Sci., 17, 583, 1978.

3. Hogan, M. J., Role of the retinal pigment epithelium in macular disease, Trans. Am. Acad. Ophthalmol. Otolaryngol., 76, 64, 1972.

4. Feeney-Burns, L., Berman, E. R., and Rothman, M. S., Lipofuscin of human retinal pigment epithelium, Am. J. Ophthalmol., 90, 783, 1980.

5. Weiter, J. J., Delori, F. C., and Dorey, C. K., Central sparing in annular macular degeneration, Am. J. Ophthalmol., 106, 286, 1988.

6. Dorey, C. K., Wu, G., Ebenstein, D., Garsd, A., and Weiter, J. J., Cell loss in the aging retina: Relationship to lipofuscin accumulation and macular degeneration, Invest. Ophthalmol. Vis. Sci., 30, 1691, 1989.

7. Berman, E.R.., Biochemistry of the retinal pigment epithelium, in The Retinal Pigment Epithelium, Zinn, K.M. and Marmor, M.F., Eds., Harvard Univ. Press, Cambridge, Mass., 1979, 83.

8. Zimmerman, W.F., Godchaux, W., and Belkin, M., The relative proportions of lysosomal enzyme activities in bovine retinal pigment epithelium. Exp. Eye Res., 36, 1983.

9. Feeney-Burns, L., Gao, C-L., and Tidwell, M. Lysosomal enzyme cytochemistry of human RPE, Bruch's membrane and drusen. Invest. Ophthalmol. Vis. Sci., 28, 1138, 1987.

10. Leibowitz, H. M., Krueger, D. E., Maunder, L. R., et al., The Framingham eye study monograph: An ophthalmological and epidemiological study of cataract, glaucoma, diabetic retinopathy, macular degeneration, and visual acuity in a general population of 2631 adults, Surv. Ophthalmol., 24 (suppl.), 335, 1980.

11. Ganley, J. P., and Roberts, J., Eye Conditions and Related Need for Medical Care Among Persons 1-74 Years of Age: United States, 1971-1972, DHHS Publ. No. (PHS) 83-1678, 1983.

12. Weiter, J. J., Delori, F. C., Wing, G. L., and Fitch, K., Relationship of senile macular degeneration to ocular pigmentation, Am. J. Ophthalmol., 99, 185, 1985.

13. Munoz, B., West, S., Bressler, N., Bressler, S., Rosenthal, F. S., and Taylor, H. R., Blue light and risk of age-related macular degeneration, Invest. Ophthalmol. Vis. Sci., 31 (suppl.), 49, 1990.

14. Gregor, Z., and Joffe, L., Senile macular changes in the black African, Br. J. Ophthalmol., 62, 547, 1978.

15. Newsome, D. A., Swartz, M., Leone, N. C., Elston, R. C., and Miller, E., Oral zinc in macular degeneration, Arch. Ophthalmol., 106, 192, 1988.

16. Bird, A., Pauleikhoff, D., Olver, J., Maguire, J., Sheraidah, G., and Marshall, J., The correlation of choriocapillaris and Bruch's membrane changes in aging, Invest. Ophthalmol. Vis. Sci., 31(suppl.), 47, 1990.

17. Handelman, G. J., and Dratz, E. A., The role of antioxidants in the retina and retinal pigment epithelium and the nature of prooxidant-induced damage, in Advances in Free Radical Biology and Medicine, Vol. 2, Pryor, W. A., Ed., Pergamon Press, New York, 1986, 1.

18. Chio, K. S., Reiss, U., Fletcher, B., and Tappel, A. L., Peroxidation of subcellular organelles: Formation of lipofuscinlike fluorescent pigments, Science, 166, 1535, 1969.

19. Bok, D., Retinal photoreceptor-pigment epithelium interactions, Invest. Ophthalmol. Vis. Sci., 26, 1659, 1985.

20. Reme, C., Autophagy in visual cells and pigment epithelium, Invest. Ophthalmol. Vis. Sci., 16, 807, 1977.

21. Feeney-Burns, L., Hilderbrand, E. S., and Eldridge, S., Aging human RPE: Morphometric analysis of macular, equatorial, and peripheral cells, Invest. Ophthalmol. Vis. Sci., 25, 195, 1984.

22. Burns, R. P., and Feeney-Burns, L., Clinico-morphologic correlations of drusen of Bruch's membrane, Tr. Am. Ophth. Soc., 78, 206, 1980.

23. Farkas, T., Sylvester, V., and Archer, D., The ultrastructure of drusen, Am. J. Ophthalmol., 71, 1196, 1971.

24. Sarks, S. H., Ageing and degeneration in the macular region: A clinico-pathological study, Brit. J. Ophthalmol., 60, 324, 1976.

25. Korte, G. E., Repucci, V., and Henkind, P., RPE destruction causes choriocapilary atrophy, Invest. Ophthalmol. Vis. Sci., 25, 1135, 1984.

26. Glaser, B. M., Campochiaro, P.A., Davies, J. L., and Sato, M., Retinal pigment epithelial cells release an inhibitor of neovascularization. Arch. Ophthalmol., 103, 1870, 1985.

27. Sarks, S. H., VanDriel, D., Maxwell, L., and Killingsworth, M., Softening of drusen and subretinal neovascularization, Trans. Ophthalmol. Soc., U.K., 100, 414, 1980.

28. Macular Photocoagulation Group, Argon laser photocoagulation for neovascular maculopathy: Three year results for randomized clinical trials, Arch. Ophthalmol., 224, 493, 1986.

29. Feeney-Burns, L., and Eldred, G. E., The fate of the phagosome: Conversion to 'age pigment' and impact in human retinal pigment epithelium, Trans. Ophthalmol. Soc. U.K., 103, 416, 1983.

30. Eldred, G. E., and Katz, M. L., Fluorophores of the human retinal pigment epithelium: Separation and spectral characterization, Exp. Eye Res., 47, 71, 1988.

31. Eldred, G. E., Vitamins A and E in RPE lipofuscin formation and implications for age-related macular degeneration, in Inherited and Environmentally Induced Retinal Degenerations, LaVail, M. M., Anderson, R. E., and Hollyfield, J. G., Eds., Alan R. Liss, New York, 1989, 113.

32. Eldred, G. E., and Katz, M. L., Vitamin E-deficiency pigment and lipofuscin (age) pigment from the retinal pigment epithelium differ in fluorophoric composition, Invest. Ophthalmol. Vis. Sci., 29(suppl.), 92, 1988.

33. Katz, M. L., Eldred, G. E., Siakotos, A. N., and Koppang, N., Characterization of disease-specific brain fluorophores in ceroid-lipofuscinosis, Am. J. Med. Genetics Suppl., 5, 253, 1988.

34. Katz, M. L., and Eldred, G. E., unpublished data, 1988.

35. Eldred, G. E., and Katz, M. L., The autofluorescent products of lipid peroxidation may not be lipofuscin-like, Free Radical Biol. Med., 7, 157, 1989.
36. Katz, M. L., and Eldred, G. E., Retinal light damage reduces autofluorescent pigment deposition in the retinal pigment epithelium, Invest. Ophthalmol. Vis. Sci., 30, 37, 1989.
37. Robison, W. G., Jr., Kuwabara, T., and Bieri, J. G., Deficiencies of vitamins E and A in the rat. Retinal damage and lipofuscin accumulation, Invest. Ophthalmol. Vis. Sci., 19, 1030, 1980.
38. Katz, M. L., Drea, C. M., and Robison, W. G., Jr., Relationship between dietary retinol and lipofuscin in the retinal pigment epithelium, Mech. Ageing Dev., 35, 291, 1986.
39. Eldred, G. E., and Katz, M. L., Possible mechanism for lipofuscinogenesis in the retinal pigment epithelium and other tissues, in Lipofuscin - 1987: State of the Art, Zs.-Nagy, I., Ed., Akademiai Kiado, Budapest and Elsevier Science Publishers, Amsterdam, 1988, 185.
40. Katz, M. L., Drea, C. M., Eldred, G. E., Hess, H. H., and Robison, W. G., Jr., Influence of early photoreceptor degeneration on lipofuscin in the retinal pigment epithelium, Exp. Eye Res., 43, 561, 1986.
41. Katz, M. L., Eldred, G. E., and Robison, W. G., Jr., Lipofuscin autofluorescence: Evidence for vitamin A involvement in the retina, Mech. Ageing Dev., 39, 81, 1987.
42. Matthes, M. T., and LaVail, M. M., Inherited retinal dystrophy in the RCS rat: Composition of the outer segment debris zone, in Inherited and Environmentally Induced Retinal Degenerations, Lavail, M. M., Anderson, R. E., and Hollyfield, J. G., Eds., Alan R. Liss, New York, 1989, 315.
43. Tsukida, K., and Ito, M., The structure of kitol, J. Nutr. Sci. Vitaminol., 26, 319, 1980.
44. Pfoertner, K.-H., Englert, G., and Schoenholzer, P., Photosensitized [4 + 2] cyclodimerizations of aromatic retinoids, Tetrahedron, 44, 1039, 1988.
45. LaVail, M. M., and Battelle, B.-A., Influence of eye pigmentation and light deprivation on inherited retinal dystrophy in the rat, Exp. Eye Res., 21, 167, 1975.
46. Rando, R. R., The chemistry of vitamin A and vision, Angew. Chem. Int. Ed., 29, 461, 1990.

FURTHER INSIGHT INTO THE SPECTRAL DEPENDENCE OF PHOTICALLY INDUCED RETINAL DEGENERATIONS

Laurence M. Rapp

Cullen Eye Institute
Baylor College of Medicine, Houston, TX 77030

The mechanisms of light-induced degeneration of the retina and retinal pigment epithelium (RPE) can be divided into three major categories. First, mechanical damage is the result of acoustic transients or shock waves produced by short pulses of light at high power density levels.[1,2] Second, thermal damage is the consequence of macromolecule denaturation when radiant exposures cause a temperature rise in excess of 10° C.[3] Third, photochemical damage refers to various cytotoxic reactions that are initiated by photosensitization and other excitation pathways.[4] One feature in common to both mechanical and thermal damage is that the primary photon absorber is thought to be melanin in the RPE and choriocapillaris.[5] In contrast, various molecules have been proposed as the chromophores mediating photochemical retinal damage including visual pigments, visual pigment bleaching products, riboflavin, flavoenzymes, cytochrome oxidase and NADH.[5-7] This chapter will review the experimental evidence suggesting that photochemical retinal damage can be further divided into separate classes. This evidence is based on differences in action spectra and histological loci indicating the involvement of more than one mediator.

Noell and coworkers[8,9] first demonstrated that photic damage to the mammalian retina can be caused by light levels that are too low to involve thermal mechanisms. In their work,[9] the action spectrum of retinal degeneration in rats was found to correspond to the effectiveness of light in eliciting visual excitation. This result was confirmed by others[10,11] and an action spectrum approximating the absorption spectrum of the rod visual pigment rhodopsin was demonstrated by Williams and Howell.[12] Further evidence that visual pigments can mediate retinal light damage was obtained by Harwerth and Sperling[13] who showed that selective sensitivity loss in two classes of monkey cones (blue- and green-sensitive) can be caused by exposure to narrow-band light corresponding to the cones' absorption maxima.

Other studies have indicated that short-wavelength light causes photochemical damage to the retina by mechanisms that do not necessarily involve visual pigment absorption. In rhesus monkeys, Ham et al.[14] examined the spectral dependence of funduscopically visible retinal lesions caused by 1000 sec exposures to monochromatic lazer lines ranging from 441 to 1064 nm. They observed a steady increase in retinal susceptibility to damage as a function of decreasing wavelength with no tendency to peak at 441.6 nm. Using both functional and histological criteria, Lawwill et al.[15] also found that blue light (457.9 lazer line) was more effective in producing retinal damage than the longer visible wavelengths. Subsequent studies by Ham et al.[16] in aphakic monkeys showed the wavelength of peak effectiveness in causing retinal damage extended into the near-ultraviolet region of the spectrum. In rodents and squirrels, photoreceptor cell degeneration was caused by exposure to near-ultraviolet light.[17-19] Examining pigmented rats, van Norren and Schellekens[21] determined that near-ultraviolet light is more effective than visible wavelengths in damaging the retina. In this same species, Rapp et al.[20] found that damage induced by ultraviolet-A light occurred independently of rhodopsin bleaching.

Various classification schemes have been offered to categorize the different types of photochemical retinal damage. Summarizing his own findings on albino rats, Noell[22] distinguished between two kinds of rhodopsin-mediated retinal damage. Using relatively high light intensities in adult animals, damage of the "first" kind resulted in the destruction of both photoreceptor and pigment epithelial cells. Damage of the "second" kind tended to occur in younger animals exposed to lower light intensities and caused the selective loss of photoreceptor cells. Taking into account the primate data, Lawwill[23] suggested that there are three distinct mechanisms of photochemical retinal damage. The first and second mechanisms involved mediation by the rod and cone visual pigments, respectively. The third mechanism referred to the short-wavelength ("blue") light effect which had been documented in rhesus monkeys. An important distinguishing characteristic of short-wavelength damage (in Lawwill's experiments) was that it occurred equally in all layers of the retina from the RPE through the nerve fiber layer. He hypothesized that short-wavelength damage was the result of the direct action of light on the mitochondria which are present in all cell layers. More recently, Kremers and van Norren[7] differentiated between two classes of photochemical damage having action spectra that correspond to either visual pigment absorption or to ultraviolet wavelengths. They pointed out that the ultraviolet action spectrum closely corresponds to the absorption spectrum of rhodopsin bleaching products, but did not exclude the possibility that melanin or mitochondrial enzymes may be mediating the damage.

One of the difficulties in attempting to identify the different mechanisms of photochemical retinal damage is the inability to extrapolate experimental findings from one animal species to another. To help resolve this problem, my laboratory developed an experimental paradigm to produce rhodopsin-mediated and short-wavelength damage in a single animal species, the Long Evans rat.[20] These animals were anesthetized and exposed to wavelength bands that were centered either at the absorption peak of rhodopsin (green; 500 nm) or in the ultraviolet-A (UVA; 360 nm) region of the spectrum. The UVA exposure caused retinal damage that was histologically dissimilar from green light. This was particularly evident at one day post-exposure. At this time-point, UVA-exposed retinas had pyknotic nuclei in both the inner and outer nuclear layers and the RPE was markedly thinned. Another interesting feature of these retinas was that their rod outer segments were remarkably well-preserved. In contrast, green light-exposed retinas showed damage that was photoreceptor cell specific. There was severe disorganization of rod inner and outer segments and some photoreceptor cell nuclei were pyknotic. RPE and inner retinal cells, however, appeared normal. Electron microscopy was helpful in further differentiating the histological characteristics of UVA and green light damage. Mitochondrial alterations consisting of severe swelling and inner membrane vesiculation were found in the rod ellipsoid region (Figure 1) and in the RPE of UVA-exposed retinas. However, the rod outer segments showed an orderly stacking of membrane discs. In green light-exposed retinas, there was severe disorientation and vesiculation of the rod outer segment disks. Photoreceptor and RPE mitochondria, however, appeared normal.

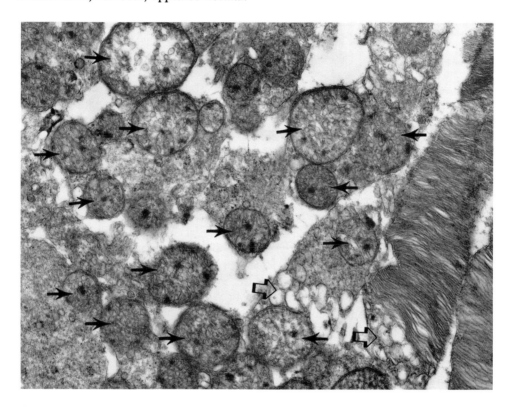

Figure 1. Electron micrograph of the rod inner segment ellipsoid region of an albino rat retina exposed to 100 μW/cm^2 of UVA light. Note the swelling and inner membrane vesiculation of the mitochondria (filled arrows) and the appearance of electron-lucent zones at the outer segment base (open arrows). ×17,200.

The observations just described depict a clear distinction between two classes of light damage. However, when considering all possible mechanisms of photochemical damage, it seems unlikely that a single process can be isolated. In support of this is the recent work of Pautler et al.[24] that showed a "blue light" action spectrum for functional damage to bovine RPE that significantly overlapped both the ultraviolet and rhodopsin-mediated action spectra of retinal damage. Thus, exposure to broad-band light (visible or ultraviolet) is likely to produce more than one subclass of photochemical damage. For example, the "first kind" of light damage described by Noell[22] was characterized using broad-band green light and involved photoreceptor and RPE destruction. Although this kind of damage was shown to be rhodopsin-mediated, it seems possible that the longer wavelength shoulder of the "blue light" action spectrum could contribute to RPE involvement via direct action on these cells. However, evidence against primary damage to RPE from these exposures comes from the finding that no significant RPE damage occurred in rats with hereditary retinal disease receiving intense light exposure at a stage when photoreceptors were missing.[22]

The "blue light" damage mechanism might also be responsible for the histopathological features that are common to ultraviolet and "white" light damage. As seen in Figure 1, UVA exposure of the pigmented rat retina caused rod inner segment vacuolization and basal rod outer segment vesiculation. These alterations closely resemble the discrete electron-lucent regions found at the rod outer segment base of rabbits exposed to high intensity "white" light.[25] Blacklight (predominately UVA) exposure of albino rats caused photoreceptor cell edema and disc separations that, at early stages, were confined to the distal tips of the rod outer segments.[18] This is precisely the same initial change reported for albino rats exposed to fluorescent (white) light.[26]

Despite significant advances, a clear understanding of the different mechanisms of photochemical retinal degeneration will require a concerted research effort. As described herein, interpretation of the existing data is confounded by inherent susceptibility differences among animal species and the considerable variation that exists among the exposure paradigms used. Nonetheless, the data provide support for a few basic principles. Regarding the photochemical mediators, there is convincing evidence that both rod and cone visual pigments can initiate damage. Furthermore, one or more short-wavelength mechanisms appear to be involved in photochemical retinal damage. Action spectrum determinations by Pautler et al.[24] suggest that the mediator(s) of "blue light" damage to the RPE may be hemoproteins such as cytochrome C oxidase. Other chromophores were suggested to mediate ultraviolet light damage since the "blue light" action spectrum did not match that of Ham et al.[14] for short-wavelength damage to the rhesus monkey retina. A recent study in my laboratory found that albino rats, which completely lack melanosomes, were readily damaged by UVA light.[27] This suggests that melanin is not the chromophore mediating ultraviolet-A retinal damage. Concerning the biological mechanisms by which absorbed light leads to cellular damage, there are an exhaustive number of reactions that have been implicated (reviewed by Noell[28]). Among them are photooxidation, retinol-induced membranolysis, enzyme inactivation, and numerous physiological responses to light that may be damaging when exposure is excessive.

In summary, 35 years (since Noell's initial discovery) of research on the photochemical mechanisms of light-induced degeneration of the retina and RPE has produced many intriguing findings. The task in the future will be to sort out the information already obtained in order to further elucidate the spectral dependence and biochemical etiology of retinal phototoxicity. Undoubtedly, continued research efforts will reveal as yet unidentified mechanisms of photochemical retinal damage.

ACKNOWLEDGEMENTS

This work was supported in part by National Institutes of Health grants EY04554 and EY02520 and Research to Prevent Blindness, Inc. The technical assistance of Barbara Tolman and Cindy Koutz is greatly appreciated.

REFERENCES

1. Cleary, S.F. and Hamrick, P.E., Laser-induced acoustic transients in the mammalian eye. J. Acous. Soc., 46, 1037, 1969.
2. Ham, W.T., Jr., Mueller, H.A., Goldman, A.I., Newman, B.E., Holland, L.M. and Kuwabara, T., Ocular hazard from picosecond pulses of ND: YAG laser radiation. Science, 185, 362, 1974.
3. Clarke, A.M., Geeraets, W.J. and Ham, W.T., Jr., An equilibrium thermal model for retinal injury from optical sources. Appl. Opt., 8, 1951, 1969.
4. Ham, W.T., Jr., Mueller, H.A., Ruffolo, J.J., Jr., Miller, J.E., Cleary, S.F., and Guerry, R.K., and Guerry, D., Basic mechanisms underlying the production of photochemical lesions in the mammalian retina. Curr. Eye Res., 3, 165, 1984.
5. Ham, W.T., Jr., Ruffolo, J.J., Jr., Mueller, H.A., and Guerry, D., The nature of retinal radiation damage: dependence on wavelength, power level and exposure time. Vis. Res., 20, 1105, 1980.
6. Noell, W.K., Possible mechanisms of photoreceptor damage by light in mammalian eyes. Vis. Res., 20, 1163, 1980.
7. Kremers, J.M. and van Norren, D., Two classes of photochemical damage of the retina. Las. Light Ophthalmol., 2, 41, 1988.
8. Noell, W.K., Aspects of experimental and hereditary retinal degeneration, in Biochemistry of the Retina, Graymore, C.N,. Ed., Academic Press, New York, 1965, 51.
9. Noell, W.K., Walker, V.S., Kang, B.S. and Berman, S., Retinal damage by light in rats. Invest. Ophthalmol. , 5, 450, 1966.
10. Gorn, R.A. and Kuwabara, T., Retinal damage by visible light. A physiological study. Arch. Ophthalmol., 77, 115, 1967.
11. Lawwill, T., Effects of prolonged exposure of rabbit retina to low intensity light. Invest. Ophthalmol., 12, 45, 1973.
12. Williams, T.P. and Howell, W.L. Action spectrum of retinal light-damage in albino rats. Invest. Ophthalmol. Vis. Res., 24, 285, 1983.

13.   Harwerth, R.S., and Sperling, H.G., Prolonged color blindness induced by intense spectral lights in rhesus monkeys. Science, 174, 520, 1974.

14.   Ham, W.T., Jr., Mueller, H.A. and Sliney, D.H., Retinal sensitivity to damage from short wavelength light. Nature, 260, 153, 1976.

15.   Lawwilll, T., Crockett, S. and Currier, G., Functional and histological measures of retinal damage in chronic light exposure. Documenta Ophthal., 15, 285, 1977.

16.   Ham, Jr., W.T., Mueller, H.A., Ruffolo, Jr., J.J., Dupont Guerry III, and Guerry, R.K., Action spectrum for retinal injury from near-ultraviolet radiation in the aphakic monkey. Am. J. Ophthalmol., 93, 299, 1982.

17.   Zigman, S. and Vaughan, T., Near-ultraviolet light effects on the lenses and retinas of mice. Invest. Ophthalmol., 13, 462, 1974.

18.   Henton, W.W. and Sykes, S.M., Recovery of absolute threshold with UVA-induced retinal damage. Physiol. Behav., 32, 949, 1984.

19.   Collier, R.J., Waldron, W.R., and Zigman, S., Temporal sequence of changes to the grey squirrel retina after near-UV exposure. Invest. Ophthalmol. Vis. Sci, 30, 631, 1989.

20.   Rapp, L.M., Tolman, B.L. and Dhindsa, H.S., Separate mechanisms for retinal damage by ultraviolet-A and midvisible light. Invest. Ophthalmol. Vis. Sci., 31, 1186, 1990.

21.   van Norren, D. and Schellekens, P., Blue light hazard in rat. Vis. Res., 30, 1517, 1990.

22.   Noell, W.K. (1980). There are different kinds of retinal light damage in the rat, in The Effects of Constant Light on Visual Processes, Williams, T.P. and Baker, B.N., Eds., Plenum Press, New York, 3.

23.   Lawwill, T., Three major pathologic processes caused by light on the primate retina: A search for mechanisms. Tr. Am. Ophthalmol. Soc., 80, 517, 1982.

24.   Pautler, E.L., Morita, M., and Beezley, P., Hemoprotein(s) mediate blue light damage in the retinal pigment epithelium, Photochem. Photobiol., 51, 599, 1990.

25.   Hoppeler, Th., Hendrickson, Ph., Dietrich, C. and Reme, Ch., Morphology and time-course of defined photochemical lesions in the rabbit retina. Exp. Eye Res., 7, 849, 1988.

26.   Kuwabara, T. and Gorn, R.A., Retinal damage by visible light. An electron microscope study. Arch. Ophthal., 79, 69, 1968.

27.   Rapp, L.M. and Smith, S.C., Evidence against melanin as the mediator of retinal phototoxicity by short-wavelength light. Exp. Eye Res., submitted.

28.   Noell, W.K., Possible mechanisms of photoreceptor damage by light in mammalian eyes. Vis. Res., 20, 1163, 1980.

PROTECTION AGAINST RETINAL LIGHT DAMAGE BY NATURAL AND SYNTHETIC ANTIOXIDANTS

D.T. Organisciak, R.M. Darrow, I.R. Bicknell, Y-L. Jiang,
M. Pickford* and J.C. Blanks*
Department of Biochemistry, Wright State University, Dayton, OH,
and
*Doheny Eye Institute, USC School of Medicine, Los Angeles, CA

I. INTRODUCTION

A central feature of all hypotheses of visual transduction is that photon absorption by rhodopsin triggers a complex cascade of molecular events which alters the ionic conductance of the photoreceptor cell.[1-6] Prolonged light exposure, however, can cause damage to the photoreceptors. It is now apparent that light damage also involves a complex series of events which depend upon the duration and intensity of light, its wavelength, and the distribution of absorbing chromophore(s) in the retina.[7-13] Because the action spectrum of light damage in the rat is identical to the rhodopsin absorption spectrum,[7,14] photoreceptor cell damage is most effectively caused by green light; the same appears to be true for the frog.[15] Retinal damage, therefore, is related to the rhodopsin content of the eye just prior to light exposure. It follows, that environmental or genetic factors that alter rhodopsin levels can also influence the extent of retinal damage.[16-20] In addition, the manner by which intense light is administered can affect the outcome of retinal light damage. Rats treated with short intermittent light doses, interrupted in each case by darkness, incur more damage than those exposed to the same light in a continuous fashion.[7,21]

It is now clear that there are two types of retinal light damage in rats, with both irreversible and reversible components.[9,22,23] Type I damage is largely irreversible and is found in long term dark reared normal rats, and in young RCS-dystrophic rats before there is a significant accumulation of rod cell debris in the inner photoreceptor cell matrix.[9,16,22] It is characterized by massive photoreceptor cell death with associated damage or loss of adjacent RPE cells. In Type I damage, loss of visual cells, visual cell DNA and rhodopsin, and altered electrophysiological responses of retina and RPE have been reported.[24,25] Type II damage, the most common form of light damage studied, is characterized by a predominant reduction in the A-wave of the ERG, and by the loss of visual cells; damage to the RPE is less severe or absent.[9,22] It is best seen in young rats reared in cyclic light, and widely studied in adult rats maintained in cyclic light environments.[9,22,26-31] The type of retinal damage and the extent of reversible or irreversible retinal changes appear to depend on the long term metabolic state of the visual cell, in addition to the level of rhodopsin and its packing density in ROS.[9,18,19,22,26-32]

Irrespective of the type of light damage, or the manner by which light is given, supplementation of rats with ascorbic acid prior to exposure reduces the extent of damage.[30,31,33] Protection is also afforded rats with reduced levels of docosahexaenoic acid (22:6) in their ROS membranes, especially when ascorbate is also given.[24,25] There is good evidence suggesting that oxidative processes are involved in light damage,[34,35] and that 22:6 is lost from ROS membranes as a result of light exposure.[30,34,35] Similarly, among the endogenous antioxidants in the rat retina, only ascorbic acid decreases as a function of exposure to intense light.[36-38] Furthermore, the loss of ROS-22:6 during intense light exposure is reduced by supplemental vitamin C.[24,30] Whether ascorbate's mechanism of action involves a direct effect on superoxide anion or singlet oxygen,[39,40] a cooperative interaction with membrane-bound vitamin E,[41-43] or an effect on a membrane receptor,[44] its high concentration in the eye suggests an antioxidative role during light exposure.

To better understand the protective role of vitamin C in the retina and the loss of ROS 22:6 during light exposure, we have compared the natural L-stereoisomer of ascorbic acid with the unnatural D-stereoisomer. Whereas L-ascorbate can function as both an enzymatic cofactor and an antioxidant, D-ascorbate, which has been shown to reduce lipid peroxidation in guinea pigs,[45] is not a cofactor for enzymatic activity in mammals. In addition, we have studied the synthetic antioxidant dimethylthiourea (DMTU), which also protects against retinal light damage in rats,[46] by comparing it to ascorbic acid protection and by measuring its effects on ROS-22:6 levels.

II. MATERIALS AND METHODS

A.   ANIMAL MAINTENANCE, ANTIOXIDANTS, LIGHT EXPOSURE

Weanling male albino Sprague-Dawley rats were obtained from Harland Inc. (Indianapolis, IN) and maintained in a weak cyclic-light environment (20-40 lux) for 12 hrs per day (lights on 08:00) or in darkness. The rats were fed ad libitum Purina Rat Chow and had free access to water. After 40 days in their respective environments the rats were injected IP, or not, with one of the antioxidants; all rats were dark adapted overnight. A second IP injection of antioxidant was given just before the animals were exposed to intense light. Typically, a dose of 500 mg/kg body wt was used,[30] but in some experiments doses of 250 mg/kg of DMTU were used. In experiments to test the combined effects of ascorbate and DMTU a third dose of L-ascorbic acid at 500 mg/kg was given just before the 4th hr of light exposure. L-ascorbic acid was obtained from Sigma Inc. (St. Louis, MO), D-ascorbic acid [D(-)-isoascorbic acid] was obtained from Fluka, Inc. (Hauppauge, NY) and DMTU was purchased from Aldrich Chemical Co. (Milwaukee, WI).

Light exposures consisted of 1-hr light: 2-hr dark periods of intermittent light, as previously described.[21] These were in green Plexiglas #2092 chambers[7] (band pass 490-580 nm), and started at 09:00. During the light periods illumination was 1750-2000 lux. Usually 3 rats were exposed per chamber (one unsupplemented, one L- or D-ascorbate and one injected with DMTU). During light treatment the animals had free access to food and water. At the end of the exposure period the rats were either placed into the dark environment for 2 additional weeks before use, or sacrificed immediately in a

CO_2 saturated chamber. All procedures employed in this study conformed to the ARVO Resolution on the Use of Experimental Animals in Research.

B.   TISSUE MEASUREMENTS

1.   Rhodopsin Determinations

As an index of the extent of retinal light damage, rhodopsin levels were measured in the eyes of experimental animals following a two week period in darkness. These were compared to the rhodopsin levels in unexposed control animals, similarly maintained. Procedures for the excision of eyes and rhodopsin measurements have been described.[24,30]

2.   ROS Fatty Acid Determinations

Immediately after the last hr of light exposure, ROS were isolated and lipids extracted.[36] Total ROS lipid fatty acid profiles were determined by gas-liquid chromatography,[24] with particular attention to the content of 22:6 fatty acids. The ratio of cholesterol to lipid phosphorus was also determined.[24,30,36]

3.   Tissue Levels of Ascorbate and DMTU

The levels of L-ascorbic acid in whole blood, retina, and RPE/choroid were determined by HPLC in rats perfused with saline prior to retinal dissection.[33] Similarly, DMTU levels in serum, retina and RPE/choroid were determined by HPLC. For these measurements, tissues were excised from perfused rats and homogenized in 50 mM potassium phosphate buffer, pH 7.8, containing 0.1 mM EDTA. Following centrifugation at 6000 xg for 10 min, the supernatants were filtered through a 0.45 μ filter and injected onto a C18 reversed phase HPLC column. DMTU was eluted with a mobile phase consisting of 95% H_2O:5% MeOH at a flow rate of 1 ml/min. Detection was by absorbance at 242 nm, with quantitation by comparison with DMTU standards of known concentration.

4.   Retinal Histology

Dark reared albino rats were exposed to light for three 1-hour intervals, interrupted by two 2-hour dark periods. A 30-minute dark recovery period was allowed after the final 1-hour light exposure. For one-half of the animals, either ascorbate or DMTU was given IP 24 hours before and just prior to light exposure. The other half of the animals served as untreated controls. The animals were sacrificed, the eyes enucleated, and placed into fixative (2% paraformaldehyde, 2.5% glutaraldehyde, 0.1M cacodylate buffered) at the end of the 30-minute recovery period. The superior and inferior temporal quadrants of each eye were embedded in epoxy resin and sectioned at 1μm thickness. The sections were stained and photographed at the light microscopic level.

III. RESULTS

A. RHODOPSIN IN LIGHT EXPOSED RATS

The protective effects of the L- or D- forms of ascorbic acid and DMTU were determined in dark- and cyclic-light-reared rats by measuring rhodopsin levels 2 wks after intermittent light exposure. As shown in Figure 1, both forms of ascorbic acid and the antioxidant DMTU reduced or prevented retinal light damage. For the dark-reared rats, DMTU treatment was more effective than either L- or D-ascorbate. After 3-1 hr light doses essentially no damage was found in the DMTU rats, whereas a 25% rhodopsin loss was measured in the ascorbate-treated animals. Unsupplemented rats, however, lost 70% of their rhodopsin as a result of 3-1 hr light exposures. After 8 doses of light, DMTU treated rats retained 70% of the control rhodopsin level (2.1 nmol/eye), while the ascorbate-treated rats had only about 40% rhodopsin remaining. Importantly, however, for all exposures both the natural L-ascorbate and the unnatural D-stereoisomer of ascorbic acid were nearly equally protective.

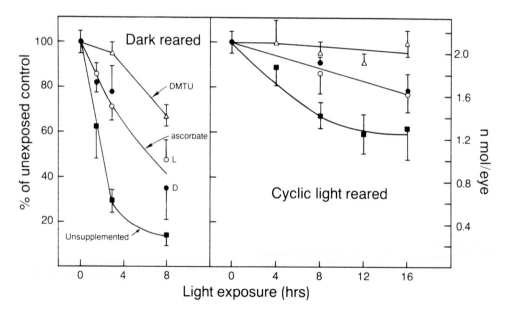

Figure 1. Rhodopsin was measured 2 wks after intermittent light exposure. Values shown are the mean ± SD for 8-12 separate determinations L = L-ascorbic acid, D = D-ascorbic acid.

Similar results were found for the cyclic-light-reared rats. Both the L- and D-ascorbate treatments provided equal protection, with rhodopsin levels intermediate between those in the unsupplemented rats and those treated with DMTU. In the cyclic-light-reared rats, however, the effect of the synthetic antioxidant was remarkable. Irrespective of the duration of light treatment, lasting for up to 48 hrs in the case of 16 light doses, DMTU provided complete protection against retinal damage. On the other hand, ascorbate protection was reduced as the duration of light exposure was extended.

B. TISSUE LEVELS OF ANTIOXIDANT

Because DMTU was so effective in reducing the extent of light damage, we determined its uptake and distribution, along with L-ascorbate, in retinal tissues. Table 1 contains the major results of these measurements.

Table 1

Tissue Distribution of L-Ascorbic Acid and DMTU[a]

	L-Ascorbic Acid (n = 4 - 20)			DMTU (n = 4 - 8)		
Time after injection[b]	Whole blood μ mol/ml	Retina n mol	RPE/Choroid n mol	Serum μ mol/ml	Retina n mol	RPE/Choroid n mol
Uninjected Control	0.03 ± 0.01	12.9 ± 1.3	2.0 ± 0.8	- 0 -	- 0 -	- 0 -
10 mins	2.3 ± 0.5	17.4 ± 1.8	7.6 ± 2.3	8.2 ± 3.0	100 ± 7.8	31.8 ± 5.7
4 or 7 hrs[c]	0.14 (2)	15.5 ± 1.9	2.4 ± 0.5	10.1± 1.7	196 ± 28.6	39.6 ± 16.3
24hrs	0.05 (2)	11.1 ± 2.0	ND[d]	2.7 ± 1.9	59.1 ± 32.2	14.8 ± 2.5

a: Results are the mean ± SD for the number of determinations in parenthesis - Rats were perfused with saline before analysis. b: IP injections 2x at 500 mg/kg 24 hrs apart. c: 4 hrs DMTU; 7 hrs L-ascorbic acid d: ND Not determined

In rats treated IP with equal doses of either of the antioxidants, both L-ascorbate and DMTU rapidly appeared in the blood, retina, and RPE/choroid. The level of DMTU in the serum was 8.2 μ mol/ml 10 min after injection and 100 nmol per retina; it was about 32 nmol in the RPE/choroid. Ascorbate levels were 2.3 μ mol/ml blood, and 17.4 and 7.6 nmol in the retina and RPE/choroid, respectively. Whereas, these levels were significantly higher than the endogenous levels of L-ascorbate present in uninjected controls, they were much lower than the DMTU levels in comparable rats. The half-life of DMTU was also longer than that of L-ascorbate. For example, DMTU levels were highest 4 hrs after injection and remained elevated for at least 24 hrs, L-ascorbate levels started to decline after only 10 min and were near control levels 24 hrs after administration. Thus, rats treated with DMTU accumulated higher levels of the antioxidant in retinal and RPE/choroid tissues, and retained higher levels for a longer period of time than ascorbate-treated rats.

C. MORPHOLOGICAL FINDINGS

To confirm the biochemical findings of reduced photoreceptor cell damage in antioxidant treated rats, the eyes from dark-reared rats were examined histologically. As shown in Figure 2, both L-ascorbate (B) treatment and DMTU (D) resulted in tissue sections with more normal morphology than those of the unsupplemented rats. (A and C)

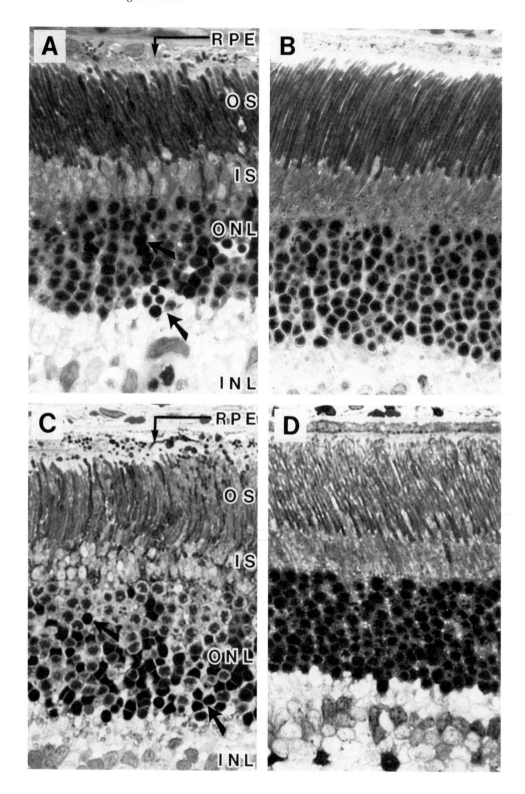

Figure 2. Light micrographs of rats exposed to three 1-hour cycles interrupted by 2-hour dark periods. A thirty minute recovery period was allowed following the final exposure before enucleation.

A: Littermate control to animal in B. The RPE is vacuolated and contains numerous phagosomes. Necrotic cells are present in the ONL (arrows). (X960). B: Ascorbate was given IP 24 hours and immediately before light exposure. Note that RPE appears normal in thickness. The ONL appears more normal than in A. (X860). C: The RPE is swolen and contains a large number of phagosomes. The OS are disorganized, and necrotic cells appear in the ONL (arrows). The IS is vacuolated. (X860). D: DMTU was injected IP 24 hours and immediately before exposure. The thickness of the RPE is normal and it contains few phagosomes. The OS, IS and ONL appear normal. (X860).

In the unsupplemented animals tissue damage typically included swelling of the retinal pigment epithelium, evidence of necrosis in the outer nuclear layer, loss of cone nuclei, distended outer segments, and the presence of a large number of phagosomes in the RPE and subretinal space. In all experimental cases, treatment with ascorbate or DMTU greatly reduced the degree of retinal damage. In general, DMTU seemed to be more effective than ascorbate. Most striking is the reduction in the number of phagosomes seen in comparison with the untreated controls.

D.   ROS FATTY ACIDS

To learn more about the effects of the antioxidants on ROS membranes we measured the levels of the major fatty acids in ROS isolated immediately after light exposure. In Table 2 the effects of antioxidant treatment have been compared for dark-reared rats following 8-1 hr light doses. As shown, both forms of ascorbate resulted in the same high level of ROS-22:6 fatty acid. Whereas 22:6 in the unsupplemented-light exposed rats was 8 mol% lower than in unexposed controls, 22:6 levels in both the L- and D-ascorbate treated rats were the same as control. Similarly, DMTU treated rat ROS retained just over 53 mol% 22:6 fatty acid. In addition, there were no significant changes in arachidonic acid (20:4), oleic acid (18:1) or the major saturated fatty acids (16:0; 18:0) in the antioxidant treated rat ROS. In the unsupplemented rats, however, ROS 16:0 was increased with respect to control, as was the mol% cholesterol. The levels of ROS-22:6 in cyclic-light- or dark-reared rats treated with DMTU before exposure to 16-1 hr light doses, were nearly the same as found in the ROS of unexposed rats (51-53 mol%).

Table 2
Major Fatty Acids in ROS from Dark Reared Rats
after 8 hrs Intermittent Light [a]

(mol %)

Fatty Acid	Unexposed (n = 10)	Unsupplemented (n = 8)	D-ascorbate (n = 4)	L-ascorbate (n = 4)	DMTU (n = 4)
16:0	12.0 ± 1.3	17.7 ± 1.9	13.4 ± 1.1	14.7 ± 2.2	12.8 ± 1.8
18:0	25.4 ± 1.8	25.4 ± 2.3	24.5 ± 1.4	25.4 ± 1.6	22.9 ± 1.2
18:1	4.2 ± 0.7	5.8 ± 1.1	2.8 ± 0.4	2.8 ± 0.9	4.3 ± 0.9
20:4	3.5 ± 0.3	4.6 ± 1.0	4.5 ± 0.3	3.8 ± 0.5	4.6 ± 0.7
22:6	51.2 ± 2.7	42.8 ± 3.1	51.2 ± 2.0	49.8 ± 3.8	53.2 ± 1.8
Cholesterol	11 ± 3	16 ± 4	11 ± 5	13 ± 6	14 ± 2

[a] ROS isolated immediately after the last hour of light exposure

E. TREATMENT WITH ASCORBATE PLUS DMTU

To determine if the ascorbic acid and DMTU effects were additive or synergistic, and because neither antioxidant completely protected dark-reared rats, we examined their combined effects on rhodopsin recovery in animals exposed to light for 8-1 hr periods. For these experiments DMTU was tested at 250 mg/kg, whereas L-ascorbic acid was given three times (500 mg/kg) to maintain higher tissue levels. As shown in Table 3, three IP doses of L-ascorbic acid or 2 injections of DMTU at one-half the normal dose resulted in a significant degree of protection. In the case, of ascorbate 59% of the control rhodopsin level was found, compared to only 18% in the uninjected rats; for DMTU the rhodopsin level was 45% of control. Together, the two anti-oxidants produced a nearly additive effect (1.7 nmol rhodopsin/eye). As expected, DMTU at the normal 500 mg dose resulted in greater protection than at the 250 mg dose. Rhodopsin recovery in this case (1.6 nmol/eye) was nearly the same as for the combined low dose DMTU and ascorbic acid. Additional ascorbic acid supplementation produced no greater rhodopsin recovery than with DMTU alone (data not shown).

Table 3
Rhodopsin Two Weeks after 8 hrs of Intermittent Light Treatment
(n mol/eye ± SD)

Unexposed control	Uninjected	DMTU[a] 2 x 250 mg/kg	AA[b] 3 x 500 mg/kg	DMTU + AA Combined	DMTU[a] 2 x: 500 mg/kg
2.2 ± 0.1 n = (8)	0.4 ± 0.1 (8)	1.0 ± 0.3 (12)	1.3 ± 0.4 (18)	1.7 ± 0.3 (10)	1.6 ± 0.1 (14)
100%	18%	45%	59%	77%	73%

a IP injection 24 hrs before and just prior to exposure: dark reared rats

b (AA) L-ascorbic acid given as above plus just before the start of 4th light cycle

IV. DISCUSSION

The results of this study support an antioxidative role for ascorbic acid and DMTU in protecting the retina from light induced damage. For ascorbate, both the natural L-stereoisomer and the unnatural D- form were equally protective (Figure 1). Ascorbate was most effective when both tissue and blood levels were high and less effective when those levels were low (Figure 1, Table 1). The degree of protection also depended on whether the rats were reared in a weak cyclic-light environment or in darkness before intense light treatment. This may relate to the different forms of light damage in the rats. Retinal damage in the dark-reared rats (Type I),[9,16,22] was extensive and protection by the antioxidants less. On the other hand, retinal damage to cyclic-light-reared rats by intermittent light was less and the protection greater. Irrespective of these differences, the similar degree of protection by L- or D-ascorbate indicates that each probably functioned as an antioxidant, as shown previously for D-ascorbate in guinea pigs[45] and as suggested for L-ascorbate in light damaged rats.[30,31,33] Thus, ascorbate does not appear to serve as an enzymatic cofactor during retinal light damage.

In the case of DMTU, retinal protection from light damage was remarkable. By either rhodopsin measurements (Figure 1) or histology (Figure 2), DMTU was more effective than ascorbic acid. In the dark-reared-DMTU-treated rats, only about 30% rhodopsin loss was measured after 8-1 hr light doses; in the cyclic-light-reared rats, protection was complete for up to 16-1 hr light doses. DMTU tissue levels were higher than ascorbate levels in comparable L-ascorbate injected rats, and the half-life of DMTU was longer (Table 1). Thus, DMTU given twice at a dose of 250 mg/kg provided a similar degree of protection to that of ascorbic acid given three times at a dose of 500 mg/kg (Table 3). Other studies have shown that DMTU is effective in reducing oxidant-induced lung injury,[47] uveitis[48] and endotoxin induced ocular inflammation[49] in experimental animals. It appears to be an efficient hydroxyl radical scavenger,[47] may interact with H_2O_2 to prevent hydroxyl radical formation,[47] and also reacts with hypochlorous acid produced by cells containing myeloperoxidase.[50]

In our study, DMTU not only reduced or prevented retinal damage, but also prevented the loss of 22:6 fatty acids from ROS membranes of light exposed rats (Table 2). This suggests that the intense light-mediated loss of 22:6 from ROS membranes occurs by an oxidative process.[24,30,34] Likewise, L- and D-ascorbic acid prevented the loss of ROS-22:6 in dark-reared rats, but retinal damage still occurred for both the ascorbate and DMTU treatments, alone or in combination, (Figure 1, Table 3). In Type I light damage, therefore, the oxidative loss of ROS-22:6 cannot be the only cause of retinal damage. On the other hand, in Type II damage (cyclic- light-reared animals) the loss of ROS-22:6 may be more causally related to the extent of retinal damage, as shown previously[24,29] and as suggested by the present work. At this time, the mechanism(s) of light damage is incompletely understood. Whether 22:6 oxidation results in the formation of a toxic photoproduct(s) or not, its loss from ROS membranes during intense light warrants further investigation.

Whatever the order of molecular events between the initial absorption of photons by rhodopsin and retinal light damage turns out to be, reactive oxygen species probably play an important role. It is tempting to speculate that the nearly simultaneous histological changes seen in the ROS, RIS, nuclear region (Figure 2), and photoreceptor synaptic terminal of intense light exposed rat retinas[7,8,23,28] may result from the diffusion of a light induced toxic substance(s). In this regard, antioxidants such as ascorbic acid and DMTU may be useful in helping to define the ultimate pathway of damaging reactions in the eye.

ACKNOWLEDGEMENTS

This work was supported by grant EY-1959 from the National Eye Institute to DTO and EY-3042 to JCB, and EY-3040 (Core Center grant to the Doheny Eye Institute).

V. REFERENCES

1. Hagins, W.A. The visual process: excitatory mechanisms in primary receptor cells. Annu. Rev. Biophys. Bioeng., 1, 131, 1972.

2. Yee, R. and Liebman P.A. Light-activated phosphodiesterase of the rod outer segment. Kinetics and parameters of activation and deactivation. J. Biol. Chem., 253, 8902, 1978.

3. Miller, W.H. Molecular mechanisms of photoreception, in Current Topics in Membranes and Transport, Vol. 15, Miller, W.H., Ed., Academic Press, New York, 1981.

4. Kuhn, H. Early steps in the light triggered activation of the cyclic GMP enzymatic pathway in rod photoreceptors, in Information and Energy Transduction in Biological Membranes, Alan R. Liss, New York, 1984. 303.

5. Brown, J.E., Rubin, L.J., Ghalayini, A.J., Tarver, A.P., Irvine, R.F., Berridge, M.J., and Anderson, R.E. Myo-inositol polyphosphate may be a messenger for visual excitation in Limulus photoreceptors, Nature, 311, 160, 1984.

6. Pugh, E.N. and Cobbs, W.H. Visual transduction in vertebrate rod and cones: A tale of two transmitters, calcium and cGMP. Vis. Res., 26, 1613, 1986.

7. Noell, W.K., Walker, V.S., Kang, B.S., and Berman, S. Retinal damage by light in rats. Invest. Ophthalmol., 5, 450, 1966.

8. Gorn, R.A. and Kuwabara, T. Retinal damage by visible light. Arch. Ophthalmol., 77, 115, 1967.

9. Noell, W.K. Possible mechanisms of photoreceptor damage by light in mammalian eyes. Vis. Res., 20, 1163, 1980.

10. Sperling, H.G. Prolonged intense spectral light effects on Rhesus retina, in The Effects of Constant Light on Visual Processes, Williams, T.P. and Baker, B.N., Eds., Plenum Press, New York, 1980. 195.

11. Lawwill, T. Effects of prolonged exposure of rabbit retina to low intensity light. Invest. Ophthalmol., 12, 45, 1980.

12. Ham, W.T., Miller, H.A., and Sliney, D.H. Retinal sensitivity to damage from short wavelength light. Nature, 260, 153, 1976.

13. Rapp, L.M. and Williams, T.P. A parametric study of retinal light damage in albino and pigmented rats, in The Effects of Constant Light on Visual Processes, Williams, T.P. and Baker, B.N., Eds., Plenum Press, New York, 1980. 133.

14. Williams, T.P. and Howell, W.L. Action spectrum of retinal light-damage in albino rats. Invest. Ophthalmol. Vis. Sci., 24, 285, 1983.

15. Kagan, V.E., Shvedova, A.A., Novikov, K.N., and Kozlov, Y.P. Light induced free radical oxidation of membrane lipids in photoreceptors of frog retina. Biochim. Biophys. Acta, 330, 76, 1973.

16. Noell, W.K. Hereditary retinal degeneration and damage by light, in Estratto dagli Atti Simposio di Oftalmologia Pediatrica Parma, Italy, 1974. 322.

17. O'Steen, W.K. Ovarian steroid effects on light-induced retinal photoreceptor damage. Exp. Eye Res., 25, 361, 1977.

18. Noell, W.K. Effects of environmental lighting and dietary vitamin A on the vulnerability of the retina to light damage. Photochem. Photobiol., 29, 717, 1979.

19. Organisciak, D.T. and Noell, W.K. The rod outer segment phospholipid/opsin ratio of rats maintained in darkness or cyclic light. Invest. Ophthalmol. Vis. Sci., 16, 188, 1977.

20. LaVail, M.M., Gorrin, G.M., Repaci, M.A., Thomas, L.A., and Ginsberg, H.M. Genetic regulation of light damage to photoreceptors. Invest. Ophthalmol. Vis. Sci., 28, 1043, 1987.

21. Organisciak, D.T., Jiang, Y-L., Wang, H-M., Pickford, M., and Blanks, J.C. Retinal light damage in rats exposed to intermittent light: Comparison to continuous exposure, Invest. Ophthalmol. Vis. Sci., 30, 795, 1989.

22. Noell, W.K. There are different kinds of retinal light damage in rats, in The Effects of Constant Light on Visual Processes, Williams, T.P. and Baker, B.N., Eds., Plenum Press, New York, 1980. 3.

23. Kuwabara, T. Retinal recovery from exposure to light. Amer. J. Ophthalmol., 70, 187, 1970.

24. Organisciak, D.T., Wang, H-M., and Noell, W.K. Aspects of the ascorbate protective mechanism in retinal light damage of rats with normal and reduced ROS docosahexaenoic acid, in Degenerative Retinal Disorders: Clinical and Laboratory Investigations, Hollyfield, J.G., Anderson, R.E., and LaVail, M.M., Eds., Alan R. Liss, New York, 1987. 455.

25. Noell, W.K., Organisciak, D.T., Ando, H., Braniecki, M.A., and Durlin, C. Ascorbate and dietary protective effects in retinal light damage of rats: Electrophysiological, histological and DNA measurements, in Degenerative Retinal Disorders: Clinical and Laboratory Investigations, Hollyfield, J.G., Anderson, R.E., and LaVail, M.M., Alan R. Liss, New York, 1987. 469.

26. Noell, W.K., Delmelle, M.C., and Albrecht, R. Vitamin A deficiency effect on retina: Dependence on light. Science, 172, 72, 1971.

27. Noell, W.K. and Albrecht, R. Irreversible effects of visible light on the retina: Role of vitamin A, Science, 172, 76, 1971.

28. Moriya, M., Baker, B.N., and Williams, T.P. Progression and reversibility of early light-induced alterations in rat retinal rods. Cell Tissue Res., 246, 607, 1986.

29. Penn, J.S., Naash, M.I., and Anderson, R.E. Effect of light history on retinal antioxidants and light damage susceptibility in the rat. Exp. Eye Res., 44, 779, 1987.

30. Organisciak, D.T., Wang, H-M., Li, Z-Y., and Tso, M.O.M. The protective effect of ascorbate in retinal light damage of rats. Invest. Ophthalmol. Vis. Sci., 26, 1580, 1985.

31. Li, Z-Y., Tso, M.O.M., Wang, H-M., and Organisciak, D.T. Amerlioration of photic injury in rat retina by ascorbic acid. Invest. Ophthalmol. Vis. Sci., 26, 1589, 1985.

32. Penn, J.S. and Anderson, R.E. Effect of light history on rod outer-segment membrane composition in the rat. Exp. Eye Res., 44, 767, 1987.

33. Organisciak, D.T., Jiang, Y-L., Wang, H-M., Bicknell, I.R. The protective effect of ascorbic acid in rats exposed to intermittent light. Invest. Ophthalmol. Vis. Sci., 31, 1195, 1990.

34. Wiegand, R.D., Giusto, N.M., Rapp, L.M., and Anderson, R.E. Evidence for rod outer segment lipid peroxidation following constant illumination of the rat retina. Invest. Ophthalmol. Vis. Sci., 24, 1433, 1983.

35. Organisciak, D.T., Favreau, P., and Wang, H-M. The enzymatic estimation of organic hydroperoxides in the rat retina. Exp. Eye Res., 36, 337, 1983.

36. Organisciak, D.T., Wang, H-M., and Kou, A.L. Ascorbate and glutathione levels in the developing normal and dystrophic rat retina: Effect of intense light exposure. Cur. Eye Res., 3, 257, 1984.

37. Hunt, D.F., Organisciak, D.T., Wang, H-M., and Wu, R.L.C. Alpha-Tocopherol in the developing rat retina: A high pressure liquid chromatographic analysis. Cur. Eye Res., 3, 1281, 1984.

38. Wiegand, R.D., Joel, C.D., Rapp, L.M., Nielsen, J.C., Maude, M.B., and Anderson, R.E. Polyunsaturated fatty acids and vitamin E in rat rod outer segments during light damage, Invest. Ophthalmol. Vis. Sci., 27, 727, 1986.

39. Nishikimi, M. Oxidation of ascorbic acid with superoxide anion generated by the xanthine-xanthine oxidase system, Biochem. Biophys. Res. Commun., 63, 463, 1975.

40. Bodannes, R.S. and Chan, P.C. Ascorbic acid as a scavenger of singlet oxygen. F.E.B.S. Letters, 105, 195, 1979.

41. Niki, E., Saito, T., Kawakami, A., and Kamiya, Y. Inhibition of oxidation of methyl linoleate in solution by vitamin E and vitamin C. J. Biol. Chem., 259, 4177, 1984.

42. Packer, J.E., Slater, T.F., and Willson, R.L. Direct observation of a free radical interaction between vitamin E and Vitamin C. Nature, 278, 737, 1979.

43. Leung, H.W., Van, M.J., and Mavis, R.D. The cooperative interaction between vitamin E and Vitamin C in suppression of peroxidation of membrane phospholipids. Biochim. Biophys. Acta, 664, 266, 1981.

44. Delclos, K.B. and Blumberg, P.M. Identification of ascorbic acid as the heat-stable factor from brain which inactivates the phorbol ester receptor. Can. Res., 42, 1227, 1982.

45. Kunert, K-J. and Tappel, A.L. The effect of vitamin C on in vivo lipid peroxidation in guinea pigs as measured by pentane and ethane production. Lipids, 18, 271, 1983.

46. Organisciak, D.T., Darrow, R.M., and Marak, G.E. Protection against retinal light damage by dimethylthiourea, Invest. Ophthalmol. Vis. Sci. (Suppl.), Vol. 31, 294, 1990.

47. Fox, R.B. Prevention of granulocyte-mediated oxidant lung injury in rats by a hydroxyl radical scavenger, dimethylthiourea. J. Clin. Invest., 74, 1456, 1984.

48. Rao, N.A., Fernandez, M.A., Sevanian, A., Romero, J.L., Till, G.O., and Marak, G.E. Treatment of experimental lens-induced uveitis by dimethylthiourea. Ophthalmic Res., 20, 106, 1988.

49. Fleisher, L.N., Ferrell, J.B., Olson, N.C., and McGahan, M.C. Dimethylthiourea inhibits the inflammatory response to intravitreally-injected endotoxin. Exp. Eye Res., 48, 561, 1989.

50. Wasil, M., Halliwell, B., Grootveld, M., Moorhouse, C.P., Hutchinson, D.C.S., and Baum, H. The specificity of thiourea, dimethylthiourea and dimethylsulphoxide as scavengers of hydroxyl radicals. Biochem. J., 243, 867, 1987.

THE INFLUENCE OF CARBOHYDRATES ON THE ASSOCIATION BETWEEN THE RETINAL PIGMENT EPITHELIUM AND NATURAL AND SYNTHETIC RHODOPSIN-CONTAINING MEMBRANES

EDWARD L. KEAN[‡], JAMES J. PLANTNER, and YOSHIAKI ITOH[*]
LABORATORY FOR EYE RESEARCH and DEPARTMENT OF BIOCHEMISTRY[‡]
CASE WESTERN RESERVE UNIVERSITY

I. ABSTRACT

A summary of research is presented which investigated the hypothesis that the carbohydrate groups of rhodopsin act as recognition signals for the interaction between rhodopsin-containing membranes and the cells of the retinal pigment epithelium (RPE). The surface orientation of the carbohydrates of rhodopsin, mannose and GlcNAc, on inverted disc membranes and rhodopsin-liposomes was shown to be such that they were available for reaction with hypothetical receptors on the RPE. Competition studies concluded that lectin-like recognition between the RPE cells of the embryonic chick maintained in cell culture and the target membranes was not involved, and in addition, galactosylation of rhodopsin did not serve as a recognition signal. Further evidence was presented demonstrating the influence of charge on the process. Evidence supporting the notion that the rhodopsin molecule, albeit at sites other than its saccharides, may be involved in the recognition process was obtained by blocking reactions with anti-rhodopsin Fab fragments.

II. INTRODUCTION

Considerable attention has been directed to the function that carbohydrate groups in glycoproteins may serve as targeting signals for cell-cell, cell-membrane, and cell-soluble macromolecule interactions.[1] In the visual system, hypotheses in this direction have stimulated both speculation and research concerning the involvement of glycoconjugates in the phagocytosis of rod outer segments (ROS) by the retinal pigment epithelium (RPE). Common to the surface of all cells is the presence of an array of glycolipids and glycoproteins. Complex carbohydrates of these types have been demonstrated on the RPE cell surface,[2] although clear evidence demonstrating their function as receptors for the shed ROS is still lacking. The initiating phase of the series of events in the phagocytic process must be the binding of the shed packet of discs to the RPE. In that rhodopsin is the major glycoprotein of the ROS, it has been suggested that the carbohydrates of this molecule, mannose and GlcNAc,[3] might serve as sites of recognition for interaction with receptors on the RPE. We have directed our attention to exploring this latter possibility. Our studies have used the RPE of the embryonic chick maintained in cell culture as the major biological tool, and inverted ROS disc membranes, intact ROS, and rhodopsin-liposomes as the target membrane systems. The influence of monosaccharides and oligosaccharides on the association of the rhodopsin-containing membranes with the RPE cells was followed by a sensitive, specific radioimmunoassay for rhodopsin.[4] Evidence was obtained[5,6] rejecting the concept that the carbohydrates of rhodopsin acted as recognition signals, and also against the proposal that the presence of galactose on this molecule served in this manner for binding to the ROS.[6] This report is a review of some of these studies, and additional evidence in this direction. Further complexities associated with these processes were revealed with the demonstration that ionic strength of the incubation medium and charge properties of the ligands strongly influenced the association between the rhodopsin-containing membranes and the cells. That the rhodopsin molecule may still serve as focus of recognition, although not through its carbohydrates, received support from experiments in which the association was blocked by pretreating rhodopsin-liposomes with anti-rhodopsin Fab fragments. In addition, recent preliminary studies have suggested the presence of rhodopsin receptors on the RPE.[7]

III. MATERIALS AND METHODS

A. ROD OUTER SEGMENTS AND DISC MEMBRANES

Rod outer segment disc membranes were isolated from fresh bovine eyes by the Ficoll procedure[8] and intact ROS isolated as described previously.[6]

B. RHODOPSIN-LIPOSOMES

Bovine rhodopsin was purified from frozen, dark-adapted retinas (Hormel Co., Austin, Minn.) as described previously[3]. Rhodopsin-liposomes were prepared by using egg phosphatidylcholine (Avanti Biochemicals, Inc., Birmingham, Ala.) and purified bovine rhodopsin (molar ratio: 100:1, respectively) as described previously.[9] The concentration of rhodopsin in the liposomes was determined from the difference in absorbance measured in the presence of hydroxylamine at 498nm before and after bleaching in 5% Triton X-100. Calculations were based on an extinction coefficient of 40,600.[10] Rhodopsin concentration was also measured by radioimmunoassay (RIA) for rhodopsin.[4]

C. CELL CULTURE

RPE cells were isolated from 7 day chick embryos and maintained in primary culture as described previously.[11] Secondary cultures were prepared from the primary cultures by dissociation with Coon's enzyme solution.[11] The cells were grown to confluency and maintained for an additional 1-2 weeks in Eagle's minimum essential medium containing 5% fetal bovine serum.

D. INCUBATION OF DISC MEMBRANES OR RHODOPSIN-LIPOSOMES WITH CULTURED RPE CELLS; ASSAYS

Cell association was measured as previously.[5] In short, immediately prior to the incubation, the growth medium was removed from the cells, and the confluent layer was washed with DPBS⁻. A suspension of ROS disc membranes or rhodopsin-liposomes in DPBS⁻ containing 5.6 mM glucose was added to the cells, and incubation carried out at 37°C or 4°C for various periods of time in the light. After incubation, the suspension was removed, the cells washed 12 times with DPBS⁻, and the monolayer removed by peeling off the entire sheet. The latter step was necessary in order to eliminate the artifactual contribution of rhodopsin-liposomes adhering to the plastic. In the presence of 1 ml of 5% Triton X-100, containing 1 mM PMSF, the cells, maintained on ice, were disrupted by sonication. The rhodopsin content of the extract was measured by RIA[4] and protein by a modification of the Lowry procedure.[12] Association was based on rhodopsin per milligram protein. Viability of the RPE cells was measured by trypan blue exclusion following incubation of parallel cultures.

E. PREPARATION OF Fab FRAGMENTS

Antibody to bovine rhodopsin was prepared from mouse ascites fluid according to the method described by Tung.[13] IgG was purified from this preparation by precipitation from 18% Na_2SO_4, resolubilization, and ion exchange chromatography on DEAE cellulose.[14] Fab fragments were prepared from the purified IgG by papain digestion and purified by DEAE cellulose chromatography.[15] The Fab fragments were shown to maintain cross-reactivity with bovine rhodopsin in the RIA assay. When assayed by Ouchterlony double diffusion, the Fab fragments cross-reacted with commercially obtained (Pel-Freeze, Rogers, Ark.) goat anti-mouse F(ab')$_2$, while no reactivity was detected when tested against goat anti-mouse Fc fragment serum (Cappel Laboratories, Malvern, Pa.).

Rhodopsin-liposomes were incubated with varying amounts of either anti-rhodopsin Fab or commercial control mouse Fab in 0.04M Na phosphate, pH 7.8, at 25° for 2 hr. The rhodopsin-liposomes were centrifuged at 100,000xg for 45 min, and the pellet resuspended in DPBS⁻ prior to incubation with RPE. Varying molar ratios of Fab/rhodopsin were present during the preincubation.

F. GALACTOSYLATION OF ROS DISC MEMBRANES

Disc membranes were galactosylated using milk galactosyltransferase and UDP[^{3}H] galactose, and analyzed as described previously.[5] Control membranes were treated in the same manner, but in the absence of the sugar nucleotide.

G. MATERIALS

The following materials were obtained from the indicated sources: Eagle's minimum essential medium with Earle's salts, fetal bovine serum, from GIBCO Laboratories, Grand Island, NY; heparin, chondroitin sulfate, fucoidin, from Sigma, St. Louis, Mo. Phosphomannan was a generous gift from Dr. M.E. Slodki of the U.S. Department of Agriculture Research Laboratory, Peoria, Ill. Neoglycoproteins were kindly donated by

Dr. Y. C. Lee, Johns Hopkins University, Baltimore, MD, and by Dr. M. Monsigny, Laboratory of Glycoconjugate Research, Universite' d'Orleans, Cedex, France.

IV. RESULTS

A. MONOSACCHARIDES AND THE BINDING OF NATURAL AND SYNTHETIC RHODOPSIN-CONTAINING MEMBRANES

1. Disc Membranes and Rod Outer Segments

a. Carbohydrate Orientation; Effect of Mannose and GlcNAc:

The intradiscal location of the carbohydrate groups of rhodopsin in native discs has been demonstrated previously.[16] Consistent with this orientation, the binding of ^{125}I-succinyl concanavalin A was enhanced 15-20 fold after freezing and thawing as compared to native membranes.[6] Discs perturbed in this manner, (F/T discs), with their carbohydrate groups now accessible to surface reactions, served as substrates to investigate the influence of exogenously added carbohydrates on their interaction with RPE cells. Saturation kinetics were observed for the association of the F/T discs with embryonic chick RPE cells, a process which was also temperature dependent; the rate at 37°C being 3.5 fold greater than at 4°C.[6]

Table 1. Effect of Monosaccharides on the Binding of Rhodopsin-Liposomes and Disc Membranes by the Chick Retinal Pigment Epithelium

Bovine ROS disc membranes (30 μM) or rhodopsin-liposomes (5.5 μM) were incubated with secondary cultures of chick embryo RPE cells in the presence of the indicated sugars. Binding was measured by RIA as indicated in Materials and Methods.

| | Binding (% of Control)[a] | |
Sugar	Disc Membranes[b]	Rhodopsin-Liposomes[c]
Glucose	148 ± 8(4)	89 ± 2(6)
Mannose	114 ± 2 (2)	97 ± 4(20))
L-Fucose	125 ± 2(2)	90 ± 5(9)
GlcNAc	74 ± 8(5)	124 ± 10(6)
Galactose	93 ± 2(2)	84 ± 2(5)
Fructose	--------	93 ± 2(3)
GalNAc	--------	91 ± 5(3)

[a] Data are presented as the mean ± S.E.M. (number of determinations)

[b] Sugars were present at a concentration of 5.6 mM during incubation at 37°C for 2 hr.

c Sugars were present at a concentration of 150 mM during incubation at 37°C for 90 min.

The first indication that available carbohydrate groups on the discs may not play a role in these processes was the observation that there was little difference in the binding between native and F/T discs. This was substantiated in a series of experiments in which discs were incubated in the presence of high concentrations of mannose and GlcNAc, the sugars in rhodopsin, as seen in Table 1. In the presence of from 200 to 2,000 fold molar excess of these sugars over that of the rhodopsin used during the incubations, there was little or no inhibition of the association of the F/T discs with the RPE cells. Similar results were obtained using rod outer segments instead of disc membranes.[6]

b. Galactosylation of Rhodopsin

The presence of trace amounts of galactosylated rhodopsin <u>in vivo</u> has been reported,[17] and the suggestion has been made that galactose might be involved as a site of recognition in the phagocytosis of ROS.[18] We have investigated this possibility by examining the effect of enzymatically galactosylating rhodopsin in purified F/T disc membranes (using the galactosyltransferase of milk) on their binding by the RPE cell, as seen in Figure 1. The results from these studies demonstrated that galactosylation of rhodopsin in the membranes did not result in an enhanced association of discs with the RPE.[6] This was true for incubations carried out at 4°C (surface binding) or at 37°C (binding plus internalization). There was actually a decrease in association compared to control disc membranes subjected to a mock galactosylation.

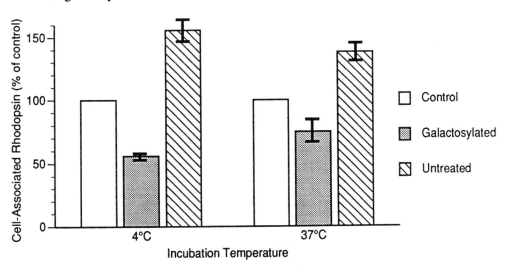

Figure 1. Effect of galactosylation of ROS disc membranes on their association with RPE cells. F/T ROS disc membranes were galactosylated as described in Materials and Methods. Control membranes were treated identically, but without UDP-galactose. The galactosylated membranes (0.12 mole galactose/mole rhodopsin) control membranes and untreated membranes were incubated at 4°C or 37°C with secondary cultures of chick embryo RPE cells for 3 hr. The equivalent rhodopsin concentration was about 20-30 μM. Following incubation, the binding by the cells was measured by RIA, as indicated in Materials and Methods.

2. Rhodopsin-Liposomes; A Synthetic Membrane System

a. Carbohydrate Orientation

Affinity purified rhodopsin incorporated into synthetic membranes in the presence of phospholipids (liposomes) was used as a substrate to explore the influence of carbohydrates on the interaction with RPE cells, in addition to the natural vesicles isolated from the retina described above. The orientation of the carbohydrate groups of rhodopsin in the liposomes was examined by following their lectin-induced aggregation.[9] Light-scattering studies using con A, succinylated con A, and wheat germ agglutinin clearly demonstrated the surface orientation of the carbohydrate groups of rhodopsin, mannose and GlcNAc, and their accessibility to reactions that take place at this locus.

b. Influence of Monosaccharides on the Association with RPE; Influence of Lectins.

In the presence of concentrations of mannose and GlcNAc of up to 33,000 fold molar excess over the rhodopsin-liposomes in the incubation (based on rhodopsin equivalents), no interference was seen in the association of the vesicles with the RPE cells (Table 1). In addition to these two sugars, a variety of other carbohydrates tested at this same high concentration did not inhibit the association of the vesicles with the cells. In addition to using RPE cells from the embryonic chick, many of these same characteristics were observed with bovine RPE cells, maintained in culture.[5]

Although endogenous lectin-like activity was not found on the RPE that mediated binding to the sugar groups of rhodopsin, the presence of exogenously added plant lectins, added at 0.28 μM concentrations, resulted in greatly enhanced binding: con A, 24 fold; WGA, 47 fold. Consistent with the lack of involvement of galactose in this process observed previously with the disc membranes, the presence of Maclura pomifera (a lectin with specificity toward α-D-galactose) did not enhance binding.[5]

c. Effect of Neoglycoproteins

Synthetic glycoproteins composed of BSA to which carbohydrates are covalently attached (neoglycoproteins) have been observed to inhibit cell-ligand interactions, even at nanomolar concentrations, where free sugars have little effect,[19] reflecting the higher binding constant of the polymer-bound saccharides. When examined in the present system at 10^{-5}M, the following neoglycoproteins showed the indicated % activity as compared to the controls: BSA,99%; BSA-galactose $_{(13)}$, 84%; BSA-mannose$_{(24)}$, 89%; BSA glucose$_{(12)}$, 81%; BSA-GlcNAc$_{(25)}$, 80%; BSA-mannose-6-phosphate$_{(16)}$, 72%. Thus, most of these compounds showed little inhibition of the binding of the rhodopsin-liposomes to the RPE cell, the greatest inhibition being shown by the mannose-6-phosphate derivative.

B. EFFECT OF ANTI-RHODOPSIN Fab

The studies described above demonstrated the relative lack of interference by carbohydrates on the association of natural and synthetic forms of rhodopsin-containing membranes with RPE cells. These findings argue against the involvement of the carbohydrate groups of rhodopsin as sites of recognition for the process of phagocytosis. This does not rule out other regions of this molecule playing such a role. We examined the possibility that if receptors for rhodopsin are present on the RPE cell, albeit recognizing sites other than the carbohydrates, blocking their access to rhodopsin on the target membranes with an antibody against rhodopsin might result in an interference in the binding process. In order to avoid the complications of multivalency and the participation of FC receptors, Fab fragments were prepared from mouse anti-bovine rhodopsin for use in these experiments. The rhodopsin-liposomes were pre-coated with this preparation and the influence of this treatment on their association with RPE cells was investigated. As seen in Figure 2, when compared with control Fab, coating the liposomes with anti-rhodopsin Fab brought about an enhanced inhibition in the association of the vesicles with the cells.[20] With decreasing ratio of Fab to rhodopsin (using a constant amount of rhodopsin-liposomes) there was relatively little inhibition by control Fab while there continued to be considerable inhibition by anti-rhodopsin Fab. Thus, at a ratio of 1:8 of Fab/rhodopsin-liposomes, there was no inhibition by control Fab, but 21% inhibition by anti-rhodopsin Fab.

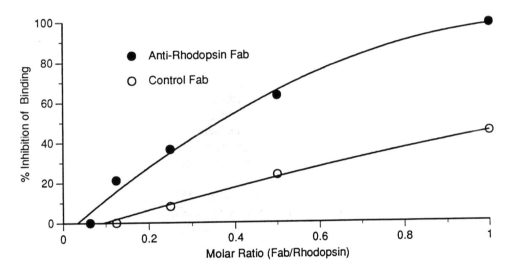

Figure 2.   Effect of pretreatment of rhodopsin-liposomes with anti-rhodopsin Fab on their association with RPE cells. Rhodopsin-liposomes were preincubated with varying molar ratios of either mouse anti-rhodopsin Fab or control mouse Fab at 25° for 2 hr., as described in Materials and Methods. After washing, the pretreated rhodopsin-liposomes were incubated with cultured chick embryo RPE cells at 37°C for 90 min., and their association with the cells was measured by RIA, as indicated in Materials and Methods. (Shirakawa and Kean, unpublished observations)

C. INFLUENCE OF CHARGE

The inhibition of binding observed above with BSA-mannose-6-phosphate suggested the possible involvement of phosphomannosyl receptors in the recognition process. Experiments were carried out which examined the effect of phosphorlyated sugars in the incubation medium. As seen in Table 2, considerable inhibition in association of the rhodopsin-liposomes with the RPE cells occurred in the presence of of mannose-6-phosphate, glucose-6-phosphate, and fructose-6-phosphate. However, when the ionic strength of the incubation medium was adjusted by removing an amount of NaCl from the DPBS⁻ buffer equal to the concentration of the sugar phosphate added, a great decrease in or elimination of the inhibition was seen. These observations suggest the influence of charge or ionic strength on the binding rather than specific phosphohexosyl recognition. The influence of charge received additional support when sulfated sugars were tested. As seen in Table 2, strong inhibition in binding was also observed in the presence of glucose-6 and glucose-3 sulfates. As observed above, the simple sugars by themselves brought about little or no inhibition.

Table 2. Effect of Sugar Phosphates and Sulfates on the Binding of Rhodopsin-Liposomes by the Chick Retinal Pigment Epithelium

Rhodopsin-liposomes (R-L) (5.5 µM) were incubated at 37°C for 90 min. with secondary cultures of chick embryo RPE cells in the presence of the indicated concentrations of the compounds listed below. Binding was measured by RIA as indicated in Materials and Methods.

Compound	Concentration (mM)	Binding of the R-L (% of Control)[a] Ionic Strength[b] Not Adjusted	Adjusted
Mannose-6-PO_4	5	$80.5 \pm 2.0(3)$	$98.0 \pm 9.8(6)$
	15	$63.8 \pm 5.5(6)$	$79.7 \pm 2.5(6)$
	50	$53.9 \pm 4.2(3)$	$91.7 \pm 0.7(2)$
Glucose-6-PO_4	5	$42.3 \pm 3.7(3)$	$94.1 \pm 4.0(3)$
	15	$55.6 \pm 5.1(3)$	$97.2 \pm 0.3(3)$
Fructose-6-PO_4	5	--------	$87.6 \pm 6.3(3)$
	15	$33.1 \pm 0.8(3)$	$87.6 \pm 4.8(3)$
Pentamannose PO_4	5	$98.3 \pm 6.6(3)$	--------
	15	$110 \pm 13.(3)$	--------
	30	$69.2 \pm 4.9(2)$	--------
Glucose-3-SO_4	5	$32.4 \pm 1.9(3)$	--------
Glucose-6-SO_4	5	$19.1 \pm 3.3(3)$	--------

[a] Data are presented as the mean ± S.E.M. (number of determinations)

[b] Ionic strength was adjusted by removing an equivalent amount of NaCl from the DPBS⁻ buffer during incubation, as described in Materials and Methods.

The influence of charge was also indicated when several polymers were examined. As seen in Table 3, strong inhibition of association was observed in the presence of several phosphorylated and sulfated polysaccharides.

Table 3. Effect of Charged Carbohydrate Polymers on the Binding of Rhodopsin-Liposomes (R-L) by the Chick Retinal Pigment Epithelium

Rhodopsin-liposomes (5.5 µM) were incubated at 37°C for 90 min. with secondary cultures of chick embryo RPE cells in the presence of the indicated concentrations of the compounds listed below. Binding was measured by RIA as indicated in Materials and Methods.

Compound	Concentration (mg/ml)	Binding of the R-L (% of Control)[a]
Phosphomannan	1	117 ± 7.2(3)
	5	44.7 ± 2.7(6)
	10	24.0 ± 0.4(2)
	15	16.0 ± 0.5(3)
Fucoidin	1	6.5 ± 3.1(5)
	10	2.5 ± 0.5(3)
Chondroitin SO_4	1	36.0 ± 11.(6)
Heparin	1	24.5 ± 3.1(2)

[a] Data are presented as the mean ± S.E.M. (number of determinations)

V. DISCUSSION

While the phenomena of the shedding of ROS and their phagocytosis by the cells of the RPE during the process of rod renewal have been well-documented, little is still known concerning the mechanisms governing these processes. Research from several laboratories has explored the initiating events, i.e., the recognition and binding of the membranes by the RPE. An approach that has guided much of this research has been to explore the involvement of carbohydrates, in analogy to their roles in other systems, as cell surface receptors, as signals for protein targeting, in cell-cell and cell-membrane interactions.[1] Hypotheses have been made invoking the participation of carbohydrates on both of the two entities involved, i.e., on the target (both natural and synthetic membranes and beads), and the RPE. The involvement of glycoprotein receptors on the RPE has received attention by several laboratories.[2, 21-23] The present studies have explored the possibility that the carbohydrates of rhodopsin played a role as recognition markers. Our studies used inverted ROS disc membranes and rhodopsin-liposomes as model systems in which rhodopsin is the major protein of the former membrane and the sole protein of the latter.

These studies concluded that the carbohydrate groups of rhodopsin do not function in this manner. Findings from several other laboratories are consistent with this conclusion. Thus, McLaughlin's laboratory showed that the uptake by normal rat RPE of mannose-coated[24] and GlcNAc-coated[25] styrene beads was less than that of uncoated beads. Philp, et al[26] reported a lack of inhibition of the phagocytosis of ROS by embryonic chick RPE in the presence of a tryptic glycopeptide prepared from rhodopsin, or high concentrations of BSA-mannose or mannan. Gregory, et al[21] observed that the free monosaccharides, mannose, fucose and galactose not only did not inhibit phagocytosis, but stimulated the process. However, Tarnowski, et al[27] reported the phagocytosis of mannan coated beads and the uptake of mannose-BSA, suggested to be due to the presence of specific mannose receptors on the RPE cell.

The lack of involvement of the saccharides of rhodopsin as recognition signals for binding and phagocytosis of ROS was also indicated by the studies of Laird and Molday.[28] They observed little or no inhibition in ROS binding or phagocytosis by bovine RPE cells in the presence of frozen/thawed disc membranes or in the presence of an excess of the peptide from the amino terminus of rhodopsin, nor when the ROS were labeled with an anti-rhodopsin monoclonal antibody or its $F(ab')_2$ fragment. However, Laird and Molday concluded in addition that the rhodopsin molecule per se does not function as a signal for binding the ROS to the RPE cell. In contrast, we have observed that treating rhodopsin-liposomes with the Fab fragment from a polyclonal antibody against rhodopsin resulted in considerable inhibition of association with RPE cells. Since the monoclonal antibody used by Laird and Molday was directed toward the amino terminus of the molecule, it remains possible that regions of rhodopsin other than the amino terminus may play a role in this process. Further studies in this regard which have been carried out suggest the presence of rhodopsin receptors on the RPE cell (Kean, et al [7]). High specificity was demonstrated toward rhodopsin in competition studies with a variety of other glycoproteins for the binding of ^{125}I-rhodopsin with embryonic chick RPE cells. Whether such components play a role in binding and phagocytosis is not known at this time.

It has been proposed and often entertained in the eye research literature that the galactosylation of rhodopsin, either transient or present on a limited population of molecules, may serve as a signal for recognition and subsequent phagocytosis of ROS by the cells of the RPE.[18] Heretofore, however, there has been no direct experimental data available to evaluate this hypothesis. Results from the experiments described here demonstrated that enzymatic galactosylation of rhodopsin in frozen/thawed disc membranes failed to enhance the binding of the discs to the RPE.

Phosphohexosyl recognition for the binding of lysosomal enzymes via the mannose-6-phosphate receptor in the Golgi apparatus is an extensively documented process.[29] Evidence has also appeared implicating a mannose-6-phosphate receptor in phagocytosis.[30] Tarnowski, et al[31] have demonstrated the presence of a mannose-6-phosphate receptor on the RPE cell, but have pointed out that this process may not be involved in normal phagocytosis of ROS. In the present report we have shown that although phosphorylated sugars can inhibit the association of rhodopsin-liposomes with the RPE cell, this effect may reflect more the influence of charge rather than an effect due to a sugar phosphate receptor since the inhibition was reduced or abolished when the ionic strength of the incubation medium was adjusted to account for the contribution of the ligand. In addition, extensive inhibition was also brought about by sulfated sugars. Gregory, et al[21] have described the inhibition by several glycosaminoglycans of the binding and phagocytosis of ROS by bovine RPE. In the present studies, these types of compounds also resulted in extensive inhibition of the binding of rhodopsin-liposomes. This effect was similar to that which occurred in the presence of the phosphorylated polysaccharide, phosphomannan, and the sulfated fucose polymer, fucoidin. Thus, as with the sugar phosphates and sulfates, these latter observations suggest that charge may play an important role in the interaction between the RPE and rhodopsin-containing membranes, in addition to the possible involvement of phosphate- or sulfate- glycosylation sequences.

VI. REFERENCES

1. Paulson, J.C., Glycoproteins: what are the sugar chains for?, TIBS, **14**, 272, 1989.
2. Colley, N.J., Clark, V.M., and Hall, M.O., Surface modification of retinal pigment epithelial cells: Effects on phagocytosis and glycoprotein composition, Exp. Eye Res., **44**, 377, 1987.
3. Plantner, J.J. and Kean, E.L., Carbohydrate composition of bovine rhodopsin, J. Biol. Chem., **251**, 1548, 1976.
4. Plantner, J.J., Hara, S. and Kean, E.L., Improved, rapid radioimmunoassay for rhodopsin, Exp. Eye Res., **35**, 534, 1982.
5. Shirakawa, H., Ishiguro, S., Itoh, Y., Plantner, J.J. and Kean, E.L., Are sugars involved in the binding of rhodopsin-membranes by the retinal pigment epithelium?, Invest. Ophthalmol. Vis. Sci., **28**, 628, 1987.
6. Lentrichia, B.B., Itoh, Y., Plantner, J.J., and Kean, E.L., The influence of carbohydrates on the binding of rod outer-segment (ROS) disc membranes and intact ROS by the cells of the retinal pigment epithelium of the embryonic chick, Exp. Eye Res., **44**, 127, 1987.
7. Kean, E.L., Gupta, P., and Lowder, E., Binding of rhodopsin by RPE cells, Invest. Ophthalmol. Vis. Sci., Supplement, **31**, 371, 1990.
8. Smith, H.G., Stubbs, G.W., and Litman, B.J., The isolation and purification of osmotically intact discs from retinal rod outer segments, Exp. Eye Res., **20**,211, 1975
9. Ishiguro, S., Shirakawa, H. and Kean, E.L., Reactivity with lectins of the saccharide components of rhodopsin in reconstituted membranes, Biochim. Biophys. Acta, **812**, 752, 1985.
10. Wald, G. and Brown, P.K., The molar extinction of rhodopsin, J. Gen. Physiol., **38**,189, 1953.
11. Kean, E.L., Hara, S. and Lentrichia, B.B., Binding of Neoglycoproteins by the chick pigment epithelium cell in culture, Vision Res., **21**, 133, 1981.

12. Markwell, M.A.K., Haas, S.M., Bieber, L.L. and Tolbert, N.E., A modification of the Lowry procedure to simplify protein determination in membrane and lipoprotein samples, Anal. Biochem., **8 7**, 206, 1978.

13. Tung, A.S., Production of large amounts of antibodies, nonspecific immunoglobulins, and other serum proteins in ascitic fluids of individual mice and guinea pigs, Methods Enz. , **9 3**, 12, 1983.

14. Mishell, B.B. and Shiigi, S.M., *Selected Methods in Cellular Immunology*, W.H. Freeman Co., San Francisco, 1980, 280.

15. Mage, M.G., Preparation of Fab fragments from IgGs of different animal species, Methods Enz., **7 0**, 142, 1980.

16. Clark, S.P., and Molday, R.S., Orientation of membrane glycoproteins in sealed rod outer segment disks, Biochem., **1 8**, 5868, 1979.

17. Smith, S.B., and O'Brien, P.J., A subset of rat rhodopsin contains galactose, Invest. Ophthalmol. & Vis. Sci., Supplement, **3 1**, 4, 1990.

18. O'Brien, P.J., Rhodopsin as a glycoprotein: a possible role for the oligosaccharide in phagocytosis, Exp. Eye Res., **2 3**, 127, 1976.

19. Schlepper-Schafer, J., Holl, N., Kolb-Bachofen, V., Friedrich, E., and Kolb, H., Role of carbohydrates in rat leukemia cell-liver macrophage cell contacts, Biol. Cell, **5 2**, 253, 1984.

20. Shirakawa, H., and Kean, E.L., Binding of rhodopsin-liposomes (RL) by retinal pigment epithelium (RPE) cells of the embryonic chick, Invest. Ophthalmol. Vis. Sci. , Supplement, **2 6**, 339, 1985.

21. Gregory, C.Y., Converse, C.A., and Foulds, W.S., Effect of glycoconjugates on rod outer segment phagocytosis by retinal pigment epithelial explants *in vitro* , Current Eye Res., **9** , 65, 1990.

22. Boyle, D.L., and McLaughlin, B.J., The effect of swainsonine on the phagocytosis of rod outer segments by rat RPE, Current Eye Res. , **9**, 407, 1990.

23. Hall, M.O., Burgess, B.L., Arakawa, H., and Fliesler, S.J., The effect of inhibitors of glycoprotein synthesis and processing on the phagocytosis of rod outer segment by cultured retinal pigment epithelial cells, Glycobiology, **1**, 51, 1990.

24. Seyfried-Williams, R., and McLaughlin, B.J., The use of sugar-coated beads to study phagocytosis in normal and dystrophic retina, Vis. Res., **2 3**, 485, 1983.

25. Tarnowski, B.I., and McLaughlin, B.J., Phagocytic interactions of sialated glycoprotein, sugar and lectin coated beads with rat retinal pigment epithelium, Current Eye Res., **6**, 1079, 1987.

26. Philp, N.J., Nachmias, V.T., Lee, D., Stramm, L., and Buzdygon, B., Is rhodopsin the ligand for receptor-mediated phagocytosis of rod outer segments by retinal pigment epithelium?, Exp. Eye Res., **4 6**, 21, 1988.

27. Tarnowski, B.I., Shepherd, V.L., and McLaughlin, B.J., Mannose-6-phosphate receptors on the plasma membrane on rat retinal pigment epithelial cells, Invest. Ophthalmol. Vis. Sci., **2 9**, 291, 1988.

28. Laird, D.W., and Molday, R.S., Evidence against the role of rhodopsin in rod outer segment binding to RPE cells, Invest. Ophthalmol. Vis. Sci., **2 9**, 419, 1988.

29. Kornfeld, S., Trafficking of lysosomal enzymes, <u>FASEB J.</u>, **1**, 462, 1987.
30. Stoolman, L.M., Tenforde, T.S., and Rosen, S.D., Phosphomannosyl receptors may participate in the adhesive interaction between lymphocytes and high endothelial venules, <u>J. Cell Biol.</u> **9 9**, 1535, 1984.
31. Tarnowski, B.I., Shepherd, V.L., and McLaughlin, B.J., Expression of mannose receptors for pinocytosis and phagocytosis on rat retinal pigment epithelium, <u>Invest. Ophthalmol. Vis. Sci.</u>, **2 9**, 742, 1988.

* Dr. Itoh's present address: Biological Laboratory, Aichi Medical College, Nagakuti, Aichi, Japan.

PROTEOGLYCANS IN THE rds MOUSE INTERPHOTORECEPTOR MATRIX BEFORE AND AFTER PHOTORECEPTOR LOSS

Akihiko Tawara* and Joe G. Hollyfield†

* Department of Ophthalmology
Kyushu University
Fukuoka 813, Japan

† Cullen Eye Institute
Baylor College of Medicine
Houston, Texas 77030, U.S.A.

The distribution of sulfated proteoglycan in the interphotoreceptor matrix (IPM) of rds mouse was examined before and after the loss of photoreceptors with electron microscopy using the cationic copper dye, Cupromeronic Blue (CmB). In the interphotoreceptor matrix (IPM) of 18-day-old rds mouse three distinct CmB-positive filaments types were observed: type A (40-55 nm long and around 5 nm in diameter), type B (up to 0.5 µm long and 5-10 nm in diameter) and type C filaments (up to 1.0 µm long and 15-25 nm in diameter). Numerous type B and type C filaments were present in the IPM. Type C filaments formed a net-like pattern around the apical aspects of photoreceptor inner segments and around the pigment epithelial microvilli. Type A filaments were located principally in the apical cytoplasm of the pigment epithelial cells and in the proximal IPM. In the 20-month-old rds mouse, where virtually no photoreceptor cells remain, only minimal CmB staining (30-40 nm long and 3-5 nm in diameter) which was different than the filament types observed in the earlier stage was evident between pigment epithelium and retina. Pretreatment with chondroitinase AC eliminated almost all CmB-positive filaments from the 18-day-old and 20-month-old mouse IPM, indicating that the CmB-positive filaments represent chondroitin-sulfate type proteoglycans. The distinct change of distribution of chondroitin sulfate-type proteoglycans in the IPM of 20 months postpartum rds was was associated with the loss of photoreceptor cells. From this study, we suggest that photoreceptors may be critically involved in the maintenance of proteoglycans in the IPM of the mouse.

I. Introduction

The interphotoreceptor matrix (IPM), located between the neural retina and the pigment epithelium, is the extracellular domain surrounding photoreceptor inner and outer segments.[1] Proteins, glycoproteins, and glycosaminoglycans (GAGs) are the major groups of maculomolecules which have been isolated from the IPM.[2,3,4] With the exception of hyaluronic acid and heparin, free GAGs do not exist but are components of proteoglycan molecules, where they are covalently linked as side chains to a core protein. Previously, we evaluated the distribution of sulfated proteoglycans in the IPM of normal adult mouse retina, and followed the appearance of these macromolecules during postnatal development using the cationic copper dyes,

Cuprolinic Blue and Cupromeronic Blue (CmB).[5,6] These dyes are highly specific stains for sulfated proteoglycans when applied at critical electrolyte concentrations. Our findings indicate that proteoglycans of the chondroitin sulfate-type are present in the mouse IPM forming complex meshwork which surrounds both rod and cone photoreceptors.[5] These components are considered to be secreted principally by the retinal pigment epithelial cells, because of abundant population of proteoglycan staining in the pigment epithelium coupled with the absence of any staining in the cytoplasm of photoreceptors and Müller cells.[6]

Retinal degeneration slow (rds), is a recessive mutation in mice which causes a progressive loss of photoreceptors commencing around 2 weeks postpartum. In rds, photoreceptor outer segments fail to develop and typical disc structures are rarely observed. By one year, virtually all photoreceptors are missing while other retinal layers are normal in appearance.[7]

In this study, we have examined the distribution of sulfated proteoglycans in the IPM of 18-day-old and 20-month-old rds mice using CmB to determine whether differences in their distribution could be detected between before and after the loss of photoreceptors.

II. Materials and Methods

Materials: CmB was provided by Dr. Tom Wickersham, Aldrich Chemical Co. (Milwaukee, WI). Chondroitinase AC was purchased from Sigma Chemical Co. (St. Louis, MO). Tissues from mice of the inbred C3H strain, which are homozygous for the rds gene (rds/rds), were provided by Dr. S. C. Sanyal.

Fixation: Eyes from 18 days and 20 months postpartum rds mice were immersed in 2% formaldehyde, 2.5% glutaraldehyde in 0.1 M phosphate buffer containing a few drops of 5% $CaCl_2$ (pH 7.4) immediately after enucleation. The anterior segment was removed in fixative. At each postpartum age, two half eyecups from 2 eyes were processed for proteoglycan staining.

Histochemical procedures: CmB staining followed the method of Scott.[8,9] All half eyecups were cut into 3 pieces prior to staining. Fixed tissues were equilibrated for one hour in several changes of 25 mM sodium acetate, 0.2 M $MgCl_2$ and 2.5% (w/v) glutaraldehyde, pH 5.7. Tissues were then placed in 0.05% CmB in the sodium acetate fixative where they remained overnight. The following morning, tissues were rinsed 3 times in fixative without the dyes, followed by 3 washes in aqueous 0.5% sodium tungstate, and 3 washes in 0.5% sodium tungstate in 50% (v/v) ethanol. Tissues were then dehydrated in graded concentrations of ethanol and embedded in Epon. Ultrathin sections were analyzed by electron microscopy, with or without uranyl acetate staining. For this analysis, sections were taken only from the posterior pole of eyecups. Filament dimensions were measured on electron micrographs printed at a final magnification 100,000 times by measuring the 30 filaments in each class.

Enzyme digestion: Two eyes from 18-day-old and one eye from 20-month-old rds mice were used for this analysis. After removal of the anterior segment, the sensory retina of 18-day-old rds mouse was gently peeled from the eye cup, and immersed in the fixative described above. The isolated retina was then cut into six pieces. Several strips, about 500 μm wide, which included retina, choroid and sclera were cut from the fixed eyecup of a 20-month-old rds mouse. Tissues were placed in 0.1 M phosphate buffer where they remained overnight. Tissues were then divided into two groups for the following treatment: Group 1; after storing in enriched Tris buffer (0.25 M Tris-HCl, 0.18 M NaCl, 0.05% BSA, 5 mM benzamidine-HCl and 0.1 M 6-amino-caproic acid, pH 8.0) for 5 hours, the tissues were incubated in 450 μl enriched Tris buffer with 50 μl of 10 U/ml chondroitinase AC for 24 hours at 37°C. Group 2; as a control, the tissues were stored in enriched Tris buffer for 5 hours, then incubated in 500 μl enriched Tris buffer with no enzyme for 24 hours at 37°C. Following these incubations, tissues were stained with CmB as described above.

III. Results

CmB staining: At 18 days postpartum rds mice, photoreceptor cells had inner segment and, a protruding cilium but outer segment membrane discs were seldom observed (Figures 1, 2). Inner segments undergoing lysis were occasionally encountered. Some presented a fragmented appearance, while others were slightly swollen and contained large vacuoles. There were many small vesicular bodies detaching from the photoreceptor and accumulating in the IPM between the inner segments and pigment epithelium (Figure 1). Microvilli from the pigment epithelium extended among the vesicular bodies toward the inner segments (Figure 1).[10,11,12,13] Some pigment epithelial cells had a very reduced apical to basal height while in other areas the pigment epithelial cells were multi-layered.

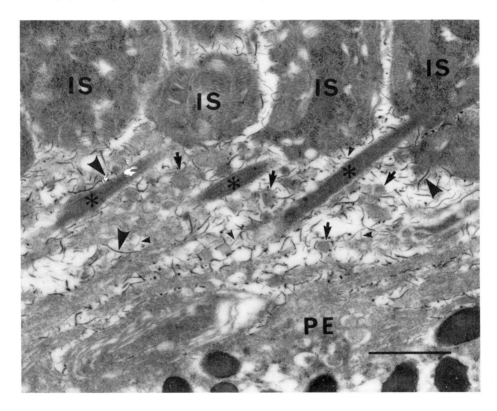

Fig. 1: Electron micrograph of the 18-day-old rds mouse retina stained with CmB. Photoreceptor inner segments (IS) has a cilium (asterisks) but no outer segment. Many vesicular bodies (arrows) are present in the IPM. There are numerous CmB-positive filaments, type C (large arrow heads) and type B (small arrow heads) in the IPM. PE: pigment epithelium.× 22,500(bar indicates 1.0 μm).

Numerous CmB-positive filaments were present in the IPM (Figures 1,2). Three types of CmB-positive filaments were present (Figure 2). These were virtually identical to the three classes of filaments we observed in the normal mouse.[6] Type A, the smallest filaments measured 40-55 nm long and about 5 nm in diameter Type B filaments, intermediate in size measured 5-10 nm in diameter. Type C, the largest filaments, with slightly curving profiles measured 15-25 nm in diameter. The lengths of type B and type C filaments were difficult to determine because their tortuous profiles were rarely fully aligned with the plane of section. Some type B filaments were observed to reach up to 0.5 μm, and type C up to 1.0 μm. Abundant type C filaments were present around pigment epithelial microvilli extending among the vesicular bodies and around the apical portion of inner segments (Figure. 1). Type C filaments appeared as long overlapping profiles with each other to form a net-like pattern. Type B and C filaments were observed throughout the IPM. Type A filaments were present in the apical cytoplasm and within microvilli of the pigment epithelial cells (Figure. 2).

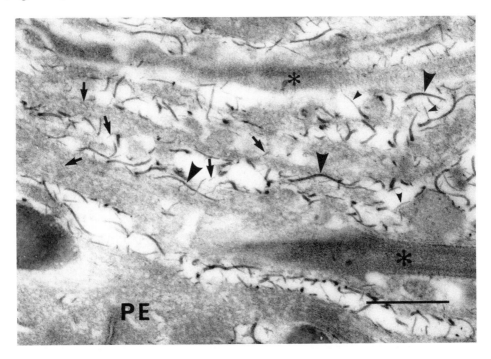

Fig. 2: Electron micrograph of the IPM around the pigment epithelium in the CmB-stained 18 days postpartum retina. Three types of filaments, type C (large arrows heads), type B (small arrow heads) and type A (arrows), are distinguished. Asterisks indicate the cilium. PE: pigment epithelium. × 45,000 (bar indicates 0.5 μm).

In 20-month-old <u>rds</u> retinas, no outer nuclear layer was present and only rarely was a single, isolated photoreceptor encountered. The pigment epithelial cells, some of which had compressed villous processes on their apical surface while others lacked, abutted closely onto the photoreceptor-free outer retinal surface (Figure 3). The extracellular space between pigment epithelium and the retina was extremely reduced at this age and contained fine CmB-positive filaments (Figure 3). Although these filaments at first appeared to represent type A filaments, by measuring it was apparent that they were thinner (3-5 nm) and shorter (30-40 nm) than type A filaments observed in the IPM and pigment epithelium at 18 days postpartum (Figure 3). The same fine filaments were observed in the extracellular space among the retinal cells located adjacent to pigment epithelium (Figure 4). No type B nor type C filaments were present within the compartment between pigment epithelium and the adjacent retina (Figure 3). In the cytoplasm of the pigment epithelial cells, only an occasional type A filament was observed (Figure 3). Numerous CmB-positive filaments were present along the basal side of the pigment epithelium in the Bruch's membrane (Figure 5). The same fine filaments were observed in the extracellular space among the retinal cells located adjacent to pigment epithelium (Figure 4). No type B nor type C filaments were present within the compartment between pigment epithelium and the adjacent retina (Figure 3). In the cytoplasm of the pigment epithelial cells, only an occasional type A filament was observed (Figure 3). Numerous CmB-positive filaments were present along the basal side of the pigment epithelium in the Bruch's membrane (Figure 5).

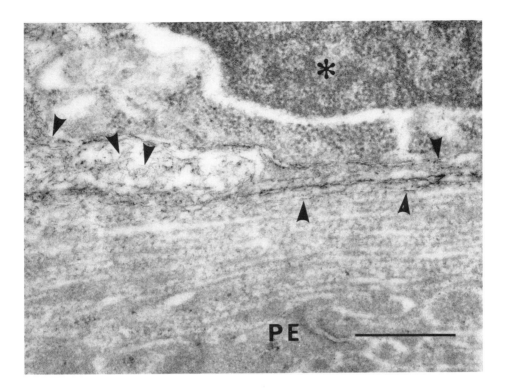

Fig. 3: Electron micrograph of the 20-month-old <u>rds</u> mouse retina stained with CmB. There is no photoreceptor cell and the pigment epithelium (PE) attaches to a cell which should be located in the inner nuclear layer in the normal retina (asterisk). Neither type C nor type B filaments, but type unknown fine filaments (arrow heads) are present in the extracellular space between pigment epithelium and the adjacent cell. Few type A filaments are seen in the cytoplasm of the pigment epithelial cell. × 55,800 (bar indicates 0.5 μm).

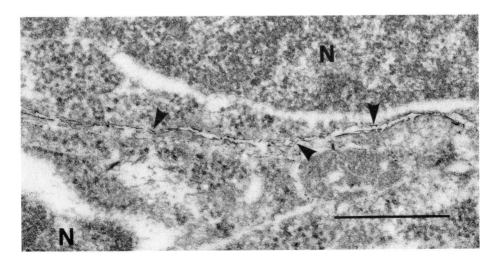

Fig. 4: Electron micrograph of the retinal cell layer adjacent to the pigment epithelium in the 20-month-old mouse retina which was stained with CmB. Fine filaments (arrow heads) which is similar to those in Fig. 3 are present in the extracellular space. N: nucleus of the retinal cell. × 63,900 (bar indicates 0.5 μm).

Enzyme digestion: In the isolated retina of 18-day-old rds mouse, which was incubated in enriched Tris buffer prior to CmB staining, photoreceptor inner segments and connecting cilia retained the morphology described above for unpeeled retinas. Many vesicular bodies remained in the IPM, although the numbers appeared to be much lower than in the IPM of unpeeled retinas. CmB-positive filaments, principally types B and C, were observed along the surface of the inner segments, cilia and vesicular bodies. Digestion with chondroitinase AC before CmB staining resulted in elimination of almost all staining from the IPM (Figure 6). On the surface of the inner segments, however, some fine CmB-positive filaments remained (Figure 6). In 20-month-old rds mouse, incubation with chondroitinase AC prior to CmB treatment resulted in a reduction but not complete elimination of staining from the space between the pigment epithelium and the retina. At the edge of the tissue block, however, filament staining were rarely observed (Figure 7), while near the center of the tissue block, some filament staining usually remained.

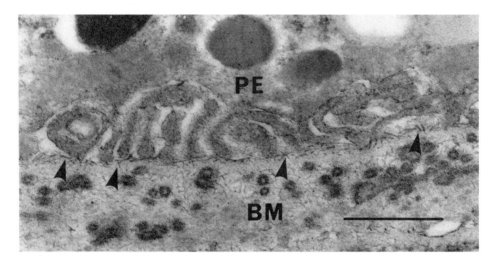

Fig. 5: Electron micrograph of the basal side of the pigment epithelium in the CmB-stained 20-month-old rds mouse retina. There are many CmB-positive filaments (arrow heads) along the basal side of the pigment epithelium (PE) in the Bruch's membrane (BM). × 54,000.

IV.   Discussion

Proteoglycans in the IPM of the rds mouse retina were evaluated histochemically, using CmB at a critical electrolyte concentration. In the IPM of 18-day-old rds mouse, where photoreceptor outer segments failed to develop and typical disc structures were rarely observed, many small vesicular bodies detached from the photoreceptor were present. At this time, three distinct types of CmB-positive filaments appeared virtually the same ones as those in the normal mouse IPM, although their pattern of distribution was different than that in the normally developed IPM.[6] Chondroitinase AC treatment removed almost all filament staining from the IPM of the 18 days postpartum rds retina, although some fine filaments remained. Whether the fine IPM filaments which continue to stain following the chondroitinase AC treatment is the results of incomplete enzyme digestion of chondroitin sulfate moieties in these IPM proteoglycans or whether they represent chondroitinase AC resistant proteoglycans cannot be conclusively defined. However, since CmB has high specificity to sulfated proteoglycans at a critical electrolyte concentration, and since filament staining in the rds IPM is quite similar to that in the normal mouse retina, which was eliminated completely by chondroitinase AC pretreatment, it is likely that those CmB-positive filaments represent sulfated, probably chondroitin sulfate-type, proteoglycans.[6]

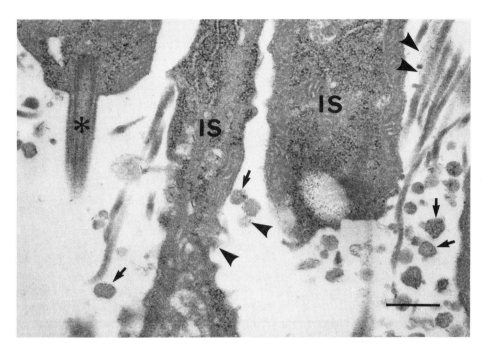

Fig. 6: The IPM of the 18-day-old <u>rds</u> mouse retina which was peeled prior to chondroitinase
AC digestion and CmB staining. Almost all the CmB-positive staining except for very
fine filaments (arrow heads) are eliminated from the IPM. Asterisk indicates the cilium.
Arrows indicate vesicular bodies. IS: inner segment. × 29,700 (bar indicates 0.5 μm).

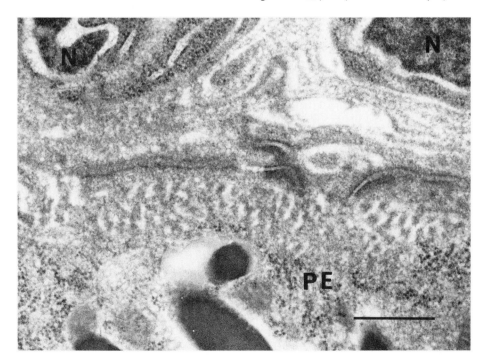

Fig. 7: Electron micrograph of the retina from the 20-month-old <u>rds</u> mouse treated with
chondroitinase AC and stained with CmB. At the edge of the tissue block, there are few
CmB-positive filaments in the area between pigment epithelium (PE) and retina, or in the
cytoplasm of the pigment epithelial cell. N: nucleus of the retinal cell. × 45,000 (bar
indicates 0.5 μm).

In 20-month <u>rds</u> retinas, which contained no photoreceptor cells, neither types A, B nor C filaments were observed in the extracellular spaces between the pigment epithelium and the adjacent photoreceptor-free retina in stark contrast to the abundant distribution of CmB-positive proteoglycans in the normal IPM.[5] Some fine staining profiles, which were smaller than any filament type observed in the IPM at 18 days retina, were present. Since these filaments showed sensitivity to chondroitinase AC, they represent chondroitin sulfate-type proteoglycans which, however, is considered to be different in structure than those in the IPM at 18 days retina. This filament type might be produced by the cells in the remaining retina, because the same filaments were present in the adjacent retinal cell layer. Only a sparse population of type A filaments was present in the pigment epithelial cells in this 20-month tissue, although numerous CmB-positive filaments were present on the basal side of this epithelial layer. These change in distribution of proteoglycans in the 20-month-old <u>rds</u> mouse retina appear to be related to the disappearance of photoreceptors, since at earlier age, while photoreceptor cells still remain, all three types of proteoglycan filaments were present. Thus, the loss of organization of proteoglycans from the IPM of <u>rds</u> appears to accompany or follow the death of photoreceptors.

In normal mouse retina, the abundant proteoglycan staining within the cytoplasm of the pigment epithelial cells associated with the Golgi apparatus and within small vesicles, in contrast with few stained profiles in the cytoplasm of photoreceptor or Müller cells suggest that the pigment epithelium may be a major site of IPM proteoglycan biosynthesis.[6] Our recent biochemical studies, however, indicates that the isolated retina can synthesize chondroitin sulfate-type proteoglycans which quickly become associated with photoreceptor outer segments.[14] Therefore, the virtual absence of organized proteoglycans in the extracellular matrix adjacent to pigment epithelium in <u>rds</u> following the loss of photoreceptors may indicate either that the continued biosynthesis, secretion and organization of proteoglycans in the IPM require a sustained cellular interaction between pigment epithelial and photoreceptor cells, or that the photoreceptors may be heavily involved in the synthesis of these components than was previously appreciated. Further studies on the regulation of biosynthesis and turnover of these components will address these issues.

V. ACKNOWLEDGMENTS

Supported by grants from the Retina Research Foundation, Houston, Texas, the National Society to Prevent Blindness, New York, New York, and the National Institutes of Health, Bethesda, Maryland. AT was supported by a postdoctoral fellowship from the Retinitis Pigmentosa Foundation Fighting Blindness, Baltimore, Maryland; JGH is the recipient of a Senior Scientific Investigator Award from Research to Prevent Blindness, New York, New York, and an award from the Alcon Research Institute, Fort Worth, Texas.

VI. REFERENCES

1 Röhlich, P. (1970). The interphotoreceptor matrix: Electron microscopic and histochemical observations on the vertebrate retina. <u>Exp. Eye Res</u>. 10,80-86.

2. Berman, E. R. and Bach, G. (1968). The acid mucopolysaccharides of cattle retina. <u>Biochem. J</u>. 108,75-88.

3. Adler, A. J. and Severin, K. M. (1981). Proteins of the bovine interphotoreceptor matrix: Tissues of origin. <u>Exp. Eye Res</u>. 32,755-69.

4. Adler, A. J. and Klucznik, K. M. (1982). Proteins and glycoproteins of the bovine interphotoreceptor matrix: Composition and fractionation. Exp. Eye Res. 34,423-34.

5. Tawara, A., Varner, H. H. and Hollyfield, J. G. (1988). Proteoglycans in the mouse interphotoreceptor matrix. I. Histochemical studies using Cuprolinic Blue. Exp. Eye Res. 46,689-704.

6. Tawara, A., Varner, H. H. and Hollyfield, J. G. (1989). Proteoglycans in the mouse interphotoreceptor matrix. II. Origin and development of proteoglycans. Exp. Eye Res. 48,815-39.

7. Sanyal, S., De Ruiter, A. and Hawkins, R. K. (1980). Development and degeneration of retina in *rds* mutant mice: Light microscopy. J. Comp. Neurol. 194,193-207.

8. Scott, J. E. (1973). Affinity competition and specific interactions in the biochemistry and histochemistry of polyelectrolytes. Biochem. Soc. Trans. 1,787-806.

9. Scott, J. E. (1980). Collagen-proteoglycan interactions. Localization of proteoglycans in tendon by electron microscopy. Biochem. J. 187,887-91.

10. Sanyal, S. and Jansen, H. G. (1981). Absence of receptor outer segments in the retina in *rds* mutant mice. Neurosci. Lett. 21,23-26.

11. Cohen, A. I. (1983). Some cytological and initial biochemical observations on photoreceptors in retinas of rds mice. Invest. Ophthalmol. Vis. Sci. 24,8832-43.

12. Jansen, H. G. and Sanyal S. (1984). Development and degeneration of retina in *rds* mutant mice: Electron microscopy. J Comp. Neurol. 224,71-84.

13. Sanyal, S., Chader, G. and Aguirre, G. (1985). Expression of retinal degeneration slow (rds) gene in the retina of the mouse. In Retinal Degeneration. Experimental and Clinical Studies. (Eds LaVail, M. M., Hollyfield, J. G., and Anderson, R. E.). Pp. 239-56 Alan R. Liss Inc. : New York.

14. Landers, R. A., Tawara, A., Varner, H. H. and Hollyfield, J. G. (1990) Proteoglycans in the mouse interphotoreceptor matrix. IV. Retinal synthesis of chondroitin sulfate proteoglycan. Exp. Eye. Res. 51 (in press).

LIGHT-INDUCED CHANGES IN THE INTERPHOTORECEPTOR MATRIX: IMPLICATIONS FOR INHERITED RETINAL DEGENERATIONS AND NORMAL PHOTORECEPTOR PHYSIOLOGY

Fumiyuki Uehara, Douglas Yasumura, Michael T. Matthes and Matthew M. LaVail

Departments of Anatomy, Ophthalmology and Beckman Vision Center
University of California, San Francisco
San Francisco, CA 94143-0730, USA

I. INTRODUCTION

The interphotoreceptor matrix (IPM) is an extracellular matrix composed of proteins, glycoproteins and proteoglycans that fills the interphotoreceptor space.[1-13] Several important interactions between photoreceptors and retinal pigment epithelium (RPE)[14] are thought to be mediated by the interphotoreceptor matrix (IPM).[1,6,15-23] Using histochemical, immunocytochemical and lectin probes for several IPM constituents, we have recently found that several IPM components in the rat undergo a major shift in distribution or molecular conformation following the transition between light and dark.[24]

In the present work, we 1) review the evidence for a light-evoked change in the IPM, including the difference in rod- and cone-associated IPM compartments; 2) consider the possible relationships of the light-evoked IPM changes with certain physiological events in normal photoreceptors; and 3) examine the light-evoked IPM changes in several different forms of inherited retinal degeneration.

II. MATERIALS AND METHODS

The IPM in the retinas of rats and mice of various genotypes and ages was examined histochemically, immunocytochemically and with lectin cytochemistry at different periods of light and dark adaptation (specific details given in the appropriate section). Before their eyes were taken for histological processing, all animals were maintained in cyclic lighting (12:12 hours light:dark) at an in-cage illumination of less than 20 ft-c for at least 1 week (but usually their entire life). The animals were killed by an overdose of carbon dioxide, after which they were quickly perfused with a paraformaldehyde-glutaraldehyde mixture. The eyes were bisected along the vertical meridian, embedded in polyester wax and sectioned at 8 μm thickness. To demonstrate various components of the IPM, the sections were stained with either the colloidal iron reaction (which binds to negatively charged molecules); antibodies to chondroitin 6-sulfate or interphotoreceptor retinoid-binding protein (IRBP); or the FITC-labeled lectins, wheat germ agglutinin (WGA; binds to sialic acid and/or N-acetyl-D-glucosamine), peanut agglutinin (PNA; binds with the Galβ1→3GalNAc sequence of carbohydrates) or Ricinus communis agglutinin-1 (RCA-1; specific for terminal β-galactose residues). These procedures are described in detail elsewhere.[4,20,24,25]

The animals examined were normal rats of the albino F344 strain, pink-eyed RCS-*rdy*[+] strain[26] and pigmented RCS-*rdy*[+]*p*[+] strain,[26] as well as Royal College of Surgeons (RCS) rats with inherited retinal dystrophy. Three different forms of inherited retinal degeneration in mice were also examined. These were the nervous,[27] Purkinje cell degeneration[27] and retinal degeneration slow[28] mutants. Normal littermate or age-matched controls were also examined. All procedures with animals conformed to the ARVO Resolution on the Use of Animals in Research and the guidelines of the UCSF Committee on Animal Research.

III. LIGHT-EVOKED CHANGES IN THE IPM

Various components of the IPM have been shown to be distributed non-uniformly in the interphotoreceptor space. For example, different staining patterns have been observed in different horizontal strata of the IPM using immunohistochemistry with antibodies against IRBP[12,29-31] and proteoglycans,[32,33] as well as by histochemistry using various cationic reagents[34] or cuprolinic blue.[35] In light-adapted rodents the histochemically demonstrable IPM has typically been observed most concentrated at the apical surface of the RPE (defined as the apical outer segment zone).[20,34] The IPM is also concentrated at the inner segment-outer segment junction (defined as the basal outer segment zone), thus leaving a relative paucity of stainable IPM in the intervening spaces alongside the outer segments (defined as the interstitial zone).[20,34] Illustrations demonstrating this heterogeneous distribution of IPM in light-adapted rats are shown with colloidal iron staining (Figure 1a), chondroitin 6-sulfate immunoreactivity (Figure 1c), WGA binding (Figure 1e) and IRBP immunoreactivity (Figure 1g). It should be noted that in light-adapted retinas, a significant amount of IPM staining is also found among the inner segments, often extending to the outer limiting membrane (Figures 1a,c,e,g).

We recently found that in dark-adapted rats, the IPM showed a remarkably different distribution.[24] Instead of the apical and basal bands of concentrated IPM staining seen in the light, the IPM in the dark was much more uniformly distributed throughout the outer segment zone, and little or no stained IPM was present in the inner segment zone (Figures 1b,d,f,h).

When the kinetics of the IPM distributional changes were examined at the onset of light in the morning, the change was rapid (Figure 2a). At 1 and 3 minutes after light onset, the dark pattern was still present. However, by 5 minutes after light onset the banded pattern typical of light-adapted retinas was evident.[24] In most retinas, the change was complete throughout the retina, whereas in some only the central portion of the retina showed the banded pattern, while the peripheral retina (which presumably received less light in those animals) still displayed the diffuse dark-adapted pattern. By 10 minutes in the light and thereafter, all retinas showed the banded light-adapted pattern throughout the retina. By contrast, a much longer time was required for the change to occur from the light-adapted IPM pattern to the diffuse dark-adapted pattern (Figure 2a). This change required 1-2 hours to complete, although the timing was less consistent from animal to animal than the more rapid dark-to-light change.

We then carried out a number of experiments designed to show whether the IPM distributional change was a light-evoked response or was driven by a light-entrained circadian rhythm,[24] like outer segment disc shedding in the rat.[36] We modified the the normal 12:12 light:dark cycle in the following ways: extended the period of the dark cycle in the morning, extended the light period in the evening, interrupted both light and dark periods with

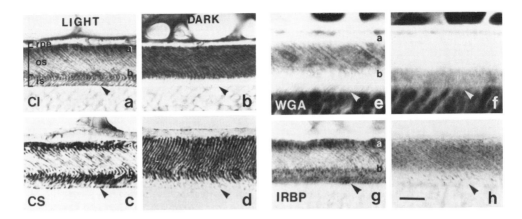

Figure 1. Light micrographs of polyester wax-embedded sections stained to demonstrate various constituents of the IPM of albino rat eyes taken either in the light (left micrograph of each pair; one or more hours into the light cycle) or in the dark (right micrograph of each pair; two or more hours into the dark cycle). **a** and **b**, colloidal iron reaction. **c** and **d**, chondroitin 6-sulfate immunoreactivity. **e** and **f**, WGA binding. **g** and **h**, IRBP immunoreactivity. In all cases in the light, the stained IPM is most concentrated at the apical region (a) of the outer segment zone (os) adjacent to the apical surface of the retinal pigment epithelium (rpe) and at the basal region (b) of the outer segment zone at the junction with the photoreceptor inner segments (is). Some stained IPM is also present between the inner segments, extending inward to the outer limiting membrane (arrowheads). In the dark, the stained IPM is uniformly distributed across the outer segment zone and little is present between the inner segments. Scale bar, 10 μm. (From Uehara et al., 1990.[24] Copyright American Association for the Advancement of Science.)

the opposite lighting at several different times, and made multiple transitions from light to dark during a single day. If the IPM changes followed a circadian rhythm, they would have occurred at the subjective on- and off-times (i.e., 7:00 a.m. and 7:00 p.m., respectively) regardless of the lighting. Instead, as shown in Figure 2b, the IPM changes followed the lighting changes in every case. Thus, the IPM distributional changes are light-evoked phenomena.

We also carried out an experiment designed to test whether the light acts directly in the eye or through a systemic factor to effect the IPM distributional change.[24] By patching one eye of anesthetized rats in the dark with black opaque tape and then exposing the rats to light, we found that the IPM in the open eye redistributed to the banded light pattern, whereas the IPM in the patched eye remained in the diffuse dark pattern (Figure 2c). Thus, the IPM change appears to be induced within the eye rather than by a systemic factor, which presumably would have affected both eyes.

The IPM has also been shown to be non-uniform in the vertical plane. The domains of the IPM that are associated with cone outer segments have been shown to differ from those associated with rod outer segments. This is based on differential sugar-specific lectin binding (i.e., cone-associated IPM binds PNA, whereas rod-associated IPM does not[37-43]) and, at least in the case of primates, antibodies to chondroitin 6-sulfate which bind specifically to the cone-associated IPM.[44] The specialized domains surrounding cones have been termed the "cone associated IPM or cell coat,"[39,41,45] the "cone matrix sheath,"[40] or the "conedom."[46]

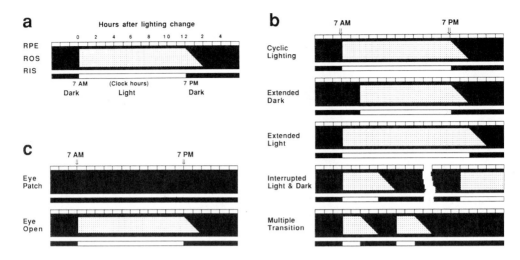

Figure 2. Diagrams illustrating (**a**) the kinetics of the light-evoked IPM distributional change, (**b**) experiments to determine whether the IPM changes were light-induced or followed a circadian rhythm, and (**c**) the results of monocular eye patching experiments. Each RPE cell represents one hour of time. The thin bar below each retinal diagram gives the lighting condition. **a**, The diffuse IPM pattern seen in the dark changes to the banded pattern rapidly (within 5 minutes) after light onset, whereas the change from the banded light pattern to the diffuse dark pattern requires 1-2 hours after light offset. **b**, The cyclic light pattern shown in Figure **2a** is repeated first. This is followed by extending the dark period 2 hours into the usual light period; extending the light 2 hours into the usual dark period; interrupting the light period 4 hours into the cycle and the dark period 1 hour into the cycle; and multiple transitions within one light period. In every case, the IPM change followed the light transition with the kinetics expected from data obtained at the normal time of light-dark transition (Figure **a**). **c**, When one eye was patched in rats, that eye showed the same diffuse dark IPM pattern throughout a light cycle, whereas the open eye of the same rats showed the expected IPM changes following light transition.

We have recently examined the cone matrix sheaths in the rat to determine whether these domains of the IPM undergo light-evoked distributional changes similar to the IPM as a whole. Using the lectins, PNA and RCA-1, which preferentially bind the cone matrix sheaths, we found no difference in binding in the light and dark (Figure 3).[25] Thus, the IPM of cone matrix sheaths appears not to undergo light-evoked changes in distribution, so those changes seen in the overall IPM (Figure 1) apparently result from changes in the rod-associated IPM alone. It should be noted, however, that there was a relatively small amount of PNA binding to the rod-associated IPM that did not show light-evoked changes in distribution (Figure 3).

If sections are pretreated with neuraminidase, the terminal sialic acid residues are removed from carbohydrates in the rod-associated IPM,[39,41-43] which exposes specific sugars recognized by PNA and RCA-1 in those regions.[47-51] Thus, when this procedure was followed, PNA and RCA-1 binding to the rod-associated IPM showed light-evoked changes, (Figure 4) similar to those seen with the other probes (Figure 1).

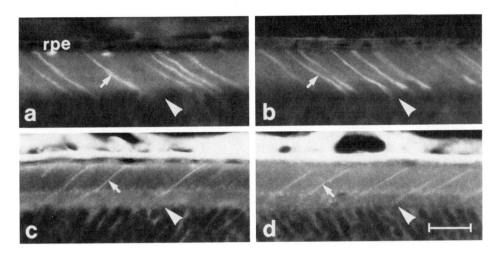

Figure 3. Light micrographs demonstrating binding of the FITC-labeled lectins, PNA (**a** and **b**) and RCA-1 (**c** and **d**) in light adapted (left column) and dark adapted (right column) rat retinas. Binding of the two lectins to the cone matrix sheaths (arrows) is the same in the light and dark. There is also a markedly less intense binding of PNA to the rod matrix domains (between the cone matrix sheaths) that shows the same distribution in the light and dark. Arrowheads, outer limiting membrane; rpe, retinal pigment epithelium. Scale bar, 20 μm. (From Uehara, et al., 1990.[25] Copyright Association for Research in Vision and Ophthalmology.)

In a recent developmental study, it was shown that the age at which the IPM obtained the capacity to undergo a light-evoked distributional change was between P14 and P16.[52] This is also the age at which a significant change in the glycoconjugates occurs in the IPM of the normally developing rat retina.[53] The terminal sialic acid residues of IPM carbohydrates around rods appear to reach their adult levels at about P16.[53] Thus, it is possible that the presence of sialic acid on the termini of sugar chains of IPM glycoconjugates may be required for the light-evoked change in the IPM to occur.[52] This possibility gains some credibility from the fact that the cone-associated IPM, which does not show light-evoked changes,[25] also contains little or no sialic acid.[47]

Factors other than sialic acid obviously may be important in determining the ability of the IPM to undergo light-evoked changes. For example, the requirement of mature, regularly aligned rod outer segments is suggested by the developmental relationship of the IPM light response and the regularly arranged, adult-like appearance of rod outer segments both of which are obtained between P14 and P16 in the rat.[52,54]

IV. PHYSIOLOGICAL RELATIONSHIPS OF THE LIGHT-EVOKED IPM CHANGE

What are the physiological events associated with light onset that could trigger the IPM light response? We have previously discussed several possible physiological events, such as alterations in ion fluxes and pH that occur in and around photoreceptors following light onset. These include 1) an increase in extracellular Ca^{2+},[55,56] 2) a decrease in extra-

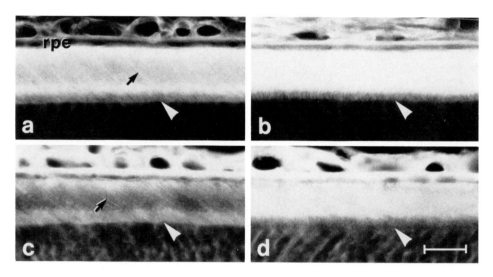

Figure 4. Light micrographs demonstrating binding of the FITC-labeled lectins, PNA (**a** and **b**) and RCA-1 (**c** and **d**) in light adapted (left column) and dark adapted (right column) rat retinas following pretreatment of the sections with neuraminidase. PNA binding in the light (**a**) is evident throughout the outer segment zone, but is most intense in the apical and basal outer segment zones and to the cone matrix sheaths that can be seen crossing the outer segment zone (arrow). In the dark (**b**), PNA binding is intense throughout the outer segment zone. RCA-1 binding in the light (**c**) is evident in the apical outer segment region, the inner segment zone and to the cone matrix sheaths (arrow). In the dark (**d**), RCA-1 binding is significantly more intense throughout the outer segment zone than in the light, but little binding is present in most of the inner segment zone. Arrowheads, outer limiting membrane; rpe, retinal pigment epithelium. Scale bar, 20 μm. (From Uehara, et al., 1990.[25] Copyright Association for Research in Vision and Ophthalmology.)

cellular $^{K+}$,[57,58] 3) an increase in the extracellular pH,[59,60] and 4) a predicted release of lactic acid by photoreceptors.[60] These changes may possibly effect an IPM distributional change by acting on the glycosaminoglycans of the IPM, which are known in other experimental systems to undergo conformational changes (reversible extension and retraction) when the pH or ionic composition of their milieu is changed.[61] The time course of each of these ionic or pH changes following light onset is rapid, less than 4 minutes, and the reverse process following light offset is much slower. Thus, for both the light and dark IPM responses, the temporal relationships of the ionic and pH changes are appropriate for effecting the IPM changes. However, the magnitude of some of the ionic changes is relatively small, and it is not known whether they are large enough to cause the changes observed in the IPM.

Another possible event is the hyperpolarization of the rod inner and outer segment that occurs following light onset. As noted above, the rod-associated IPM is bound by the lectin, WGA, and by RCA-1 following sialic acid removal by neuraminidase, indicating that this region of the IPM is composed predominantly of highly negatively charged sialoglycoconjugates of the serum or N-glycoside type. An increase in the negative charge of the rod outer segments during hyperpolarization may repel the negatively charged IPM surrounding it. The result might be the accumulation of IPM at the apical surface of the RPE as seen in the light-adapted state (Figure 1); however, since the inner and outer segments are isopotential, this would not explain the accumulation at the basal outer segment region (Figure 1). The increase in negative charge of the inner and outer segments apparently does not repel the PNA-binding IPM of the mucin or O-glycoside type found in the cone-associated IPM (Figure 3). It is clear that the physiological events that trigger the IPM light response remain to be identified.

What is the possible role(s) or physiological consequence(s) of the light-evoked IPM change in distribution? We have previously suggested that the gross distributional changes in the proteoglycans and acidic glycoproteins during the light response may facilitate the transfer of substances between photoreceptors and the RPE.[24] For example, a close temporal relationship exists between the IPM changes and the movement of vitamin A between the photoreceptors and RPE during the visual pigment cycle during light and dark adaptation. In both the rapid light response and slower dark response, the vitamin A movement occurs almost simultaneously with or soon after the IPM change.[24,62] Although it has been thought that the retinoid-binding protein, IRBP, may transport vitamin A between the photoreceptors and RPE,[8,10,11] this view has recently been challenged.[63] Regardless of whether it serves an active role in vitamin A movement, IRBP avidly binds retinoids.[8,10,11,63] Our current findings suggest that IRBP may assist in the movement of retinoids in a passive manner. Immediately following light onset, vitamin A is released from the photoreceptors, and IRBP is in a position to bind it, since the protein is uniformly distributed throughout the IPM in the dark (Figure 1h). The IRBP (along with the bound retinoids) then becomes concentrated at the RPE cell surface due to the IPM light response (Figure 1g), which would presumably facilitate the transfer of bound vitamin A to the RPE.

The changes in IPM distribution and concentration following the onset of light may influence the transfer of substances between photoreceptors and the RPE in other ways, as well. For example, changes in chondroitin sulfate concentration (e.g., Figures 1c,d) may effect the diffusion of substances through the IPM.[64] In addition, changes in the IPM concentration during the IPM light response may also influence the rate of water flux across the interphotoreceptor space, as well as the degree of hydration of the IPM, and therefore the diffusion rates across the matrix.[24]

It is also probable that redistribution of the highly negatively charged IPM following light onset (or light offset) has an effect on the electrophysiological properties of photoreceptors. An ionic change in the extracellular space that presumably accompanies the IPM distributional change would influence the dark current, and thereby the physiological properties of the photoreceptors. If a small spot of retina were illuminated, then it is probable the change in electronegativity of the IPM in the illuminated spot would cause a change in the adjacent photoreceptor cells, with a decreasing degree of action proportional to the distance away from the illuminated spot.

In this regard, it is important to recall that the cone-associated IPM is not rich in sialoglycoconjugates, and the cone matrix constituents do not show a light-evoked distributional change (Figure 3). Therefore, the O-linked glycoconjugates of the cone matrix sheath may insulate the cone photoreceptors from the extracellular changes that could otherwise alter the physiological properties of the cells, such as those discussed above for the rod photoreceptors. These hypotheses on the influence of light-evoked IPM light changes on the electrophysiological properties of the photoreceptor cells remain to be tested experimentally.

V. LIGHT-EVOKED IPM CHANGES AND INHERITED RETINAL DEGENERATIONS

The IPM has been shown to have an abnormal distribution in several forms of inherited retinal degeneration. The first observation of an IPM abnormality in an hereditary retinal degeneration was in the RCS rat,[20] which showed 1) an almost complete absence of the normal apical band of IPM adjacent to the RPE; 2) a paucity of IPM in the outer segment debris membranes which accumulate due to a phagocytosis defect in the RPE;[65,66] and 3) an excessive accumulation of IPM in the basal outer segment region. These changes occur about one week before overt signs of photoreceptor cell death, so it has been suggested the IPM abnormalities may play a role in photoreceptor cell death.[20] IPM changes at later stages of the RCS disorder have also been characterized.[67]

<u>nr</u> mice

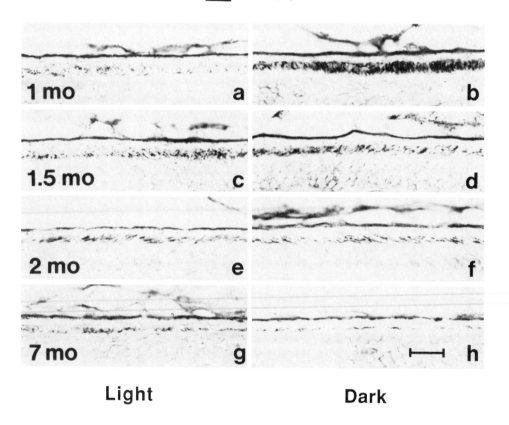

Light   Dark

Figure 5. Light micrographs showing the colloidal iron reaction in polyester wax sections of light adapted (left column) and dark adapted (right column) *nr* mice at different ages as shown on the micrographs. At 1 month of age (**a** and **b**), the IPM light response is clearly seen. Most significantly, the IPM fills the outer segment zone in the dark (**b**) but not in the light (**a**). Subtle light-dark differences are seen at 1.5 months (**c** and **d**), but not at older ages (**e**, **f**, **g** and **h**). Scale bar, 15 μm.

<u>pcd</u> (albino) mice

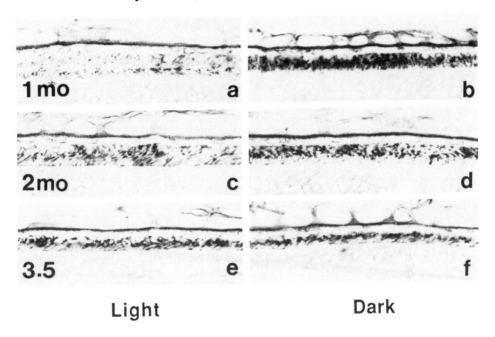

Light   Dark

Figure 6. Light micrographs showing the colloidal iron reaction in polyester wax sections of light adapted (left column) and dark adapted (right column) *pcd* mice at different ages. At 1 month of age (**a** and **b**), the IPM light response is clearly seen. Most significantly, the IPM fills the outer segment zone in the dark (**b**) but not in the light (**a**). The response is still present at 2 months of age (**c** and **d**), but not at older ages (**e** and **f**). Same magnification as Figure 5.

We have recently examined the developing RCS rat retina histochemically to determine if and when differences occur from normal rats in the IPM light response.[52] We found that the light-evoked change shown previously in adults first appeared between P14 and P16 in both normal and RCS rats. The response was lost in RCS rats between P20 and P25, a time when the outer segment zone is rapidly losing its organized structure and significant numbers of pyknotic photoreceptor nuclei have begun to appear. These findings suggested that for the IPM light response to occur, mature, organized photoreceptor outer segments are required. Moreover, the disruption of the IPM light response may contribute to the accumulation of IPM in the basal outer segment zone and thereby to photoreceptor cell death in RCS rats.[52]

The IPM in several murine forms of inherited retinal degeneration have been examined, although only at a relatively few ages.[68] For example, the retinas of nervous mice (gene symbol, *nr*) at 4-5 months of age have a cytopathological structure similar to that of younger RCS rats,[27] and they show an IPM distribution similar to that in the RCS rat.[68] The retinas of retinal degeneration slow (*rds*) mice have no outer segments,[69] and at P12 through 3-4 months of age show a massive accumulation of IPM.[68] The retinas in both of these mutants degenerate slowly over the course of a year.[70]

<u>rds</u> mice

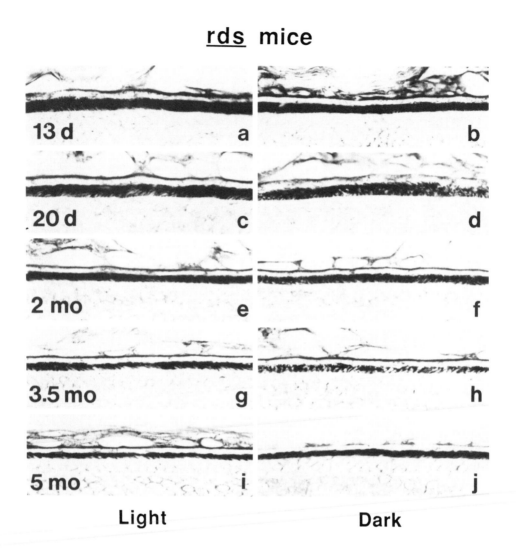

Light   **Dark**

Figure 7. Light micrographs showing the colloidal iron reaction in polyester wax sections of light adapted (left column) and dark adapted (right column) *rds* mice at different ages. At all ages, the abundant IPM fills the interphotoreceptor space and no difference in IPM distribution is seen in the light and dark. Same magnification as Figure 5.

We have now examined the retinas of *nr* and *rds* mice at several ages to test the hypothesis that normal, mature photoreceptor outer segments are required for the light-evoked distributional changes to occur in the IPM. In addition, we examined retinas of the cerebellar mutant mouse, Purkinje cell degeneration (*pcd*), which also shows a photoreceptor degeneration[27,71,72] that is similar in overall time course to *nr* and *rds*.[70]

In *nr* mice at 1 month of age, the IPM light response could be seen; it was somewhat equivocal at 1.5 months; and it was absent at 2 and 7 months of age (Figure 5). Although the outer segments are somewhat disorganized at 1 month of age, the outer segment zone becomes highly disorganized between 1 and 2 months of age in *nr* mice.

In albino *pcd* mice (the *pcd* mutation maintained on the albino BALB/c strain), the IPM light response was found at 1 month of age; it was evident at 2 months of age, but not as complete as at 1 month; and it was absent at 3.5 months of age (Figure 6). The outer segments become shorter and more disorganized between 1 and 3.5 months of age, although they are not completely normal at 1 month of age.[71,72]

In *rds* mice at all ages examined (i.e., P13 through 5 months), the abundant IPM showed no difference between the light and dark (Figure 7).

The data on the three murine forms of retinal degeneration are consistent with the hypothesis generated from observations on the RCS rat[52] that normal, mature photoreceptor outer segments are required for the light-evoked IPM distributional change to occur. It should be noted, however, that the IPM light response was evident in *nr* mice at 1 month of age (and possibly at 1.5 months) and in *pcd* mice at 1 month of age (and probably at 2 months). At these ages, the photoreceptor outer segments are already somewhat disrupted, but they are clearly in a much more normal configuration than at later ages. Furthermore, there is little information on the physiological status of the photoreceptor cells in these mice (or in *rds* mice) at the ages examined. Thus, we cannot rule out the involvement of photoreceptor inner segments, photoreceptor cells, in general, or even the RPE in regulating the IPM light response.

Does the loss of the IPM light response lead to photoreceptor degeneration? The loss of a light response apparently does not play the initial role in the death of photoreceptors, since many die before the loss of the IPM light response occurs. However, if the redistribution of IPM is important in the normal transfer of substances between the photoreceptors and RPE, it is possible that loss of the IPM light response may play a role in the slow, progressive loss of photoreceptors at later ages. It is remarkable that the three forms of murine retinal degeneration that are genetically and cytopathologically distinct all show virtually the same time course in late stages of the diseases.[70] It is possible that the genetically induced causes of the retinal degenerations lead only to the initial loss of photoreceptor cells. This is consistent with the somewhat different initial rates of photoreceptor cell loss in the different diseases.[73] There may be some common factor that dictates the rate of photoreceptor cell loss at later ages. Although there may be others, the loss of the IPM light response is one candidate for such a hypothetical factor.

VI. ACKNOWLEDGEMENTS

We thank N. Lawson and G. Riggs for technical and secretarial assistance. This work was supported in part by NIH Research Grants EY01919, EY06842, Core Grant EY02162 and funds from the Retinitis Pigmentosa Foundation Fighting Blindness, Research to Prevent Blindness and That Man May See, Inc. Dr. LaVail is the recipient of a Research to Prevent Blindness Senior Scientific Investigators Award.

VII. REFERENCES

1. Sidman, R. L., Histochemical studies on photoreceptor cells, *Ann. N.Y. Acad. Sci.*, 74, 182, 1958.
2. Zimmerman, L. E., Applications of histochemical methods for the demonstration of acid mucopolysaccharides to ophthalmic pathology, *Trans. Am. Acad. Ophththalmol. Otolaryngol.*, 62, 697, 1958.
3. Berman, E. R. and Bach, G., The acid mucopolysaccharides of cattle retina, *Biochem. J.*, 108, 75, 1968.
4. Röhlich, P., The interphotoreceptor matrix: electron microscopic and histochemical observations on the vertebrate retina, *Exp. Eye Res.*, 10, 80, 1970.
5. Bach, G. and Berman, E. R., Amino sugar-containing compounds of the retina I. Isolation and identification, *Biochim. Biophys. Acta*, 252, 453, 1971.
6. Feeney, L., Synthesis of interphotoreceptor matrix. I. Autoradiography of ^{3}H-fucose incorporation, *Invest. Ophthalmol.*, 12, 739, 1973.
7. Feeney, L., The interphotoreceptor space. I. Postnatal ontogeny in mice and rats, *Dev. Biol.*, 32, 101, 1973.
8. Lai, Y.-L., Wiggert, B., Liu, Y. P. and Chader, G. J., Interphotoreceptor retinol-binding protein: possible transport vehicle between compartments of the retina, *Nature*, 298, 848, 1982.
9. Adler, A. J. and Klucznik, K. M., Proteins and glycoproteins of the bovine interphotoreceptor matrix: composition and fractionation, *Exp. Eye Res.*, 34, 423, 1982.
10. Adler, A. J. and Martin, K. J., Retinol-binding proteins in bovine interphotoreceptor matrix, *Biochem. Biophys. Res. Comm.*, 108, 1601, 1982.
11. Liou, G. I., Bridges, C. D. B., Fong, S.-L., Alvarez, R. A. and Gonzalez-Fernandez, F., Vitamin A transport between retina and pigment epithelium-an interstitial protein carrying endogenous retinol (interstitial retinol-binding protein), *Vision Res.*, 22, 1457, 1982.
12. Bunt-Milam, A. H. and Saari, J. C., Immunocytochemical localization of two retinoid-binding proteins in vertebrate retina, *J. Cell Biol.*, 97, 703, 1983.
13. Uehara, F., Muramatsu, T. and Ohba, N., Two-dimensional gel electrophoretic analysis of lectin receptors in the bovine interphotoreceptor matrix, *Exp. Eye Res.*, 43, 227, 1986.
14. Steinberg, R. H., Research update: report from a workshop on cell biology of retinal detachment, *Exp. Eye Res.*, 43, 695, 1986.
15. Zimmerman, L. E. and Eastham, A. B., Acid mucopolysaccharide in the retinal pigment epithelium and visual cell layer of the developing mouse eye, *Am. J. Ophthalmol.*, 47, 488, 1959.
16. Zimmerman, L. E., Acid mucopolysaccharides in ocular histology and pathology, *Inst. Medicine Chicago, Proceedings*, 23, 267, 1961.
17. Hall, M. O. and Heller, J., Mucopolysaccharides of the retina, in *The Retina*, Straatsma, B., Hall, M., Allen, R. and Crescitelli, F., Eds., Univ. of Calif. Press, Los Angeles, 1969, 211.
18. Zauberman, H., Measurement of adhesive forces between the sensory retina and the pigment epithelium, *Exp. Eye Res.*, 8, 276, 1969.
19. Feeney, L., The interphotoreceptor space. II. Histochemistry of the matrix, *Dev. Biol.*, 32, 115, 1973.
20. LaVail, M. M., Pinto, L. H. and Yasumura, D., The interphotoreceptor matrix in rats with inherited retinal dystrophy, *Invest. Ophthalmol. Vis. Sci.*, 21, 658, 1981.

21. Adler, A. J. and Evans, C. D., Proteins of the bovine interphotoreceptor matrix: retinoid binding and other functions, in *The Interphotoreceptor Matrix in Health and Disease*, Bridges, C. D. and Adler, A. J., Eds., Alan R. Liss, Inc., New York, 1985, 65.

22. Bridges, C. D. and Adler, A. J., *The Interphotoreceptor Matrix in Health and Disease*, Alan R. Liss, Inc., New York, 1985.

23. Besharse, J. C., Iuvone, P. M. and Pierce, M. E., Regulation of rhythmic photoreceptor metabolism: a role for post-receptoral neurons, in *Progress in Retinal Research*, Osborne, N. and Chader, G., Eds., Pergamon Press, Oxford, 1988, 21.

24. Uehara, F., Matthes, M. T., Yasumura, D. and LaVail, M. M., Light-evoked changes in the interphotoreceptor matrix, *Science*, 248, 1633, 1990.

25. Uehara, F., Yasumura, D. and LaVail, M. M., Rod- and cone-associated interphotoreceptor matrix in the rat retina, *Invest. Ophthalmol. Vis. Sci.*, (In press), 1991.

26. LaVail, M. M., Photoreceptor characteristics in congenic strains of RCS rats, *Invest. Ophthalmol. Vis. Sci.*, 20, 671, 1981.

27. Mullen, R. J. and LaVail, M. M., Two new types of retinal degeneration in cerebellar mutant mice, *Nature*, 258, 528, 1975.

28. Sanyal, S., De Ruiter, A. and Hawkins, R. K., Development and degeneration of retina in rds mutant mice: light microscopy, *J. Comp. Neur.*, 207, 193, 1980.

29. Gonzalez-Fernandez, F., Landers, R. A., Glazebrook, P. A., Fong, S.-L., Liou, G. I., Lam, D. M. K. and Bridges, C. D. B., An extracellular retinol-binding glycoprotein in the eyes of mutant rats with retinal dystrophy: development, localization, and biosynthesis, *J. Cell Biol.*, 99, 2092, 1984.

30. Eisenfeld, A. J., Bunt-Milam, A. H. and Saari, J. C., Immunocytochemical localization of interphotoreceptor retinol-binding protein in developing normal and RCS rat retinas, *Invest. Ophthalmol. Vis. Sci.*, 26, 775, 1985.

31. Chader, G. J., Interphotoreceptor retinoid-binding protein (IRBP): a model protein for molecular biological and clinically relevant studies, *Invest. Ophthalmol. Vis. Sci.*, 30, 7, 1989.

32. Porrello, K. and LaVail, M. M., Immunocytochemical localization of chondroitin sulfates in the interphotoreceptor matrix of the normal and dystrophic rat retina, *Curr. Eye Res.*, 5, 981, 1986.

33. Porrello, K., Yasumura, D. and LaVail, M. M., Immunogold localization of chondroitin 6-sulfate in the interphotoreceptor matrix of normal and RCS rats, *Invest. Ophthalmol. Vis. Sci.*, 30, 638, 1989.

34. Porrello, K. and LaVail, M. M., Histochemical demonstration of spatial heterogeneity in the interphotoreceptor matrix of the rat retina, *Invest. Ophthalmol. Vis. Sci.*, 27, 1577, 1986.

35. Tawara, A., Varner, H. H. and Hollyfield, J. G., Proteoglycans in the mouse interphotoreceptor matrix. I. Histochemical studies using cuprolinic blue, *Exp. Eye Res.*, 46, 689, 1988.

36. LaVail, M. M., Rod outer segment disc shedding in rat retina: relationship to cyclic lighting, *Science*, 194, 1071, 1976.

37. Johnson, L. V., Hageman, G. S. and Blanks, J. C., Restricted domains of interphotoreceptor matrix ensheath vertebrate cone photoreceptors, *J. Cell Biol.*, 99, 61, 1984.

38. Johnson, L. V., Hageman, G. S. and Blanks, J. C., Restricted extracellular matrix domains ensheath cone photoreceptors in vertebrate retinae, in *The Interphotoreceptor Matrix in Health and Disease*, Bridges, C. D. and Adler, A. J., Eds., Alan R. Liss, Inc., New York, 1985, 33.

39. Sameshima, M., Uehara, F. and Ohba, N., Specialized interphotoreceptor matrices around cones and rods, as revealed by ferritin-conjugated lectin cytochemistry, *Acta Soc. Ophthalmol. Jpn.*, 89(Suppl), 137, 1985.
40. Johnson, L. V., Hageman, G. S. and Blanks, J. C., Interphotoreceptor matrix domains ensheath vertebrate cone photoreceptor cells, *Invest. Ophthalmol. Vis. Sci.*, 27, 129, 1986.
41. Sameshima, M., Uehara, F. and Ohba, N., Specialization of the interphotoreceptor matrices around cone and rod photoreceptor cells in the monkey retina, as revealed by lectin cytochemistry, *Exp. Eye Res.*, 45, 845, 1987.
42. Hollyfield, J. G., Rayborn, M. E., Landers, R. A. and Myers, K. M., Regional variations in insoluble IPM domains surrounding both rod and cone photoreceptors in the human retina, *Invest. Ophthalmol. Vis. Sci.*, 31(Suppl), 72, 1990.
43. Kirchoff, M. A., Anderson, K., Johnson, L. V. and Hageman, G. S., Composition and distribution of insoluble interphotoreceptor matrix constituents, *Invest. Ophthalmol. Vis. Sci.*, 31(Suppl), 153, 1990.
44. Hageman, G. S. and Johnson, L. V., Condroitin-6 sulfate glycosaminoglycan is a major constituent of primate cone photoreceptor matrix sheaths, *Curr. Eye Res.*, 6, 639, 1987.
45. Uehara, F., Sameshima, M., Muramatsu, T. and Ohba, N., Affinity isolation of cone outer segments using a peanut agglutinin-nitrocellulose sheet, *Exp. Eye Res.*, 43, 687, 1986.
46. Hollyfield, J. G., Varner, H. H., Rayborn, M. E. and Osterfeld, A. M., Attachment of the retina to the pigment epithelium: Linkage through the conedom, an extracellular matrix sheath associated uniquely with cone photoreceptors, in *Extracellular and Intracellular Messengers in the Vertebrate Retina*, Redburn, D. A. and Pasantes-Morales, H., Eds., Alan R. Liss, Inc., New York, 1989, 1.
47. Uehara, F., Muramatsu, T., Sameshima, M., Kawano, K., Koide, H. and Ohba, N., Effects of neuraminidase on lectin binding sites in photoreceptor cells of monkey retina, *Jpn. J. Ophthalmol.*, 29, 54, 1985.
48. Kivelä, T. and Tarkkanen, A., A lectin cytochemical study of glycoconjugates in the human retina, *Cell Tissue Res.*, 249, 277, 1987.
49. Molday, L. L. and Molday, R. S., Glycoproteins specific for the retinal rod outer segment plasma membrane, *Biochim. Biophys. Acta*, 897, 335, 1987.
50. Cohen, D. and Nir, I., Cytochemical characterization of sialoglycoconjugates on rat photoreceptor cell surface, *Invest. Ophthalmol. Vis. Sci.*, 28, 640, 1987.
51. Polans, A. S. and Burton, M. D., Sialoglycoproteins of the frog rod outer segment plasma membrane, *Invest. Ophthalmol. Vis. Sci.*, 29, 1523, 1988.
52. Uehara, F., Yasumura, D. and LaVail, M. M., Development of light-evoked changes of the interphotoreceptor matrix in normal and RCS rats with inherited retinal dystrophy, *Exp. Eye Res.*, (In press), 1991.
53. Uehara, F., Yasumura, D. and LaVail, M. M., Lectin binding of the interphotoreceptor matrix during retinal development in normal and RCS rats, *Curr. Eye Res.*, 9, 687, 1990.
54. Weidman, T. A. and Kuwabara, T., Development of the rat retina, *Invest. Ophthalmol.*, 8, 60, 1969.
55. Gold, G. H. and Korenbrot, J. I., Light-induced calcium release by intact retinal rods, *Proc. Natl. Acad. Sci. USA*, 77, 5557, 1980.
56. Gold, G. H., Plasma membrane calcium fluxes in intact rods are inconsistent with the "calcium hypothesis", *Proc. Natl. Acad. Sci. USA*, 83, 1150, 1986.
57. Oakley, B., II and Green, D. G., Correlation of light-induced changes in retinal extracellular potassium concentration with c-wave of the electroretinogram, *J. Neurophysiol.*, 39, 1117, 1976.

58. Steinberg, R. H. and Oakley, B., II, Light-evoked changes in $[K^+]_o$ in retina of intact cat eye, *J. Neurophysiol.*, 44, 897, 1980.
59. Borgula, G. A. and Steinberg, R. H., Light-evoked changes of $[H^+]$ in the retina of the intact cat eye, *Invest. Ophthalmol. Vis. Sci.*, 25 (Suppl), 289, 1984.
60. Borgula, G. A., Karwoski, C. J. and Steinberg, R. H., Light-evoked changes in extracellular pH in frog retina, *Vision Res.*, 29, 1069, 1989.
61. Comper, W. D. and Laurent, T. C., Physiological function of connective tissue polysaccharides, *Phys. Rev.*, 58, 255, 1978.
62. Dowling, J. E., The chemistry of visual adaptation in the rat, *Nature*, 188, 114, 1960.
63. Ho, M.-T. P., Massey, J. B., Pownall, H. J., Anderson, R. E. and Hollyfield, J. G., Mechanism of vitamin A movement between rod outer segments, interphotoreceptor retinoid-binding protein, and liposomes, *J. Biol. Chem.*, 264, 928, 1989.
64. Comper, W. D., Lisberg, W. and Veis, A., Diffusion potentials of polyelectrolytes and their possible relationship to biological electrochemical phenomena, *J. Colloid Interface Sci.*, 57, 345, 1976.
65. Bok, D. and Hall, M. O., The etiology of retinal dystrophy in RCS rats, *Invest. Ophthalmol.*, 6, 649, 1969.
66. LaVail, M. M., Sidman, R. L. and O'Neil, D. A., Photoreceptor-pigment epithelial cell relationships in rats with inherited retinal degeneration. Radioautographic and electron microscope evidence for a dual source of extra lamellar material, *J. Cell Biol.*, 53, 185, 1972.
67. Porrello, K., Yasumura, D. and LaVail, M. M., The interphotoreceptor matrix in RCS rats: histochemical analysis and correlation with the rate of retinal degeneration, *Exp. Eye Res.*, 43, 413, 1986.
68. LaVail, M. M., Yasumura, D. and Porrello, K., Histochemical analysis of the interphotoreceptor matrix in hereditary retinal degenerations, in *The Interphotoreceptor Matrix in Health and Disease*, Bridges, C. D. and Adler, A. J., Eds., Alan R. Liss, Inc., New York, 1985, 179.
69. Sanyal, S. and Jansen, H. G., Absence of receptor segments in the retina of *rds* mutant mice, *Neurosci. Let.*, 21, 23, 1981.
70. LaVail, M. M., Analysis of neurological mutants with inherited retinal degeneration, *Invest. Ophthalmol. Vis. Res.*, 21, 638, 1981.
71. Blanks, J. C., Mullen, R. J. and LaVail, M. M., Retinal degeneration in the *pcd* cerebellar mutant mouse. II. Electron microscopic analysis, *J. Comp. Neur.*, 212, 231, 1982.
72. LaVail, M. M., Blanks, J. C. and Mullen, R. J., Retinal degeneration in the *pcd* cerebellar mutant mouse. I. Light microscopic and autoradiographic analysis, *J. Comp. Neur.*, 212, 217, 1982.
73. LaVail, M. M., unpublished observations, 1990.

THE CHOROIDAL MICROVASCULATURE OF SPONTANEOUSLY DIABETIC RATS: STRUCTURE AND LUMINAL SURFACE PROPERTIES OF THE CHORIOCAPILLARIS ENDOTHELIUM

Ruth B. Caldwell[*] and Malinda E.C.Fitzgerald[‡]

[*]Department of Anatomy
The Medical College of Georgia
Augusta, GA 30912

[‡]Department of Anatomy and Neurobiology
The University of Tennessee
Memphis, TN 38163.

In diabetic rats, choroidal permeability to albumin is increased, basement membranes are thickened, and anionic charge sites at the choriocapillaris abluminal surface are decreased. In other vascular beds, permeability differences are correlated with differences in luminal membrane microdomains as indicated by altered distribution of luminal membrane anionic charge. To see whether or not the choroidal microvasculature shows changes in luminal surface charge distribution or other structural features during diabetes, we studied spontaneously diabetic and control rats using ultrastructural tracers and morphometric techniques. Rats were first injected with horseradish peroxidase and then perfused with aldehydes. Next, tissue sections were incubated with cationized ferritin, reacted to visualize peroxidase, and prepared for electron microscopic study. This analysis showed that cellular elements and extracellular matrix material in the interstitial stroma were increased in the diabetic rats. In addition, peroxidase uptake, ferritin binding, and numbers of fenestrations were reduced in many vessels of the diabetic rats as compared with the controls. However, variability was very high in the diabetic rats and differences between groups on the quantitative measures were not statistically significant.

I. INTRODUCTION

The effects of diabetes on the choriocapillaris are largely unknown. Biochemical studies in diabetic rats have shown increased choroidal permeability to albumin, but the cellular location of this effect is unclear.[1] In addition, basement membranes of choriocapillaris vessels and Bruch's membrane are thickened and anionic charge sites at the abluminal surface of choriocapillaris endothelial cells are decreased, but the effects of these changes on vascular function are unknown.[2-4] We therefore studied the effects of diabetes on the endothelial cell properties thought to be important in determining transcellular permeability -- luminal membrane microdomains.

The endothelial cells of the choriocapillaris contain large numbers of fenestrations, the majority of which face towards Bruch's membrane and the retinal pigment epithelium, suggesting that these cells are uniquely specialized for the exchange of fluid and metabolites between the blood and the pigment epithelium. Despite these fenestrations, however, permeability of the choriocapillaris to high molecular weight protein tracers is limited as compared with other fenestrated vascular beds.[5-9] Such differential permeability of fenestrated microvascular endothelial cells has been suggested to depend on the relative density of fenestrations, channels, and vesicles and on the biochemical composition of their diaphragms.[10-13] Support for this idea comes from studies using selective enzyme treatments and cationized ferritin or lectin-ferritin binding techniques. These studies suggest that endothelial cell luminal membranes microdomains in the choriocapillaris differ from those of more permeable fenestrated endothelia.[14,15] To see whether or not alterations in luminal membrane microdomains occur during diabetes, we studied the choriocapillaris endothelium of spontaneously diabetic and control rats using electron microscope morphometry and cationized ferritin and horseradish peroxidase tracer techniques.

II. METHODS

(A). ANIMALS
A total of 23 spontaneously diabetic rats (BB-Wor-Utm, 4 - 18 mos old) and diabetes prone controls (normoglycemic litter mates) were used. Animals were monitored daily for glycosuria and growth. Diabetic rats received daily injections of PZI insulin, with the dose adjusted according to maintain hyperglycemia, but prevent ketosis.[2] Rats were maintained on a 12 hr alternating light - dark cycle (illumination ~ 5 lux). All experiments were conducted during the light period.

(B). PROTOCOL
Anesthetized rats were injected intravenously with a mixture of methylsergide maleate and diphenhydramine HCl (1 mg/kg) to inhibit histamine and serotonergic responses to horseradish peroxidase. Five minutes later, HRP (100 mg/kg) was administered intravenously. After 30 min, animals were intracardially perfused with physiological saline (0.9% NaCl) followed by 2% paraformaldehyde/2% glutaraldehyde/ 0.5% acrolein fixative in 0.1M sodium cacodylate buffer, pH 7.4 as described previously.[16] Retina-choroid tissue sections were prepared and incubated in cationized ferritin (CF, 5mg/ml 0.1 M sodium cacodylate, 37°C 1 hr) as described.[16] After CF incubation, sections were reacted with hydrogen peroxide in the presence of diaminobenzidine (DAB) for peroxidase localization, and tissue was processed routinely for electron microscopy.

(C). QUANTITATIVE ANALYSIS
The following parameters were analyzed quantitatively: number of fenestrations and channels per 100 µm of luminal membrane, proportion of fenestrations facing the pigment epithelium, HRP uptake, cationized ferritin labeling of fenestration and channel diaphragms and of the plasma membranes, luminal surface area of the vessels, and relative diameter of the spaces between the vessels. For this analysis, adjacent 0.5 µm thick and 70 nm thin sections of the choriocapillaris were studied from nine diabetic and seven control rats. The relative breadth of Bruch's membrane occupied by choriocapillaris vessels and intervessel pillars were determined using a light microscope equipped with a drawing tube. Drawings were made of the choriocapillaris and diameter of vessels and intervessel pillars were determined using a computer assisted digitizing tablet. The other measurements were made at the electron microscopic level. For this analysis, 10 randomly chosen vessels were photographed from each animal at a magnification of 6,000X. For most vessels a photomontage of overlapping micrographs was necessary in order to cover the entire

vessel. These photomontages were used for measuring luminal surface area, calculating surface density of fenestrations and channels, and evaluating ferritin labeling on fenestral diaphragms. Luminal surface area was measured using a microcomputer and digitizing tablet and the number of fenestrations and channels/100 µm of luminal membrane were determined. CF labeling of fenestral and channel diaphragms was determined using an eyepiece reticule. In addition, the number of HRP labeled organelles/µm (HRP density) was determined for each vessel. For analysis of plasma membrane CF binding, random areas within each vessel where the luminal membrane was cut in cross section and well focused were photographed at 50,000X. These micrographs were coded and two observers evaluated them empirically according to the density of CF particles. Vessels with three or more uniform rows of CF particles were rated as having "high binding", those with one to two continuous rows of CF particles were rated as having "moderate binding", and those with a single discontinuous row of particles were rated as having "low binding" (see Figure 2).

(D). CONTROL STUDIES
Control studies of endogenous peroxidase activity and possible effects of HRP on CF labeling were done as described previously.[16] In other control experiments the histamine and serotonin inhibitors were omitted to evaluate possible effects of HRP-induced alterations on pinocytotic uptake and CF binding.

III. RESULTS

(A). MORPHOLOGY
The diabetic rat choroid and choriocapillaris showed basal laminae thickening as reported previously (data not shown).[2-4] Areas of basal lamina duplication were also observed (Figure 1).[2,3] Areas of basal lamina duplication were also present in the control rats, but were less elaborate than those in the diabetic rats (data not shown). Another alteration in the diabetic rats was an increase in cells and cell processes in the intercapillary spaces (Figure 1a). The identity of these cells is unknown, but their small size and the pattern of their nuclear chromatin were similar to those in endothelial cells. Pale cytoplasm and swollen endoplasmic reticulum in some intercapillary space cells (Figure 1a) and clusters of cellular debris in other areas suggested that some of these cells were degenerating.

(B). HRP UPTAKE
In diabetic rats HRP reaction product was present intracellularly in vesicles, multivesicular bodies, and lysosomes (Figure 1b). Reaction product was also present extracellularly, decorating the basal laminae of the choriocapillaris endothelium and the pigment epithelium as well as the extracellular matrix material and cell processes in the pericapillary spaces (Figure 1b). The same pattern of HRP distribution seen in the diabetic rats was observed in the normoglycemic control rats except that the amount of HRP reaction product bound to matrix material and cell membranes in the intercapillary space was lower due to the smaller amount of extracellular matrix material and cellular processes as compared with diabetic rats (data not shown). Quantitative analysis showed moderate levels of HRP uptake in the diabetic rats treated with inhibitors of HRP-induced vascular alterations. Number of labeled organelles per cell profile was lower in many vessels of the diabetic rats (mean $\pm$ S.D. = 12.8 $\pm$ 1.5) than in the control vessels (17.5 $\pm$ 6.7). However, variability was high and the difference was not statistically significant. The untreated rats were not analyzed quantitatively.

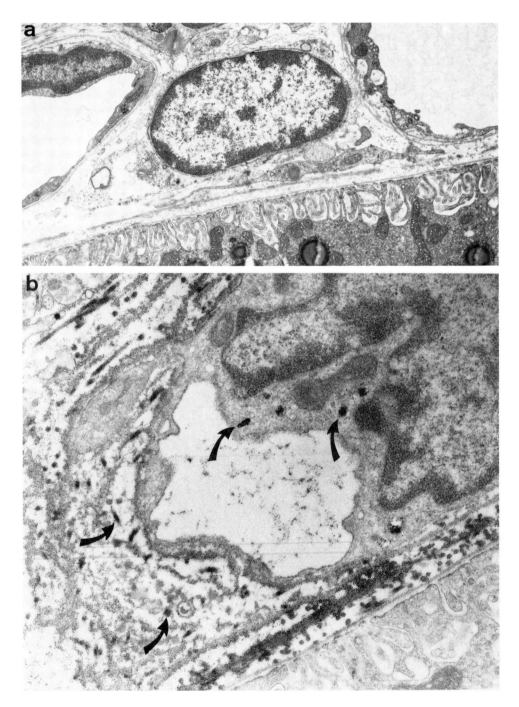

Figure 1: Numerous cell processes and an abnormal cell with pale cytoplasm and swollen endoplasmic reticulum occupy the intercapillary space in a diabetic rat (a). HRP reaction product (arrows, b) stains the duplicated basal lamina and other extracellular matrix material around a choriocapillaris vessel in a diabetic rat and is present intracellularly within vesicles, multivesicular bodies, and lysosomes. (a = ×8,600; b = 16,550).

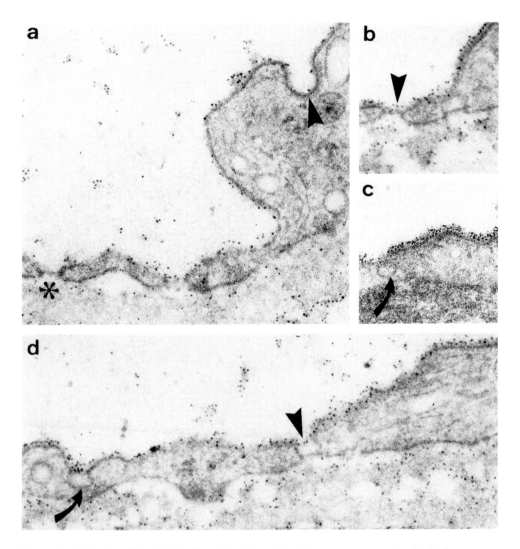

Figure 2: Cationized ferritin binding sites (arrowheads) are present on luminal plasma membranes; coated vesicles (a); and diaphragms of fenestrations (a, b), channels (b, d) and uncoated vesicles (d). Most uncoated vesicles (arrow, d) and a few fenestral diaphragms (asterisk, a) are unlabeled. Some control and most diabetic vessels had "low binding" (a). Few vessels in either group had "high binding" (b). Most control and some diabetic vessels had "moderate binding" (b, d). (×64,500).

(C). <u>CATIONIZED FERRITIN BINDING</u>

In both diabetic and control rats, cationized ferritin binding sites were present on the luminal plasma membrane, in coated vesicles, and on the diaphragms of most fenestrations, channels, and uncoated vesicles (Figure 2). Ferritin particles were almost never seen within uncoated vesicles (Figure 2c, d). Unlabeled diaphragms were sometimes seen (Figure 2a). The relative density of ferritin labeling was somewhat variable and labeling in a few vessels of the control rats and many of the vessels of the diabetic rats was relatively sparse with a single layer of ferritin particles interrupted by intervals of unlabeled

TABLE 1

Analysis of Luminal Membrane CF Binding Patterns[a]

Group	Low binding	Moderate binding	High binding
Diabetic (+ inhibitor)	56 ± 49	28 ± 31	15 ± 25
Diabetic (- inhibitor)	65 ± 42	16 ± 14	18 ± 31
Control (+ inhibitor)	30 ± 13	52 ± 3	17 ± 14

[a]Values are expressed as the percentage (mean + S.D) vessels classified as belonging to each category of CF labeling. Diabetic rats had been hyperglycemic for 4 - 7 months. Rats treated with inhibitors of HRP-induced permeability increases (+ inhibitor) and untreated (- inhibitor) rats were analyzed. When a composite value for all vessels was calculated for each rat, differences between groups were not statistically significant ($p > 0.05$, ANOVA).

TABLE 2

Fenestration and Channel Diaphragms Labeled with CF[a]

Group	Fenestral diaphragms	Channel diaphragms
Diabetic (+ inhibitor)	91 ± 7	90 ± 9
Diabetic (- inhibitor)	88 ± 5	96 ± 4
Control (+ inhibitor)	94 ± 2	98 ± 4

[a] Values are expressed as percent labeled diaphragms (mean ± S.D). Groups are as described in Table 1. Values are not significantly different ($p > 0.05$, ANOVA).

membrane (Figure 2a). The majority of vessels in the control animals had "moderate binding" with one to two relatively continuous rows of ferritin particles on their plasma membranes (Figure 2b, d). Vessels with "high binding" with two to three continuous layers of ferritin particles were rare in both groups (Figure 2c). Quantitative analysis showed that the majority of vessels in diabetic rats had "low binding" while in the control rats the majority of the vessels had moderate CF binding. However, the differences between groups was not significant due to high variability within the diabetic rats (Table 1). CF binding on the diaphragms of the fenestrations and channels was similar in the diabetic and control rats. In all three groups, the majority of the diaphragms were labeled with one or more ferritin particles (Table 2). Slightly more diaphragms were labeled in control rats than in either of the two diabetic groups, but the difference was not statistically significant (Table 2).

(D). MORPHOMETRIC STUDIES

Choriocapillaris luminal surface area in the younger diabetic animals was similar to that in the controls (Table 3). In the older rats, larger vessels were more common in the control rats, but group differences were not statistically significant. Because the accumulations of cellular processes and extracellular matrix material between choriocapillaris endothelial cells in the diabetic rats (see Figure 1) suggested that the area of intervessel stroma might be increased, we measured the relative diameters of the vessels and intervessel spaces in thick sections from diabetic and age-matched control rats. This analysis showed that some areas in the diabetic rats were larger than those in the controls, but again, due to variability between subjects, the differences were not statistically significant (Table 3). The density of fenestrations within the choriocapillaris endothelial cells was low in many vessels of the diabetic rats. However, variability was high in both diabetic and control rats and the differences were not significant. The density of the transendothelial channels in the vessels of the older diabetic rats was significantly reduced as compared with the younger diabetic rats, but differences between diabetic and control rats were not statistically significant (Table 3).

TABLE 3

Quantitative Analysis of Choriocapillaris Morphology [a]

Group	Luminal surface area (in μm)	Intervessel spaces (% total length)	Channels[b] (#/100 μm)	Fenestrations (#/100 μm)
Young Diabetic	36 ± 6	27 ± 5	10 ± 5	61 ± 14
Control	33 ± 4	24 ± 8	7 ± 2	92 ± 14
Old Diabetic	37 ± 10	22 ± 6	4 ± 2	78 ± 11
Control	44 ± 9	20 ± 2	5 ± 2	84 ± 36

[a] Values are expressed as means $\pm$ standard deviation. Young diabetic rats had been hyperglycemic for ≤ 4 mos. Old diabetic rats had been hyperglycemic for ≥ 9 mos. [b] Channels were reduced in the old diabetic rats as compared with the young diabetic group ($p < 0.05$, ANOVA). Other differences were not significant ($p > 0.05$, ANOVA).

IV. DISCUSSION

In summary, the main differences between the diabetic and control animals evident in this study were that the choriocapillaris intercapillary stroma of the diabetic rats contained increased amounts of extracellular matrix material as compared with the controls and that abnormal cells which sometimes appeared to be degenerating were present in the intervessel spaces. Extracellular matrix material increases are well known in diabetes, but to our knowledge this is the first report of cellular degeneration in the choriocapillaris of diabetic rats. The identity of the abnormal cells is unknown. They are similar in size to endothelial cells or pericytes. However, it is unlikely that either of these cell types is degenerating in view of our data showing normal capillary morphology and a previous morphometric study which found no difference in pericyte distributions between control and diabetic rats in the choriocapillaris after nine months of diabetes.[17] Further experiments using immunolocalization techniques are necessary to identify these cells conclusively.

In terms of their luminal surface properties, while many individual vessels of the choriocapillaris in diabetic rats appeared abnormal, showing low levels of HRP uptake, sparse patterns of CF binding, and relatively few fenestrations, other vessels in the same animals remained relatively normal. Thus, when composite values were calculated for each animal and groups were compared statistically using analysis of variance, the values in the diabetic rats were not significantly different from the controls. This observation was unexpected. Extracellular matrix alterations are known to have a strong influence on structure and function of other cell types in vitro and in vivo studies showing changes in choriocapillaris structure in association with extracellular matrix alterations during development and disease suggest that they also affect the endothelium of the choriocapillaris.[18] However, even though extracellular matrix changes are a consistent finding in diabetic rats,[2-4] our study suggests that many endothelial cells in the choriocapillaris of spontaneously diabetic rats remain relatively normal.

The variability in the effects of diabetes seen in this study is consistent with observations in human diabetics. Intersubject variability is a well-known feature of clinical diabetes, where some patients develop proliferative diabetic retinopathy while others never progress from background retinopathy, and others appear to be unaffected. Variability is also seen in breakdown of the blood-retinal barrier, where increased albumin permeability has been observed in some eyes from human diabetic donors while other eyes with other signs of diabetic retinopathy remain normal in terms of albumin permeability.[19,20] If variability during diabetes is also high between vessels from the same individuals as suggested by our data and by clinical studies showing focal blood-retinal barrier leakage to fluorescein in diabetic patients,[21] analysis of large quantities of tissue samples from large numbers of subjects will be necessary to demonstrate reliable differences between diabetic and normal eyes. This may not be possible using electron microscope morphometry because no matter how well controlled the sampling procedures, only a tiny fraction of the total retinal tissue can be analyzed. Similar sampling difficulties could account for some of the apparent contradictions between data resulting from studies of the inner retinal vessels in diabetic rats, where some workers find apparent permeability increases, while others report no change from control retinas. [22-26]

In addition to the sampling problems inherent in studies of diabetic tissues, it is also possible that the non-specific tracers used in the present study are not sufficiently sensitive to detect alterations in the diabetic microvessels. In an earlier study of the retinal microvasculature of spontaneously diabetic rats, using the same techniques as in the present study, we found that some morphologically altered vessels in the diabetic rats had increased pinocytotoic uptake and reduced and patchy CF binding as compared with control rats.[16] However, when large numbers of vessels were analyzed quantitatively and average values similar. In contrast with the latter results, studies using lectin ferritin probes and similar analytic techniques showed statistically significant changes in luminal membrane microdomains of the retinal vessels in the outer retina that were not evident with cationized ferritin.[27] Thus, studies using the more sensitive lectin ferritin techniques might demonstrate alterations not evident in the present study.

While our study showed no statistically significant differences between diabetic and normal rats in luminal membrane properties, we did observe differences between choriocapillaris and inner retinal vessels in luminal surface microdomains. In the choriocapillaris endothelial cells most uncoated vesicles are unlabeled following cationized ferritin incubations, whereas in the inner retinal vessels many of the uncoated vesicles are labeled.[16] The larger population of positively charged or uncharged vesicles could provide a means for transcellular transport of negative plasma proteins such as albumin by the choriocapillaris and may account for albumin permeability observed in the normal choroid and choriocapillaris.[28]

V. ACKNOWLEDGEMENTS

Excellent technical assistance was provided by Libby Perry, Darlene Moes, and Li Yan Ye. Supported by research grants from the National Eye Institute NIH-EY-04618 and The Juvenile Diabetes Foundation, International. MECF was supported by a postdoctoral fellowship from the Neuroscience Center for Excellence at The University of Tennessee, Memphis.

VI. REFERENCES

1. Williamson, J.R., Chang, K., Tilton, R.G., Prater, C., Jeffrey, F.R., Weigel, J., Sherman, W.R., Eades, D.M. and Kilo, C., Increased vascular permeability in spontaneously diabetic BB/W rats and in rats with mild versus severe streptozotocin-induced diabetes. Prevention by aldose reductase inhibitors and castration, <u>Diabetes,</u> 36, 813, 1987.

2. Caldwell, R.B., Slapnick, S.M. and McLaughlin, B.J., Decreased anionic sites in Bruch's membrane of spontaneous and drug-induced diabetes. <u>Invest. Ophthalmol. Vis. Sci.</u> 27, 1691, 1986.

3. Hori, S., Nishida, T., Mukai, Y., Pomeroy, M. and Mukai, N., Ultrastructural studies on choroidal vessels in streptozotocin-diabetic and spontaneously hypertensive rats, <u>Res. Comm. Chem. Path. Pharm.</u>, 1980, 29, 211.

4. Vinores, S.A., Campochiaro, P.A., May, E.E. and Blaydes, S.H., Progressive ultrastructural damage and thickening of the basement membrane of the retinal pigment epithelium in spontaneously diabetic BB rats, <u>Exp. Eye Res.</u>, 1988, 46, 545.

5. Pino, R.M. and Essner, E., Structure and permeability to ferritin of the choriocapillary endothelium of the rat eye, <u>Cell Tissue Res.</u>, 1980, 208, 21.

6. Pino, R.M. and Essner, E., Permeability of rat choriocapillaris to hemeproteins. Restriction of tracers by a fenestrated endothelium, <u>J. Histochem. Cytochem.</u>, 1981, 29, 281.

7. Essner, E. and Gordon, S.R., Observations on the permeability of the choriocapillaris of the eye, <u>Cell Tissue Res.</u>, 1983, 231, 571.

8. Pino, R.M. and Thouron, C.L., Vascular permeability in the rat eye to endogenous albumin and immunoglobulin G (IgG) examined by immunohistochemical methods, J. Histochem. Cytochem., 1983, 31, 411.

9. Pino, R.M., Restriction to endogenous plasma proteins by a fenestrated capillary endothelium: an ultrastructural immunocytochemical study of the choriocapillary endothelium, Am. J. Anat., 1985, 172, 279.

10. Milici, A.J., L'Hernault, N. and Palade, G.E., Surface densities of diaphragmed fenestrae and transendothelial channels in different murine capillary beds, Circ. Res., 1985, 56, 709.

11. Simionescu, N., Transcytosis and traffic of membranes in the endothelial cell, in, International Cell Biology, ed. Scherger, H.G. Springer-Verlag, Berlin, 1981, 657.

12. Simionescu, N., Simionescu, M. and Palade, G.E., Differentiated microdomains on the luminal surface of the capillary endothelium. I. Preferential distribution of anionic sites, J. Cell Biol., 1981, 90, 605.

13. Simionescu, M., Simionescu, N. and Palade, G.E., Biochemically differentiated microdomains of the cell surface of capillary endothelium, Ann. NY Acad. Sci., 1982, 401, 605.

14. Pino, R.M., The cell surface of a restrictive fenestrated endothelium, Cell Tissue Res., 1986, 243, 145.

15. Pino, R.M., The cell surface of a restrictive fenestrated endothelium II. Dynamics of cationic ferritin binding and the identification of heparin and heparan sulfate domains on the choriocapillaris, Cell Tissue Res., 1986, 243, 157.

16. Fitzgerald, M.E.C. and Caldwell, R.B., The retinal microvasculature of spontaneously diabetic BB rats: Structure and luminal surface properties, Microvasc. Res., 1990, 39, 15.

17. Tilton, R.G., LaRose, L.S., Kilo, C. and Williamson, J.G., Absence of degenerative changes in retinal and uveal capillary pericytes in diabetic rats, Invest. Ophthalmol. Vis. Sci., 1986, 27, 716.

18. Burns, M. S., Bellhorn, R. W., Korte, G. E. and Heriot, W. J., Plasticity of the retinal vasculature, in Progress in Retinal Research, vol. 5, eds. Osborne, N. and Chader, G., ,Vol. 5, Pergamon Press Ltd., Oxford, 1986, 253.

19. Vinores, S.A., Gadegbeku, C., Campochiaro, P.A. and Green, W.R., Immunohistochemical localization of blood-retinal barrier breakdown in human diabetics, Am J. Path., 1989, 134, 231.

20. Vinores, S.A., McGehee, R., Lee, A., Gadegbeku, C., Orman, W. and Campochiaro, P.A., Ultrastructural localization of blood-retinal barrier breakdown sites in diabetic and galactosemic rats and in human diabetics, Invest. Ophthalmol. Vis. Sci., 1990, 31(Suppl), 196.

21. Bek, T. and Lund-Anderson, H., Localised blood-retinal barrier leakage and retinal light sensitivity in diabetic retinopathy, Brit. J. Ophthalmol., 1990, 74, 388.

22. Ishibashi, T., Tanaka, K. and Taniguchi, Y., Disruption of blood-retinal barrier in experimental diabetic rats: An electron microscopic study, Exp. Eye Res., 1980, 30, 401.

23. Ishibashi, T., Tanaka, K. and Taniguchi, Y., Electron microscopic examination of retinal vascular changes in diabetic rats, Japan Medical Research Foundation, Tokyo, 1983, 1, 455.

24. Kirber, W.M., Nichols, C.W., Grimes, P.A., Wingrad, A.I. and Laties, A.M., A permeability defect of the retinal pigment epithelium. Occurrence in early streptozotocin diabetes, Arch. Ophthalmol., 1974, 98, 725.

25. Wallow, I.H.G. and Engerman, R.L., Permeability and patency of retinal blood vessels in experimental diabetes, Invest. Ophthalmol. Visual Sci., 1977, 16, 447.

26. Wallow, I.H.L., Posterior and anterior permeability defects/ Morphological observations on streptozotocin-treated rats, Invest. Ophthalmol. Visual Sci., 1983, 24, 1254.

27. Fitzgerald, M.E.C. and Caldwell, R.B., Lectin-ferritin binding on spontaneously diabetic and control rat retinal microvasculature, Curr. Eye Res., 1989, 8, 271.

28. Roque, R.S., Caldwell, R.B. and Hassell, J.R., Permeability and extracellular matrix alterations during retinal microvascular transformation, J. Cell Biol., 1990, 111, 148a.

SECTION III

RETINAL AND PIGMENT EPITHELIAL CELL TRANSPLANTATION

This section consists of studies aimed at one form of potential therapy for inherited retinal degenerations, retinal or retinal pigment epithelial (RPE) cell transplantation. The strategy of this approach is, quite simply, to replace genetically affected cells with genetically normal cells. The section begins with a historical perspective on ocular transplantation and is followed by six chapters on retinal or photoreceptor transplantation and two on RPE cell transplantation.

The studies on retinal or photoreceptor cell transplantation are marked by differences in experimental approach. They include transplantation of whole retinal expanses, dissociated whole retina, dissociated photoreceptor cells alone, and intact sheets of retina or photoreceptors. Despite these differences, most of the studies show observations of photoreceptor and retinal development of the transplanted tissue and integration of the grafted tissue into the host retina. In addition, evidence is presented for projection of transplanted retinal cells (using retinal grafts) to the superior colliculus. Moreover, in experiments where intact sheets of photoreceptors are transplanted into light-damaged retinas mostly devoid of photoreceptors, the transplants appear to mediate cortically recorded visual evoked responses and pupillary light reflexes. Although many of the results in these chapters are preliminary, taken together they indicate significant promise for the developing field of retinal and photoreceptor cell transplantation.

The two chapters on RPE cell transplantation build on the remarkable finding in 1988 that, when normal RPE cells are transplanted into the eyes of RCS rats with inherited retinal dystrophy, they rescue photoreceptors from degenerating. The first chapter provides data on optimal conditions for RPE cell transplantation, the prevention of secondary vascular changes in transplanted eyes, and the application of RPE transplantation to an age-related form of retinal degeneration. The second presents a refined method of RPE cell transplantation in rabbit eyes.

HISTORICAL ASPECTS OF RETINAL TRANSPLANTATION

Dean Bok, Department of Anatomy and Cell Biology, Department of Ophthalmology and Jules Stein Eye Institute, Center for the Health Sciences, University of California, Los Angeles, CA 90024

Our organizers have asked me to present some of the history of retinal transplantation as a prelude to the new information that we will be receiving on retinal transplantation at this symposium. The subject of interest today deals with the intraocular transplantation of neurosensory retina and of the retinal pigment epithelium, sometimes the two combined. I will therefore place most of my emphasis on that subject.

I. TRANSPLANTATION OF THE RETINA.

Efforts at transplantation of the neurosensory retina have involved its placement in various parts of the brain as well as the eye. As has been pointed out in one of the publications of del Cerro and associates,[1] scientists have been transplanting tissues into the eye for over a hundred years (as early as 1873 by van Dooremaal)[2] and the variety of transplanted tissues is impressive. The work that I encountered in my my graduate school histology course, namely that of Markee[3,] left a lasting impression upon me. Markee studied uterine endometrial changes in the late menstrual phase by implanting bits of endometrium from monkeys into their anterior eye chambers. The implants became vascularized and the vascular response to changes in hormonal levels could be studied for hours by looking through the transparent cornea. However, if one reviews all intraocular transplantation studies of central nervous tissue prior to 1985, only one report deals with the implantation of retinal tissue. This is the work of Royo and Quay in 1959.[4] These authors transplanted relatively undifferentiated rat fetal retinal tissue (neurosensory retina plus retinal pigment epithelium [RPE]) at embryonic day 16 into the maternal rat's anterior chamber and thereafter studied the development of the retina histologically. The implanted retinas developed a histiotypic organization to some extent, including the formation of rudimentary photoreceptors, although these quickly fell behind in development. The implants migrated through the pupil and became firmly attached to the posterior surface of the host's iris. Slowly, components of the cellular mass migrated around the lens and, during this process, the ganglion cells sent fibers to the host's retina. The transplants formed rounded rosette-like masses with the rudimentary photoreceptors located on the internal surface of the mass and projecting their processes internally. The RPE, rather than maintaining its association with the photoreceptors, appeared to contribute to the formation of a stratified squamous epithelium adjacent to the transplant. Surprisingly, the hyaloid artery was reformed as a result of these implants and the migrating neurons from the implant followed its path toward the retina.

I have described these results in some detail because, as you will hear today, we have not made a great deal of progress with respect to the transplantation of fetal neurosensory retina as far as the morphological outcome is concerned. Rosette formation remains a problem and the issue of connectivity between implant and host retina remains unresolved as does functional activity of the implants.

In 1985 the laboratories of del Cerro and Turner reported their initial studies on the intraocular transplantation of undifferentiated retina. The initial work of del Cerro and associates closely approximated the original work of Royo and Quay in 1959 except that the donors were not the direct offspring of the hosts and transplants were performed across rat strains.[1,5] In some respects the results were similar but there were notable exceptions. Contrary to the results of Royo and Quay, the differentiating implants did not migrate through the pupil and beyond. Instead, when implantation occurred it was always to the cornea and sometimes to the anterior iris as well, where it remained fixed. del Cerro et al.[1] did not observe migration of ganglion cell axons toward the posterior pole and questioned whether the reported migration of ganglion cells beyond the lens was a correct interpretation by Royo and Quay. Indeed, due to their improved histological methods (electron microscopy was not a standard method in 1959), del Cerro et al. were able to more accurately identify the details of the cellular response. Photoreceptor differentiation was severely impaired beyond the induction of cilia and a few outer segment discs, a phenomenon which has been uniformly observed in a myriad of reports where experimental conditions lead to the separation of neurosensory retina from RPE. Essentially, the photoreceptors do not differentiate beyond the ciliary stage reported in the early tissue culture studies of LaVail and Hild.[6] However a more recent study by Ninomiya reports that co-transplantation of incompletely-differentiated tecta and retina into syngenic rats dramatically improves survival rates for the implant.[7]

At about the same time that del Cerro and associates were implanting whole retinal tissue into the anterior chamber, Turner and his collaborators were placing transplants into fresh or healed lesion sites in the neurosensory rat retina.[8,9] Taking the cue from CNS transplantation studies in other systems in which wound repair was the objective, Turner and Blair made wounds in the dorsal retinas of rats by penetrating eyewall incisions.[8] They then positioned incompletely-differentiated neurosensory retinal fragments from neonatal rats of the same strain into these lesion sites either immediately following the lesion or after wound healing was complete. In both cases, a 90-100% survival rate was reported. The implanted retinas continued to differentiate into their histotypical, layered structure although this, like all other reported cases of transplantation of completely-differentriated retina, was complicated by rosette formation. The plexiform layers of the retina appeared to integrate with the host retina, ie. retinal layers peripheral and central to the graft that were diminished in thickness due to the lesion, appeared to thicken when a graft was present. No functional studies were performed to determine whether the grafts had sufficient connectivity with the host to subserve vision.

Silverman and Hughes have used yet a different route for neurosensory retinal transplantation.[10] They vibratome-sectioned the photoreceptor layer from 8-day old rat retinas and, with the aid of a gelatin substrate, inserted the transplant transcorneally, behind the iris, penetrating the neurosensory retina at the ora serrata, and guiding the transplant from that point through the subretinal (retinal ventricular) space toward the posterior pole. The hosts in this case were rats whose rods had previously been eliminated by light damage. Transplants examined up to four weeks post-transplantation clearly indicated success in placement of the transplant. Some areas showed a flat transplant with no obvious outer segments, however all transplants exhibited some degree of rosette formation. In 33% of cases, this involved more than half of the transplant. The only attempt to test functional integrity in this case was the demonstration that the transplant contained opsin as exhibited by immunocytochemistry. In spite of the claim by Silverman and Hughes that this indicated active opsin biosynthesis, it is known that the normal 8-day old rat retina (the age at which the donor tissue was taken) contains rudimentary outer segments and is actively engaged in opsin synthesis. Silverman and Hughes have subsequently performed some radioactive 2-deoxyglucose studies on similar transplants which suggest that the cells can be stimulated to take up this metabolic marker.[11]

At this point it is appropriate to emphasize the critical need for better functional testing of retinal transplants. Transplantation of retinas into nonocular sites has preceeded intraocular transplantation studies and the tests for function performed in these studies are to be emulated. McLoon and Lund[12] were successful in transplanting fetal rat retinas (13-15 days gestation) near the superior colliculus of neonatal rats. As was the case for intraocular transplants, the retinas developed somewhat histotypically but also suffered from rosette formation and lack of well-developed outer segments. However, the transplants sent projections to brain nuclei which are normally retinorecipient such as the superior colliculus and lateral geniculate nucleus. Subsequently, Klassen and Lund were able to demonstrate the functional integrity of some of these connections[13]. Initially, one of the eyes from the neonatal host was removed prior to transplantation of the fetal retina. After five months, they severed the optic nerve of the remaining eye, taking care to leave intact the sympathetic outflow from the third cranial nerve. Removal of overlying structures and illumination of the retinal transplant dramatically revealed an intact, albeit sluggish pupillary reflex.

Subsequent studies have shown that the same results can be obtained when the fetal rat retina is transplanted to the adult brain.[14] Functional testing at this level of elegance is required for intraocular transplants.

II. TRANSPLANTATION OF THE RETINAL PIGMENT EPITHELIUM

Gouras and associates were the first to initiate intraocular RPE transplantation.[15] Their initial studies focused on the prospect of acutely removing resident RPE cells from the recipient and replacing them with those of a donor. The experimental animals used in the early experiments were owl monkeys whose vitreous is liquid and therefore easy to remove. Employing an "open-sky" surgical approach, a 250^0 circumferential cut was made along the cornea just anterior to the limbus. Following intracapsular lens removal and aspiration of the liquid vitreous, the neurosensory retina was cauterized along three sides of a rectangular area, cut through the cauterized zone and folded away to expose the underlying epithelium. Thereafter, the RPE was trypsinized and removed from the exposed area and replaced by cultured human RPE cells that had been labeled in vitro with ^{3}H-thymidine. The animals were positioned to allow sedimentation and attachment of the RPE cells over the denuded area. No attempt was made to reattach the neurosensory retinas and, following wound closure, the animals were allowed to survive as long as seven days after transplantation. The transplants were monitored histologically and by tissue autoradiography. These studies clearly demonstrated that, within two hours of transplantation, cultured RPE cells are capable of attaching to denuded Bruch's membrane. The presence of ^{3}H-thymidine-labeled cells left no doubt as to the exogenous origin of the cells. There was, however, early evidence for reaction to these interspecies grafts. Transplantation periods longer than 3 days resulted in evidence for invasion by cells of the immune system. Also, the transplanted cells appeared to proliferate in uncontrolled fashion, forming multiple layers.

Aside from the immune response, this highly-invasive method of RPE transplantation had, as acknowledged by the authors, the obvious disadvantage of the interruption of retinal circuitry and the ultimate need for reattachment of the neurosensory retina. Gouras and associates therefore developed a closed-eye method for RPE transplantation involving a pars plana approach.[16] Additionally, these studies involved rabbit to rabbit grafting of

RPE cells. By means of a pars plana incision, a cannula filled initially with suspended RPE cells followed by a bolus of balanced salt solution (BSS) was inserted to a point 2 to 3 disc diameters from the optic nerve and a hole was formed in the neurosensory retina by a stream of BSS ejected from the cannula. Subsequently, patches of RPE were denuded with a similar stream of fluid. In the process, a small bleb detachment was produced under the neurosensory retina and, when all of the BSS was expelled, the suspended RPE cells, initially loaded into the cannula were deposited under the bleb. After 24 to 48 hours, the neurosensory retina spontaneously reattached. Once again, ^{3}H-thymidine tracer studies verified the fact that some of the cells that attached to Bruch's membrane were exogenous in origin. Transplanted cells began their attachment to Bruch's membrane by one hour and were mixed with native cells dislodged by the procedure. The transplanted cells appeared to be involved in the phagocytosis of outer segment debris within 24 hours of transplantation. This approach involved procedures that were clearly less traumatic to ocular tissues and appeared to lessen the inflammatory response. Some disadvantages in this approach were listed by the authors, namely the prospect of producing hemorrhage of the neurosensory retina in primates which, unlike rabbits, have a vascular retina, the prospect of inadvertently seeding the vitreal surface of the retina with RPE cells which could lead to proliferative vitreal retinopathy (PVR) and the production of a retinal hole which could also lead to complications including retinal tears, PVR and detachment.

Li and Turner, in 1988, reported transplantation of rat RPE cells by an external route which did not interrupt the integrity of the neurosensory retina.[17] RPE cells were freshly isolated from 6-8 day-old pigmented Long Evans rats and transplanted onto Bruch's membrane of albino Sprague Dawley rats ranging in age from 10 postnatal days to adulthood. The endogenous melanin in the donor cells or the fluorescent stain, Nuclear Yellow served as a marker for injected cells. A small incision was made through the sclera and choroid of the host eye and dispersed cells were injected with a syringe. Following wound closure, the eyes were examined histologically and ultrastructurally at periods ranging from 24 hrs to 3 months after transplantation. In separate experiments, trypan blue injection along with the RPE cells indicated that many of the resident cells were damaged. This suggested that attachment of the grafted cells was probably enhanced via denuding of Bruch's membrane by the jet stream of vehicle emanating from the syringe needle. The transplanted cells developed a normal relationship with Bruch's membrane and photoreceptors. There was no obvious immune rejection of the transplanted cells after three months even though two different strains of rat were employed in these studies.

Turner and associates took advantage of the opportunity to use their RPE transplantation methods in RCS rats whose RPE is virtually incapable of phagocytosing outer segment discs and is known to be the site of expression of the gene defect responsible for this reduced phagocytosis.[18,19] Li and Turner initiated experiments to determine whether normal RPE cells transplanted into the subretinal space of RCS rats during the early stages of disease could replace endogenous, defective cells thereby preventing photoreceptor degeneration.[20] Twenty-six day-old, pink-eyed RCS rats were used as hosts and pigmented, 6-8 day-old Long Evans rats provided the donor cells. The host retinas were examined at 60 postnatal days when the outer nuclear layer is normally reduced to 1-2 cells. Areas of retina containing transplanted RPE cells maintained an outer nuclear layer thickness of 10-11 cells, comparable to that which existed at the time of transplantation. Thus the transplanted RPE cells appeared to rescue their underlying photoreceptors. As was the case in earlier and subsequent studies by Li and Turner there was no morphological evidence of tissue rejection in the host animals.[17] Sheedlo et al. and Lopez et al. subsequently extended these observations to 3 and 4 months respectively.[21,22]

When Mullen and LaVail reported their classic chimaeric rat experiments, they carefully noted a disparity between the number of normal RPE cells present in a given area of retina and the number of underlying photoreceptors rescued.[19] The area of rescue extended well beyond the normal RPE cell boundaries. They postulated that a trophic factor might be operative in these areas in addition to the removal of outer segment discs by normal RPE cells. Li and Turner also observed that the area of photoreceptor rescue was not commensurate with the small number of cells delivered to the subretinal space.[20]

Silverman and Hughes,[23] prompted by these observations, performed some important sham transplantations that gave further credence to the prospect of a role for trophic factors in photoreceptor rescue. They administered saline injections to 25 day-old RCS rats using the surgical approach of Li and Turner.[17] Additionally, they used their own transcorneal approach to sham-operate a group of 31 day-old RCS rats.[10] In this case, only the gelatin insert without tissue was placed in the subretinal space. Two months after surgery, the retinas were examined histologically, a time when photoreceptor nuclei should have been reduced to a single row, provided the normal course of degeneration had taken place. Areas receiving saline injections or gelatin inserts showed significant preservation in outer nuclear layer thickness (8-10 nuclei). The authors also claimed that there was little or no debris buildup in the treated regions and concluded from these observations that photoreceptor rescue in the RCS rat does not require the injection of normal PRE cells. However, the cytological detail provided by their frozen sections did not warrant this conclusion in this reviewer's opinion. Evidence for permanent rescue of photoreceptors would require proof that there was no outer segment debris and that normal RPE phagocytic function had been restored. It is clear from this study nonetheless that factors in addition to the introduction of normal RPE cells are operative during the response of the photoreceptors to RPE transplantation. Considerable insight into this question will be given during this symposium by the work of Faktorovitch et al.[24] which suggests that fibroblast growth factor b might be a trophic factor involved in the rescue phenomenon. Single injections of this growth factor provide long-term survival of RCS photoreceptors. The debris layer persists nonetheless in these animals, indicating that the growth factor itself does not restore full phagocytic function.

This brings us to the state of matters regarding retinal transplantation as currently published. We are fortunate to have as participants at this symposium, nearly all of the investigators currently involved in retinal transplantation studies. Their recent accomplishments will now be presented for your consideration.

III. REFERENCES

1. del Cerro, M., Gash, D.M., Rao, G.N., Notter, M.F., Wiegand, S.J., Sathi, S. and del Cerro, C., Retinal transplants into the anterior chamber of the rat eye, *Neuroscience*, 21, 707, 1987.
2. Van Dooremaal, J.C., De ontwikkeling van levende weefsels op vreemden boden *Hoogeschool*, 3, 77, 1873.
3. Markee, J.E., Menstruation in intraocular endometrial transplants in the rhesus monkey, *Contrib. Embryol.*, 28, 219, 1940.
4. Royo, P.E. and Quay, W.B., Retinal transplantation from fetal to maternal mammalian eye, *Growth*, 23, 313, 1959.
5. del Cerro, M., Gash, D.M., Gullapalli, N.R., Notter, M.F., Wiegand, S.J. and Gupta, M., Intraocular retinal transplants, *Invest. Ophthalmol. Vis. Sci.*, 26, 1182, 1985.
6. LaVail, M.M. and Hild, W., Histotypic organization of the rat retina in vitro, *Z. Zellforsch.*, 114, 557, 1971.

7. Ninomiya, S., Morphological changes of embryonic retina and tectum transplanted into the anterior eye chamber of adult rats, *Acta Societ. Ophthalmol. Jap.*, 93, 475, 1989.

8. Turner, J.E. and Blair, J.R., Newborn rat retinal cells transplanted into a retinal lesion site in adult host eyes, *Dev. Brain Res.*, 391, 91, 1986.

9. Laedtke, T.W. and Turner, J.E., Embryonic retinal grafts have a beneficial effect on the damaged host retina, *Brain Res.*, 500, 61, 1989.

10. Silverman, M.S. and Hughes, S.E., Transplantation of photoreceptors to light-damaged retina, *Invest. Ophthalmol. Vis. Sci.*, 30, 1684, 1989.

11. Silverman, M.S. and Hughes, S.E., Light dependent activation of light-damaged retina by transplanted photoreceptors, *Invest. Ophthalmol. Vis. Sci. (Suppl.)* 30, 208, 1989.

12. McLoon, S.C. and Lund, R.D., Specific projections of retina transplanted to rat brain., *Exp. Brain Res.*, 40, 273, 1980.

13. Klassen, H. and Lund, R.D., Retinal transplants can drive a pupillary reflex in host rat brains, *Proc. Natl. Acad. Sci. U.S.A.*, 84, 6958, 1987.

14. Klassen, H. and Lund, R.D., Retinal graft-mediated pupillary responses in rats: restoration of a reflex function in the mature mammalian brain. *J. Neurosci.*, 10, 5789, 1990.

15. Gouras, P., Flood, M.T., Kjeldbye, H., Bilek, M.K. and Eggers, H., Transplantation of cultured human retinal epithelium to Bruch's membrane of the owl monkey eye. *Curr. Eye Res.*, 4, 253, 1985.

16. Lopez, R., Gouras, P., Brittis, M. and Kjeldbye, H., Transplantation of cultured rabbit retinal epithelium to rabbit retina using a closed-eye method, *Invest. Ophthalmol. Vis. Sci.*, 28, 1131, 1987.

17. Li, L. and Turner, J.E., Transplantation of retinal pigment epithelial cells to immature and adult rat hosts: short and long-term survival characteristics, *Exp. Eye Res.*, 47, 771, 1988.

18. Bok, D. and Hall, M.O., The role of the pigment epithelium in the etiology of inherited retinal dystrophy in the rat, *J. Cell Biol.*, 49, 664, 1971.

19. Mullen, R.J. and LaVail, M.M., Inherited retinal dystrophy: primary defect in pigment epithelium determined with experimental rat chimeras, *Science*, 192, 799, 1976.

20. Li, L. and Turner, J.E., Inherited retinal dystrophy in the RCS rat: Prevention of photoreceptor degeneration by pigment epithelial cell transplantation, *Exp. Eye Res.*, 47, 911, 1988.

21. Sheedlo, H.J., Li, L. and Turner, J.E., Functional and structural characteristics of photoreceptor cells rescued in RPE-cell grafted retinas of RCS dystrophic rats, *Exp. Eye Res.*, 48, 841, 1989.

22. Lopez, R., Gouras, P., Kjeldbye, H., Sullivan, B., Repucci, V., Brittis, M., Wapner, F. and Goluboff, E., Transplanted retinal pigment epithelium modifies the retinal degeneration in RCS rats, *Invest. Ophthalmol. Vis. Sci.*, 30, 586, 1989.

23. Silverman, M.S. and Hughes, S.E., Photoreceptor rescue in the RCS rat without pigment epithelium transplantation. *Curr. Eye Res.*, 9, 183, 1990.

24. Faktorovitch, E.G., Steinberg, R.H., Yasamura, D., Matthes, M.T. and LaVail, M.M., Basic fibroblast growth factor delays photoreceptor degeneration in inherited retinal dystrophy, *Nature (In press)*, 1990.

ULTRASTRUCTURE OF LONG TERM RETINAL CELL TRANSPLANTS TO RAT RETINA

Berndt Ehinger[+], Charles L. Zucker[*], Anders Bergström[+], Magdalene Seiler[*], Robert B. Aramant[*], Björn Gustavii[#], and Alan R. Adolph[*]

[*]Eye Research Institute, Boston (MA, USA) and Departments of [+]Ophthalmology and [#]Gynecology, University of Lund, (Sweden).

KEY WORDS

Retinal cell transplants, homografts, xenografts, retinal fetal cells, synapses, electron microscopy.

SUMMARY

The development of 5 rat homotransplants and 5 human xenotransplants to rat eyes have been examined in the electron microscope. The rat homotransplants were of 9 to 10 weeks total age after conception in four cases and 20 weeks in one case. They were at stage E15 when transplanted. The human transplants were examined at 30 to 41 weeks after conception when examined. The human fetal retinas (6-12 weeks post-conception) were obtained from elective abortions. Transplants developed both in the epiretinal and subretinal space. Xenotransplanted rats were immunosuppressed with Cyclosporin A.

The transplants from both species developed according to their intrinsic, genetically determined timetable. The development was heterogeneous with some parts showing almost normal differentiation and others little. Rat subretinal transplants were more developed than epiretinal grafts, but only epiretinal grafts have so far been seen to make contacts with the host retina. Photoreceptor cells developed with both inner and outer segments and synaptic terminals. In regions corresponding to the inner plexiform layer, the adult complement of synapses was seen, including advanced features like serial synapses as well as a few reciprocal synapses at the bipolar cell dyads. Incompletely differentiated synapses of both the amacrine and bipolar cell types were often observed, especially in the rat epiretinal transplants. Ganglion cell processes could not be identified with certainty.

Transplant cells touched host photoreceptor cells and pigment epithelium without any obvious specializations. Graft cells were occasionally found in the host retina, and nerve cell processes were observed to cross the membrane separating the transplant and host.

INTRODUCTION

It has been known for more than two decades that embryonic retina can survive transplantation and continue to develop in a new location[1]. Only within the last few years has it become conceivable that retinal transplantation offers the possibility to replace failing neurons. Immature retinal cells have been successfully transplanted to adult retina in a few mammalian species[2-7], and xenografts have also been successful (mouse to rat, fetal human retinal cells to adult rat retina[8,9]. Transplantation of mature retinal cells has also been reported[10,11]. Because the cells develop no faster than their intrinsic, genetically determined timetable, transplants of human origin need to remain in the host eye up to approximately the normal, full term, human gestational age.

The development of synapses and other ultrastructural features of human retinal cell transplants have hitherto not been studied, and there are only few reports on the ultrastructure of transplanted rat retinal cells. To establish to which extent the transplants form the same type of contacts as in the normal development and whether they make contacts with the host retina, we have examined the ultrastructure of transplants of fetal retina from both rats and humans to adult rat retina. The rat transplants were studied after 7 to 8 weeks (four eyes) and, in one case, 19 weeks. The human transplants were left in place for 30 - 41 weeks of total age post-conception to ensure that significant development be observable. All the synapse types seen in normal retinas were found in the transplants, and neuronal processes were seen to cross the border between the transplant and the host retina.

MATERIALS AND METHODS

A. HUMAN XENOTRANSPLANTS

With due permits, human embryos were obtained from elective abortions with the informed consent of the women seeking abortion. The fetal retinas were dissected from the surrounding tissues in sterile phosphate buffered saline, which also was used as the injection vehicle. Adult female albino Sprague-Dawley rats received unilateral retinal grafts by injecting a few μl of embryonic tissue into a small lesion made by cutting through sclera, choroid, and retina 1-2 mm behind the equator[11]. One donor retina was used for several host eyes, and pieces of peripheral and central donor retina were randomly mixed in the transplants. The xenotransplanted animals were immunosuppressed with Cyclosporin A as described elsewhere[9,12]. They were also given tetracycline (Terramycin[(R)], 100 mg/l) in their drinking water *ad libitum* to prevent infections. The eyes of the host animals were fixed <u>in situ</u> by an injection of a small volume (0.1 - 0.4 ml) of 2% osmium tetroxide in cacodylate buffer (see Ehinger et al.[12]).

The xenograft survival figures are from 74 consecutive operations with human tissue (see Table 1). Grafts from five eyes (obtained at 30-41 weeks age after conception) were used for the EM analysis of the long term development of the transplants. One was subretinal and four were epiretinal.

B. RAT HOMOTRANSPLANTS

Rat homotransplants were produced in rats with the same method as the human xenotransplants. Transplants from five eyes have been examined in the electron microscope, four from transplants taken 8 weeks after the transplantation and one taken 19 weeks after the transplantation. All were transplanted at stage E15. Three transplants were subretinal and two were epiretinal.

RESULTS

A. HUMAN XENOTRANSPLANTS

Human fetal retina has been available at ages ranging from about 4 weeks after conception up to about 14 weeks. There was no clear-cut difference in the survival rate with transplants of different donor ages. However, the total time in the host strongly influenced graft survival (Table 1) with a success rate of approximately 80% at short survival times which fell to about 30% in the longest experiments.

TABLE 1

Human xenografts to rat eyes. Transplant survival at different times after transplantation

Age of transplant tissue when fixed (days)	Number of hosts examined	Number of surviving transplants	Percentage of hosts with surviving transplants
50-99	41	34	83
100-149	17	11	65
150-199	14	11	79
200-249	17	9	53
250-305	29	8	28

Light microscopically, the grafts were seen to consist of cell layers organized in rosettes with photoreceptor cells pointing inward into the lumen of the rosette as previously described[9]. A rosette is a lumen surrounded by an innermost layer of photoreceptor cells and, to varying degrees, by other retinal layers. There is also an outer limiting membrane (i.e. a zone of tight junctions between the cells) at the level of the photoreceptor cells. Rods and cones were seen to form the most central cell layer of the rosettes. Often, a concentric neuropil similar to the normal outer plexiform layer

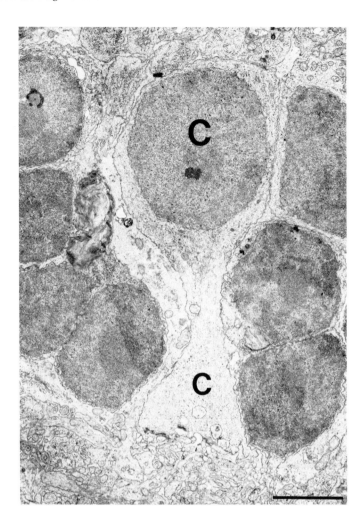

Figure 1. Low power micrograph of a part of a rosette in a human xenotransplant to a rat eye. A well developed cone with a large and relatively pale cell nucleus and a well developed synaptic terminal is seen, surrounded by rod nuclei. The total age of the transplant after conception was 30 weeks. Calibration bar = 5 μm.

was seen around the rosette. The space between the rosettes was filled with cells similar to those of the inner nuclear layer and with regions with neuropil resembling the inner plexiform layer. Interspersed amongst such relatively well differentiated regions, parts containing only poorly differentiated cells were also found. There was no well-developed ganglion cell layer, nor was there any well organized inner limiting membrane.

Electron microscopically, cones were clearly discernible in addition to numerous rods in most of the rosettes (Figure 1). Photoreceptor outer segments often were present in the center of rosettes. Although usually distorted, outer segments with nearly normal appearance have been observed.

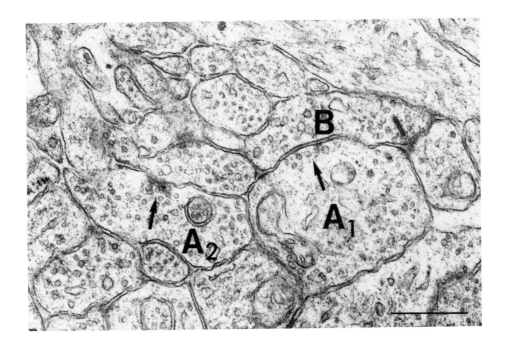

Figure 2. Region corresponding to the inner plexiform layer in a human xenotransplant (30 weeks total age after conception). A bipolar cell process (B) with a prominent synaptic ribbon is seen engaged in a dyad synapse with two amacrine cell processes, one of which (A1) makes a reciprocal synapse back onto the bipolar cell process (arrow). A different amacrine cell process (A2) makes a synapse (arrow) onto an amacrine cell process. Calibration bar = 0.5 μm.

In certain regions of the transplants, well developed cone and rod terminals were numerous and showed invaginations of processes of both the horizontal cell type and the bipolar cell type. Numerous synaptic vesicles filled the photoreceptor terminals and synaptic ribbons were prominent at the invaginations. There was a presynaptic arciform density, and both the pre- and postsynaptic membranes showed increased electron density as in the fully developed photoreceptor synapse. Other regions of the transplants were less well developed, and many of the photoreceptor terminals then had poorlydefined structural features.

In regions homologous to the inner plexiform layer, synapses of the conventional type (thought to represent amacrine cell synapses) were relatively common (Figure 2).

They made contacts with bipolar cell processes (Figure 2) and amacrine cell processes as well as many processes that could not be positively identified. Serial synapses with other amacrine cells were common (Figure 2) and reciprocal synapses have been observed. Infrequently, amacrine cells making synapses on small spines or thin inter-varicose processes were seen.

Bipolar cell processes in the inner plexiform layer are characterized by their high number of synaptic vesicles and ribbon synapses, arranged in dyads, and such processes were often observed (Figure 2). Ribbon synapses were frequently seen in a so-called monad arrangement, i.e., with only one postsynaptic process.

When identifiable, the postsynaptic elements in a dyad were always amacrine cell processes, but in a quarter to a fifth of the cases, we could not determine the nature of one of the postsynaptic processes because it did not contain any synaptic vesicles or any other characteristic amacrine cell marker. We cannot exclude that such unidentified postsynaptic processes originate in ganglion cells. Sometimes, the postsynaptic amacrine cell processes formed reciprocal synapses back onto the bipolar cell (Figure 2).

There were usually no structural specializations or changes in the parts where the grafts contacted the retina, pigment epithelium, or Bruch's membrane of the host. However, cells with structural characteristics of transplanted cells have a few times been seen in the host, introduced from an epiretinal graft through a break in the inner limiting membrane. Similarly, cells from subretinal grafts have been seen to intermingle with the host cells at the light microscopical level.

The inner surface of epiretinal grafts never had the organization typical of the inner limiting membrane. However, in both sub- and epiretinal grafts, the interior of the graft contained short (50-200 μm) pieces of basal membrane associated with collagen-like fibrils and Müller cell processes. The epiretinal grafts contacted the inner limiting membrane of the host retina without any specializations in the cells or processes. Small breaks in the host inner limiting membrane were common, and transplant cells (identified by their size, shape and of their nuclei density) could then be seen to reach into the host retina in the region. In other places, nerve cell processes crossed the border between host and graft[12].

B. RAT HOMOTRANSPLANTS

Like the human xenotransplants, the rat transplants were regularly found to contain regions that resembled the normal layers in the adult retina. Subretinal grafts were generally better differentiated than epiretinal grafts. The description given here is based on the appearance of subretinal grafts and differences between the two types will be noted separately.

The cells in the transplants were often arranged in rosettes. Photoreceptor inner and outer segments with connecting cilia and basal bodies were well developed. The photoreceptor terminals tended to be either clustered or aligned with each other, frequently exhibiting one or several synaptic ribbons with postsynaptic processes arranged in a triadic configuration (Figure 3). Occasionally, synaptic ribbons were found within photoreceptor terminals without any direct association with the cell membrane or any postsynaptic processes. At the junction of host and graft, host photoreceptor outer segments directly overlying the graft were somewhat distorted but intact. Although these outer segments may directly oppose the graft with no obvious

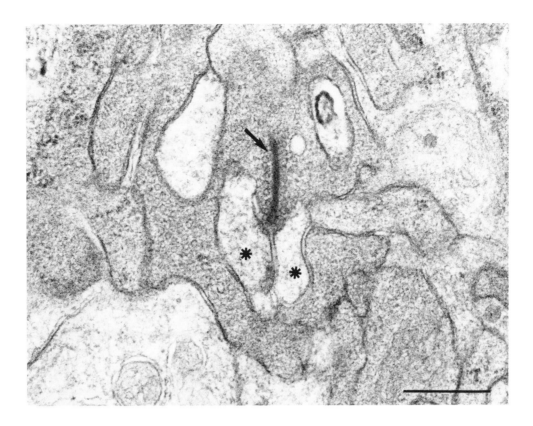

Figure 3. Electron micrograph of an outer plexiform region in a rat subretinal homotransplant (50 days post transplant survival) with a well developed photoreceptor terminal. A synaptic ribbon (arrow), surrounded by a halo of vesicles is presynaptic to two well defined laterally positioned postsynaptic processes, possibly of horizontal cell origin (asterisks). Such a configuration is typical of normal adult retinas. Calibration bar = 0.5 μm.

separating membrane, little or no integration was usually observed.

Regions corresponding to the inner plexiform layer exhibited a relatively high synaptic density which was consistent from region to region. Most, but not all synaptic terminals were well filled with conventional synaptic vesicles. Occasionally, small and large dense-cored vesicles could be seen. Amacrine-to-amacrine and amacrine-to-bipolar synapses were common, sometimes in both serial and reciprocal configurations. Bipolar ribbon synapses were also common, often having postsynaptic processes in a typical dyadic arrangement. Ribbon synapses with only one postsynaptic element (monadic synapses) and cell processes with synaptic ribbons not connected to the cell membrane were infrequently present. A few gap junctions have been identified, involving amacrine cell processes (Figure 4).

Discrete regions resembling the outer and inner plexiform layers were less regularly found in epiretinal transplants. Although rosettes were common, their borders tended not to be as sharply delineated as in subretinal transplants. Regions

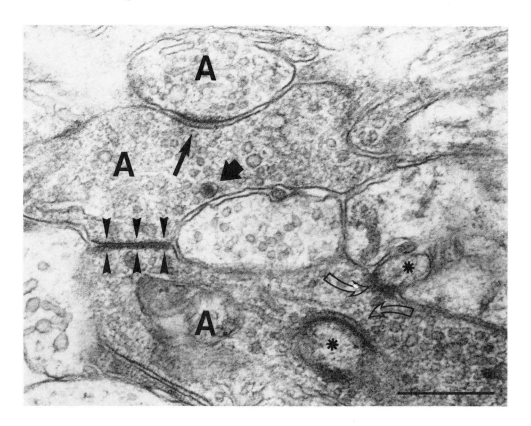

Figure 4. Region corresponding to the inner plexiform layer in a rat epiretinal homotransplant (54 days post transplant survival). Several synaptic vesicle filled amacrine cell processes (A) are seen. A large dense-cored vesicle (large arrow) is also shown. Two of the amacrine cell processes are connected via a gap junction (arrowheads) while these processes also make synaptic contacts with another amacrine cell process (thin arrow) and two dendritic spines (open arrows, asterisks). Calibration bar = 0.5 μm.

analogous to the outer plexiform layer were less common than in the subretinal transplants, with occasional photoreceptor terminals tending to be incorporated into general neuropil areas. When present, photoreceptor terminals were less likely to be contacted by clearly defined postsynaptic elements than in subretinal transplants. In epiretinal transplants, the synaptic ribbons sometimes appeared to be condensed, abnormally folded, or were displayed as two or three segments lying next to each other. Often, they showed no direct contact with the cell membrane. Within rosette cores, photoreceptor inner and outer segments were found only at a low density and were poorly developed. The cores could be densely filled with microvillus processes from Müller cells radiating out of a well defined tight junctional "outer limiting membrane".

The neuropil regions corresponding to the inner plexiform layer regions tended to be quite variable in epiretinal transplants, with many areas of rather poor structural integrity. Even in the better areas, many amacrine cell terminals appeared as "ghosts", exhibiting a sparse cytoplasm with an exceptionally low density of synaptic vesicles. Small clusters of vesicles were found at synaptic areas in these terminals. Other amacrine cell terminals appeared more normal, with a good complement of synaptic vesicles, some of which may be of the small or large dense-cored type. Bipolar cell terminals showed significant variability in ribbon placement and postsynaptic elements. Some terminals were relatively normal, but monadic arrangements were common, and ribbons not showing any direct contact with the cell surface were very common.

Epiretinal grafts appeared to interact with the host more readily than the subretinal transplants. Sites of integration seemed to occur centered around the site of a blood vessel growing out from the host into the graft. In these areas, IPL-like neuropil from the graft juxtaposed freely with the host such that it was nearly impossible to distinguish host from graft.

DISCUSSION

At the time of surgery, the youngest human transplants (6-7 weeks after conception) consists of a neuroepithelium only (see, e.g., Spira and Hollenberg[13]). The oldest transplants are only slightly more developed at the time of transplantation. An outer plexiform layer has just begun to appear in the central part of the retina, but photoreceptor cells and the other layers are not identifiable until several weeks later[13-15]. It is important to keep in mind that most descriptions of the development of the retina refer to its central parts. The periphery lags behind with as much as six weeks. Since the transplant tissue was taken from both central and peripheral donor retina and therefore presumably often contained randomly mixed pieces of central and peripheral donor retina, it is to be expected that a single transplant can exhibit different stages of development. The rat retina is also quite undeveloped at stage E15 (see Perry and Walker[16]).

In normal adult rat or human retina, all neuron types are readily identified by electron microscopy, with the exception of ganglion cells and interplexiform cells. This was also found in the grafts analyzed in these studies. Rods (and cones in the human xenotransplants) were directly identifiable because of the localization of the nucleus and the appearance of the synaptic pedicles.

Like in normal adult human retina, horizontal cell perikarya were not easily distinguished from bipolar cell perikarya in the transplants. However, horizontal cell processes were readily identified in the invaginations of the photoreceptor pedicles. Therefore, horizontal cells do occur in the present long-term transplants, which agrees well with light microscopical observations in rat homotransplants[17].

Bipolar and amacrine cell processes are easily identified in the inner plexiform layer by their distinctive synapses, and both types were seen in abundance in the transplants. Ganglion cells and their processes are much harder to identify unequivocally even in the normal adult retina. Results in other studies have suggested that it is questionable whether ganglion cells develop in grafts[17]. In the current study, processes were seen in bipolar cell dyads that could have been ganglion cell processes. However, since positive ultrastructural methods were not available for identifying ganglion cells, it remains undetermined whether ganglion cells survive or mature in the transplants.

At the time of transplantation, synapses normally have just begun to form in the human retina[13,14], and photoreceptor outer segments have not appeared. On the other hand, all the synapse types of the adult retina were seen in the long-term grafts of this study. Clearly, despite the disruption of the tissue at transplantation and the foreign environment in the host eye, the transplanted cells have matured and have developed various contacts. Not only did all major synapse types develop, but there were also signs of more advanced circuitry in the form of reciprocal synapses involving two amacrine cell processes or a bipolar and an amacrine cell process.

The human grafts always contained well-developed regions together with regions containing only poorly differentiated cells with relatively few processes, and a similar observation was made in a previous study[9]. There were no obvious morphologic reasons for this variability, but one possible reason is the mixing of peripheral and central retinal cells with different degrees of maturation at the time of transplantation[9].

The difference in the degree of development noted in epiretinal and subretinal rat transplants is interesting. Not only did the rosettes appear less well developed in the epiretinal transplants, but they also seemed to contain fewer well developed neuron processes in the regions corresponding to the outer and the inner plexiform layers. On the other hand, the subretinal grafts were not observed to make contacts with the host retina (in both human xenotransplants and rat homotransplants), whereas contacts were seen between the host and epiretinal transplants.

The work summarized here has thus shown that in both homo- and xenotransplants to rat host retinas, embryonic retinal cells continue to differentiate, forming their normal synaptic contacts with each other. The graft and the host are apparently also able to form cellular contacts of different types with each other, but so far, this is still a limited and irregular phenomenon with unknown control.

ACKNOWLEDGEMENTS

This study was supported by the Retinal Transplant Program of the Eye Research Institute and by grants from the Swedish Medical Research Council (project 14X 2321), the Segerfalk Foundation, the Crafoord Foundation, the T and R Söderberg Foundation, the Kronprinsessan Margaretas Arbetsnämnd, Dr. S. Williams and the Faculty of Medicine at the University of Lund. We are grateful to Dr. J. E. Dowling, Harvard University, for providing access to his electron microscopy facilities and to Sandoz for supplying Sandimmun[(R)]. The technical assistance of Nike Beckmann is gratefully acknowledged.

REFERENCES

1.   Royo, P. E., Quay, W. B., Retinal transplantation from fetal to maternal mammalian eye, Growth, 23, 313, 1959.

2.   Turner, J. E., Blair, J. R., Newborn rat retinal cells transplanted into a retinal lesion site in adult host eyes, Dev. Brain Res., 26, 91, 1986.

3.   Aramant, R., Seiler, M. and Turner, J. E., Donor age influences on the success of retinal grafts to adult rat retina, Invest. Ophthalmol. Visual Sci., 29, 503, 1988.

4. Del Cerro, M., Notter, M. F., Wiegand, S. J., Jiang, L. Q. and Del Cerro, C., Intraretinal transplantation of fluorescently labeled retinal cell suspensions, Neurosci. Lett., 92, 21, 1988.

5. Del Cerro, M., Notter, M. F. D., Del Cerro, C., Wiegand, S. J., Grover, D. A. and Lazar, E., Intraretinal transplantation for rod-cell replacement in light-damaged retinas, J. Neur. Transplant., 1, 1, 1989.

6. Seiler, M., Aramant, R., Ehinger, B. and Adolph, A. R., Transplantation of embryonic retina to adult retina in rabbits, Exp. Eye Res., 51, 225, 1990.

7. Gouras, P., Lopez, R., Du, J, Gelandze, M., Kwun, R., Brittis, M., Kjeldbye, H., Transplantation of retinal cells, Neuro-ophthalmology, 10, 165, 1990.

8. Aramant, R., Turner, J. E., Cross-species grafting of embryonic mouse and grafting of older postnatal rat retinas into the lesioned adult rat eye: the importance of cyclosporin A for survival, Brain Res., 469, 303, 1988.

9. Aramant, R., Seiler, M., Ehinger, B., Bergström, A., Gustavii, B., Brundin, P. and Adolph, A. R., Transplantation of human embryonic retina to adult rat retina, Restor. Neurol. Neurosci., 2, 9, 1990.

10. Silverman, M. S., Hughes, S. E., Transplantation of photoreceptors to light-damaged retina., Invest. Ophthalmol. Vis. Sci., 30, 1684, 1989.

11. Silverman, M. S., Hughes, S. E., Photoreceptors transplantation in inherited and environmentally induced retinal degeneration: anatomy, immunohistochemistry and function, in Inherited and Environmentally Induced Retinal Degenerations, LaVail, M. M., Ed., Alan R. Liss, Inc., New York, 1989, 687.

12. Ehinger, B., Bergström, A., Seiler, M., Aramant, R. B., Zucker, C. L., Gustavii, B. and Adolph, A., Ultrastructure of human retinal cell transplants with long survival times in rats, Exp. Eye Res., in press, 1991.

13. Spira, A. W., Hollenberg, M. J., Human retinal development: Ultrastructure of the inner retinal layers, Developmental Biol., 31, 1, 1973.

14. Hollenberg, M. J., Spira, A. W., Early development of the human retina, Can. J. Ophthalmol., 7, 472, 1972.

15. Johnson, A. T., Kretzer, F. L., Hittner, H. M., Glazebrook, P. A. and Bridges, C. D., Development of the subretinal space in the preterm human eye: ultrastructural and immunocytochemical studies, J. Comp. Neurol., 233, 497, 1985.

16. Perry, V. H., Walker, M., Morphology of cells in the ganglion cell layer during development of the rat retina., Proc. R. Soc. Lond., (Biol) 208, 433, 1980.

17. Aramant, R., Seiler, M., Bergström, A., Adolph, A., Ehinger, B. and Turner, J., Neuronal markers in rat retinal grafts, Brain Res., 53, 47, 1990.

TRANSPLANTING EMBRYONIC RETINA TO THE RETINA OF ADULT ANIMALS

Robert Aramant,[#] Magdalene Seiler,[#]
Berndt Ehinger,[*] Anders Bergström,[*] Alan R. Adolph,[#]
Björn Gustavii,[+] and Patrik Brundin[x]

[#]Eye Research Institute, Boston, MA, and Departments of
[*]Ophthalmology, [+]Gynecology and [x]Med. Cell Research, University of Lund, Sweden.

KEY WORDS

Retinal transplants, embryonic retina, CNS transplants, lamination, homografts, xenografts, immunohistochemistry, cryopreservation, RPE.

I. INTRODUCTION

Retinal transplantation (transplantation of retinal cells or retinal pigment epithelial (RPE) cells to the posterior pole of the eye) is an exciting new research field.[1-8] Most studies have been done in animal models, but xenografting of human tissue has been reported by several groups.[1,2,9-12] The ultimate goals are to replace damaged host cells, restore eyesight, or prevent retinal degeneration in humans. Transplantation of embryonic retinal tissue provides an excellent model to study retinal development.

Donor retinal or RPE cells have been transplanted as dissociated cells,[1,2,4,13-15] tissue aggregates,[3,6,7,9,16,17] or whole sheets [5,12,18] to the subretinal or epiretinal space of adult host animals. A subretinal transplant is located between the host retina and RPE; an epiretinal transplant faces the vitreous. Transplantation of retina aggregates to a retinal lesion site is most successful when immature donor tissue is used, e.g., embryonic up to newborn retina in the rat [16,17]. However, a whole sheet of the photoreceptor layer of the adult retina [18] or a suspension of dissociated adult rat rods mixed with RPE cells [8] can be transplanted successfully to the subretinal space, using an anterior approach. Various studies have shown that healthy RPE cells transplanted to RCS (Royal College of Surgeons) rats can slow down photoreceptor degeneration [14,15,19] (see also Gouras et al., and Turner et al., this volume).

In this paper, we review our studies based on transplanting embryonic retinal aggregates to the epiretinal or subretinal space of adult host animals. The method was modified after Turner and Blair,[3] and has been described in detail elsewhere.[7] In the dorsal part of the eyeball, a small incision is made through the sclera, choroid, and retina, and closed with 10-0 sutures. The donor tissue is taken up into a custom-made glass needle and injected into the retinal lesion site.

II. CHARACTERISTICS OF RETINAL GRAFTS

A. SURVIVAL OF TRANSPLANTS

In the rat, a broad range of donor ages, from embryonic day (E) 13 to post-natal day (P) 1, can be used successfully for transplantation of retinal aggregates to an adult host retina.[16,17] Grafts derived from older post-natal donor ages (P4-10) show more signs of cell death (with replacement by connective tissue), P14 grafts degenerate completely, and P21 epiretinal grafts elicit an immune response [17]. If the donor cells are derived from a different species, the transplants will not survive unless the host is immunosuppressed.[9,20] Donor cells from the same species, irrespective of the strain from which they are derived, will survive as long as embryonic or early post-natal tissue is used.

B. LAMINATION

During transplantation, the donor tissue is disrupted. The tissue fragments then fuse to form a graft. Each graft is individual. The transplants can have different shapes, from a flat to a round form, and are organized in folded sheets and rosettes. A rosette is defined as a lumen surrounded by an outer limiting membrane, photoreceptors, and other retinal layers. The immature donor retinas contain mostly or exclusively neuroepithelial cells, depending on the donor age.

In the host retina, the immature transplanted retinal cells continue to develop, forming all retinal layers and most cell types. However, an inner limiting membrane and Müller cell endfeet are never seen on the vitreous surface of the transplants (see section III.A of this chapter); and, to date, we have no evidence of the presence of ganglion cells in the graft (see also section III.B. of this chapter). An example of the lamination of a rat E19 retinal graft is shown in **Figure 1**. The extent of lamination (formation and separation of retinal layers in the transplant) depends on the donor age.[17] Although P1 donor retinas can form successful grafts, they are less laminated than grafts derived from embryonic donor tissue.[21]

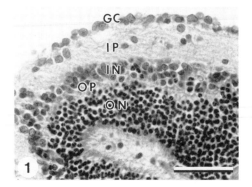
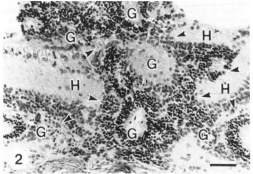

Figure 1: **Lamination** of rat retinal graft (E19 donor, 4 weeks after transplantation). A large rosette contains most retinal layers, but there is no inner limiting membrane on vitreous surface. Photoreceptor inner and outer segments can be seen in lumen of rosette. GC = ganglion cell layer; IP = inner plexiform layer; IN = inner nuclear layer; OP = outer plexiform layer; ON = outer nuclear layer. (The same labelling applies to the other figures.) 8 μm paraffin section. Hematoxylin & eosin. Bar = 50 μm.

Figure 2: **Integration** of rat retinal graft (G) with host retina (H) (E13 donor, 4 weeks after transplantation). This transplant is in the epiretinal and subretinal space. No glial barrier can be seen between host and graft (arrowheads). 8 μm paraffin section. Hematoxylin & eosin. Bar = 50 μm.

C. SUBRETINAL VERSUS EPIRETINAL SPACE

Our experiments over the years [20,22] have shown that graft viability differs between epiretinal and subretinal grafts, especially when fragile donor tissue (e.g., early embryonic retina, cryopreserved or dissociated cells) is used for transplantation. Such tissue is more likely to survive in the subretinal space and usually has fewer signs of cell death (degenerating cells or holes). This indicates that the subretinal space is a more favorable environment than the epiretinal space for this grafting model. There are several possible explanations for this: (a) donor cells are kept together by the narrow space, (b) the adjoining host RPE produces the interphotoreceptor matrix (IPM), and possibly trophic substances promoting graft survival and differentiation, (c) the blood vessels in the adjoining host choroid can provide nutrients, and (d) the subretinal space might be more immunologically privileged than the vitreous.

II. THE CAPACITY OF ADULT RETINA TO ACCEPT TRANSPLANTED EMBRYONIC CNS CELLS

A. INTEGRATION OF RETINAL TRANSPLANTS

Retinal transplants can fuse with the cut edges of the host retina so that no glial barrier exists between host and graft. In contrast to this, neural transplants in the brain are often encapsulated by a glial barrier.[23] An example of the integration of an E13 rat retinal graft is demonstrated in **Figure 2**. The lack of a glial barrier also has been noted in an immunohistochemical study [24,25] using glial-cell specific antibodies for GFAP (glial fibrillary acidic protein), S-100 (a Ca^{2+}-binding protein), and vimentin. This study indicated that host glial cells started to invade the transplant two days after transplantation.[24]

B. INTEGRATION OF EMBRYONIC BRAIN TRANSPLANTS

Results from previous studies [6,22] indicated that retinal ganglion cells did not survive or mature in retinal transplants. We tried to promote the survival and differentiation of retinal ganglion cells in retinal grafts by cografting rat E13 retina with tectal anlage. As a control, retina was cografted with cerebellar anlage.[26] Cografting retina with tectum did not affect retinal grafts; no ganglion cells could be identified in the grafts. However, the interesting result in this study was that brain grafts (tectum or cerebellum) survived, grew, fused extraordinarily well with the host retina (see **Figure 3**), and contained many neuronal fibers. There was unusual, extensive neurofilament staining in the inner plexiform layer of the host retina near and several millimeters away from the grafts (see **Figure 4**) which was not seen in the normal retina. This indicated neuronal outgrowth from the brain grafts or ingrowth of retinal neurons, presumably amacrine or bipolar cells, to the brain grafts. Injection of horseradish peroxidase (HRP) into tectal or cerebellar grafts in retinal wholemounts in vitro indicated that there is an outgrowth of fibers from both types of grafts onto the surface or into the inner plexiform layer of the host retina; tectal grafts formed terminal-like structures with swellings in the inner plexiform layer near the inner nuclear layer more frequently than did cerebellum grafts.[27]

C. RETROGRADE TRACING FROM HOST BRAIN

In a pilot study,[28] fluorogold was injected bilaterally into the superior colliculus of rats with long-term (6 and 11 months) P1 retinal transplants to retrogradely label the host ganglion cells and to determine whether any label could be found in the grafts. The animals were sacrificed 10 days after injection of the tracer. Fluorescence microscopy of retina sections showed selective labelling of most ganglion cells in the host retina. In the grafts (3 in total), many cells were stained with different labelling intensities, and many fibers were labelled (example in **Figure 5**). Since no amacrine cells had been labelled in the host retina, a trans-synaptic transport of the dye to the transplant was unlikely. These results raise the interesting possibility that the grafts may have sprouted fibers up to the host brain. This issue will be explored in further experiments.

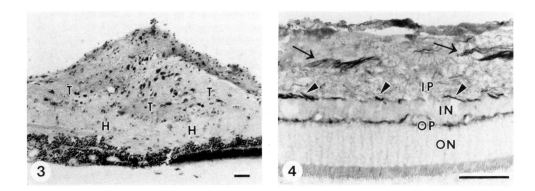

Figure 3: **Integration of embryonic tectal graft** (T) with host retina (H) (E13 donor, 4 weeks after transplantation). The transplant, containing large and small neurons, has grown on top of the host retina. No glial barriers can be seen. 8 μm paraffin section. Hematoxylin & eosin. Bar = 50 μm.

Figure 4: **Abnormal neuronal fibers** (arrowheads) of a host retina with an embryonic tectal transplant, in the inner plexiform layer at the border of the inner nuclear layer. Host ganglion cell axons (arrows) appear to be oriented toward the tectal graft which is outside the figure on the right side. (An extension of the graft is seen on top of the retina.) These results indicate neuronal outgrowth from or toward the tectal graft. 8 μm cryostat section, stained for **neurofilament 200**. Bar = 50 μm.

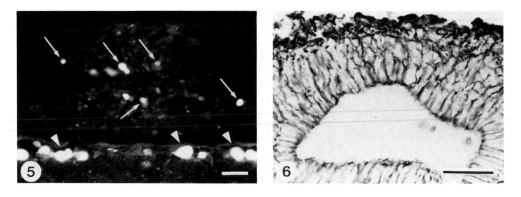

Figure 5: **Connectivity:** Retinal graft (G), P1 donor, on top of host retina (H), 11 months after transplantation. The host superior colliculus had been injected bilaterally with **fluorogold**. The animal was sacrificed 10 days after the injection. Host retinal ganglion cells (arrowheads) and cells in the graft (arrows) are specifically labelled. Since no amacrine cells had been labelled in the host retina, a trans-synaptic transport of the dye into the graft is unlikely. 10 μm paraffin section. Bar = 50 μm.

Figure 6: **Glial cells** in human retinal graft (total age: 25 weeks). Retinal donor cells derived from a human embryo of 8-weeks postconceptional age were xenografted to rat retina. The radial fibers of Müller cells can be seen in a large rosette, but there is no continuous inner limiting membrane on the vitreous surface. Staining for **vimentin**. 8 μm cryostat section. Bar = 50 μm.

TABLE 1[*]

Antibodies Used to Identify Cell Types in Retinal Transplants

Cell type	Immunoreactivity in normal retina	Immunoreactivity in transplant
A. Glial cells		
Müller cells	+ vimentin	+
	+ S-100	+
	+ CRALBP [32]	+ near host
	− GFAP	+ same as injured retina
Astrocytes	+ vimentin	+
	+ S-100	+
	+ GFAP	+
B. Inner retinal layers		
Ganglion cells - axons	+ NF (160, 200)	− not found (rat, rabbit)
- axons + dendrites	+ MAP 1A	(+) only few small cells (rabbit)
- axons, soma, IPL	+ Thy-1 (OX-7)	(+) no cells stained, but faint staining in IPL
- soma, IPL	+ NSE	(+) some small cells stained (could be amacrine cells?)
Amacrine cells - soma and fibers	+ HPC-1 [33] (mostly IPL)	+
- cholinergic	+ ChAT [34]	+ disturbed fiber lamination
- dopaminergic	+ TH [35]	+ - " - - " - - " -
- GABAergic	+ GAD [36]	+ - " - - " - - " -
	+ somatostatin-28	+ - " - - " - - " -
	+ NSE	+
C. Outer retinal layers		
Horizontal cells	+ HPC-1 [33]	+
- processes	+ NF (160, 200)	+ in OPL of rosettes
- processes	+ vimentin	+ (rat only)
- processes + soma	+ MAP 1A (rabbit only)	+ (in rabbit grafts)
Bipolar cells	+ PKC	+ (so far, rabbit only)
Rods	+ rhodopsin [45,63]	+
	+ S-antigen [43]	+
	+ α-transducin [44]	+
Cones	+ NSE	+ (rabbit and human grafts)
(blue ?) cones	+ S-antigen [43]	+ (human grafts)

---

[*]　List of abbreviations: see end of this chapter

III. CELL TYPES AND LAYERS IN RETINAL TRANSPLANTS

Using immunohistochemistry for cell-type specific antigens,[29-31] (review) we have investigated the presence and distribution of retinal cell types in grafts. In most cases, the HRP Elite-ABC kit (Vector Labs, Burlingame, CA) was used for the detection of the primary antibody. The immunohistochemical methods have been published in detail elsewhere.[6,7,9] The experiments are summarized in **Table 1**.

A. GLIAL CELLS

The time course of expression of different glial markers was studied by immunohistochemistry for S-100 (a Ca^{2+}-binding protein), GFAP (glial fibrillary acidic protein), and vimentin.[24,25] This study showed that glial cells in rat E15 retinal transplants develop approximately according to a normal timetable. At about 3 weeks after transplantation (corresponding to P14), Müller cells in the transplants turn reactive (GFAP-positive). This response indicated that the transplant presented an abnormal situation for the Müller cells. Starting two days after transplantation, host-derived glial cells appeared to invade the transplants. No inner limiting membrane with Müller cell endfeet could be seen on the vitreous surface of the grafts. In contrast, the morphology of Müller cells in the outer nuclear layer and at the outer limiting membrane appeared to be normal. This finding was confirmed using additional antibodies, e.g., against vimentin [29] and against CRALBP (cis-retinaldehyde binding protein) [32] in grafts of different species (rat, rabbit,[7] human - see section IV.C of this chapter). **Figure 6** shows vimentin staining in a human xenograft.

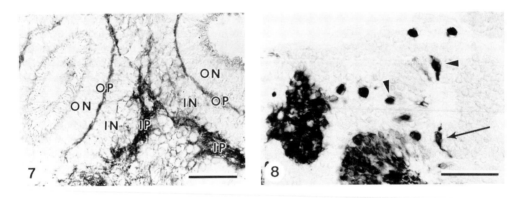

Figure 7:   **Lamination** of area in human retinal graft (8-week-old donor, total age: 25 weeks), stained with monoclonal antibody **HPC-1**. In 2 rosettes, the inner and outer plexiform layers and cell bodies in the inner nuclear layer and ganglion cell layer are specifically stained. 8 μm cryostat section. Bar = 50 μm.

Figure 8:   **Photoreceptors** in human retinal graft (7-week-old donor, total age: 37 weeks), stained with monoclonal antibody for **S-antigen**. In two rosettes, most outer nuclear cells are immunoreactive, whereas one rosette (on the right) contains only a few stained cells, both rods (arrowheads), and one cone (arrow). This indicates different degrees of maturation in the graft. 8 μm paraffin section. Bar = 50 μm.

B. INNER RETINAL LAYERS

Embryonic rat retinal transplants have been studied at different times after transplantation using the neuronal marker antibody HPC-1,[33] and antibodies against neurofilament (NF) 160 kD,[29] ChAT (choline actyltransferase),[34] TH (tyrosine hydroxylase) [35], GAD (glutamic acid decarboxylase),[36] and somatostatin-28 (see

Table 1).[6] In this study, no surviving or mature retinal ganglion cells were detected in the grafts, but different types of **amacrine cells** were seen. The lamination of the inner plexiform layer was disturbed completely in the grafts. **Figure 7** shows the lamination of a human retinal graft stained with the antibody HPC-1, which labelled the inner and outer plexiform layers.

We have also used other cell markers for **retinal ganglion cells**: antibodies against the neuronal surface glycoprotein Thy 1.1,[37,38] the microtubule-associated protein (MAP) 1A,[39] NF 200 kD,[29] and neuron-specific enolase (NSE), which marks ganglion cells as well as amacrine cells. The antibody OX-7 against Thy 1.1 faintly labelled the inner plexiform layer of P1 rat retinal grafts but did not label cells.[40] An antibody against MAP 1A stained a few small cells in the ganglion cell layer of rabbit retinal grafts.[41] These studies do not exclude the possibility that some small ganglion cells survived in the grafts, but it appears that large ganglion cells do not survive or mature.

C. OUTER RETINAL LAYERS

Horizontal cells are immunoreactive for different antigens (see Table 1).[29,30] In a time-course study of rat retinal grafts, we found that horizontal cells appeared to mature in the transplants 1 week later than in the normal retina as seen by immunohistochemistry for NF 160 kD.[6] NF-immunoreactive horizontal cells were found in the outer plexiform layer of rosettes when inner and outer nuclear layers were completely separated. NF-stained horizontal cells, but not retinal ganglion cells, were also found in rabbit retinal grafts.[7]

We have begun to study the development of **photoreceptors** in transplants (see Table 1) by immunohistochemistry.[31 (review)] Rods and a subpopulation of cones which have been suggested to be blue-sensitive [42] are immunoreactive for S-antigen. An antibody against S-antigen,[43] an important protein for the phototransduction process, was used to identify **rods** and some cones in transplants of human embryonic retina (see section IV.C).[9] In such transplants, **cones** (identifiable by an antiserum against NSE) are always found near the outer limiting membrane in rosettes and surrounded by rods, which stain (partially or completely, depending on maturation) for S-antigen,[43] rod α-transducin (a membrane-bound G-protein),[44] and rhodopsin.[45] This staining pattern indicates that the cells in the outer nuclear layer are arranged in the correct orientation. **Figure 8** shows an example of immunostaining for S-antigen in a human retinal graft. Antibodies for S-antigen,[43] rod α-transducin,[44] and rhodopsin [45] also stain photoreceptors in rat and rabbit retinal grafts.[41] These results show that photoreceptors in the transplants contain several key proteins essential for processing light. However, graft photoreceptors are usually less immunoreactive for rod α-transducin than host photoreceptors. In large human retinal transplants, immunoreactivity for photoreceptor-specific antigens is found more frequently in rosettes near the host retina.

IV. XENOGRAFTING OF HUMAN EMBRYONIC RETINA

A. BACKGROUND

The development of human embryonic CNS tissue has been studied in several xenograft models in experimental animals.[46-48] These studies provided the basis for attempts to transplant brain cells as a cure for various human degenerative disorders, e.g., Parkinson's disease.[49 (review)] Only a few xenograft studies have been done in the retina-to-retina transplantation model. Mouse embryonic retina has been transplanted to the retina of adult immunosuppressed rats,[20] and a sheet of adult human photoreceptor layer has been grafted to the retina of light-damaged rats.[18] Mouse retinas also have been transplanted routinely to the brain of newborn rat hosts, which are not yet immunocompetent.[50 (review)]

B. MATERIAL AND METHODS

Human embryonic tissue (3-10 weeks post-conceptional age) was obtained from elective abortions. The retinas were transplanted to the eyes of immunosuppressed normal rats. The transplants were analyzed after different survival times up to a total age of 37 weeks (total age = donor age + survival time after transplantation). The differentiation of the transplants was evaluated by histology and by immunohistochemistry for S-antigen.[9] The transplants have been characterized further by immunohistochemistry for other photoreceptor and glial markers.[51] Human retinal transplants have also been studied by electron microscopy [52] (see also Ehinger et al., this volume).

C. RESULTS

The transplanted immature retinal cells differentiated according to the human developmental timetable. Development of **glial cells** was seen relatively early (at 16 weeks total age) with faint vimentin staining. **Figure 6** shows vimentin stained-Müller cells in a transplant at 25 weeks total age. At this stage, graft glial cells were stained with the same intensity as the host retina. The differentiation of **inner retinal layers** has been partially characterized by staining with the monoclonal antibody HPC-1.[33] Plexiform areas in the grafts were stained faintly at 15-16 weeks total age and clearly at 25 weeks (**Figure 7**).

Developing cones, round cell bodies near the developing outer limiting membrane, were seen in the earliest stage studied (13 weeks total age). Expression of S-antigen in graft **photoreceptors** (rods and a subpopulation of cones [42]) was first observed at a total age of 20 weeks. Other rod photoreceptor markers, such as α−transducin and rhodopsin, were also seen for the first time at 20 weeks total age. Some cones stained for NSE already at a total age of 19 weeks. However, in the inner nuclear layers, a few neurons were faintly immunoreactive for NSE before cones were labelled. Older transplants contained progressively more photoreceptors in the outer nuclear layers.

There were areas of different maturation in the grafts, probably because pieces of central and peripheral retina were randomly mixed during transplantation. During normal human development, the central retina matures about 6 weeks before the peripheral retina.[9 (for review)] Another reason for this could be the influence of the host retina; often photoreceptors appeared to be more mature in rosettes near the host retina. **Figure 8** shows S-antigen staining in a human xenograft of 37 weeks total age.

V. CRYOPRESERVATION

A bank of freeze-stored donor tissue would free transplantation research from depending on the availability of fresh donor tissue. Using different rat donor ages (E13, E16, E19, and E22), we compared the success rates of retinal transplantation between cryopreserved and fresh donor tissue.[21, 53] Rat embryonic retinas were frozen in a medium containing 10% dimethylsulfoxide (DMSO) and stored in liquid nitrogen for 4 and 8 months. After rapid thawing and washing, cryopreserved retinas were then grafted to adult rat retina. The host animals were sacrificed 4 weeks after transplantation. Fresh donor retinas, corresponding in age to the experimental cryopreserved tissues, were transplanted as a control.

In this study, the development of the transplants was evaluated using a scoring system, modified from two protocols [16,17] based on criteria of size (volume), viability (absence or signs of degenerating cells), extent of lamination (development of retinal layers), and integration (fusion with the host). The scores of the different experimental groups were compared statistically.

Successful grafts were achieved with all donor ages, but the degree of **lamination** decreased significantly ($p<0.001$) in cryopreserved grafts compared with fresh tissue grafts. The scores of size and viability of cryopreserved grafts were lower than those of grafts of fresh tissue, but not significantly. There was no difference in graft integration with the host between the different experimental groups. Epiretinal cryopreserved grafts were significantly ($p<0.001$) less viable (contained more degenerating cells and holes) than subretinal cryopreserved grafts. However, between fresh epiretinal and fresh subretinal grafts, there was no difference in viability. Overall, the best survival rate and lamination of cryopreserved grafts was achieved with donor age E16. Fresh E22 (P1) grafts, although not as well laminated as grafts of other donor ages, were better laminated than E16 cryopreserved grafts.

There are several possible explanations for the reduced lamination of cryopreserved grafts. It has been observed in several studies [54-56] that cryopreserved embryonic neuronal tissue is very **fragile** and has a tendency for **fragmentation**. Freezing and thawing might change the membrane lipoproteins affecting the adhesion between the cells. The cryoprotectant DMSO can be toxic to cells and, therefore, has to be removed rapidly.

In conclusion, embryonic retina stored for 8 months in liquid nitrogen can be successfully transplanted to rat retina. In spite of the exposure to cryoprotectant procedures and the long storage, the transplanted fragile embryonic retinal cells form transplants and differentiate to different retinal cell types and layers. Cryopreserved transplants integrate as well with the host retina as transplants derived from fresh tissue.

VI. COGRAFTS OF RETINA AND RPE

The RPE cells are important for the normal differentiation and layer formation of the neural retina *in vitro*.[57-59] They are necessary for the survival and differentiation of photoreceptor cells *in vivo*.[60]

Using a modification of the transplantation method of Turner and Blair,[3] we have shown previously that embryonic rabbit retina can be transplanted to adult rabbit retina. Although the cells continue to differentiate after transplantation, forming most retinal layers, the survival rate of long-term transplants is low, and they are not well laminated.

To improve this retina-to-retina grafting model, we studied whether cografting RPE cells with retina had an effect of on retinal transplants.[61,62] Pigmented rabbit E16 retina was dissected either with or without attached RPE and transplanted onto the retinas of young adult rabbit hosts. Each host received a retina-only transplant in one eye, and a retina/RPE cograft in the other. Animals were sacrificed 4, 8, and 12 weeks after transplantation.

After 4 weeks, large epiretinal or subretinal grafts were seen in both experimental groups. The survival rate decreased considerably 8 and 12 weeks after transplantation. Cografting of retina with RPE resulted in transplants with better lamination than in retina-only transplants. Transplanted RPE cells were organized in clusters of cells surrounded by a basal lamina, often associated with blood vessels. In cografts of retina and RPE, all retinal cell layers could be observed, including an inner limiting membrane with Müller cell endfeet and an apparent ganglion cell layer (see **Figure 9**). The inner limiting membrane developed near RPE cell clusters inside the graft. Only occasionally were RPE cells found inside rosettes, with little or no contact with graft photoreceptor cells. In retina-only grafts, no inner limiting membrane was seen, and the other retinal layers were not as well developed as those in retina/RPE cografts (see **Figure 10**).

The degree of lamination resembling a normal retina, with an inner limiting membrane and Müller cell endfeet, has not been seen before in this retina-to-retina transplantation model. Cografting of rabbit embryonic RPE cells and retina apparently promotes the lamination of retinal transplants.

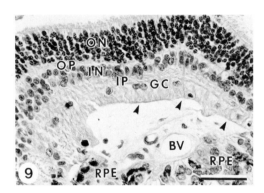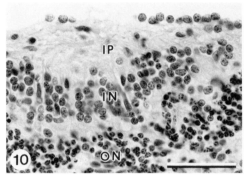

Figure 9: **Cograft of rabbit embryonic retina and RPE cells:** rabbit E16 donor, 8 weeks after transplantation. Area of transplant shows almost complete lamination, including an inner limiting membrane with Müller cell endfeet (arrowheads), facing transplanted RPE with a blood vessel (BV). 8 μm paraffin section. Bar = 50 μm.

Figure 10: **Rabbit retinal transplant without RPE cells:** rabbit E16 donor, 8 weeks after transplantation. Although some degree of lamination can be seen, inner and outer nuclear layers are not separated completely. No inner limiting membrane is found on the vitreous surface. 8 μm paraffin section. Bar = 50 μm.

VII. CONCLUSIONS

Retinal transplants derived from aggregated immature donor tissue rearrange themselves after grafting into folded sheets and rosettes. Most cell types and all layers (corresponding to those in the normal retina) are found in transplants of embryonic retina except for retinal ganglion cells and an inner limiting membrane. The grafts fuse with the host retina so that no glial barriers exist between host and graft. Inter-species grafting has been successfull with mouse and human donor retinas transplanted to rat hosts. Embryonic cryopreserved rat donor tissue stored for a long time can be transplanted successfully. After cografting embryonic retina with RPE, we found that retinal grafts can contain an inner limiting membrane and an apparent ganglion cell layer, which are not seen in grafts of retina alone.

VIII. ACKNOWLEDGMENTS

The authors wish to thank Ann M. Potter for her excellent technical assistance, and the following researchers for providing us with antibodies: Dr. C.J. **Barnstable**, New Haven, CT (HPC-1);[33] Dr. L.A. **Donoso**, Philadelphia, PA (monoclonal antibody against S-antigen);[43] Dr. K.R. **Fry**, Houston, TX (monoclonal antibody AB-5, not yet tested); Dr. B.K.K. **Fung**, Los Angeles, CA (monoclonal antibody against rod α-transducin);[44] Drs. G. **Garwin**, J. **Saari**, Seattle, WA (rabbit antiserum against CRALBP);[32] Dr. R.S. **Molday**, Vancouver, Canada (monoclonal antibodies against rhodopsin: rho 4D2, 1D4);[45] Dr. W. **Oertel**, Munich, F.R.G. (sheep antiserum against GAD);[36] Drs. J.J. **Plantner**, E. **Kean**, Cleveland, OH (rabbit antiserum against rhodopsin);[63] Dr. P. **Salvaterra**, Duarte, CA (monoclonal antibody against ChAT);[34] and Dr. P.R. **Vulliet**, Davis, CA (monoclonal antibody against TH).[35]

ABBREVIATIONS

ChAT	=	choline acetyl transferase	IPM	=	interphotoreceptor matrix
CNS	=	central nervous system	MAP	=	microtubule-associated protein
CRALBP	=	cis-retinaldehyde binding protein	NF	=	neurofilament
DMSO	=	dimethyl sulfoxide	NSE	=	neuron-specific enolase
E	=	embryonic day (day of gestation)	ON(L)	=	outer nuclear layer
GABA	=	γ-amino-butyric acid	OP(L)	=	outer plexiform layer
GAD	=	glutamic acid decarboxylase	P	=	post-natal day (after birth)
GC(L)	=	ganglion cell layer	PKC	=	protein kinase C
GFAP	=	glial fibrillary acidic protein	RCS	=	Royal College of Surgeons
HRP	=	horseradish peroxidase	RPE	=	retinal pigment epithelial cells
IN(L)	=	inner nuclear layer	TH	=	tyrosine hydroxylase
IP(L)	=	inner plexiform layer			

REFERENCES

1. Gouras, P., Flood, M.T., and Kjeldbye, H., Transplantation of human retinal cells to monkey retina, *An. Acad. Brasil. Cienc.*, 56, 431, 1984.

2. Gouras, P.G., Flood, M.T., Kjeldbye, H., Bilek, M.K., and Eggers, H., Transplantation of cultured human retinal epithelium to Bruch's membrane of the owl monkey's eye, *Curr. Eye. Res.*, 4, 253, 1985.

3. Turner, J.E., and Blair, J.R., Newborn rat retinal cells transplanted into a retinal lesion site in adult host eyes, *Dev. Brain Res.*, 26, 91, 1986.

4. Del Cerro, M., Notter, M.F.D., Wiegand, S.J., Jiang, L.Q., and Del Cerro, C., Intraretinal transplantation of fluorescently labeled retinal cell suspensions, *Neurosci. Lett.*, 92, 21, 1988.

5. Silverman, M.S., and Hughes, S.E., Transplantation of photoreceptors to light-damaged retina, *Invest. Ophthalmol. Vis. Sci.* 30, 1684, 1989.

6. Aramant, R., Seiler, M., Ehinger, B., Bergström, A., Adolph, A.R., and Turner, J.E., Neuronal markers in rat retinal grafts, *Dev. Brain. Res.*, 53, 47, 1990.

7. Seiler, M., Aramant, R., and Ehinger, B., Transplantation of embryonic retina to adult retina in rabbit, *Exp. Eye Res.*, 51, 225, 1990.

8. Gouras, P., Du, J., Gelanze, M., Lopez, R., Kwun, R., Kjeldbye, H., and Kauffmann, D., Survival and synapse formation of transplanted rat rods, *Invest. Ophthalmol. Vis. Sci.*, 31 (ARVO Suppl.), 595, 1990.

9. Aramant, R., Seiler, M., Ehinger, B., Bergström, A., Gustavii, B., Brundin, P., and Adolph, A.R., Transplantation of human embryonic retina to adult rat retina, *Restor. Neurol. Neurosci.*, 2, 9, 1990.

10. Del Cerro, M., Lazar, E., Grover, D.A., Gallagher, M.J., Sladek, C.D., Chu, J., and Del Cerro, C., Intraocular transplantation and culture of human embryonic retinal cells, *Invest. Ophthalmol. Vis. Sci.*, 31 (ARVO Suppl.), 593, 1990.

11. Lopez, R., Gouras, P., Kjeldbye, H., Sullivan, B., Brittis, M., and Das, S.R., Transplantation of human RPE cells into the monkey, *Invest. Ophthalmol. Vis. Sci.*, 31 (ARVO Suppl.), 594, 1990.

12. Silverman, M.S., Kaplan, M.J., Valentino, T.L., and Lee, C.M., Transplantation of human and non-human primate photoreceptors to damaged primate retina, *Invest. Ophthalmol. Vis. Sci.*, 31 (ARVO Suppl.), 594, 1990.

13. Lopez, R., Gouras, P., Brittis, M., and Kjeldbye, H., Transplantation of cultured rabbit retinal epithelium to rabbit retina using a closed-eye method, *Invest. Ophthalmol. Vis. Sci.*, 28, 1131, 1987.

14. Li, L.-X., and Turner, J.E., Inherited retinal dystrophy in the RCS rat: prevention of photoreceptor degeneration by pigment epithelial cell transplantion, *Exp. Eye Res.*, 47, 911, 1988.

15. Lopez, R., Gouras, P., Kjeldbye, H., Sullivan, B., Repucci, V., Brittis, M., Wapner, F., and Goluboff, E., Transplanted retinal pigment epithelium modifies the retinal degeneration in the RCS rat, *Invest. Ophthalmol. Vis. Sci.*, 30, 586, 1989.

16. Blair, J.R., and Turner, J.E., Optimum conditions for successful transplantation of immature rat retina to the lesioned adult retina, *Dev. Brain. Res.*, 36, 257, 1987.

17. Aramant, R., Seiler, M., and Turner, J.E., Donor age influences on the success of retinal transplants to adult rat retina, *Invest. Ophthalmol. Vis. Sci.*, 29, 498, 1988.

18. Silverman, M.S., and Hughes, S.E., Photoreceptor transplantation in inherited and environmentally induced retinal degeneration: anatomy, immunohistochemistry and function, in *Inherited and Environmentally Induced Retinal Degeneration*, LaVail, M.M., Ed., Alan R. Liss, New York, 1989, 687.

19. Sheedlo, H.J., Li, L., and Turner, J.E., Functional and structural characteristics of photoreceptor cells rescued in RPE-cell grafted retinas of RCS dystrophic rats, *Exp. Eye Res.*, 48, 841, 1989.

20. Aramant, R., and Turner, J.E., Cross-species grafting of embryonic mouse and grafting of older postnatal rat retinas into the lesioned adult rat eye: the importance of Cyclosporin A for survival, *Dev. Brain. Res.*, 41, 303, 1988.

21. Aramant, R., Seiler, M., and Adolph, A.R., Cryopreservation and transplantation of immature rat retina into adult rat retina, manuscript in preparation, 1990.

22. Aramant, R., and Seiler, M., unpublished observations, 1987 - 1990.

23. Azmitia, E.H., and Whitaker, P.M., Formation of a glial scar after microinjection of fetal neurons into the hippocampus or midbrain of the adult rat: an immunohistochemical study, *Neurosci. Lett.*, 38, 145, 1983.

24. Seiler, M., and Turner, J.E., The activities of host and graft glial cells following retinal transplantation into the lesioned adult rat eye: developmental expression of glial markers, *Dev. Brain Res.*, 43, 111, 1988.

25. Seiler, M., and Turner, J.E., Host and graft glial cell activities following retinal transplantation to the adult rat eye, in *Neurobiology of the Inner Retina*, Weiler, R., Osborne, N.N., Eds., Springer, Berlin, 1989, 481.

26. Aramant, R., Seiler, M., and Adolph, A.R., Cografts of retina and tectum or cerebellum to adult rat retina, *Soc. Neurosci. Abstr.*, 14, 1276, 1988.

27. Stirling, R.V., Aramant, R., Seiler, M., and Adolph, A.R., In vitro labelling to demonstrate connection between host retina and fetal tectum or cerebellum grafts in adult rats, *Soc. Neurosci. Abstr.*, 15, 308, 1989.

28. Aramant, R., unpublished data, 1988.

29. Shaw, G., and Weber, K., The structure and development of the rat retina: an immunofluorescence microscopical study using antibodies specific for intermediate filament proteins, *Eur. J. Cell Biol.*, 30, 219, 1983.

30. Barnstable, C.J., Blum, A.S., Devoto, S.H., Hicks, D., Morabito, M.A., Sparrow,J.R., and Treisman, J.E., Cell differentiation and pattern formation in the developing mammalian retina, *Neurosci. Res.*, 8 (Suppl.), S27, 1988.

31. Shallal, A., McKechnie, N.M., and Al-Mahdawi, S., Immunochemistry of the outer retina, *Eye*, 2 (Suppl.), S180, 1988.

32. Saari, J.C., Bunt-Milam, A.H., Bredberg, D.L., and Garwin, G.G., Properties and immunocytochemical localization of three retinoid-binding proteins from bovine retina, *Vision Res.*, 24, 1595, 1984.

33. Barnstable, C.J., Hofstein, R., and Agakawa, K., A marker of early amacrine cell development in rat retina, *Dev. Brain Res.*, 20, 286, 1985.

34. Houser, C.R., Crawford, G.D., Barber, R.P., Salvaterra, P.M., and Vaughn, J.E., Organization and morphological characteristics of cholinergic neurons: an immunocytochemical study with a monoclonal antibody to choline acetyltransferase, *Brain Res.*, 266, 97, 1983.

35. Hall, F.L., and Vulliet, P.R., Immunocytochemical localization of tyrosine hydroxylase in the growth cones of PC 12 cells, *Proc. West Pharmacol. Soc.*, 30, 45, 1987.

36. Oertel, W.H., Schmechel, D.E., Tappaz, M.L., and Kopin, I.J., Production of a specific antiserum to rat brain glutamic acid decarboxylase by injection of an antigen-antibody complex, *Neuroscience*, 6, 2589, 1981.

37. Barnstable, C.J., and Dräger, U.C., Thy-1 antigen: a ganglion cell specific marker in rodent retina, *Neuroscience*, 11, 847, 1984.

38. Perry, V.H., Morris, R.J., and Raisman, G., Is Thy-1 expressed only by ganglion cells and their axons in the retina and optic nerve? *J. Neurocytol.*, 13, 809, 1984.

39. Okabe, S., Shiomura,Y., and Hirokawa, N., Immunocytochemical localization of microtubule-associated proteins 1A and 2 in the rat retina, *Brain Res.*, 483, 335, 1989.

40. Aramant, R., unpublished data, 1987.

41. Seiler, M., and Aramant, R., unpublished data, 1990.

42. Müller, B., Peichl, L., De Grip, W.J., Gery, I., and Korf, H.-W., Opsin and S-antigen-like immunoreactions in photoreceptors of the tree shrew retina, *Invest. Ophthalmol. Vis. Sci.*, 30, 530, 1989.

43. Donoso, L.A., Merryman, C.F., Edelberg, K.E., Naids, R., and Kalsow, C., Retinal S-antigen in the developing retina and pineal gland: a monoclonal antibody study, *Invest. Ophthalmol. Vis. Sci.*, 26, 561, 1985.

44. Navon, S.E., and Fung, B.K., Characterization of transducin from bovine retinal rod outer segments. Use of monoclonal antibodies to probe the structure and function of the subunit, *J. Biol. Chem.*, 263, 489, 1988.

45. Hicks, D., and Molday, R.S., Differential immunogold-dextran labeling of bovine and frog rod and cone cells using monoclonal antibodies against bovine rhodopsin, *Exp. Eye Res.*, 42, 55-71, 1986.

46. Clarke, D.J., Brundin, P., Strecker, R.E., Nilsson, O.G., Björklund, A., and Lindvall, O., Human fetal dopamine neurons grafted in a rat model of Parkinson's disease: ultrastructural evidence for synapse formation using tyrosine hydroxylase immunocytochemistry, *Exp. Brain Res.*, 73, 115, 1988.

47. Nilsson, O.G., Brundin, P., Widner, H., Strecker, R.E., and Björklund, A., Human fetal forebrain neurons grafted to the rat hippocampus produce an organotypic cholinergic innervation pattern, *Brain Res.*, 456, 193, 1988.

48. Redmond, D.E., Naftolin, F., Collier, T.J., Leranth, C., Robbins, R.J., Sladek, C.D., Roth, R.H., and Sladek, J.R., Cryopreservation, culture and transplantation of human fetal mesencephalic tissue into monkeys, *Science*, 242, 768, 1988.

49. Lindvall, O., Transplantation into the human brain: present status and future possibilities, *J. Neurol. Neurosurg. Psychiatry* (Suppl.), p. 39, 1989.

50. Lund, R.D., Hankin, M.H., Sefton, A.J., and Perry, V.H., Conditions for optic axon outgrowth, *Brain Behav. Evol.*, 31, 218, 1988.

51. Seiler, M., Aramant, R., Ehinger, B., Bergström, A., and Adolph, A.R., Immunohistochemistry of human embryonic retina transplanted to adult rat retina, *Soc. Neurosci. Abstr.*, 16, 1283, 1990.

52. Ehinger, B., Bergström, A., Seiler, M., Aramant, R.B., Zucker, C.L., Gustavii, B., and Adolph, A.R., Ultrastructure of human retinal cell transplants with long survival times in rats, *Exp. Eye Res.*, in press.

53. Seiler, M., Aramant, R., and Adolph, A.R., Transplantation of cryopreserved embryonic retina into adult rat retina, Abstr. for IIIrd International Symposium on Neural Transplantation, Cambridge, U.K., *Restor. Neurol. Neurosci.*, p. 30, 1989.

54. Jensen, S., Sørensen,T., Møller, A.G., and Zimmer, J., Intraocular grafts of fresh and freeze-stored rat hippocampal tissue: a comparison of survivability and histological and connective organization, *J. Comp. Neurol.*, 227, 558, 1984.

55. Sørensen, T., Jensen, S., Møller, A., and Zimmer, J., Intracephalic transplants of freeze-stored rat hippocampal tissue, *J. Comp. Neurol.*, 252, 468, 1986.

56. Collier, T.J., Redmond, D.E.,Jr., Sladek, C.D., Gallagher, M.J., Roth, R.H., and Sladek, J.R., Intracerebral grafting and culture of cryopreserved primate dopamine neurons, *Brain Res.*, 436, 363, 1987.

57. Vollmer, G., Layer, P.G., and Gierer, A., Reaggregation of embryonic chick retina cells: pigment epithelial cells induce a high order of stratification, *Neurosci. Lett.* 48, 191, 1984.

58. Liu, L., Cheng, S.-H., Jiang L.-Z., Hansmann, G., and Layer, P., The pigmented epithelium sustains cell growth and tissue differentiation of chicken retinal explants in vitro, *Exp. Eye Res.*, 46, 801, 1988.

59. Layer, P.G., and Willbold, E., Embryonic chicken retinal cells can regenerate all cell layers in vitro, but ciliary pigmented cells induce their correct polarity, *Cell Tissue Res.*, 258, 233, 1989.

60. Hollyfield, J.G., and Witkovsky, P., Pigmented retinal pigment epithelium involvement in photoreceptor development and function, *J. Exp. Zool.*, 189, 257, 1974.

61. Seiler, M., Aramant, R., Bergström, A., and Adolph, A.R., Cografting retina and retinal pigment epithelium into adult rabbit retina, *Invest. Ophthalmol. Vis. Sci.*, 31 (ARVO Suppl.), 596, 1990.

62. Seiler, M., Aramant, R., Bergström, A., and Adolph, A.R., Co-transplantation of embryonic retina and retinal pigment epithelial cells to rabbit retina: the importance of retinal pigment epithelial cells for retinal differentiation, manuscript in preparation, 1990.

63. Plantner, J.J., Hara, S., and Kean, E.L., Improved rapid immunoassay for rhodopsin, *Exp. Eye Res.*, 35, 543, 1982.

LONG TERM STATUS OF TRANSPLANTED PHOTORECEPTORS

P. Gouras, J. Du, R. Lopez, R. Kwun, H. Kjeldbye
Edward S. Harkness Eye Institute
Columbia University
635 W. 165 Street
New York, N. Y. 10032 U.S.A.

The fact that retinal cells are capable of being enzymatically dissociated from each other and kept viable in vitro suggests the possibility of using them in appropriate ways to substitute for either absent or defective cells in otherwise blind retinas. We began this research with retinal epithelial cells [1], which are perhaps the most tractable to work with and over the past several years have been attempting a similar strategy with photoreceptor cells. [2-4] The photoreceptor cells are the most intriguing because they are invariably affected by all processes that damage their satellite nourishing cells, the epithelium and Muller cells. They are the critical link in vision interfacing the external world with an enormous neural machine that is rendered ineffective in their absence. The possibility of reconnecting them to this system, which we presume is still capable of functioning, is tantalizing for its possibilities.

At least four teams are active in this area. Each has been using a different strategy. We have concentrated on isolating a single type of cell, either retinal epithelial [5] or photoreceptor [2] and in certain cases a mixture of these two. A solution of isolated cells is relatively easy to introduce into the subretinal space by microtechniques. [6,7] Del Cerro and associates [8,9] have been also using microinjection techniques to introduce dissociated populations of all retinal cells, a technique we believe to be somewhat more complicating for interpreting results but may be more agreeable to the transplants. Silverman and Hughes [10,11] have been slicing through the receptor layer and introducing an entire segment containing mainly photoreceptors, as an integrated element, into the subretinal space. This has the advantage of preserving orientation but requires more extensive and potentially more traumatic surgery. Aramant et al [12,13] have been introducing small segments of embryonic retina into the subretinal space. This has the advantage of exploiting the viability of fetal tissue but shares some of the handicaps of the previous method.

None of these groups have demonstrated unequivocally that these transplanted photoreceptors can function and/or form synapses with host retinal neurons. Silverman and Hughes [11] have reported that their transplants will mediate light-induced changes in 2-deoxy-glucose metabolism and at this meeting reported light evoked electrical responses from eyes with transplants. The problem with such light-induced mass responses is that most of the animal models of retinal degeneration have some residual degree of visual function which could be responsible for these effects.

It would be useful to be able to locate and identify the transplanted photoreceptors at the electron microscopic (EM) level so that one can carefully examine their ultrastructural status. The markers used so far have been fluorescent stains [9,10] which are useful at the light but not at the EM level. They have another disadvantage; they could be incorporated by host cells, especially if the transplanted receptors degenerate and release their stain.

We have been using two markers for transplanted photoreceptors, which can be identified by EM and which are less prone to masquerade host as donor cells by artefactual uptake of stain. One is ^{3}H-thymidine which is incorporated into the nucleus of a dividing cell and provides good spatial resolution in an autoradiographic emulsion. About 50% of the rods in myomorphic retina divide during the first week after birth. Therefore by injecting ^{3}H-thymidine subcutaneously on a daily basis during this period about 50% of the rods can be labelled. Figure 1 illustrates such labelled rat rods transplanted to the subretinal space of adult rats of the Royal College of Surgeon's (RCS) strain

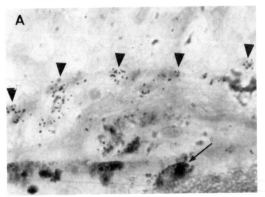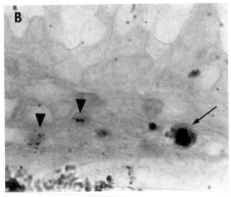

Figure 1 Light microscopic autoradiographs of five (A) and seven (B) month old RCS rat retina showing the radiolabeled nuclei of rods transplanted to three retinas one and three months before, respectively. The arrowheads point out the radiolabel in the nuclei of the rods. The arrows point out pigmented retinal epithelial cells transplanted with the rods.

one and three months previously. The RCS rats were five to seven months old when sacrificed, a time when virtually all of the rods in their retinas had degenerated. The transplanted rod nuclei are easily distinguishable in the autoradiographs by the "buck shot" like pattern of black grains over their nuclei. In order to track the transplant site ophthalmologically and histologically we have also mixed some dissociated retinal pigmented epithelial cells (RPE) with the rods at a ratio of 1 RPE/10 rods. These also

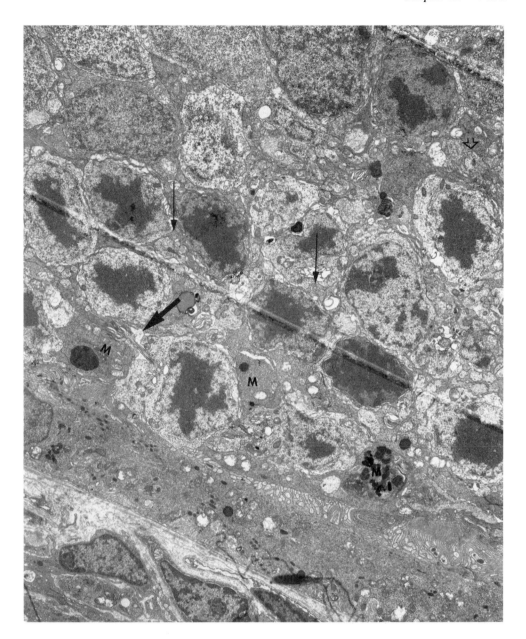

Figure 2. Electron micrograph of the adult RCS rat retina
in which rods have been transplanted two weeks previously.
The rods were identified by light microscopic
autoradiography. The thick arrow points to an outer segment
connected to an inner segment by a cilium. The thin arrows
point out other cilia. The open arrow (upper right) points
out a rare synapse found in this area. A macrophage (M)
opposes the small outer segment, seen at high power in Figure 3.

mark the transplant site and are arrowed in Figure 1.

Figure 2 illustrates the EM view of a group of transplanted rods, identified in a nearby section by light

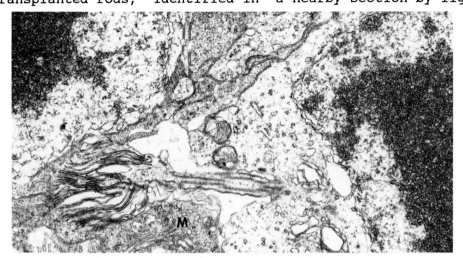

Figure 3. Electron micrograph of the primitive outer segment found among rod nuclei, transplanted two weeks earlier to an adult (4 1/2 month old) RCS rat retina. A macrophage process (M) is in close contact with the outer segment.

microscopic autoradiography. These rods have been transplanted to the adult RCS rat retina two weeks previously. There are a number of factors which also make them appear unusual in this retina. There are many more rods than are seen in the adult RCS retina. They are degenerate, however. There is virtually no outer segment material and little evidence of synaptic organelles. There is one primitive outer segment seen, connected to its cell body; it is oriented away rather than toward the epithelial layer. Figure 3 illustrates this at higher magnification. There is an outer segment connected to a cilium which in turn is connected to the inner segment and the cell body of the rod. The outer segment is in contact with two other cells, one appears to be the cell body of a neighboring rod; the other appears to be the process of a macrophage, which has insinuated between the epithelial layer and the outer segment. It is possible that positional effects play a role in the proper survival of these rods and their highly specialized outer segment. We are attempting to understand this by observing what constellation of structures in the environment leads to better survival of outer segments in some transplanted rods than in others.

In many cases, especially at one month after transplantation, we see numerous rod spherule synapses in the transplant areas. Figure 4 illustrates an example of this in an adult RCS rat retina, one month after transplantation. The rod nucleus, labeled R in Figure 4 was from a group that had been identified as transplants by

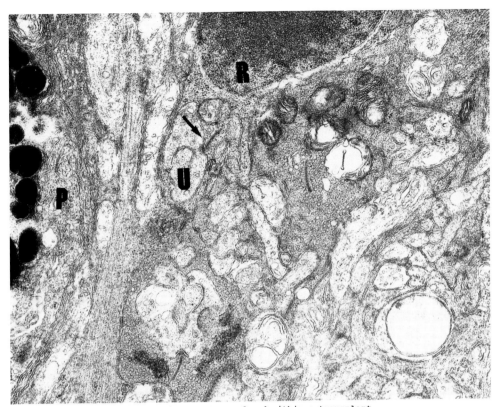

Figure 4. Synaptic structures found within a transplant
area found in the adult RCS rat retina, one moth after
transplantation surgery. The rod nucleus (R) was among a
cluster of rod nuclei identified by light microscopic
autoradiography in an adjacent thick section. The pigment
cell (P) is a co-transplanted retinal epithelial cell that
also identifies the transplant site. A synapse is found in
the cytoplasm of the rod cell (R) making contact with an
unidentified cell (U). Other synapses can be seen in this area.

light microscopic autoradiography. There are several
synaptic ribbons near this nucleus and one (on the left,
arrowed) is adjacent to a synapse with an unidentified cell.
Synapses are found in the outer plexiform layer of the RCS
retina [14] so that it is difficult to know whether we are
dealing with newly formed synapses from transplanted rods or
residual synapses in the degenerating RCS retina. The one
illustrated in Figure 4 has a lot of circumstantial evidence
implying that is belongs to a transplanted rod. The synapse
is in the vicinity of a nucleus which is in a group labeled
by ^{3}H-thymidine. Whether this particular nucleus had such a
label is unknown in this electron micrograph. The rod
nucleus which seems to belong to this synapse is next to a
pigmented epithelial cell which was co-transplanted with the
rods. The retina has no pigmented cells otherwise.
Therefore circumstantially the evidence suggests the synapse
belongs to a transplanted rod. It is not sufficient,
however. In order to be certain that we have such a synapse
it is essential to have an EM marker for the rod spherule,
itself.

Such a marker has now become available. A transgenic mouse has been created with the E. coli Lac Z gene for galactosidase in tandem with a bovine rhodopsin promoter inserted into its genome.[15] Many of the rods of these mice express this bacterial galactosidase in their cytoplasm, which permits their identification by the X-gal stain. The reaction product of this histochemical stain is visible by electron microscopy. Figure 5 illustrates this product in the inner segment, perinuclear, and spherule cytoplasm of

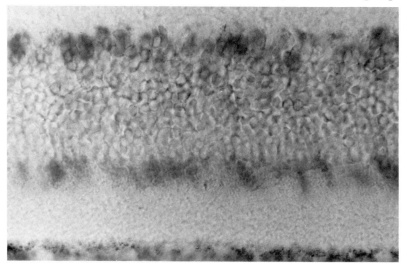

Figure 5. Light micrograph of the X-gal reaction products visible as an aqua-marine stain in the inner segment, perinuclear zone and synaptic terminal of these transgenic rods in this mouse retina. The melanin in the pigmented epithelial layer is brownish. In black and white the distinction between melanin and X-gal stain is lost.

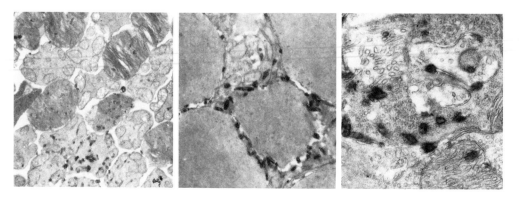

Figure 6. Electron micrograph of the X-gal stain in the inner segment (A), perinuclear cytoplasm (B) and rod spherule (C).

such rods by light microscopy. Figure 6 shows the comparable EM view of the reaction product in the inner segment (A), perinuclear cytoplasm (B) and rod spherule (C). By this means it should be possible to determine whether transplanted rods possess synapses in the host retina.

Figure 7 illustrates our preliminary attempts to use this technique by transplanting these transgenic rods to the retina of adult C3H mice. There are considered to be nuclei of transplanted rods because such an abundance of nuclei is

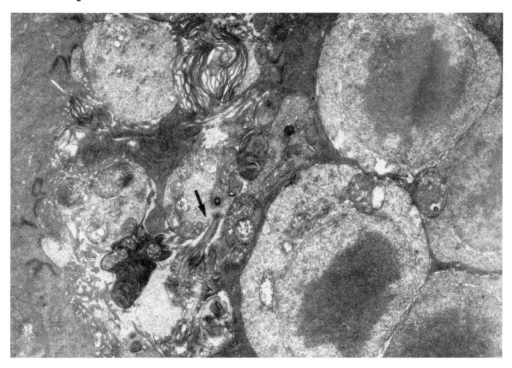

Figure 7. Rods transplanted to the subretinal space of the adult C3H mouse retina. An outer segment with a cilium connected to a rod is arrowed.

only seen in the transplant area. In addition there is outer segment material and a primitive outer segment connected to an inner segment (arrow), structures not seen at this late stage of degeneration in the C3H mouse. One of the nuclei in this cluster stained positive for galactosidase, which is illustrated in Figure 8; arrowheads identify the galactosidase product. In addition there is a synapse in the neighborhood of the nucleus (open arrow) but there is no reaction product in the cytoplasm of this structure. The galactosidase is not expressed by all rods and not as much in some rods as in others. There is a new strain of mice which express the galactosidase in every rod (J. Nathans, personal communication), which should expedite our attempts to link transplanted rods with their putative synapses.

An additional problem with this research is whether the synapses are on to host or donor cells. The methods we use,

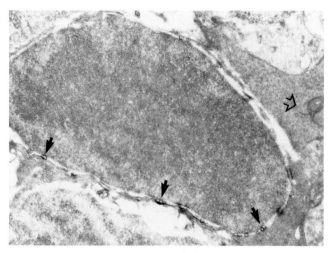

Figure 8. A transgenic rod identified by X-gal particles in
the perinuclear cytoplasm (arrows); the stain is relatively
weak in this transplanted rod. A synapse (open arrow) is
visible above.

which are based on those, pioneered by Anderson et al [16]
dissociate rods from contacts with other retinal cells.
We have examined samples by electron microscopy and they do
not show any evidence of cellular elements other than those
of the rods (we have not yet identified a cone). One does
see, however occasional structures which may be from other
retinal cells in our light microscopic view of the samples;
these structures should ultimately be detectable by EM.
Therefore the possibility exists that some of these
postsynaptic cells are from the donor rather than the host
and experiments will eventually have to be done to rule out
this possibility. One approach is to transplant these rods
to the vitreal chamber where there are no host neurons and
determine whether synapses are also found here.

In these experiments we have observed that within
minutes after introducing the rods to the subretinal space
of the host retina, macrophages appear and begin
phagocytizing outer segment debris, presumably broken off in
the surgery (Figure 9). We have the impression that
macrophages will not phagocytize healthy rods and outer
segments connected to these rods but this impression is
unproven.

The fact that macrophages are attracted to the
subretinal space by intraretinal surgery and are capable of
phagocytizing outer segment debris may be pertinent to the
saving of rods by sham surgery [17] and basic fibroblastic
growth factor. [18] Figure 10 shows rod saving produced in
the RCS rat by an injection of saline; it also shows a large
number of macrophages in the subretinal space. Figure 11
reveals the EM view of these macrophages, illustrating
phagosomes in their cytoplasm (arrow). Therefore
macrophages can compensate for the deficiency seen in the
RCS mutant, the failure of RPE to phagocytize outer segments
[19] this could explain, at least in part, why factors other
than transplanted normal RPE [7,20,21] can save RCS rods from
degeneration.

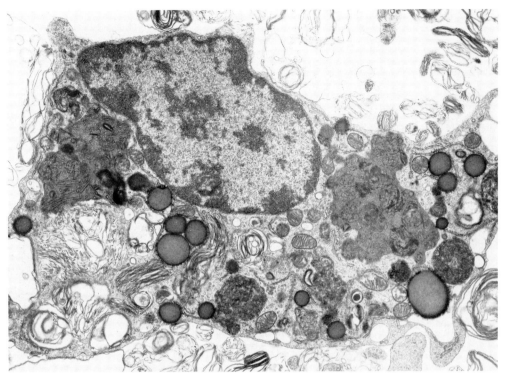

Figure 9. Electron micrograph of a macrophage within the
subretinal space of the RCS rat within one hour after
transplantation of photoreceptors. Numerous outer segment
phagosomes can be seen in its cytoplasm.

DISCUSSION

Transplanted, adult rods can survive for at least three
months in a foreign host retina. These rods are somewhat
abnormal, having extremely small, if any, outer segments.
The reason for this deficiency is unknown. It may be due to
their orientation and positioning relative to the retinal
epithelium and/or the Muller cells. Further experimentation
should elucidate this.

Most remarkable is the suggestive evidence that
transplanted rods may be able to form synapses in the host
retina. The evidence for this important conclusion must be
strengthened by unequivocal demonstration, at the EM level,
that these rod spherules making postsynaptic contacts with
other retinal cells belong unambiguously to the transplants.
The problem is that there are some residual host synapses
still present in the degenerate retinas we are examining. A
label such as galactosidase in transgenic mouse rods seems
capable of providing such information.

A second question that arises, if the first hypothesis
is correct, is the synaptic target of this rod synapse.
Does it belong to the host or the donor? It is not yet
apparent what the best strategy is for determining the

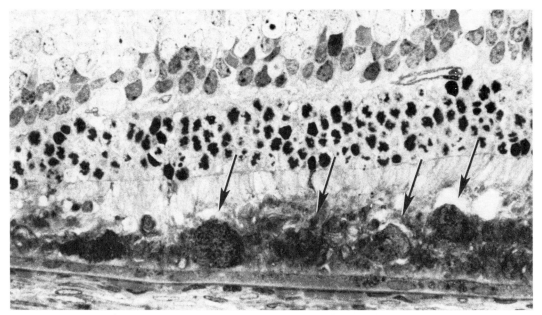

Figure 10. An example of photoreceptor saving in the RCS rat two months after the injection of saline into the subretinal space. The rat was two and a half months old when sacrificed; at this time less than one row of rod nuclei are found in the control eye or elsewhere in this retina. Numerous macrophages (arrows) are seen in the subretinal space.

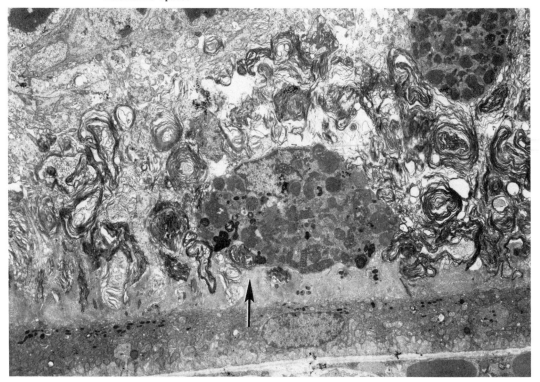

Figure 11. Electron micrograph of one of the macrophages arrowed in Figure 10. Outer segment material (arrow) are seen in its cytoplasm.

answer to this question but it seems less useful to try to answer it until the first question is unequivocally answered.

Photoreceptor transplantation appears to have a future. It has the promise of teaching us a lot about the cell biology of photoreceptors and their supporting structures and their relationship to receptor disease. How quickly it will be useful for restoring vision to blind eyes will depend upon the support the researchers are able to receive, those already intensively active and productive in this field and others being lured into it.

Supported by NIH Grant EY 03854, The G. Harold and Leila Y. Mathers Charitable Foundation, Research to Prevent Blindness Inc., The Howard Hughes Medical Institute and Alcon Research Institute.

REFERENCES

1. Gouras P, Lopez R: Transplantation of Retinal Epithelial Cells. Invest Ophthalmol Vis Sci 30:1681-1683, 1989.

2. Gouras P, Lopez R, Kjeldbye H, Sullivan B, Brittis M: Hyperphagocytosis of outer segments by normal RPE transplanted to the subretinal space of RCS rats. Invest Ophthal Vis Sci suppl 30:209, 1989.

3. Gouras P, Lopez R, Du J, Gelanze M, Kwun R, Kjeldbye H: Transplantation of Retinal Cells. Neuro-Ophthalmology 10:165-176, 1990.

4. Gouras P, Du, Gelanze M, Kwun R, Kjeldbye H, Lopez R: Transplantation of Photoreceptors Labeled with Tritiated Thymidine into the RCS rat. Invest Ophthalmol Vis Sci (in press), 1991.

5. Gouras P, Lopez R, Brittis M, Kjeldbye HM, Fasano MK: Transplantation of cultured retinal epithelium. in Retinal Signals System, Degenerations and Transplants Agardh E. and Ehinger B., Eeds., Elsevier, Amsterdam 1986, 271-286.

6. Lopez R, Gouras P, Brittis M, Kjeldbye H: Transplantation of cultured rabbit retinal epithelium to rabbit retina using a closed eye method. Invest Ophthal Vis Sci 28: 1131-1137, 1987.

7. Gouras P, Lopez R, Brittis M, Kjeldbye H, Sullivan B: The experimental route to curing a rat retinal dystrophy by transplantation. Fifth International Retinitis Pigmentosa Congress Proceedings (Favilla I, ed) pp. 267-276. Australian RP Foundation, 1988.

8. del Cerro M, Notter MFD, Wiegand SJ, Jiang LQ, del Cero C: Intraretinal transplantation of fluorescently labeled retinal cell suspensions. Neurosci Lett 91:21-26, 1988.

9. del Cerro M, Notter MFD, del Cerro C, Wiegand SJ, Grover DA, Lazar E: Intraretinal transplantation for rod-cell replacement in light-damaged retinas. J Neuro trspl. 1:1-10, 1989.

10. Silverman MS, Hughes SE: Photoreceptor transplantation in inherited and environmentally induced retinal degeneration: anatomy, immunohistochemistry and function. Prog in Clin and Biol Res 314:687-709, 1989.

11. Silverman MS, Hughes SE: Transplantation of photoreceptors to light-damaged retina. Invest. Ophthalmol Vis Sci 30:1684-1690, 1989.

12. Aramant R, Seiler M, Ehinger B, Bergstrom A, Gustavii B, Brundin P, Adolph A: Xenografting human fetal retina to adult rat retina. Invest Ophthalmol Vis Sci 32(4):594, 1990.

13. Aramant R, Seiler M, Ehinger B, Bergstrom A, Gustavii B, Brundin P, Adolph AR: Transplantation of human embryonic retina to adult rat retina. Neurol Neurosci (in press) 1990.

14. LaVail MM, Sidman M, Rausin R, Sidman RL: Discrimination of light intensity by rats with inherited retinal degeneration. Vis Res 14:694-702, 1974.

15. Zack D, Bennett J, Want Y, Davenport C, Gearhart J, Nathans J: Photoreceptor specific expression of beta-galactosidase in the retina of transgenic mice carrying a rhodopsin promoter/Lac Z construct. Invest Ophthal Vis Sci 32(4):76, 1990.

16. Townes-Anderson E, Dacheaux RF, Raviola E: Rod photoreceptors dissociated from the adult rabbit retina. J Neurosci 8:3420-331, 1988.

17. Silverman MS, Hughes SE: Photoreceptor rescue in the RCS rat without pigment epithelium transplantation. Curr Eye Res 9:283-191, 1990.

18. Faktorovich EG, Steinberg RH, Yasamusa D, Matthes MT, LaVail MM: Photoreceptor degeneration in inherited retinal dystrophy delayed by basic fibroblastic growth factor. Nature 347:83-86, 1990.

19. Kwun R, Du J, Gelanze M, Lopez R, Kjeldbye H, Gouras P: Subretinal saline injection, macrophage invasion and prolonged photoreceptor survival in the RCS rat. Invest. Ophthalmol Vis Sci Suppl 30:595, 1990.

20. Li XL, Turner JE: Inherited retinal dystrophy in the RCS rat. Photoreceptor rescue by RPE cell transplantation. Exp Eye Res 47:911-917, 1988.

21. Lopez R, Gouras P, Kjeldbye H, Sullivan B, Reppucci V, Brittis M, Wapner F, Goluboff E: Transplanted retinal Pigment epithelium Modifies the Retinal Degeneration in the RCS Rat. Invest Ophthalmol Vis Sci 40:586-588, 1989.

DEVELOPMENT OF ROD AND CONE PHOTORECEPTOR CELLS IN INTRARETINAL GRAFTS.

Manuel del Cerro, Jeffrey Kordower*, Eliot Lazar, John A. Olschowka, Donald Grover, and Coca del Cerro

Departments of Neurobiology and Anatomy, and Ophthalmology, University of Rochester Medical School, Rochester, New York, and Department of Neurological Sciences*, Rush Presbyterian Medical Center, Chicago, Illinois, 60612.

Initial results from this study have been reported in abstract form[1] and discussed in a review by del Cerro[2].

I. INTRODUCTION

Transplantation of embryonic retina into unrelated adult hosts, which was originally performed in our laboratory[3] is now a well established experimental procedure. In spite of all the progress in the field, however, the potential of grafted embryonic retinal cells to provide the host retina with rod and cone photoreceptor cells has, to date, not been satisfactorily established.   It is the purpose of this paper to present data obtained by performing retinal homo-grafts and xeno-grafts into rats eyes, which suggests that cone photoreceptors, as well as rod cells, can be succesfully grafted into the adult host retina.

II. MATERIALS AND METHODS

A. DONOR TISSUE FOR HOMOGRAFTS:

Zero to 2 day-old (PN 0-2) Fischer 344 rat pups were used to provide donor tissue. These rats were decapitated prior to enucleation and the eyes removed and placed in cold calcium-magnesium free balanced salt solution. The neural retinas were dissected free from the pigment epithelium, trimmed into small fragments, and used to make single-cell suspensions as described below.

B. CELL DISSOCIATION PROCEDURE:

Donor retinas were placed in a Petri dish with cold CMF buffer with 0.1% glucose, 100 µg/ml Streptomycin, and 2.5 µg/ml Fungizone. After 2-3 changes of fresh buffer, the tissue was cut into small pieces and transferred to a conical sterile centrifuge tube containing CMF with 0.02% EDTA. After incubation in trypsin and DNAse the tissue fragments were dissociated by repeated aspiration cycles through a Pasteur pipette. The cells were centrifuged for 5 minutes at 900 rpm, at 10° C, and the resulting pellet suspended in 1 ml of Hanks balanced salt solution. Aliquots were used to make cell counts and to determine viability using both a hemocytometer and the Trypan Blue exclusion procedure. Cell viability varied in the different runs between 85% and 95%. The final concentration of 6×10^5 cells / µl was adjusted with cold CMF.

C. DONOR TISSUE FOR XENOGRAFTS:

Two Cebus Apella monkeys were obtained from the Manheimer Primatological Foundation (Hamsted, Fla.) as part of a primate neural transplantation program. The fetuses were embryonic day 60 and E 90 as determined by timed breeding (full gestation is 165 days for Cebus monkeys). The pregnant dams were anesthetized with isoflourane (3% for induction; 1% for maintenance). The fetuses were then removed via Cesaerean section. The eyes were enucleated and collected in a Petri dish containing ice-cold calcium-magnesium-free balanced salt solution (CMF). The eyes were then placed under a stereo microscope while still in cold CMF, and the cornea, the iris, the lens, and most of the vitreous body were removed. At this point, the neural retina was gently separated from the pigment epithelium, and cut away from the optic nerve head. Minute tissue fragments were dissected with microscissors and loaded into a microsyringe for transplantation.

Eight male albino Fisher 344 rats per fetal donor were used as hosts for this study. The rats, which were 60 days old at the beginning of the experiment, were individually caged using a twelve hour on, twelve hour off illumination schedule. Food and water were available ad libitum.

Animal maintenance, handling, and surgical procedures (for monkeys and rats) were performed in strict compliance with NIH and institutional policies for humane treatment of research animals.

D. HOSTS FOR HOMO- AND XENOGRAFTS:

Groups, each consisting of 8 male albino Fischer 344 rats, were used as hosts for this study. Four groups were used for the homografts and two for the xenografts. In each case, the rats, which were 60 days old at the beginning of the experiment, were kept in a darkened room for three days. During that period, a 15 Watt incandescent lamp covered by a dark red filter, Kodak Wratten Series 1, was turned on briefly, once a day, for animal feeding and handling. Just prior to the end of the dark adaptation period, the animals were anesthetized, and dilating drops (2.5% Neo-synephrine, phenylephrine hydrochloride, and 1% Mydriacyl, tropicamide) were placed on their eyes. The rats were then indivudually housed in plastic cages illuminated by fluorescent light tubes suspended at 25 cm above the cages. Light intensity measured at the bottom of the cage by a Sekonik L-428 light meter was 3500 lux, or approximately 300 foot candles (1 footcandle = 0.0929 lux). The animals were kept in this environment for 4 weeks with water and food available ad libitum. Food pellets were offered in containers resting on the cage floor. At the end of the exposure period, the rats were exposed for one week to a regimen of 12 hour light and 12 hour darkness using a light intensity of 14 foot candles, in order to allow for stabilization of the retinal lesions. After this period, they were used as hosts for transplantation. In each group, four animals received transplants in both eyes, and four were transplanted in one eye only.

The host rats were anesthetized with intramuscular injections of ketamine (Ketalar, Parke Davis) 150 mg/ 100 g body weight, and xylazine (Rompun, Haver-Lockhart), 30 mg/ 100 g body weight. In addition to general anesthesia, topical ocular anesthetic drops (Proparacaine hydrochloride, Alcaine, Alcon, Forth Worth, TX) were applied. The eyelids were kept open with the aid of microserafines.

E. TRANSPLANTATION PROCEDURE:

Dissociated cells, adjusted to the final concentration of 600,000/ µl, were injected into the eyes of intact anesthetized hosts. The injection was performed using a 30 gauge needle fitted to a microliter syringe containing the cell suspension. By gently rotating the globe with a fine toothed forceps the best exposure was obtained. Using a Hamilton microsyringe, the cells were delivered at a point just posterior to the equator of the eye at the 12 o'clock meridian. The penetration of the needle was limited to approximately 1 mm, in order to favor the release the cells within the thickness of the host retina (Lazar and del

Cerro, 1990). Over a period of approximately 2 minutes, a two µl injection of suspended cells was transplanted.

F. POST-TRANSPLANTATION SURVIVAL AND CLINICAL STUDIES:
Survival times ranged from 10 to 90 days post-transplantation. The animals received several direct and indirect funduscopic examinations during this period.

G. IMMUNOSUPPRESION:
Daily intraperitoneal injections of Cyclosporin A (Sandoz, East Hannover, N.J.) were administered at a dose of 10 mg/ kg to the xenograft hosts throughout the course of the experiment.

H. HISTOLOGICAL TECHNIQUES:
At the end of the survival period, the rats were again anesthetized and the eyes were enucleated, hemisected, and kept overnight at 4°C under fresh fixative. At this point the nasal and temporal halves of the hemisected eyes were observed under an Olympus SZH stereo microscope. After post-fixation in a chromate-osmium tetroxide solution and embedding in epoxy resins, 1 µm thick sections of the tissue were cut and stained with Stevenel Blue[4] for study by light microscopy. Ultrathin sections were cut with a diamond knife and then contrasted with lead acetate[5].

I. QUANTITATIVE DETERMINATIONS:
Computer-assisted identification of photoreceptor cell nuclei was performed, and quantitative data were gathered, using a computer based morphometry program (IBAS) working on line with the light microscope.

III.   RESULTS

A. HOMOGRAFTS:

I. Host retinas
Histologically, the photoreceptor cell population of animals exposed to continuous fluorescent illumination differed dramatically from that of sex and age-matched controls (Figures 1 and 2). The irradiated hosts showed complete absence of photoreceptor inner and outer segments throughout the retina. A few dystrophic rod cells consisting of a small spherical soma and a rudimentary pedicle were found forming a single, discontinuous row in the retinal periphery. Quantitative observations underlined the severity and extensive nature of the damage. They indicated that the number of rod cell nuclei identifiable by either visual observation of 1µm thick sections, or by computer assisted image analysis of this material was reduced to near extinction, particularly in the equatorial region and the central retina (Figure 2).

II. Survival and Growth of the Transplants
In the grafted retinas, computer-assisted cell identification showed clusters of photoreceptor cells forming an irregular outer nuclear layer (Figure 3). As previously described[6], electron microscopic observation of these retinas consistently showed clusters of rod cells with inner segments, basal bodies, and 9+0 type cilia. Outer segments formed in many of the rosettes but tended to be defective, consisting of collections of irregular cisternae. Both conventional and ribbon synapses were present in large numbers within the patches of plexiform layer which developed around the clusters of transplanted photoreceptors. Quantitative analysis of the synaptic connectivity present in the normal,irradiated, and grafted retinas demonstrated highly significant differences.

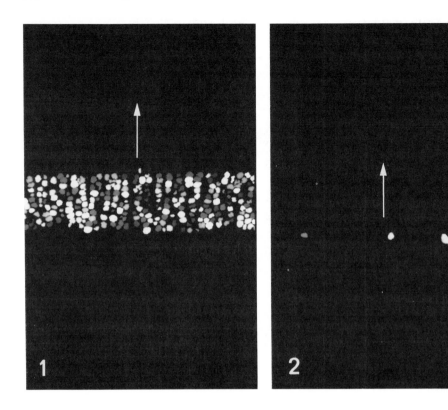

FIGURES 1and 2: Digitalized images of photoreceptor cell nuclei as identified in plastic sections by the IBAS image analyzer, working on line with a bright field light microscope. Arrows indicate the direction of the outer neuroretinal surface.

FIGURE 1:
Digitalized image indicating the distribution and numbers of photoreceptor cell nuclei in the equatorial retina of a normal Fisher 344 rat.

FIGURE 2:
Digitalized image indicating the distribution and numbers of photoreceptor cell nuclei in the equatorial retina of a Fisher 344 rat submitted to the effects of continuous fluorescent light. Overall, only about 1% of the photoreceptor cell population survives irradiation.

Integration of the transplant within the host retina was revealed by physical continuity, common vascularization, and a consistent lack of glial barriers around the transplants.

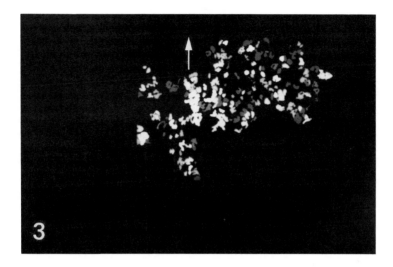

FIGURE 3:
Digitalized image of photoreceptor cell nuclei as identified in plastic sections by the IBAS image analyzer, using a bright field light microscope. Arrows show the direction of the outer neuroretinal surface. This photo indicates the distribution and number of photoreceptor cell nuclei in the equatorial retina of a Fisher 344 rat subjected to continuous fluorescent light and then grafted with a suspension of retinal cells at this site. There is a substantial repopulation of photoreceptor cells around the transplantation point.

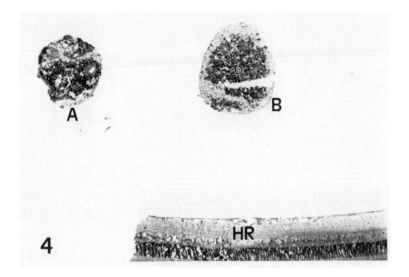

FIGURE 4:
Light micrograph of a transplant from E60 Cebus apella monkey retina to Fisher 344 rat. The graft has overgrown the host retina, and extends into the vitreous in the form of a "Y"-shaped structure. The two circular areas represent sections through the tips of the horns.

B. XENOGRAFTS:

Microscopic examination of the monkey donor retinas showed differentiation of an inner limiting membrane, a fiber layer, and a layer of retinal ganglion cells in the inner region. There was, however, an accentuated lack of differentiation in the outer region, which was occupied primarily by a neuroblastic population. The cells forming this layer still retained a high degree of mitotic activity.

Light and electron microscopic observations showed the survival of the transplanted cells and their regrouping into histogenetically differentiated structures. The grafted cells associated themselves into solid patches of tissue which closely integrated with the host retina. Not only did they fill the space created by the needle track, but they usually overgrew the boundaries of the host retina, and actually extended into the vitreous cavity (Figure 4). The bulk of the graft was formed by photoreceptor cells with their typical nuclear and cytoplasmic characteristics. These cells were often grouped into rosettes (Figure 5). Two differences were observable between the grafts originating from the two donors. One was that those grafts growing from the youngest (E 60) fetus grew more vigorously and formed a more laminated structure. The second difference noted was that grafts originating from the (E 90) fetus exhibited much clearer differentiation of cone-cell photoreceptors (Figures 6A and 6B).

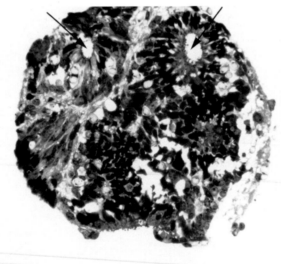

5

FIGURE 5:
High power micrograph of the graft section seen at the left of the field in Figure 4. The graft is predominantly populated by photoreceptor cells; two rosettes formed by such cells are indicated by arrows.

All the grafts, regardless of donor age, had some laminar differentiation external to the rosettes (Figure 5). Profiles of Müller cell processes as well as some conventional synaptic terminals were identifiable within the plexiform layer. The photoreceptors developing within the graft retained some of their normal polarity. It was possible to identify cone and rod-cell inner segments projecting into the lumina of the rosettes (Figures 6A and 6B). In some instances, outer segments which had formed and remained in place in the absence of any direct contact with the host retinal pigment epithelium were observed.

The transplants from both monkey fetuses were well accepted by the host throughout the survival period, as was demonstrated by the fact that there were no histologically demonstrable host reactions to the implants. In fact, there was a remarkable absence of macrophages around the grafts.

IV. DISCUSSION

The results from this study are of interest in several aspects. Firstly, they provide evidence that both rod and cone photoreceptors can be found in intraocular grafts of fetal retina. Secondly, they unequivocally prove the suitability of embryonic non-human primate neural retina as xenograft material. Finally, they indicate that a relatively advanced embryonic stage is not an absolute impediment to the survival, growth, and differentiation of dissociated neuroretinal cells of primate origin. In the following paragraphs, we shall discuss the implications of these findings.

Although a considerable body of evidence indicates that retinal cells can be successfully transplanted into the adult eye as heterografts,[2] intraocular retinal xenografts have received only limited attention. Retinal xenografting into the rodent CNS has been performed, and has provided important results regarding CNS plasticity and immunological interactions at the brain level.[7] Reports concerning intraocular retinal xenografting are, however, very limited to date. Aramant and Turner[8] transplanted embryonic mouse retinas into the site of minute surgical lesions made in adult rat retinas. This paradigm involved species less phylogenetically diverse than the ones used for our study. Also in that case, both the donor and the host animals had retinas in which the rod photoreceptors are overwhelmingly predominant.

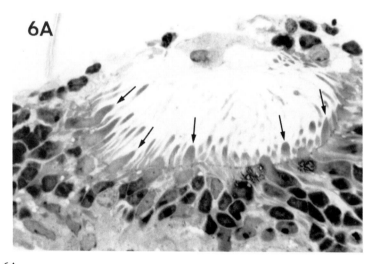

FIGURE 6A:
Light micrograph of transplant from E90 Cebus apella monkey retina into an adult Fisher 344 rat. The graft extends into the vitreal cavity. A rosette formed by photoreceptor cells shows structures with the morphological features of cone-cell inner segments projecting into the lumen (arrowheads).

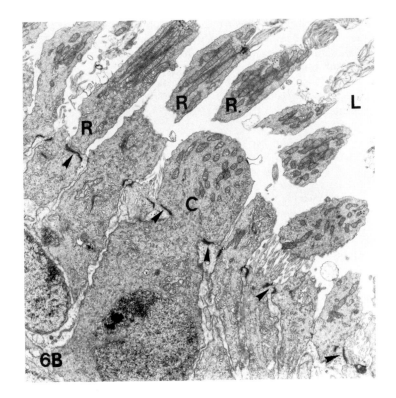

FIGURE 6B:
Panoramic electron micrograph through the rosette seen in Figure 6A. Cone and rod inner segments (C and R) project into the lumen (L). Intercellular junctions form a rudimentary outer limiting membrane (Arrowheads).

The observations from this study confirm and expand upon previous ones regarding the exceptionally wide "window of opportunity" enjoyed by the developing retina with regards to intra-ocular grafting into adults. As previously found in the case of the immature rat retina[7,8,9] and more recently in the human fetal retina,[6] it is clear that a relatively advanced developmental stage is not an absolute impediment to the survival, growth, and differentiation of transplanted neuroretinal cells. The sum of this evidence places the immature neural retina into a rather unique position among CNS regions when used as donor tissue. An impressive amount of data accumulated during the last decade indicates that CNS cells must be transplanted at the earliest possible embryonic stage if they are to survive grafting into the CNS of adult or perinatal hosts. Why, then, does the retina appear to escape this general rule?

Explanted into an extraneous environment, cone cells in particular developed inner segments which exhibited the basic morphology of the primate photoreceptors developing *in situ*. This result is of particular interest within the realm of retinal transplantation studies, since up to this time only rod cells have been reported to be successfully transplanted. Cone cells are the key photoreceptor element for primate vision. Evidence of successful grafting of these cells, even under the relatively adverse conditions of a xenograft, raises the hope that retinal transplantation may be a useful technique to repair damaged retinas in higher animals and humans.

VI. REFERENCES

1. Kordower, J. H. and del Cerro, M. (1989) Fetal monkey retina transplanted into adult rat eyes. Soc. Neurosc. Abs. 15: 1368.
2. del Cerro, M. (1990) Retinal Transplants. Progr. Retinal Res. 9: 229-272.
3. del Cerro, M., Gash, D.M., Rao, G.N., Notter, M.F., and Ishida, N. (1984) Intraocular retinal transplants. Invest. Ophthalmol. Vis. Sc. 25: 62 (abstr.).
4. del Cerro, M., Cogen, J. and del Cerro, C. (1980) Stevenel Blue, an excellent stain for optical microscopy study of plastic embedded tissues. Microscop. Acta 83: 117-121.
5. Venable, J.H. and Cogeshall R. (1965) A simplified lead citrate stain for use in electron microscopy. J. Cell Biol. 25: 407-408.
6. del Cerro, M., E. Lazar, D. A. Grover, M. J. Gallaher, C. D. Sladek, J. Chu and C. del Cerro (1990) Intraocular transplantation and culture of human embryonic retinal cells. Invest. Ophthalmol. Vis. Sc. 31: 593 (Abs.)
7. Young, M. J., K. Rao, and R. Lund (1989) Integrity of the blood-brain barrier in retinal xenografts is correlated with the immunological status of the host. J. Comp. Neurol., 283: 107-117.
8. Aramant, R. and Turner, J. E. (1988) Cross-species grafting of embryonic mouse and grafting of older postnatal rat retinas into the lesioned adult eye: the importance of cyclosporin A for survival. Devel. Brain Res. 41: 303-307.

VII. ACKNOWLEDGMENTS

This work was partially supported by National Eye Institute grant #05262, the Rochester Eye Bank, and a generous private donation.

INTRARETINAL TRANSPLANTATION: AN EXTERNAL, MULTISITE APPROACH

Eliot S. Lazar and Manuel del Cerro

Departments of Neurobiology and Anatomy, and Ophthalmology,
University of Rochester Medical School,
Rochester, New York.

Some results from this work have been presented in abstract form [1].

I. INTRODUCTION

Since our original presentation on intraocular retinal transplantation [2], the procedure for retinal grafting has undergone constant evolution, swiftly proceeding to new frontiers. A common feature to all of the retinal transplantation techniques described to date is that they require entering the eye surgically, through either a trans-scleral or trans-corneal route. This requirement necessarily carries with it all the inherent risks and possible complications of surgery, such as vitreous loss, cataract formation, and intraocular infection. Because of this, these approaches have discouraged attempts to implant multiple grafts into a single eye. We are continually attempting to devise a more effective retinal transplantation technique. Here, we describe a method which avoids these restrictions and permits multi-site intraocular grafting in a safe, easy, and reliable fashion. This procedure which is virtually free of complications, avoids the need for surgically entering the globe and therefore makes it possible to perform multiple simultaneous grafts into the intact eye. The technique, initially tested on rodent eyes, has already been used for grafting cells into monkey retinas.

II. MATERIALS AND METHODS

A. DONOR CELLS:

Second-trimester human embryonic retinal cells obtained from electively aborted embryos aged 13 to 17 weeks were used as donor tissue. Procurement of the donor cells was in strict accordance with scientific and ethical guidelines, which included institutional review and approval of the experimental protocol. In all cases, maternal consent was given only after the decision to have an elective abortion was made.

B. CELL PREPARATION:

The eyes were obtained less than one hour after fetal death, and collected in either calcium-magnesium free medium or in human plasma, at 4 º C. Operating with the aid of a surgical microscope, the eyes were dissected open. The retinas were cleanly cut away, free of contamination from either the vitreous or the retinal pigment epithelium. Isolated retinas were trimmed into small fragments, and then placed into ice cold medium. Mechanical dissociation was used to obtain suspensions of retinal cells and cell clusters. Dissociation was achieved by aspirating the retinal fragments through a 27 gauge hypodermic needle and then injecting them through the same needle. By varying the needle gauge as well as the number of aspiration-ejection cycles it is possible to maintain fine control over the final degree of cell dissociation.

C. HOSTS AND ANAESTHESIA:

Young male adult rats of the Wistar strain served as hosts. Two to three groups of six rats each were used per experiment. The animals were anesthetized with a mixture of chloral hydrate and sodium pentobarbital (Chloropent, Henry Schem Inc. Port Washington, NY) at a dose of 3 ml/Kg. Topical 1% Alcaine drops (Propaine Hydrochloride, Alcon, Fort Worth, Texas) were also used as a topical anaesthetic. The eyes were dilated pre-operatively with one drop each of 1% neo-synephrine and 1% mydriacyl (Alcon, Fort Worth, Texas).

D. DELIVERY SYSTEM AND TRANSPLANTATION PROCEDURE:

For most experiments, a 27 gauge Butterfly needle, tightly sheathed in plastic, with 1.2-1.4 mm of the needle tip remaining exposed, was connected to a Hamilton microliter syringe (Hamilton, Reno, Nevada) prior to the procedure. The plastic sheath placed on the needle acts as an adjustable regulator. By setting it at the appropriate depth, depending on the animal model being used, it serves to limit the depth of penetration and provides protection against over-penetration. The plastic sheath can be regulated so that a sufficient portion of the needle tip is left exposed to reach the subretinal space without actually penetrating the retina. This adaptation prevents large retinal holes or tears. Presently, a multi-purpose surgical instrument based on these principles is under design in our laboratories.

The microliter syringe is preloaded with a suspension of neuroretinal cells. After the animal is appropriately anesthetized, collibri forceps (Storz, St. Louis, Mo.) are used to firmly grasp the sclera at the limbus and rotate the globe anteriorly. Then, using a stereo microscope for direct visualization, the needle is manually inserted through the sclera and gently rotated until the tip can be directly viewed through the retina. Then, the tip is advanced further so as to slightly elevate the retina, while the plastic protective sheath prevents over penetration of the needle and perforation of the neuroretina. At this point, with the bevel of the needle facing the globe, the injection of cells is made. Following the injection, the needle is quickly withdrawn and the procedure repeated in the same eye, at a point 180 degrees opposite to the first injection site. Typically, two micro-injections are made into the equatorial region of each eye. One is made superiorly at the 12 o'clock position and the other at the 6 o'clock position inferiorly. As many as four penetrations have been performed in a single rat eye, and up to six into the lower hemisphere of a monkey eye. The needle is quickly withdrawn following each injection, and after the experiment is completed, a topical lubricant is placed on the cornea to prevent drying.

E. CONTROL INJECTIONS:

In order to obtain instant, permanent, and multilevel visualization of the spread of the injected fluid, colloidal carbon [3,4] was used to perform control injections in a fashion identical to the retinal transplantation procedure described. The injections were prepared in a 1:4 dilution with saline. In this experiment, one group of 6 animals served as the control, and each received colloidal carbon (Biological India Ink, Pelikan, West Germany) injections.

F. IN VIVO EXAMS:

All surgery was performed using a stereo-microscope fitted with a 35mm photographic camera as well as videotaping apparatus. Indirect and direct ophthalmoscopy was routinely performed on all the transplant recipients. This allowed us to constantly monitor the growth and condition of the transplants. Photographs were taken through the microscope using a motorized Nikon camera or using a Kowa camera in conjunction with the indirect ophthalmoscope.

G. SURVIVAL TIMES AND HISTOLOGICAL PROCEDURES:

Survival times for the animals receiving retinal cell injections ranged from 3 to 90 post-transplantation days (PTD). Control animals, who received injections of colloidal carbon were sacrificed three days following intraocular injections. The eyes were enucleated and the animals sacrificed under deep anesthesia.

The eyes were enucleated and fixed in 6% glutaraldehyde in cacodylate buffer for 24 to 48 hrs. They were then rinsed in buffer and split along a sagital axis, extending from the cornea to the optic nerve. The hemisected eyes were examined and photographed under a stereomicroscope, and were then embedded in plastic (Eponate 12. Ted Pella, Redding, CA). One um thick sections were cut and stained with Stevenel Blue [5,6] for light microscopic study. Ultrathin sections were cut with a diamond knife for electron microscopic studies. They were then stained with lead acetate[7] and studied under a Zeiss 10 electron microscope operating at 80 kv.

Some of the retinas injected with colloidal carbon were dissected free and prepared as flat-mounts in order to better evaluate the extent of diffusion of the injected fluid throughout the host retina.

III. RESULTS

Intraoperative results from the set of control experiments using colloidal carbon, plainly demonstrated that the carbon is injected precisely into the sub-retinal space. The entire procedure could be viewed directly under the operating microscope. It was possible to see how the needle penetrated the sclera and elevated the retina. Following this, the bevel was turned in order to lie it in apposition to the retina, an orientation which assured proper localization of the injected material. At this point, the injection was carried out (Diagrams 1 and 2). As the 2 µl of fluid were injected, the colloidal carbon was readily seen spreading throughout the retina. The material quickly fanned out and covered anywhere from 60 to 120 degrees per injection. The colloidal carbon dramatically illustrates the wide diffusion of the injected fluid over the surface of the host retina (Figures 1 and 2).

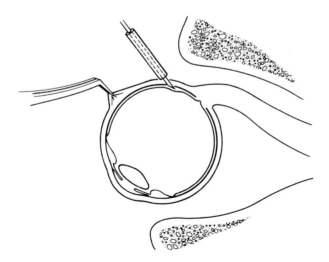

DIAGRAM 1:

Diagram illustrating how a collibri forceps is used to pull the globe far anteriorly, thus exposing the posterior pole of the retina. One can transplant cells at numerous sites in the retina utilizing this technique.

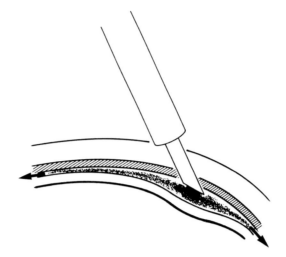

DIAGRAM 2:
Schematic demonstrating the spread of injected material immediately upon completion of the injection. Note how widely it spreads throughout the tissue.

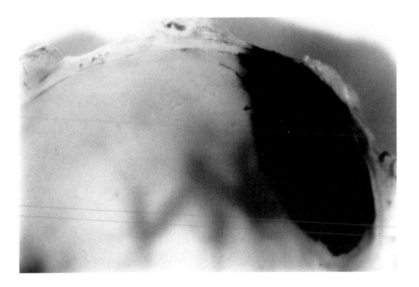

FIGURE 1:
This photograph demonstrates a hemisected eye in which the retina has been injected with two microliters of colloidal carbon in order to demonstrate the efficacy of the technique. The carbon has permeated the tissue and is densely filling the retina, and clearly the material can be seen to have diffused widely.

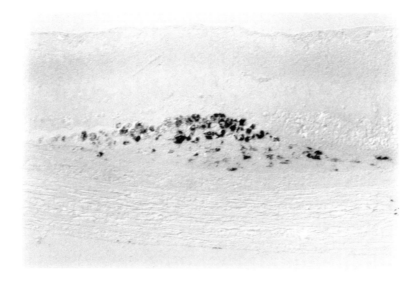

FIGURE 2:
In this histological section, the retina has received an injection of colloidal carbon. Note that the colloidal carbon is scattered throughout the subretinal space.

The carbon also serves as a control for the transplantation of living cells. This demonstrates that it is possible to access any portion of the retina, even as far posteriorly as the region around the optic nerve head, in a safe and reliable manner.

Histological observations correlated quite well with those made by biomicroscopy. Sections of the eyes injected with the tracer and from those injected with suspensions of living human fetal retinal cells showed considerable dispersion of the injected material, which spread onto the outer retinal surface from the subretinal injection point. Colloidal carbon injections in particular, dramatically illustrate the vast surface of the host retina which is covered by even a single injection. When a flat mount is made of the same preparation, it indicates the wide diffusion of the carbon granules throughout the retina. Histological specimens involving colloidal carbon injections clearly shows intraretinal colloidal carbon material scattered throughout.

In experiments where living human fetal retinal cells were grafted in rats or mice, the same pattern of distribution was observed as those seen in control injections where colloidal carbon was introduced into the subretinal space. Typically, the penetration point was marked by a comparatively larger cluster of cells (Figure 3). From here outwards, a multitude of smaller cells clusters were found at distances more than 2000 μm from the penetration point.

The growth and differentiation of the grafts compared favorably with those seen in transplants using traditional surgical approaches. The human cells survived well and most of them accumulated into clusters exhibiting rosette formation. In keeping with the protracted development of the human neural retina, intense mitotic activity continued within the graftedcell population for periods of up to two months post-transplantation, the longest time period examined to date.

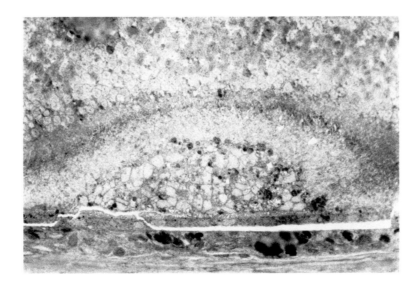

FIGURE 3:
Using the procedure described, retinal cells were transplanted into the rat retina, and the host eyes then enucleated. This section shows that the labeled donor cells are well incorporated into the host retina. The technique which we are describing does minimal damage to either the donor cells or the host retina.

The host retina, including the retinal pigment epithelium showed a remarkable lack of reaction to the mechanical disturbance introduced by the injection or the presence of grafted cells.

Clinical observations have confirmed the atraumatic nature of this technique. The wound is self-sealing, thus requiring no surgical closure. There was no no vitreal loss at the time of injection and postoperative examinations showed no corneal opacities, no lenticular changes, a normal optic nerve head, and an intra-ocular pressure which remained stable throughout. Indirect ophthalmoscopy was negative for signs of hemorrhage, neo-vascularization, uveitis or ocular infection in the eyes of approximately one hundred rats, twenty mice, and two monkeys transplanted to date using this procedure.

IV. DISCUSSION

Our initial retinal transplantation experiments [8] were performed using glass micropipettes attached to a microliter syringe. A preliminary incision was made through the sclera, and the transplant was then performed. This technique, although very effective in the rodent model, proved to be difficult and time consuming with severe limitations on the accuracy of the level of penetration. Additionally, suturing of the minute incision was associated with complications such as retinal detachments, subretinal hemorrhages, and formation of intravitreal membranes. A modified approach was developed [9] which avoided suturing, decreased the formation of pre-retinal membranes, and sharply reduced the incidence of hemorrhaging. It did not, however, eliminate them in their entirety.

The techniques for intraretinal transplantation in the reported literature to date by other groups also require surgically opening the globe. Lopez et. al. [10] used a technique which requires making a pars plana incision and inserting a micropipette through the globe into the subretinal space. The method involves forming a retinal detachment in order to properly place the transplant. They noted that " there are a number of potential pitfalls associated with this technique." They remark that the host epithelium must first be detached, a procedure which in man is associated with subretinal neovascularization. In addition they notice,"It may be difficult to be certain that no cells enter the vitreous cavity."

Turner et al. [11] have shown their technique via a diagrammatic format. They first make an incision into the globe with a blade. They then excise sclera/ choroid prior to performing their transplantations. Following the injection of material, the incision must be closed surgically with suture material. These authors do not discuss the rate of post-surgical complications attending the procedure.

Silverman and Hughes [12] reported using a technique which also involves a preliminary incision prior to implantation of tissue. They employ a transcorneal approach to the subretinal space. This involves making a transverse incision through the corneal-limbal junction and then traversing the entire globe, via the subretinal space, in order to reach the posterior pole. The extent or frequency of ocular complications associated with this technique has not been reported.

We therefore felt the need for devising a more expeditious and efficient means of transplantation, one that would make multi-site grafting not only possible but virtually free from surgical complications. Only through a quick and atraumatic method did we feel that we could limit the complications, as well as the cellular response. As our goal, we set out to formulate a means which would be uncomplicated and quick, but at the same time guarantee that the cells would be delivered intraretinally at multiple points, in a safe and reliable manner.

A closed eye method of transplantation is highly desirable as it avoids the need for surgically opening the eye and thus makes it feasible and practical to perform multiple simultaneous grafts into an intact globe. For the first time, we have photographically demonstrated a retinal transplantation procedure (Lazar and del Cerro, submitted for publication).

The procedure is quick and efficient and provides the added advantage of having multi-site delivery of cells over a wide surface area. This vastly improves the odds for success in any transplantation performed. Perhaps even more significantly, it is a relatively benign procedure. Because it is quick, there is only a need for brief anaesthesia, which still further limits the complication rate. The rapid transplantation of cells also greatly diminishes the risk of infection or post-operative complications. And, the simplicity of the procedure, an intraocular injection, means that the risk of intraoperative complications should be minimal. In all the cases which we have performed on both rodents and primates [13], we have had no intra-operative or post-operative complications. That, in and of itself, is a reason to consider this a preferred method of intraocular transplantation.

Because of its technical simplicity and safety, as well as the area of the retina which is covered during its application, this method can be easily and effectively performed. Many different applications of such methodology can be envisioned. The field of retinal transplantation can certainly benefit from a safe and reliable means of cell placement. This is our ultimate goal, and by performing it in the most mechanically simple and efficient way, we are maximizing the chances of a successful transplant.

This is a method has undergone extensive testing in our laboratory. It can now be said with certainty that the cells are being delivered at the desired subretinal or intraretinal locations under direct visual control by the operator.

VI. REFERENCES

1. Lazar E and del Cerro M: A new procedure for retinal transplantation. ARVO meeting, Sarasota Florida, May 1990. Invest. Ophthalmol. Vis. Sci. 31: 593, 1990 (Abstr.).

2. del Cerro M, Gash DM, Rao GN, Notter MFD, Wiegand SJ, and Ishida N: Intraocular retinal transplants. ARVO Meeting, Sarasota, Florida, May, 1984. Invest. Ophthalmol. Vis. Sci. 25: 62, 1984 (Abstr.).

3. del Cerro M, Grover DA, Dematte JE, and Williams, WM: Colloidal carbon as a combined ophthalmoscopic and microscopic probe of the retinal-blood barrier integrity. Ophthalmic Res. 17: 34, 1985.

4. Triarhou L and del Cerro M: Colloidal carbon as a multilevel marker for experimental lesions. Experientia 41: 620,1985.

5. del Cerro M, Cogen M J, and del Cerro C: Stevenel Blue, an excellent stain for opticalmicroscopy study of plastic embedded tissues. Microscop. Acta 83: 543, 1980.

6. del Cerro M, Standler M, and del Cerro C: High resolution optical microscopy of animal tissues by the use of sub- micrometer thick sections and a new stain. Microscop Acta 83: 117, 1980.

7. Venable, J and Cogeshall R: A simplified lead citrate stain for use in electron microscopy. J Cell Biol 25: 407, 1965.

8. del Cerro M, Gash D.M, Notter M, Rao G N, Wiegand S, Jiang L, and del Cerro C: Transplanting strips of immature retinal tissue and suspensions of dissociated retinal cells into normal and extensively damaged eyes. Ann of N.Y. Acad of Sci 495: 692, 1986.

9. del Cerro M, Notter M, del Cerro C, Wiegand S, Grover D, and Lazar E: Intraretinal Transplantation for rod-cell replacement in light-damaged retinas. J. of Neur Transpl 1:1, 1989.

10. Lopez R, Gouras P, Brittis M, and Kjeldbye H: Transplantation of cultured rabbit retinal epithelium to rabbit retina using a closed eye method. Invest Ophthalmol Vis Sci 28: 1131, 1987.

11. Sheedlo H, Li L, and Turner J: Functional and structural characteristics of photoreceptor cells rescued in RPE-cell grafted retinas of RCS dystrophic rats. Exp. Eye Res. 48: 841, 1989.

12. Silverman M, and Hughes, S: Transplantation of Photoreceptors to Light- Damaged Retina. Invest Ophthalmol Vis Sci 30: 1684, 1989.

13. del Cerro M, Lazar E, Grover D, Gallagher M, Sladek C, Chu J, and del Cerro C: Intraocular Transplantation and culture of human embryonic retinal cells. ARVO meeting, Sarasota Florida, May 1990. Invest. Ophthalmol. Vis. Sci. 31: 593, 1990 (Abstr.).

VII. ACKNOWLEDGEMENTS

Supported by NEI grant #05262, a generous private donation, and the Rochester Eye Bank.

PHOTORECEPTOR TRANSPLANTATION TO DYSTROPHIC RETINA

Martin S. Silverman[1,2], Stephen E. Hughes[1], Tony L.Valentino[3] and Yao Liu[2]

[1]Central Institute for the Deaf; [2]Department of Ophthalmology and Visual Sciences, Washington University Medical School, St. Louis MO; [3]Department of Biology, St. Louis University, St. Louis, MO.

I. INTRODUCTION

In this chapter we will briefly outline our approach to the transplantation of photoreceptors to dystrophic retina. This approach uses novel techniques that allow intact sheets of isolated photoreceptors to be transplanted to their appropriate site in an effort to reconstruct host retina lacking photoreceptors. The anatomical and physiological basis for, as well as behavioral evidence of, the recovery of visual sensation resulting from photoreceptor transplantation is presented. In addition, we will report new results that show that a number of problems with retinal cell or tissue transplantation once thought to be rather difficult to solve are being overcome.

II. HARVESTING AND TRANSPLANTING INTACT SHEETS OF PHOTORECEPTORS TO DYSTROPHIC RETINA

A. GENERAL PREMISE

In several retinal degenerative diseases select populations of cells are lost. For instance, in macular degeneration and retinitis pigmentosa retinal photoreceptors degenerate while other cells in the retina, as well as the retina's central connections, can be maintained.[1-3]

It was our hypothesis that in instances where photoreceptors were selectively lost some degree of vision might be restored by the transplantation of photoreceptors.[4-6] The most appropriate method to reconstruct the retina lacking photoreceptors clearly would be to replace only the retinal photoreceptors and not to transplant retinal fragments or mixed cell suspensions as had been reported previously.[7-12]

Not only would the non-photoreceptor cells within the transplants be unnecessary, but they could interfere with the reassociation with and reinnervation of the host's retina by the transplanted photoreceptors. This interference could be physical, displacing the photoreceptor elements away from the host postsynaptic targets, or competitive, since transplanted horizontal and bipolar cells would likely compete with the host horizontal and bipolar cells for innervation by the transplanted photoreceptors. This potential for interference with reconstruction of the dystrophic retina would be increased by the propensity of retinal cell transplants to form rosette formations (the disruption of the laminar retinal layers into circular enclosures with the photoreceptors forming the innermost layer of the enclosure) (see Heading III, Section A). Rosette formation within retinal cell transplants would tend to entrap and insulate the transplanted photoreceptors from the host retina. This entrapment could in turn facilitate synaptic connectivity between transplanted photoreceptors and cotransplanted horizontal and bipolar cells while preventing apposition and synapse formation between the transplanted photoreceptors and the host retinal tissue. Therefore, by eliminating extraneous and potentially interfering non-photoreceptor cells from the transplant, apposition of the transplanted photoreceptors to the host retina is maximized and unwanted intra-transplant synaptic connectivity is avoided, facilitating the possibility of appropriate reinnervation of the host retina by the transplanted photoreceptors.

Other characteristics of retinal photoreceptors influenced the development of our technique. For instance, photoreceptors are highly polarized cells with their outer segments directed toward the pigment epithelium and the synaptic terminals facing the inner nuclear layer (INL). Retinal dissociation techniques previously developed for the isolation of photoreceptors [13] result in the loss of the normal organization of the photoreceptors. Photoreceptor transplants made from dissociated photoreceptors form a disorganized mass (eg, multiple rosettes are formed, unpublished observations) which reduces the likelihood of correct apposition to and reinnervation of the host retina as well as apposition to the host retinal pigment epithelium. Furthermore, normal visual acuity requires that the photoreceptor elements be configured in a regular lattice arrangement.[14,15] We therefore reasoned it would be advantageous to maintain the isolated photoreceptors in an organized ONL structure to maximize coherent transduction of the visual image. For these reasons, we devised a new method of isolating the intact ONL in which the polarity and organization of the photoreceptors are maintained (see Figure 1).[4,6,16]

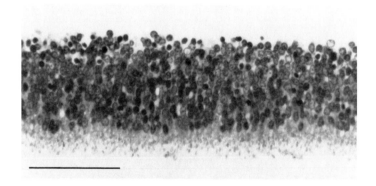

FIGURE 1. Isolation of intact ONL. Intact ONL isolated from developing retina of the 8-day-old rat after 1 day in culture. The ONL was isolated by removing the inner retinal layers with a vibratome. The isolated ONL is maintained as a flat sheet. Note that ONL organization is intact, with the photoreceptor cells showing columnar stacking and maintenance of a bacillary layer consisting of developing inner and outer segments. Bar = 100 μm.

In order to reconstruct the dystrophic retina lacking photoreceptors it would also be necessary to devise methods by which a portion of the isolated intact ONL could be transplanted to the appropriate position in the eye, adjacent to the retina's outer plexiform layer (OPL). In addition it would be necessary that this method allow the polarity and organization of the transplanted ONL to be maintained. The injection techniques for transplanting retinal fragments;[10] or cell suspensions [9,17,18] into the eye would not be appropriate since the organization and correct orientation of the transplanted photoreceptors would be lost.

We therefore devised methods for transplanting the isolated photoreceptors that maintained the organization and correct polarity of the transplant and allowed for correct positioning of the ONL adjacent to the host retina's OPL. Using these techniques, we have shown that photoreceptors can be transplanted to retina in which the host's photoreceptors are lost due to an environmental cause (constant light) [4-6] or inherited deficits (the rd mouse and the RCS rat).[6,19] Furthermore, transplanted photoreceptors possess basic characteristics of normal photoreceptor cells, eg., staining positive for opsin and maintaining an intercellular organization and apposition to the host retina that is similar to that seen in the normal ONL.

In the course of investigating the possibility of a critical period for the transplantability of photoreceptors we found that photoreceptors could be transplanted either when developing or when mature.[6,16,20] Not only can mature rat photoreceptors be transplanted, but we have shown that mature photoreceptors from human donors can be transplanted to rats as well.[6,16,20] The ability of mature photoreceptors to be transplanted is significantly different from other CNS neurons, which must be immature in order to be transplanted.[22] At present, the reason for this difference is not known but has obvious importance for retinal transplantation as well as neural transplantation research in general.

B. METABOLIC MAPPING STUDIES

In our photoreceptor transplants we saw physical apposition of the transplanted photoreceptors to the host OPL.[4-6,16] With this result two important questions could now be addressed: are the transplanted photoreceptors capable of light transduction, and if so, are they able to activate the host retina?

In preliminary metabolic mapping studies using the 2-deoxyglucose (2DG) autoradiographic technique, we have shown that transplanted photoreceptors not only respond to light stimulation but also activate the host's dystrophic retina in a light-dependent manner that closely resembles the activation pattern seen in normal retina.[6] While these studies need greater elaboration, the results indicate that the 2DG method can be used to study functional aspects of the reconstructed retina.

Although activation of the host retina by the transplanted photoreceptors was seen with deoxyglucose mapping, the nature of this activation was unclear. Specifically, did such activation represent a nonsynaptic modulation of neurotransmitter release by the transplanted photoreceptors, or did the transplanted cells form synapses with elements of the host retina?

C. SYNAPTIC CONNECTIONS

To help answer this question, we analyzed the reconstructed retinas at the ultrastructural level for structures that are indicative of photoreceptor synapses (eg, synapses containing a presynaptic ribbon structure). In the residual OPL (Figure 2A) in areas of the host retina that did not receive a photoreceptor transplant, ribbon-type synaptic connections were extremely rare (mean of 5.5 per 100 μm distance along the OPL) and were seen in association with residual cones. However, in the OPL in areas of the host retina that was apposed to the photoreceptor transplant, ribbon-type synapses were much more comparable in number (44.3 per 100 μm distance along the OPL 2 or 4 weeks after transplantation) and form as those seen in the OPL of normal retinas. These synapses are characteristic of those formed by rod photoreceptors, with an electron-dense ribbon surrounded by a cluster of vesicles (Figure 2B, C). The number found compares to 60 ribbons per 100 μm reported from normal rat eyes by Eisenfeld and coworkers.[23]

In addition to ribbon synapses, the transplanted photoreceptors also display inner segments, connecting cilia, and outer segment membranes (Figure 3).[24,25] The survival of and synapse formation by transplanted photoreceptors has been recently corroborated by Gouras and coworkers.[17]

These data suggest that transplanted photoreceptors can form new synapses with host retinal cells, indicating that the light-dependent activation we have reported may, at least in part, be synaptically mediated. However, at least two additional explanations for the presence of synapses must be considered. First, could we have inadvertently included a few horizontal and bipolar cells along with the transplanted photoreceptors? If this were the case, the synaptic connections that we saw might be between photoreceptors and cotransplanted horizontal or bipolar cells. Although the purity of the transplants is excellent (see Figure 1) and the large number of synapses found mitigate against this argument, it is still possible that we are viewing synaptic connections between cotransplanted cells.

Second, it is possible that the synapses we are seeing might be those of the few residual photoreceptors that remain after phototoxic light exposure and are not those from the transplanted photoreceptors. This is somewhat unlikely since ribbon synapses are very rare in unreconstructed areas of the host retina while they are quite numerous in reconstructed

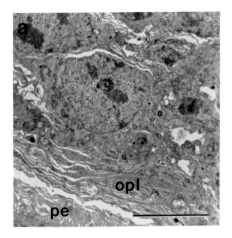
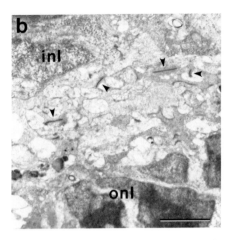
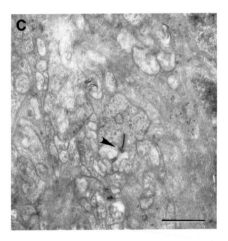

FIGURE 2.   Ultrastructure of reconstructed retina.

A. In light-damaged control eyes, the OPL is substantially reduced, with ribbon synapses being scarce or absent. The INL has become apposed to the pigment epithelium (PE).   Bar = 5 μm.

B. In the reconstructed retina, a new OPL has formed and is visible at the interface of the transplanted ONL and the host INL. Synaptic ribbons are visible (arrows), indicative of photoreceptor synapses that appear comparable to those in the normal OPL. The transplanted photoreceptors are at the bottom of the field. Synapses persist in the reconstructed retina for at least 6 months, the longest survival time so far examined in this study. Bar = 2 μm.

C. Ribbon synapse (arrow) from the OPL of reconstructed retina. The normal triad rod spherule structure, which includes a presynaptic ribbon structure, an arciform density and processes invaginating into the spherule can be clearly seen. Bar = 1 μm.

areas. In addition, the ribbon synapses seen in the reconstructed areas were almost completely of the rod type (only one ribbon seen within a presynaptic profile and dense cytoplasm characteristic of a rod synapse), while those in the nonreconstructed areas were more like those associated with cones (frequently more than one ribbon per presynaptic terminal and electron-lucent cytoplasm).

Nevertheless, it is important to develop methods that will allow us to determine definitively whether these ribbon synapses are truly formed between transplanted photoreceptors and host neurons.

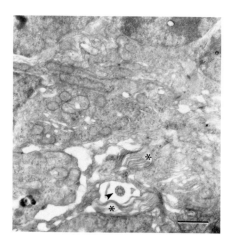

FIGURE 3.   Outer segment disks. Outer segment disks (*) can be seen within the transplanted tissue. In addition, connecting cilia are now evident (arrow). The pigment epithelium is toward the lower left. Two weeks post-transplantation. Bar = 1 μm.

III. PRESENT ISSUES IN RETINAL CELL TRANSPLANTATION

A number of issues in retinal cell transplantation have been problematic or are unresolved. They are summarized and discussed below:

• All retinal transplants so far conducted show some degree of rosette formation or distortion in the organization of the transplant.

• Photoreceptors, whether transplanted alone or with other retinal cells, do not show normal inner and outer segment growth and their apposition to the retinal pigment epithelium.

• No physiological evidence has demonstrated that retinal or photoreceptor transplants made to the eye can activate the central visual system of the blinded host.

• There have been no reports of behavioral evidence that light sensitivity or visual function is restored after retinal cell transplantation to the dystrophic retina.

A . ROSETTE FORMATIONS

A major problem with transplanting retina or photoreceptors to the retina is the formation of rosettes (the disruption of the laminar retinal layers into circular enclosures) following transplantation. All previous retinal transplants reported show considerable rosette formation or distortion in the organization of the transplant.[7-10,26] As noted earlier, rosette formations may limit the functionality of the transplant. Even our technique of transplanting an intact planar portion of the ONL, while eliminating most rosettes, often results in at least some rosette formation within the transplant (see Figure 4).[5,6]

We wished to determine whether components of the inner retina that are eliminated by isolating the ONL have an effect on the subsequent organization of the ONL after

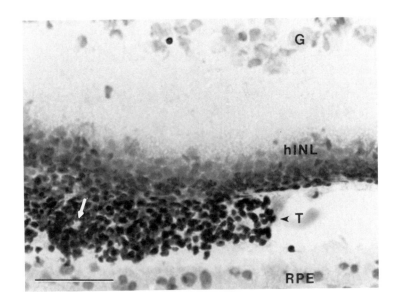

FIGURE 4.   Neonatal (8 day old) photoreceptors transplanted to host retina lacking photoreceptors. Sheets of photoreceptors transplanted to their normal position adjacent to the dystrophic host retina maintain a degree of their normal organization, but this organization can be disrupted by the formation of rosettes (arrow). In addition these transplants show very few inner and outer segments. In this and all subsequent photomicrographs transplants were made for two weeks. G = ganglion cell layer; h INL = host inner nuclear layer; T = transplanted photoreceptors; RPE = host retinal pigment epithelium. Cryostat section; H&E stain. Bar = 50 μm.

transplantation. For example, the Muller cells send processes through the ONL which may act as scaffolding to maintain the intercellular organization of this layer. While we see new Muller cell processes invading the donor ONL from the host tissue, there is an obligatory period of time when the transplanted ONL does not contain Muller cell processes. During this time, or during the regrowth of new Muller cell processes into the transplanted ONL, intercellular organization may be susceptible to rearrangement, resulting in the formation of rosettes.

In order to determine whether components of the inner retina could effect the maintenance of the organization of the transplanted ONL, two different strategies were followed. In the first, the ganglion cell layer was removed from the neonatal retina prior to transplantation. These transplants resulted in an obvious improvement in the organization of the transplanted ONL (Figure 5) with no rosettes evident. The second strategy involved transplanting intact retina (no cells layers removed). Both neonatal (Figure 6) and mature (Figure 7) retina were employed, and both yielded improvements in the organization of the ONL over that found in transplants made with isolated ONL. The mature transplants provided better preservation of the ONL structure.

In these experiments it was not our intent to restore the functionality of the host's dystrophic retina. In these transplants a considerable amount of retinal tissue is intervening between the transplanted photoreceptors and their synaptic targets within the host OPL. With this arrangement it is unlikely that appropriate connections between the transplanted photoreceptors and the host's OPL would occur.

It was our intent, however, to determine if components within the inner portion of the retina were important for the expression of inner and outer segments and for improvement in the organization in the transplanted ONL. We have found that if inner portions of the retina are included in the transplant, our transplant method results in the reduction or elimination of rosette formation.

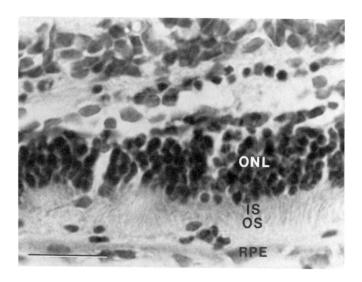

FIGURE 5. Transplantation of neonatal retina minus ganglion cell layer. Transplanted neonatal retina in which the ganglion cell layer was removed prior to transplantation to adult dystrophic retina shows a recognizable photoreceptor ONL. Inner segments (IS) and outer segments (OS) are clearly seen apposed to the host RPE. Some deformity of the transplanted ONL is seen, but the organization is clearly better (no complete rosettes are seen) than with transplantation of the isolated ONL as seen in Figure 4. Furthermore, inner and outer segments must have grown following transplantation since at the time of transplantation (8 days postnatal) inner and outer segments are not well developed. Paraffin section; H&E stain. Bar = 25 μm.

B. INNER AND OUTER SEGMENTS

Photoreceptors, whether transplanted alone or with other retinal tissue, demonstrate abnormally low expression of photoreceptor inner and outer segments. Those present have in most instances lost their normal orientation and apposition to the host RPE and instead are found within the rosette enclosures (see Figure 4).[5,6,8-10,26] Because the normal organization of outer segments is toward the adjacent RPE, the aberrant organization within the transplant is clearly inappropriate and may limit the usefulness of the transplanted photoreceptors. While photoreceptors lacking outer segments are still capable of phototransduction, they are certainly required for the normal level of light sensitivity.[27]

Our transplantation procedure allows for the normal apposition of the outer segments to the RPE, which has been shown to facilitate outer segment growth.[28,29] We have found that if portions of the inner retina are transplanted along with the intact sheet of photoreceptors, apparently normal expression of inner and outer segments occurs (see Figures 5, 6).[20] These outer segments label positive for opsin (see Figure 7).

Unexpectedly, transplants of mature retinal tissue display better maintenance of ONL organization and the expression of inner and outer segments than immature retinal tissue. Further research is necessary to investigate the anatomical, biochemical and functional characteristics of these transplants to determine more precisely what elements in the adjoining cotransplanted retina are mediating this improvement in the morphological characteristics of the transplanted photoreceptors.

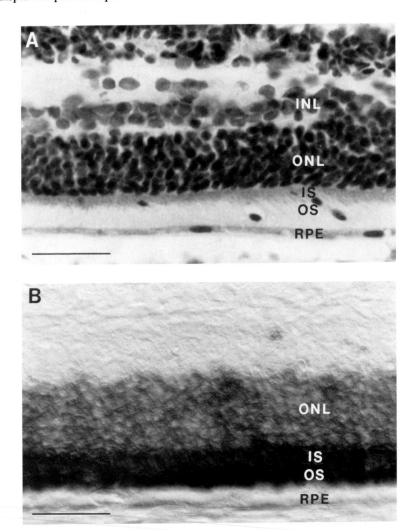

FIGURE 6.   Transplantation of intact neonatal retina.

A   The organization of the photoreceptor layer is well maintained, showing no rosette formations and inner and outer segments are clearly seen apposed to the host RPE. INL = transplanted inner nuclear layer; ONL = transplanted photoreceptor layer; IS = inner segments; OS = outer segments RPE = host retinal pigment epithelium. Paraffin section; H&E stain. Bar = 25 μm.

B   Adjacent section immunohistochemically reacted for antibody Ret P-1 specific for opsin (provided by C. Barnstable) showing the characteristic heavy staining of photoreceptor inner and outer segments. Nomarski optics. Bar = 25 μm.

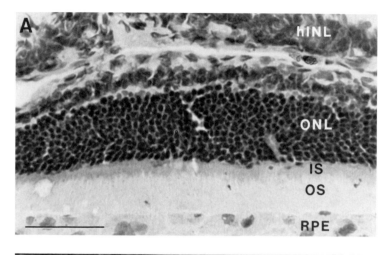

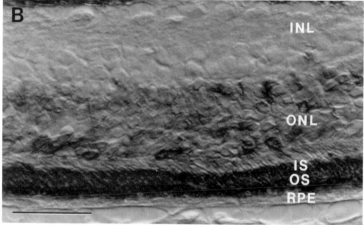

FIGURE 7.   **Transplantation of intact mature retina.**

A   The organization of the photoreceptor layer is well maintained and is comparable to the organization seen in neonatal rat retina (see Figure 6) with no rosette formations and inner and outer segments clearly apposed to the host RPE. Atrophy of inner portion of the transplanted retina is evident. Cryostat section; H&E stain. h INL = host inner nuclear layer. Bar = 50 μm.

B   Transplanted intact mature retina immunohistochemically reacted for opsin showing characteristically heavy staining of photoreceptor inner and outer segments. Paraffin section photographed using Nomarski optics. Bar = 25 μm.

C. LIGHT EVOKED BRAIN ACTIVITY FROM THE RECONSTRUCTED EYE.

No physiological evidence has demonstrated that retinal or photoreceptor transplants to the eye could activate the central visual system of the blinded host. That is, there have been no reports of light-evoked brain responses elicited from the reconstructed eye. This of course would be necessary for the transplants to be useful in restoring vision.

In the initial assessments of the functional characteristics of the transplanted photoreceptors noted above we found that transplanted photoreceptors activate the host's dystrophic retina in a light-dependent manner that closely resembles the activation pattern seen in normal retina.[6,30] These results, together with our finding of evidence for synaptic connectivity between the transplanted photoreceptors and the host retina, suggest that light-evoked activity within the central nervous system should be elicited by stimulation of the reconstructed retina.

With this in mind, we have initiated experiments directed toward determining if the reconstructed retina can produce a light-evoked response in the visual cortex. Adult light-damaged albino rats received a photoreceptor transplant (8 day old donor) in one eye while the fellow eye received a sham transplant (gelatin substrate only). One month post-transplantation, skull screws were bilaterally implanted over the representation of the inferior visual field of the visual cortex. This recording site was chosen to coincide with the retinotopic area (superior aspect of the retina) to which the transplants were made. VEP responses were elicited by strobe flash test stimuli. Responses were recorded contralateral to the stimulated eye. We found that the reconstructed retina can produce a light-evoked response in the visual cortex, whereas the unreconstructed fellow eye showed little or no response to the same light stimulus (see Figure 8).

These results indicate that light-evoked activity can in fact be recorded in the visual cortex with light stimulation of the reconstructed retina.

D . BEHAVIORAL EVIDENCE FOR VISUAL FUNCTION

There have been no reports of behavioral evidence that light sensitivity or any degree of visual function is restored after retinal cell transplantation to the dystrophic retina.

With the indications noted above that neural activity is generated in the central nervous system by the photoreceptor transplant in the reconstructed retina, the question arises as to whether this neural activity can be processed properly by the central nervous system to produce an appropriate behavioral response to the sensory stimulus. Previous studies have shown that neural transplants can restore appropriate behavioral activity.[31]   Klassen and Lund [32,33] have shown that neural transplants can restore a pupillary reflex driven by intracranially transplanted retinas, thus demonstrating that neural transplants consisting of sensory tissue are capable of mediating a behaviorally appropriate response to sensory stimulation.

1.Pupillary Reflex

The pupillary reflex (tonic constriction of the pupil to continuous light) may be an efficient method of noninvasively determining a number of characteristics of the transplanted photoreceptors and the reconstructed retina. For instance, it could be used to determine:

a.   the presence of a functional transplant.
b.   the development or time course for transplant-mediated light sensitivity, i.e., how long after transplantation does it take for the transplant to activate the host retina?
c.   the stability of the transplant over time.

We have found the eye that received the photoreceptor transplant showed a normal pupillary reflex while the sham operated eye showed a much attenuated response that was aberrant in form (a small pupillary dilation to continuous light) (Figure 9). Specifically, light induced a tonic constriction of the pupil of about 1 mm in the reconstructed eye. We compared the responses of the experimental rats to those of normal albino rats and light-damaged albino rats. To the same continuous light, the normal albino rats showed a tonic construction of the pupil of 1.5 mm, whereas the unoperated, light-damaged animals showed a small but consistent pupillary dilation in response to continuous light. This abnormal response has been termed the pupillary escape [34] and is seen clinically in cases of retinal or optic nerve degeneration.[35] Trejo and Cicerone [36] also saw a similar aberration of the pupillary reflex in the adult RCS rat at ages when most of the photoreceptors have degenerated.

These results show that the reconstructed retina can produce a pupillary reflex

A

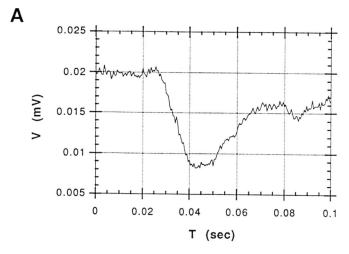

B

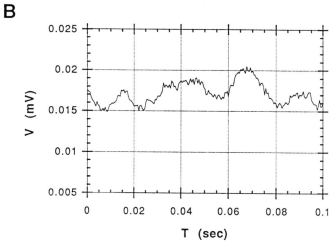

FIGURE 8   Cortical-Evoked Potential

A. Light-evoked response recorded from the visual cortex contralateral to the eye receiving a photoreceptor transplant. A prominent positive-going response (positive recorded going down) is seen at 40 msec. following flash onset. The waveform and latency of the response closely resembles the P2 response seen in normal rats. Average of 100 traces.

B. VEP recording from the visual cortex contralateral to the sham operated eye. Little or no response is seen in the cortex elicited from the sham operated eye. Average of 100 traces. Comparison of traces A and B suggests that light-dependent activation of the retina reconstructed by photoreceptor transplantation can evoke responses in the visual cortex.

comparable to the normal animal, while the light-damaged, sham operated eye shows an attenuated and aberrant reflex that is comparable to the unoperated light-damaged animal. These results indicate that transplanted photoreceptors can reconstruct the light-damaged retina to produce a behaviorally appropriate response to light.

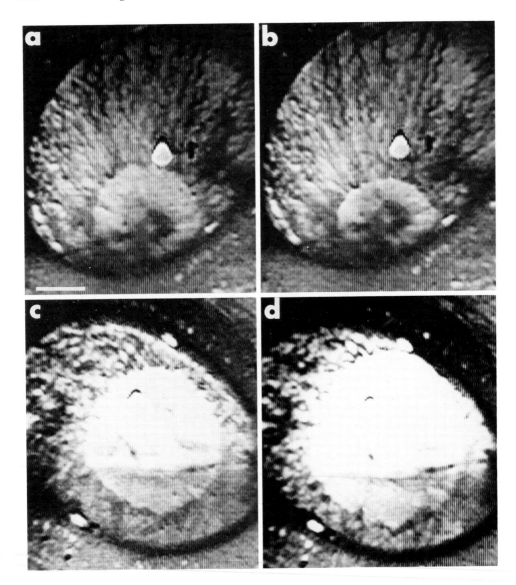

FIGURE 9. Pupillary responses from light-damaged and reconstructed retina.

Panels A and B are photographs, taken from the video monitor, of a light-damaged eye in which the retina was reconstructed by photoreceptor transplantation. Panel A shows the iris at light onset while panel B shows the same eye at 5 seconds later. Comparison of panels A and B demonstrates a normal pupillary constriction mediated by light. Bar = 1 mm for all panels.

Panels C and D show the fellow light-damaged eye that received sham surgery. Panel C shows the iris at light onset and panel D shows the iris 5 seconds later. Comparison of panels C and D show an increase in pupil size with light. This response is aberrant in form and is similar to the pupillary escape phenomenon seen clinically in cases of retinal or optic nerve degeneration. Pupillary escape is also seen in unoperated rats that have lost most of their photoreceptors due to constant light exposure.

Because the pupillary reflex has been used to accurately measure visual acuity, [37-39] it may be possible to determine aspects of the development and degree of pattern vision gained after photoreceptor transplantation. While this measure may be used in the low acuity system of the rat, it would be of considerably greater value for noninvasive behavioral measures of visual acuity in the monkey following photoreceptor transplantation. To further extend the utility of this work, adaptation of the photoreceptor transplantation technique to the primate eye is currently being pursued. [40]

IV. SUMMARY

We have investigated the possibility of reconstructing retina in model systems where photoreceptor degeneration is either inherited (the rd mouse and the RCS rat) or is environmentally induced (constant illumination in the albino rat) through transplantation of immature (8 day old) or mature rodent photoreceptors as well as mature human photoreceptors. To this end, we have devised methods for isolating the ONL from the retina and transplanting the resulting photoreceptor layer to the subretinal space of mature rodents. In all groups, the retina reattaches to the back of the eye with the transplanted photoreceptors interposed between the retina and the underlying tissues. For all groups, the transplanted photoreceptors survive transplantation for as long as has been investigated (rd mouse, 3 months; RCS rat, 9 months; constant illumination/albino, 12 months), integrate with the host's retina and are immunohistochemically reactive for opsin. Furthermore, using metabolic mapping techniques and visually evoked response recordings we have shown that transplanted photoreceptors can activate the host's reconstructed retina and the central visual system in a light-dependent manner.

In ultrastructural studies of the reconstructed retina a new outer plexiform-like layer is visible at the interface of the transplanted ONL and the host INL. Ribbon synapses are evident within this OPL. These synapses are characteristic of those formed by rod photoreceptors, displaying an electron-dense ribbon surrounded by a cluster of vesicles. Ribbon synapses are found only rarely in control light-damaged retina. These results suggest that synaptic connections between transplanted photoreceptors and host cells are made, indicating that the light-dependent activation we have reported may be, at least in part, be synaptically mediated.

A major problem with photoreceptor and retinal transplants in general has been the formation of rosettes and the incomplete formation and organization of photoreceptor inner and outer segments. However, we have recently found that if portions of the inner retina are transplanted along with the intact sheet of photoreceptors, apparently normal expression of inner and outer segments occurs. When this tissue is transplanted using our methods to maintain the polarity and organization of the tissue, normal apposition of the outer segments to the retinal pigment epithelium is achieved and rosette formation is eliminated.

With indications that neural activity is generated in the central nervous system by the photoreceptor transplant and the reconstructed retina, the question arises as to whether this activity can be processed properly by the central nervous system to produce an appropriate behavioral response to the sensory stimuli. We have found that retinas reconstructed with photoreceptor transplants show a comparatively normal pupillary reflex to light, whereas the fellow dystrophic eye shows only a minimal reflex that is aberrant in form. This finding demonstrates for the first time that neural transplantation can reconstruct the host's own sensory end organ - in this case the retina - to restore an appropriate behavioral response (i.e., the pupillary reflex) to sensory stimuli.

Our findings show that developing as well as mature photoreceptors, including mature human photoreceptors, can be transplanted to form a new ONL with mature, damaged retina. The reconstructed retina is able to activate the central visual pathway in a light-dependent manner which in turn is processed appropriately to produce a normal behavioral response. To further extend the utility of this work, adaptation of the photoreceptor transplantation technique to the primate eye is currently being pursued.

V. ACKNOWLEDGMENTS

The authors wish to thank C. Barnstable for gifts of antibody and J. Lett for excellent technical assistance. Supported by NIH grant 1 R01 EY-07547 and grants from the National Retinitis Pigmentosa Foundation Fighting Blindness, Inc. and Retinitis Pigmentosa International.

REFERENCES

1. Gartner, S. and Henkind, P., Aging and degeneration of the humna macula. 1. Outer nuclear layer and photoreceptors, *Brit. J. Ophthalmol.*, 65, 23, 1981.
2. Flannery, J.G., Farber, D.B., Bird, A.C., and Bok, D., Degenerative changes in a retina affected with autosomal dominant retinitis pigmentosa, *Invest. Ophthalmol. Vis. Sci.*, 30, 19, 1989.
3. Sarks, S.H. and Sarks, J.P., Age-related macular degeneration: atrophic form, in *Retina,* Ryan, S., Ed., C.V. Mosby, St. Louis, 1989.
4. Silverman, M.S. and Hughes, S.E., Transplantation of retinal photoreceptors to light-damaged retina. *Invest. Ophthalmol. Vis. Sci.* (Suppl.), 28, 288, 1987.
5. Silverman, M.S. and Hughes, S.E., Transplantaiion of photoreceptors to light-damaged retina. *Invest. Ophthalmol. Vis. Sci.* 30, 1684, 1989.
6. Silverman, M.S. and Hughes, S.E., Photoreceptor transplantation in inherited and environmentally induced retinal degeneration: anatomy, immunohistochemistry and function, in *Inherited and Environmentally Induced Retinal Degenerations*, LaVail, M.M., Ed., Alan R. Liss, Inc., New York, 1989, 687.
7. Royo, P.E. and Quay, W.B., Retinal transplantation from fetal to maternal mammalian eye, *Growth* , 23, 313, 1959.
8. del Cerro, M., Gash, D.M., Rao, G.N., Notter, M.F., Wiegand, S.J., and Gupta, M., Intraocular retinal transplants, *Invest. Ophthalmol. Vis. Sci.,* 26, 1182, 1985.
9. del Cerro, M., Notter, M.F., Weigand, S.J., Jiang, L.Q., and del Cerro, C., Intraretinal transplantation of fluorescently labeled retinal cell suspensions, *Neurosci. Lett.*, 92, 21, 1988.
10. Turner, J.E. and Blair, J.R., Newborn rat retinal cells transplanted into retinal lesion site in adult host eyes, *Dev. Brain Res.*, 26, 91, 1986.
11. Blair, J.R., and Turner, J.E., Optimum conditions for successful transplantation of immature rat retina to the lesioned adult retina, *Dev. Brain Res.*, 36, 257, 1987.
12. Aramant, R., Seiler, M., and Turner, J.T., Donor age influences on the success of retinal transplants to adult rat retina, *Invest. Ophthalmol. Vis. Sci.*, 29, 498, 1988.
13. Lolley, R.N., Lee, R.H., Chase, D.G., and Racz, E., Rod photoreceptor cells dissociated from mature mice retinas, *Invest. Ophthalmol. Vis. Sci.*, 27, 285, 1986.
14. Hirsh, J. and Hylton, R., Quality of the primate photoreceptor lattice and limits of spatial vision, *Vision Res.*, 24, 347, 1984.
15. Wilson, H.R., Levi, D., Maffei, L., Rovamo, J., and DeValois, R., The perception of form: retina to striate cortex, in *Visual perception: The neurophysiological foundations*, Spillmann, L. and Werner, J. S., Eds., Academic Press, Inc., San Diego, 1990, 231.
16. Silverman, M.S. and Hughes, S.E., Transplantation of retinal photoreceptors to light-damaged retina: survival and integration of receptors from a range of postnatal ages. *Soc. Neurosci. Abstr.* 13, 1301, 1987.
17. Gouras, P., Du, J., Gelanze, M., Lopex, R., Kwun, R., Kjeldbye, H. and Kauffmann, D., Survival and synapse formation of transplanted rat rods, *Invest. Ophthalmol. Vis. Sci.* (Suppl.), 31, 595, 1990.
18. Lazar, E. and del Cerro, M., A new procedure for retinal transplantation, *Invest. Ophthalmol. Vis. Sci.* (Suppl.), 31, 593, 1990.

19. Hughes, S.E. and Silverman, M.S., Transplantation of retinal photoreceptors to dystrophic retina, *Soc. Neurosci. Abstr.* 14, 1277, 1988.

20. Liu, Y., Silverman, M.S., and Hughes, S.E., Photoreceptor inner and outer segments in transplanted retina, *Soc. Neurosci. Abstr.* 16, 405, 1990.

21. Silverman, M.S. and Hughes, S.E., Transplantation of human photoreceptors to light-damaged retina. *Soc. Neurosci. Abstr.* 14, 1278, 1988.

22. Das, G.D., Neural transplantation in mammalian brain, in *Neural Tissue Transplantation Research,* Wallace, R.B. and Das, G.D., Eds., Springer-Verlag, New York, 1983, 1.

23. Eisenfeld, A.J., LaVail, M.M., and LaVail, J.H., Assessment of possible transneuronal changes in the retina of rats with inherited retinal dystrophy: cell size, number of synapses, and axonal transport by retinal ganglion cells, *J. Comp. Neurol.,* 223, 22, 1984.

24. Hughes, S.E., Valentino, T.L., and Silverman, M.S., Transplanted photoreceptors form synapses in light-damaged retina, *Invest. Ophthalmol. Vis. Sci. (Suppl.),* 31, 594, 1990.

25. Valentino T.L., Hughes S.E., and Silverman M.S., Transplanted photoreceptors form synapses in reconstructed RCS rat retina, *Soc. Neurosci. Abstr.,* 16, 405, 1990.

26. Seiler, M, Aramant, R., and Ehinger, B., Transplantation of embryonic retina to adult retina in rabbit, *Exp. Eye Res.,* 51, 225, 1990.

27. Pu, G.A. and Masland, R.H., Biochemical interruption of membrane phospholipid renewal in retinal photoreceptor cells, *J. Neurosci.,* 4, 1559, 1984.

28. Anderson, D.H., Guerin, C.J., Erickson, P.A., Stern, W.H., and Fisher, S.K., Morphological recovery in the reattached retina, *Invest. Ophthalmol. Vis. Sci.,* 27, 168, 1986.

29. Guerin, C.J., Anderson, D.H., Fariss, R.N., and Fisher, S.K., Morphological recovery in the reattached retina, *Invest. Ophthalmol. Vis. Sci.,* 30, 1708, 1989.

30. Silverman, M.S. and Hughes, S.E., Light dependent activation of light-damaged retina by transplanted photoreceptors, *Invest. Ophthalmol. Vis. Sci. (Suppl.),* 30, 208, 1989c.

31. Bjorklund, A. and Stenevi, U., *Neural Grafting in the Mammalian CNS,* Elsevier, Amsterdam, 1985.

32. Klassen, H. and Lund, R.D., Retinal transplants can drive a pupillary reflex in host rat brains, *Proc. Natl. Acad. Sci. USA,* 84, 6958, 1987.

33. Klassen, H. and Lund, R.D., Anatomical and behavioral correlates of a xenograft-mediated pupillary reflex, *Exp. Neurol.,* 102, 102, 1988.

34. Lowenstein, O. and Loewenfeld, I.E., Effect of various light stimuli, in *The Eye,* Davson, H. P., Ed., Academic Press, New York, 1969, 274.

35. Levatin, P., Pupillary escape in disease of the retina or optic nerve, *Arch. Ophthalmol.,* 62, 768, 1959.

36. Trejo, L.J. and Cicerone, C.M., Retinal sensitivity measured by the pupillary light reflex in RCS and albino rats, *Vision Res.,* 22, 1163, 1982.

37. Slooter, J. and van Noren, D., Visual acuity measured with pupil responses to checkerboard stimuli, *Invest. Ophthalmol. Vis. Sci.,* 19, 105, 1980.

38. Barbur, J.L. and Forsyth, P.M., Can the pupil response be used as a measure of the visual input associated with the geniculo-striate pathway?, *Clin. Vision Sci.,* 1, 107, 1986.

39. Barbur J.L., Thompson W.D., Pupil response as an objective measure of visual acuity, *Ophthalmol. Physiol. Opt.,* 7, 425, 1987.

40. Silverman, M.S., Kaplan, H.J., Valentino, T.L., and Lee, C.M., Transplantation of human and non-human primate photoreceptors to damaged primate retina, *Invest. Ophthalmol. Vis. Sci. (Suppl.),* 31, 594, 1990.

RPE TRANSPLANTS IN ANIMAL MODELS OF INHERITED RETINAL DYSTROPHY AND AGING

Sheedlo, H.J., Gaur, V., Li, L., Seaton, T.D., Stovall, S., Yamaguchi, K. and Turner, J.E.

Departments of Neurobiology and Anatomy and Ophthalmology, Bowman Gray School of Medicine, Winston-Salem, NC

I. INTRODUCTION

The Royal College of Surgeons (RCS) dystrophic rat has proven an excellent model system to investigate photoreceptor cell (PRC) degeneration. In retinas of these rats, PRCs begin to degenerate in postnatal week three.[1,2,3] Although the cause of PRC degeneration is not known, retinal pigment epithelial (RPE) cells have been implicated due to their defective phagocytosis of shed rod outer segments.[4,5] Over the past three years, two laboratories have reported successful arresting of PRC degeneration by transplantation of normal healthy RPE cells into dystrophic retinas.[6,7] In some of these studies, cessation of PRC loss was demonstrated for as long as 6 months in RPE-transplanted dystrophic retinas.[8,9] Also, PRC survival was detected directly beneath and lateral to the RPE transplant.[10] This later observation suggested a trophic relationship between transplanted RPE cells and PRCs. In fact, a large body of evidence is now accumulating which demonstrates the existence of RPE cell trophic factors and their effects on PRC survival and development.[11]

Rescued PRCs in RPE-transplanted retinas of RCS dystrophic rats express the photopigment opsin, as shown by immunocytochemistry. Also, the membrane-bound enzyme sodium ion, potassium ion stimulated-adenosine triphosphatase was detected along inner segments of rescued PRCs beneath RPE-cell transplants in dystrophic retinas.[12] Interestingly, dense immunostain for this enzyme was also detected in thinning retinas of one-year-old RCS dystrophic rats.[13] To further characterize the functional status of the rescued PRCs, it would be important to measure mRNA levels for opsin in these transplanted dystrophic retinas. Measurements of opsin mRNA levels have been used to demonstrate the intact nature of PRCs.

Pathological changes involving vessels of the retina are either the primary manifestation of, or a coexisting component in many of the most devastating sight compromising and blinding diseases known. In proliferative diabetic retinopathy, the leading cause of adult onset blindness, abnormal growth of new vessels from the retinal vasculature into the vitreous cavity and subsequent hemorrhage is a primary mechanism of visual dysfunction. In age-related macular degeneration, the major cause of blindness in the elderly, new vessel growth from the choroidal blood supply into the subretinal space and hemorrhage may lead to sensory retinal detachment and loss of sight.[14] Examples like these make apparent the need for a better understanding of the mechanisms and relationships of retinal vasculature abnormalities. In RCS dystrophic rats, there is a decline in the retinal vessel density with loss of normal structure of the deep bed beginning at about three months, with accompanying neovascularization of the RPE cells. With the development of the RPE cell transplantation technique, with concomitant PRC rescue, the possibility exists that these transplants may protect the retinal vessels.

Age-related retinal degeneration occurs naturally in human as well as animal eyes.[15,16,17] The RPE is involved in this effect due to the gradual failure of cell function resulting from stress caused by the high cellular activity and its exposure to toxic factors.[18,19] This gradual loss of RPE function may be a principal cause of some human degenerative macular and peripheral retinal diseases, especially the senile forms. Although several studies have shown that RPE-cell transplantation arrested PRC loss in retinas of RCS dystrophic rats, it is also possible that RPE transplants may delay the degenerative aging process in normal, non-diseased retinas. To test this concept, young, healthy RPE cells could be transplanted into aging eyes, to determine what, if any, effect these transplanted cells have on the host PRCs during the aging process. The appropriate model to utilize in this study would be Fischer-344 rats, which undergo dramatic degenerative ocular changes with aging.[20]

In this paper we will show that transplants of young RPE cells were essential to affect maximum PRC rescue in retinas of RCS dystrophic rats and rescued PRCs expressed message for the photopigment opsin. Also, RPE transplants prevented the formation of abnormal retinal vessels in RCS dystrophic rats. Furthermore, RPE cell transplants delayed PRC loss in a rat retinal aging model.

II. MATERIALS AND METHODS

A.   ANIMALS

The source of RPE cells were 6-9 day-old Long Evans, RCS normal congenic (RCS-rdy$^+$p$^+$) and dystrophic (RCS-rdy$^-$), non-pigmented Sprague-Dawley and adult Long Evans rats. The RPE cell transplanted and sham-control rats were tan-hooded RCS dystrophic or Fischer-344 rats. Age-matched Sprague-Dawley rats served as controls in the RPE optimal conditions and retinal vessel study.

Tan-hooded RCS dystrophic rats were transplanted at 17 and 26 days in the RPE optimal conditions study. RCS dystrophic rats were transplanted with normal RPE cells at 17-19 days for the opsin mRNA study, while in the retinal vessel investigation, these rats were transplanted at 26 days. Three-month old albino male Fischer-344 rats were used as hosts in the retinal aging study.

B.   RPE CELL ISOLATION

RPE cells were isolated from 6-9 day-old pigmented Long Evans and RCS congenic control and non-pigmented Sprague-Dawley rats according to a previously described procedure.[21,22] Briefly, whole eyes were treated with collagenase/hyaluronidase (#1) for 40-60 minutes, then trypsin (#2) for 50 minutes, all at 37°C. The sclera/choroid was then carefully peeled away, leaving the RPE attached to the retina. After incubation in growth medium (MEM/F12 + 20% fetal calf serum + gentamicin + kanamycin), the RPE detached from the retina as a sheet. The RPE sheets were incubated with trypsin, then dissociated into a single cell suspension. The cells were concentrated by centrifugation to 30,000-120,000 cells/μl for transplantation. The isolation of RPE cells from adult eyes was accomplished by the whole-eye technique or an eye-cup method. The incubation times were increased when using the whole-eye method to 150 minutes for solution #1 and 120 minutes for solution #2. In the eye-cup method, the cornea, lens and vitreous were removed, then the neuroretina was carefully peeled away, leaving the RPE attached to Bruch's membrane. The eye-cup was incubated in trypsin for 30 minutes at 37°C, then RPE cells were brushed from the membrane, collected and concentrated to 60,000 cells/μl. All cells were suspended in calcium ion, magnesium ion-free Hanks' balanced salt solution (CMF-HBSS), which was also injected for the sham controls.

C.   TRANSPLANTATION

A previously published technique was used for transplantation of RPE cells and vehicle injections into the subretinal space of young rats.[6,12,22] Briefly, after exposing the dorsal eye surface and excising the superior rectus muscle, a small incision (<1mm) was made between the two vorticose veins. In the Fischer-344 rat study, an incision was made close to the limbus in order to target the subretinal space in the peripheral retina. At the lateral edge of the incision, 1 or 4μl of RPE cell suspension was injected with a 32 gauge needle attached to a 10μl Hamilton syringe. For sham controls, 1, 4 or 10μl of CMF-HBSS was similarly injected.

D.   MICROSCOPIC ANALYSIS

For light microscopy, eyes of RPE-transplanted, sham-control and non-treated control rats were immersion fixed with Bouin's fixative for 5 hours. After trimming the eye to include the area of interest, the eyes were embedded in paraffin. The paraffin-embedded eyes were sectioned at 8μm, then stained with hematoxylin-eosin (H&E).

E.   RNA EXTRACTION AND NORTHERN BLOTTING

RPE-transplanted, non-treated and sham-control dystrophic rats were sacrificed with an overdose of sodium pentobarbital and the eyes were rapidly enucleated using RNase-free surgical instruments. Eyes were then shock frozen with liquid nitrogen and stored until use. Total RNA was isolated from frozen retinas by extraction in guanidium isothiocyanate.[23] Purified RNA was electrophoresed in a 1.1% agarose-formaldehyde gel and blotted onto a nytran nylon membrane. The blots were hybridized with a 1.64 kilobase bovine cDNA probe.[24]

F.   RETINAL VESSEL PREPARATION

A previously described staining method for blood vessels in flat preparations of ocular tissues was used in this study.[25] Rats, RPE-transplanted and controls, were injected with horseradish peroxidase (HRP), 500 mg/kg body weight, through the saphenous or tail vein while under anaesthesia. Fifteen minutes later, the rats were sacrificed with an overdose of sodium pentobarbital and the eyes were enucleated, then fixed in 2.5% glutaraldehyde for 2 hours. During fixation, the retina was removed from choroid and the choroid from the sclera. After rinsing in buffer, the eye tissues were treated for 24 hours with 0.05% diaminobenzidine (DAB) in 0.05M

Tris-HCl, pH 7.6. The following day, the tissue was incubated for 3 hours with 0.05% DAB + 0.05% hydrogen peroxide. Then the tissue was immersed and preserved in 100% glycerol, flat mounted and coverslipped prior to analysis.

G.   MORPHOMETRIC ANALYSES

All measurements were made from H&E-stained paraffin sections using the Jandel Video Analysis (JAVA) system, except for the retinal vessel study which used flat mount preparations. For the RPE optimal conditions study, the central region of the RPE-cell transplant in dystrophic retinas and respective regions of sham and non-treated dystrophic and control Sprague-Dawley retinas were used to measure outer nuclear layer (ONL) thicknesses. In the retinal vessel study, blood vessel length and density were measured from areas beneath and lateral to the RPE-cell transplant and in respective areas of sham-injected dystrophic and Sprague-Dawley retinas. In the retinal aging study, measurements of the ONL, outer (OPL) and inner (IPL) plexiform layers and inner nuclear layer (INL) were made 250μm from the ora serrata, to include a 50μm distance. The Students t test was used in comparison of two groups, while analysis of variance (ANOVA) was used to compare more than two groups.

III. RESULTS

A.   RPE OPTIMAL CONDITIONS STUDY

Transplantation of healthy RPE cells isolated from early postnatal Long Evans (LE) and RCS normal congenic rats into the subretinal space of RCS dystrophic rats affected a similar PRC rescue response. No significant difference in ONL thickness was detected in these two transplantation groups up to one year after transplantation. Healthy RPE transplants were shown to rescue PRCs for at least one year after grafting. The gradual decline in ONL thickness seen between 6 months and one year coincided with the normal age-related loss of PRCs as seen in age-matched Sprague-Dawley rats. Also, dystrophic retinas transplanted with RPE cells from neonatal pigmented RCS dystrophic rats (DRPE) affected PRC survival for one month post-transplantation, although this rescue effect was decreased between postnatal day 60 (P60) and P120. However, the pigmented dystrophic RPE cells appeared to survive for up to 4 months. Injection of 1μl of control vehicle into the subretinal space of RCS dystrophic rats caused a slight PRC rescue effect about one month after injection. However, by 4 months, the ONL thickness was significantly reduced and by 6 months, no PRCs were detected (Figure 1). Larger injection volumes (4 and 10μl) did not affect a greater increase in ONL thickness.

Comparison of PRC rescue in retinas of RCS dystrophic rats at different ages was performed to determine the critical period at which maximal rescue could be affected. Transplantation on day 17 affected PRC rescue to a greater degree than at day 26. However, transplantation at P38, P43 and P48 caused little, if any, PRC rescue. The reason for this latter result may be that PRC degeneration is greatly accelerated at P38 and later.

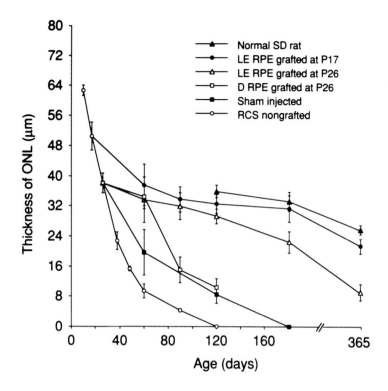

Figure 1. Outer Nuclear Layer (ONL) Thickness of RPE-Transplanted, Sham-Control and Non-Treated Retinas of RCS Dystrophic Rats.

Also, the age of the transplanted RPE cells was an important factor in PRC rescue. The ONL thickness in retinas of RCS dystrophic rats transplanted at P17 and P26 with early postnatal Long Evans RPE was significantly greater that those retinas transplanted with adult RPE cells, when examined at 2 and 4 months.

Furthermore, the number of rescued PRCs appeared to be dependent on the concentration of transplanted RPE cells. The PRC rescue response was maximized when 60,000-120,000 cells/μl were transplanted, while transplantation of 30,000 cells/μl caused a significantly diminished PRC rescue response.

B.   OPSIN mRNA STUDY

RNA preparations were analyzed by Northern blotting of transplanted retinas at P32 and P109, which corresponded to about 15 and 90 days post-transplantation. RNA preparations from retinas of Long Evans rats at P17 and P77, non-treated retinas of RCS dystrophic rats at P18 and P105 and sham-injected dystrophic retinas at P105 were used as controls. Rat retinal opsin mRNA was detected in four transcripts, 2, 2.8, 3.7 and 5.5 kilobases. Opsin mRNA levels of retinas of Long Evans rats were unchanged between P17 and P77. In contrast, retinas of RCS dystrophic rats showed a progressive decrease in opsin mRNA and, by P105, the message was not detected. However, the RPE-transplanted dystrophic retinas showed high levels of opsin mRNA as late as 3 months post-transplantation, although opsin mRNA was not detected in sham-injected dystrophic retinas at P90.

C.   RETINAL VESSEL STUDY

The deep vessel beds of RPE-cell transplanted (at P26) retinas of 4 month-old RCS dystrophic rats were significantly denser (29.8 ± 1.1 mm/mm^2), than that measured in either the non-treated (18.6 ± 2.1) or sham control (22.7 ± 1.7) dystrophic retinas, although somewhat less dense than that seen in retinas of age-matched Sprague-Dawley rats (33.8 ± 2.4). Also, the numbers of neovascularization profiles in the mid-peripheral retina were significantly greater in the non-treated (9.1 ± 1.4/mm^2) and sham control (7.8 ± 0.7) dystrophic retinas, when compared to RPE-cell transplanted dystrophic retinas (0.65 ± 0.3). Neovascularization profiles were not seen in retinas of 4 month-old Sprague-Dawley rats.

D.   RETINAL AGING STUDY

The numbers of cells in both the ONL and INL were significantly greater in RPE-transplanted retinas of Fischer-344 rats when transplanted at 3 months, as contrasted to both non-treated and sham-control retinas of these rats, from 3 to 9 months post-transplantation. Also, no difference was apparent when contrasting the effects of pigmented or non-pigmented transplanted RPE cells. However, during the 9-month post-transplantation period, a general decrease in cell number in both layers was observed in the transplanted and control groups. Most importantly, the transplantation of young RPE cells into eyes of 3 month-old Fischer-344 rats delayed the onset of age-related retinal cell loss by 3 months (Figure 2).

The thickness of the OPL and IPL of RPE-cell transplanted retinas of Fischer-344 rats were significantly greater than in control retinas during the 9-month post-transplantation period. The OPL thickness of the transplanted retinas was stabilized 3 to 6 months after transplantation, while the thickness in the control groups decreased 3 months after transplantation, then stabilized. The IPL thickness in transplanted retinas remained somewhat stable over the 9 month post-transplantation period, while in control retinas, a steady decrease in thickness was observed.

IV. DISCUSSION

This study clearly showed that long-term PRC rescue in retinas of RCS dystrophic rats required healthy RPE transplants and the transplantation needed to be performed at early stages of the disease process. The short-term effect on PRC survival by transplantation of pigmented dystrophic RPE cells may have resulted from a combination of pigmentation in the transplanted RPE cells and the effect of surgery and injection. An earlier report showed that eye pigmentation could slow the PRC degeneration in RCS rats, when compared to pink-eyed RCS rats, by about 10 days in the posterior retina and 30-35 days in the far peripheral retina of the superior half of the eye.[26] The amount of pigmentation in the transplanted RPE cells does not appear to be responsible for long-term PRC rescue, because PRC loss was still observed in dystrophic RPE-transplanted retinas even though many melanosomecontaining transplanted dystrophic RPE cells remained attached to Bruch's membrane. In contrast, retinas transplanted with RCS congenic and Long Evans RPE cells maintained a stable PRC layer 3 months post-transplantation.

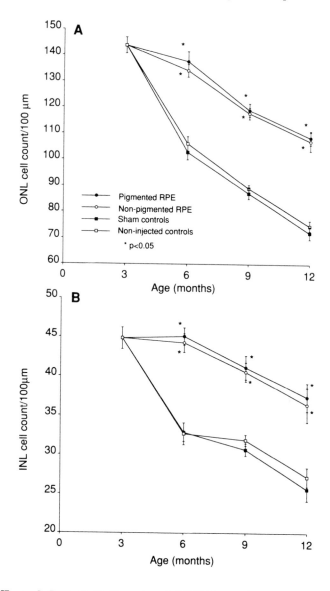

Figure 2. ONL and INL Cell Counts of RPE-Transplanted and Sham-Control Retinas of Fischer-344 Rats.

Injection of increased volumes (4 and 10µl) of vehicle had no beneficial rescue effect on PRCs beyond the area of the needle track. In turn, this sham effect was not only transient but incomplete since intact outer segments were not seen during the short 1-2 month cell body survival period. The reasons for the short-term PRC rescue effect caused by vehicle injection remain to be determined. It is possible that the debris material was washed away,[27] thus removing a barrier for normal metabolic exchange.[28] Also, trauma resulting from the incision may cause a release of factors which affect transient PRC survival.[29] In addition, macrophage proliferation within the subretinal space may, in part, be involved in this process.[30] It should be noted that every effort was made to minimize trauma to the retina during the transplantation procedure, thus we observed few macrophage-like cells in retinas transplanted with RPE cells, even when isolated from Long Evans rats, or in sham-injected retinas. Therefore, cross-strain RPE cells can also be used effectively in retinal transplantation without an adverse immune response or RPE rejection.

The ONL thickness decrease seen in both non-diseased and RPE-transplanted dystrophic retinas from 6 to 12 months may be due to the normal aging process. An earlier study has shown that retinas of 6 month-old Sprague-Dawley rats had normal retinal characteristics, but a decrease in retinal thickness, especially in the ONL, occurred at later time periods, which was attributed to age-related cell death.[31]

The greater and long-lasting effects of transplanted early-postnatal RPE, when compared to adult RPE, may have resulted from the higher proliferative activity of younger RPE cells. For example, the number of binuclear tetraploid RPE cells peaked in the first 15 days after birth, but stabilized at about the fifth month.[32] This may explain, in part, the moderate PRC rescue found when adult RPE cells were transplanted into dystrophic retinas, as seen in this study and in another laboratory.[7]

Normal levels of opsin mRNA were detected in retinas of 17 day-old Long Evans and RCS dystrophic rats. Although, following the onset of retinal degeneration in RCS rats, there was a progressive decline in the opsin mRNA levels. However, RPE transplantation in dystrophic retinas affected photoreceptor cell survival as late as 3 months post-transplantation, as opsin mRNA was detected in these retinas. In the sham-injected retinas, opsin mRNA was detected above levels in non-treated retinas; however, these retinas exhibited a continuous decline of opsin mRNA and, by P90, no message was detected. This data further corroborate our morphometric observations concerning the transient and incomplete nature of the vehicle injection effects when contrasted to the long-lasting and robust rescue caused by RPE cell transplants.

For the first time, transplants of RPE cells in retinas of RCS dystrophic rats have been shown to prevent the normal decrease in the density of the deep bed of the retinal vasculature. The normal vascular architecture was also spared and neovascularization, which normally develops in these dystrophic retinas, was inhibited. Injection of vehicle into dystrophic retinas (sham controls) caused no protective effects relating to vascular bed integrity or neovascularization profiles. These results suggest that the RCS dystrophic rats may serve as a model for the study of the relationship between the RPE and retinal vasculature.

The fact that the ONL and INL cell counts were similar in both the non-pigmented and pigmented RPE-transplanted retinas of Fischer-344 rats would suggest that the sparse light-shielding pigment of the RPE cells transplants does not play a major role in protecting the peripheral retina from degeneration. However, in pigmented RPE, melanosomes appear to offer some protection by delaying or reducing the phenomenon, although age-related changes are eventually measurable.[33,34]   Based on these results, the delay of retinal degeneration in the Fischer-344 rat may be related to the age differences between the donor and host RPE cells, which may indicate a decreased capacity of the aging host RPE to support photoreceptor cells.   The aging study reveals for the first time that the degenerative process in the aging peripheral retina of Fischer-344 rats can be successfully delayed by the transplant of healthy young RPE cells.   These results suggest that RPE cells are in some way directly involved in the retinal aging process and the Fischer-344 rat model may be an excellent model for testing this hypothesis.

V. REFERENCES

1.   Bourne, M.C., Campbell, D.A. and Tansley, K., Hereditary degeneration of the rat, Br. J. Ophthalmol., 22, 613, 1938.
2.   Dowling, J.E. and Sidman, R.L., Inherited retinal dystrophy in the rat, J. Cell Biol., 14, 73, 1962.
3.   LaVail, M.M., Analysis of neurological mutants with inherited retinal degeneration, Invest. Ophthalmol. Vis. Sci., 21, 638, 1981.
4.   Bok, D. and Hall, M.O., The role of pigment epithelium in the etiology of inherited retinal dystrophy in the rat, J. Cell Biol., 49, 664, 1971.
5.   Chaitin, M.H. and Hall, M.O., Defective ingestion of rod outer segments by cultured dystrophic rat pigment epithelial cells, Invest. Ophthalmol. Vis. Sci., 24, 812, 1983.
6.   Li, L. and Turner, J.E., Inherited retinal dystrophy in the RCS rat: Prevention of photoreceptor degeneration by pigment epithelial cell transplantation, Exp. Eye Res. 47, 911, 1988.
7.   Lopez, R., Gouras, P., Kjeldbye, H., Sullivan, B., Reppucci, V., Brittis, M., Wapner, F. and Goluboff, E., Transplanted retinal pigment epithelium modifies the retinal degeneration in the RCS rat, Invest. Ophthalmol. Vis. Sci., 30, 586, 1989.
8.   Blair, J.R., Gaur, V., Laedtke, T.W., Li, L., Liu, H., Sheedlo, H.J., Yamaguchi, K., Yamaguchi, K. and Turner, J.E., In oculo transplantation studies involving the neural retina and its pigment epithelium, Prog. Retinal Res., in press.
9.   Li, L., Sheedlo, H.J. and Turner, J.E., Long-term rescue of photoreceptor cells in the retinas of RCS dystrophic rats by RPE cell transplants, Prog. Brain Res., 82, 179, 1990.
10.   Sheedlo, H.J., Li, L. and Turner, J.E., Photoreceptor cell rescue at early and late RPE-transplantation periods during retinal disease in RCS dystrophic rats, J. Neural Transplant., in press.
11.   Spoerri, P.E., Ulshafer, R.J., Ludwig, H.C., Allen, C.B. and Kelley, K.C., Photoreceptor cell development in vitro: Influence of pigment epithelium conditioned medium on outer segment differentiation, Eur. J. Cell Biol., 46, 362, 1988.
12.   Sheedlo, H.J., Li, L. and Turner, J.E., Functional and structural characteristics of photoreceptor cells rescued in RPE-grafted retinas of RCS dystrophic rats, Exp. Eye Res., 48, 841, 1989.

13. Sheedlo, H.J., Li, L. and Turner, J.E., (Na$^+$ + K$^+$)-ATPase and opsin in retinas of RCS dystrophic rats: Time course study, Curr. Eye Res., 8, 741, 1989.

14. Matthews, M.T. and Bok, D., Blood vascular abnormalities in animals with inherited retinal degeneration, in Retinal Degeneration: Experimental Clinical Studies, LaVail, M.M., Hollyfield, J.G. and Anderson, R.E., Eds., Alan R. Liss, Inc., New York, 1985, 209.

15. Gartner, S. and Kenkind, P., Aging and degeneration of the human macula, Br. J. Ophthalmol., 65, 23, 1981.

16. Marshall, J., Grindle, J., Ansell, P.L. and Borwein, B., Convolution in human rods: An ageing process. Br. J. Ophthalmol., 63, 181, 1979.

17. Lai, Y.L., Jacoby, O. and Jonas, A.M., Age-related and light-associated retinal changes in Fischer rats, Invest. Ophthalmol. Vis. Sci., 17, 634, 1978.

18. Dorey, C.K., Wu, G., Ebenstein, D., Garsd, A. and Weiter, J.J., Cell loss in the aging retina: Relationship to lipofuscin accumulation and macular degeneration, Invest. Ophthalmol. Vis. Sci., 30, 1691, 1989.

19. Hogan, M.J., Role of retinal pigment epithelium in macular disease, Trans. Amer. Acad. Ophthalmol. Otolaryngol., 76, 64, 1972.

20. Shinowara, N.L., London, E.D. and Rapoport, S.I., Changes in retinal morphology and glucose utilization in aging albino rats, Exp. Eye Res., 34, 517, 1982.

21. Mayerson, P.L., Hall, M.O., Clark, V. and Abrams, T., An improved method of isolation and culture of rat retinal pigment epithelial cells, Invest. Ophthalmol. Vis. Sci., 26, 1599, 1985.

22. Li, L., and Turner, J.E., Transplantation of retinal pigment epithelial cells to mature and adult rat hosts: Short and long term survival characteristics, Exp. Eye Res., 47, 771, 1988.

23. Chirgwin, J.M., Przybyla, A.E., MacDonald, R.J. and Rutter, W.J., Isolation of biologically active ribonucleic acid from sources enriched in ribonuclease, Biochem., 18, 5294, 1979.

24. Nathans, J. and Hogness, D.S., Isolation, sequence analysis and intron-exon arrangement of the gene encoding bovine rhodopsin, Cell, 34, 807, 1983.

25. Raviola, P. and Freddo, T.F., A simple staining method for blood vessels in flat preparations of ocular tissues, Invest. Ophthalmol. Vis. Sci., 19, 1518, 1980.

26. LaVail, M.M. and Battelle, B., Influence of eye pigmentation and light deprivation on inherited retinal dystrophy in the rat, Exp. Eye. Res., 21, 167, 1975.

27. Silverman, M.S. and Hughes, S.E., Photoreceptor rescue in the RCS rat without pigment epithelium transplantation, Curr. Eye Res., 9, 183, 1990.

28. El-Hafnawi, E., Pathomorphology of the retina and its vasculature in hereditary retinal dystrophy in RCS rats, in Research in Retinitis Pigmentosa, E. Zrenner, H. Krastel and H.H. Goebel, Eds., Pergamon Journals, Ltd., London, 1987, 417.

29. Faktorovich, E.G., Steinberg, R.H., Yasumura, D., Matthes, M.T. and LaVail, M.M., Photoreceptor degeneration in inherited retinal dystrophy delayed by basic fibroblast growth factor, Nature, 347, 83, 1990.

30. Kwun, R., Du, J., Gelanze, M., Lopez, R., Kjeldbye, H. and Gouras, P., Subretinal saline injection, macrophage invasion and prolonged photoreceptor survival in the RCS rat, Invest. Ophthalmol. Vis. Sci., 31(abst), 595, 1990.

31. Cano, J., Machado, A. and Reinoso-Suayez, J., Morphological changes in the retina of ageing rats, Arch. Gerontol. Geriatr., 5, 41, 1986.

32. Stroeva, O.G. and Mitashov, V.I., Retinal pigment epithelium: Proliferation and differentiation during development and regeneration, Internat. Rev. Cytol., 83, 221, 1983.

33. Katz, M.L. and Robison, W.G., Age-related changes in the retinal pigment epithelium of pigment rats, Exp. Eye Res., 38, 137, 1984.

34. Katz, M.L., Drea, C.M., Eldred, G.E., Hess, H.H. and Robison, W.G., Influence of early photoreceptor degeneration of lipofuscin in the retinal pigment epithelium, Exp. Eye Res., 43, 561, 1986.

TRANSPLANTATION OF RETINAL PIGMENTED EPITHELIAL CELLS ON BRUCH'S MEMBRANE IN THE RABBIT

KATSUHIRO YAMAGUCHI,[1,2] KEIKO YAMAGUCHI,[1,2]
RICHARD W. YOUNG,[1,3] VINOD P. GAUR,[1] JAMES E. TURNER[1,2]
DEPARTMENTS OF [1]NEUROBIOLOGY AND ANATOMY,
[2]OPHTHALMOLOGY, AND [3]COMPARATIVE MEDICINE,
BOWMAN GRAY SCHOOL OF MEDICINE,
WAKE FOREST UNIVERSITY, WINSTON-SALEM, NORTH CAROLINA, USA

I. INTRODUCTION

Retinal pigmented epithelial (RPE) cell transplantation has been proposed as a possible treatment of human inherited retinal eye disease.[1,2] Studies have demonstrated photoreceptor cell rescue by transplanting healthy RPE cells into the Royal College of Surgeons rat, a model of inherited retinal dystrophy due to RPE dysfunction.[1,3] This was the first indication that RPE cell transplantation could halt photoreceptor cell degeneration. The ramifications of this finding in human retinal disease showed the need for a surgical technique of RPE cell transplantation that would be applicable to the human eye. Many interesting papers have been written on the subject of retinal pigmented epithelial (RPE) cell transplantation over the past few years.[1,2,4,5] These techniques for delivering of donor RPE cells to the subretinal space of host retinas have fallen short of a direct application to the human patient because postoperative complications such as retinal detachment, proliferative vitreoretinopathy, and hemorrhage have not been addressed. With this in mind, we felt the need to devise a complete vitreoretinal surgical technique for the transplantation of donor RPE cells into the host subretinal space with an experimental duration sufficient to judge the nature of postoperative recovery.

A more comprehensive surgical technique described in this chapter utilizes vitrectomy, endocautery, and sulfur hexafluoride (SF_6) expanding gas in an effort to prevent hemorrhage, retinal detachment and proliferative vitreoretinopathy. Under these conditions, the postoperative inflammation is quite minimal using the technique as described later in the text. We have noted this benign postoperative condition for up to three weeks. We will present histological and ultrastructural evidence that our technique establishes a normal relationship between transplanted donor RPE cells and host photoreceptor cell outer segments, neighboring host RPE cells and Bruch's membrane. These findings represent a successful transplant which is viable for the three week duration of our study.

II. Materials and Methods

A. RPE ISOLATION AND LABELING

Pigmented adult rabbits were obtained as donors of RPE cells. The donor rabbits were euthanized by lethal injection of sodium pentobarbital, the eyes were enucleated and placed in Hank's balanced salt solution (HBSS) containing gentamicin and kanamycin. The anterior segment and vitreous were removed and placed into fresh HBSS with 0.25% trypsin and incubated at 37°C for 15 minutes. After incubation, the neural retina was removed and using gentle aspiration the RPE cells were aspirated off Bruch's membrane with a sterile pipette and suspended in minimal essential medium (MEM) with 20% rabbit serum to neutralize the trypsin and to prevent RPE cell clumping. The cells were then washed three times in calcium-magnesium free HBSS (CMF-HBSS). The cell suspension was then pelleted by centrifugation, placed in CMF-HBSS and briefly stored at 4°C until needed for transplantation.

Because RPE cells from pigmented rabbits were used for grafting, and the host rabbits were albino, it was easy to identify and distinguish the grafted cells from those of the host. However, to exclude the possibility that the pigmented RPE cells in the host subretinal space represented the host RPE cells which had phagocytized the transplanted RPE cells, we have used a cell labeling procedure. Pigmented RPE cells prior to transplantation were cultured in the presence of a 10mM solution of 5-bromodeoxyuridine (Brdu). The cells were light protected and allowed to proliferate for at least two cell divisions. On the day of the transplantation, the cells were lifted off the culture dishes using 0.01% trypsin solution, washed several times in CMF-HBSS and prepared as a cell suspension for injection into the subretinal space. After the transplantation, the retinal tissues were fixed in Karnovsky's fixative and embedded in paraffin. Sections 6-8 μm thick were cut and reacted with anti-Brdu monoclonal antibody. The pigmented cells showing nuclear labeling were identified as transplanted cells.

B. SURGICAL TECHNIQUE

Host animals were selected based on a lack of pigmentation, facilitating the observation of pigmented cells being transplanted onto a nonpigmented background. With this criteria in mind, male New Zealand white rabbits were used. These animals were anesthetized using intramuscular injections of tiletamine hydrochloride plus zolazepam hydrochloride (Telazol[R], A. H. Robins, Richmond, VA) and xylazine (Rompun[R], Harver, Shawnee, KS). Periorbital fur was clipped away and the entire area including the cornea and conjunctiva was prepared for surgery using a 1:50 dilution of providone-iodine solution and water as an antiseptic.

The surgery was conducted under sterile conditions in an animal surgery facility, using an operating microscope. The animal was placed on a heating pad in a lateral recumbent position beneath the operating microscope exposing the eye to view. After draping the field, a lateral canthotomy was done and a wire lid speculum was sutured in place. Traction sutures were placed around the superior and inferior rectus muscles and nictitating membrane. Following a peritomy, sclerotomies were performed at the superonasal, superotemporal and inferotemporal quadrants 1 mm posterior to the limbus. At the inferotemporal sclerotomy site, an infusion cannula was placed and sutured to the sclera. This cannula maintains intraocular pressure during the time when open sclerotomies are performed. A hand held 20-gauge fiberoptic light guide was placed into one sclerotomy which illuminated the intraocular structures during the procedure. In the other remaining sclerotomy, a hand held SITE[R] vitreous cutter was placed. Both instruments must be directed posteriorly to avoid touching the posterior of the lens, which would lead minimally to a postoperative cataract. A special contact lens designed for vitreoretinal procedures was placed on the cornea to facilitate the visualization of the ocular fundus. Using a bimanual technique, a nearly complete vitrectomy was performed, taking into account the very confined area bound by the conical posterior aspect of the lens and the fragile retina below.

Following the vitrectomy, the vitreous cutter was removed and a endocautery probe was introduced through the same scleral stoma. The probe was placed approximately two disc spaces superior to the optic disc and thermoenergy was applied to the retina to produce a retinal stoma. The infusion solution was then lowered relative to the eye to assist in detaching the retina surrounding the retinal hole. Gentle suction applied above the retinal stoma using the SITE[R] hand piece extended the zone of retinal detachment beyond the area produced by endocautery alone. Areas of bare Bruch's membrane were created by this procedure[5].

Brdu labeled RPE cells were then introduced through the retinotomy site and into the subretinal space using a 32-gauge, blunt-tipped microneedle attached to a 10 μl Hamilton glass syringe. Sufficient numbers of RPE cells were delivered, 40 to 50 μl, under the detached retina so the entire area of detachment was covered with pigmented cells. Any reflux of RPE cells coming from the retinal hole was removed with gentle suction from the vitrectomy instrument. Once the transplantation was completed, the infusion pressure was increased to a normal level. Both superior sclerotomies were closed with 8-0 nylon suture. The cannula was removed and the sclerotomy was closed as previously stated. Enough sulfur hexafluoride (100% SF_6) (Matheson, Cucamonga, Ca.) was injected into the vitreous cavity via the pars plana to restore normal intraocular pressure and apply mild tamponade to the detachment site.

The preceding technique was performed on the host eyes two weeks apart in order to obtain eyes at two data points, 1 week and 3 weeks, at the end of the study period. By providing lag time between surgeries, the postoperative eye has enough time to absorb the expanding gas before the next surgery is performed. This allowed the experimental animal to maintain vision throughout the study. The rabbits were observed daily for signs of inflammation. The rabbits were examined by indirect ophthalmoscopy, beginning four to five days postoperatively following the absorption of the expanding gas.

The host rabbits were given daily oral doses of cyclosporin A (Sandoz, Basel, Switzerland) at 10 mg/kg throughout the three week study. All animals were maintained in a 12-hour light/ dark cycle provided by cool-white fluorescent light. Host animals were killed with a lethal injection of sodium pentobarbital and the eyes were enucleated, processed and examined with light and transmission electron microscopy as well as immunostaining using anti-Brdu antibody. NIH guidelines were upheld with respect to treatment and euthanasia of all animals.

III RESULTS

During the first postoperative week, minor corneal edema and occasional aqueous flare were noted. Congestion of conjunctival and limbal vessels were the only prolonged finding. Because the expanding gas (SF_6) remained in the eye for four to five days after surgery, observation of the fundus was difficult. Once the gas was absorbed, the fundus could be examined by indirect ophthalmoscopy. A patchy black area beneath the reattached retina denoted the transplanted RPE cells as seen in Figure 1, which was three weeks following surgery. The photograph was taken following enucleation and removal of the anterior segment. Transplanted RPE cells appear as a dark mosaic pattern in the retina (arrow).

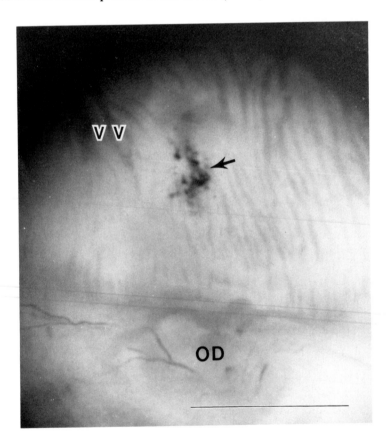

Figure 1. OD = optic disc, VV = vortex vein. (Bar = 1 mm)

In this study, sixteen of the twenty host eyes had normal gross appearing retinas at the time of tissue trimming and preparation. The four abnormal eyes had peripheral retinal tears near the infusion cannula which seems to have lead to permanent retinal detachments. Despite these peripheral detachments the transplanted sites in most cases appeared to be spared and therefore seems not to have contributed to the retinal detachments.

Histologic sections showed that the transplanted RPE cells formed a monolayer beneath the reattached retina. There was mild gliosis at the site of the retinal endocauterization and the retinal stoma was filled with glial cells. We observed no obvious rejection of the transplanted RPE cells. No inflammatory cells or macrophages were noted within the subretinal space or choroid. Pigment containing RPE cells were dispersed among the nonpigmented host RPE cells with the transplanted areas. Melanin pigment was located in the apical cytoplasmic regions of RPE cells which were also attached to Bruch's membrane as seen in Figure 2 under light microscopy. Note the pigment granules accumulated at the apical portion of the cells (arrow) seen on Bruch's membrane.

We have performed a labelling study to establish that the pigmented cells were in fact the transplanted RPE cells. The pigmented cells were labeled with 5-bromodeoxyuridine and confirmed to be the transplanted cells by fluorescence immunocytochemistry using the anti-Brdu antibody. The Brdu label was restricted to the nuclei of the pigmented cells.

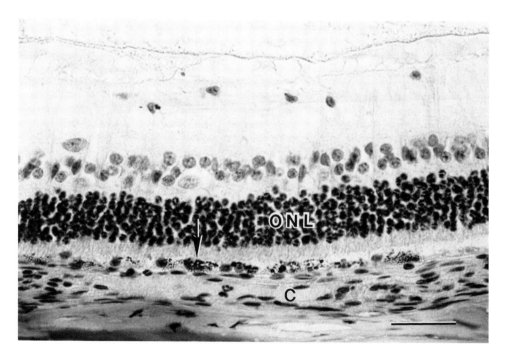

Figure 2 ONL= outer nuclear layer; C=choroid (Bar= 50 μm).

Electron microscopy further confirmed our observation that RPE cells with melanin granules were attached to Bruch's membrane. Three weeks after transplantation surgery, no significant histological changes were seen, Figure 3. The RPE cells, containing melanin pigment granules (arrowheads) primarily in the apical portion of the cell, were attached to Bruch's membrane (*). Note the relationship of the grafted RPE cell microvilli (Mv) to the host photoreceptor cell rod outer segment (OS) Also note the presence of junctional complexes (arrow) between the transplanted donor cell and the adjacent cell and basal infoldings (BI) on Bruch's membrane.

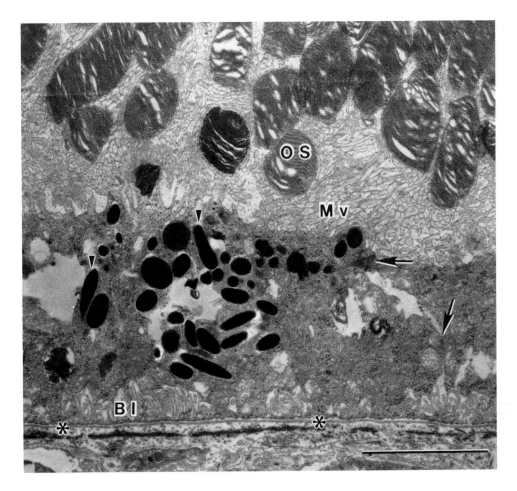

Figure 3 Mv= microvilli; OS= outer segment; BI= basal infoldings (Bar= 5 μm).

IV DISCUSSION

The hypothesis that the transplantation of retinal pigmented epithelial cells as a possible treatment for certain human eye disease has been proposed.[1,5] Members of our laboratory have recently demonstrated photoreceptor cell rescue in an animal model for inherited retinal dystrophy by transplantation of healthy RPE cells.[1,3] This was confirmed by others in a subsequent study.[6] For the retinitis pigmentosa disorders, there is no evidence that vision might be rescued by RPE cell transplantation because these disorders are considered to be both RPE and photoreceptor cell related[7] and little is known about their pathogenesis as well as the RPE cell role in retinal dystrophic disease. When considering the specialization of RPE cells in maintaining a healthy retinal tissue,[8-10] we anticipate that RPE cell transplantation may be a potential treatment for some retinal dystrophies and degenerations. Because of the increasing clinical evidence of RPE cell involvement, age-related macular degeneration of the senile type could potentially be included in this group of treatable diseases by RPE cell transplantation.[11] As the disease progresses, the patient's RPE cells and retina degenerate within the macular region producing loss of the central visual field. Degenerative changes in the RPE cells are primarily responsible for abnormal material accumulating beneath its basement membrane forming exudative drusen. Disciform lesions may result from alterations in Bruch's membrane and accumulations of debris between the retinal pigmented epithelium and the choroid. In addition, lipofuscin accumulations in the RPE cell of the aged and the retinitis pigmentosa patient has been recognized.[12,13] As they increase in number, these lipofuscin accumulations may lead to cell insufficiency and possible cell death. It is feasible that such a lesion could be treated by transplanting young, healthy RPE cells into the lesion sites.

In an earlier report, Gouras *et al* transplanted cultured human RPE cells onto Bruch's membrane of the owl monkey through an anterior open eye approach.[4] Later, a closed-eye method for transplantation of RPE cells was established by Lopez *et al* and Lane *et al* using the pars plana approach.[2,5] These were studies of short duration and used no methods for the prevention of postoperative complications such as retinal detachment and proliferative vitreoretinopathy. The present study has described a more complete vitreoretinal surgical technique for the transplantation of donor pigmented rabbit RPE cells into the subretinal space of host non-pigmented rabbits which optimizes surgical recovery and integrates donor RPE cells among host cells. We have demonstrated the presence of structures indicating the functionality of the transplanted cells; such as microvilli, relationships between RPE cells and photoreceptor cell outer segments, basal infoldings on Bruch's membrane and tight junctions with adjacent host cells. Use of the Brdu label procedure allowed a positive identification of the pigmented cells to be of donor origin. Although we were able to identify the transplanted cells in most instances, some unlabeled pigmented cells were also observed. We are currently in the process of determining the proportion of cells labeled by our *in vitro* Brdu incorporation procedure and evaluating the application of such a labeling procedure. Therefore, we present our comprehensive surgical technique as a basic approach for further studies.

VI. REFERENCES

1.   Li, L. and Turner, J.E., Inherited retinal dystrophy in the RCS rat: Prevention of photoreceptor degeneration by pigment epithelial cell transplantation, Exp. Eye Res., 47, 911, 1988.

2.   Lane, C., Boulton, M. and Marshall, J., Transplantation of retinal pigment epithelium using a pars plana approach, Eye, 3, 27, 1989.

3.   Sheedlo, H.J., Li, L. and Turner, J.E., Functional and structural characteristics of photoreceptor cells rescued in RPE-cell grafted retinas of RCS dystrophic rats, *Exp. Eye Res.*, 48, 841, 1989.

4.   Gouras, P., M.T. Flood, H. Kjeldbye, M.K. Bilek and Eggers, H., Transplantation of cultured human retinal epithelium to Brush's membrane of the owl monkey's eye, Current Eye Res., 4, 253, 1985.

5.   Lopez, R., P. Gouras, M. Brittis and Kjeldbye, H., Transplantation of cultured rabbit retinal epithelium to rabbit retina using a closed-eye method, Invest. Ophthalmol. Vis. Sci., 28, 1131 1987.

6.   Lopez, R., P. Gouras, H. Kjeldbye, B. Sullivan, V. Reppucci, M. Brittis, F. Wapner and Goluboff, E., Transplanted retinal pigment epithelium modifies the retinal degeneration in the RCS rat, Invest. Ophthalmol. Vis. Sci., 30, 586, 1989.

7.   Marshall, J. and Heckenlively, J.R., Pathologic findings and putative mechanisms in retinitis pigmentosa, in Retinitis Pigmentosa, Heckenlively, J.R., Ed., J.B. Lippincott Co., Philadelphia, 1988, 37.

8.   Young, R.W., Cell death during differentiation of the retina in the mouse, J. Comp. Neurol., 229, 362, 1984.

9.   Adler, R. Trophic interactions in retinal development and in retinal degenerations: in vivo and in vitro studies, in The Retina. A Modelfor Cell Biology Studies Part I, Adler, R., and Farber, D., Eds., Academic Press, Inc., Orlando, 1986, 111.

10.   Hewitt, A.T., Lindsey, J.D., Carbott, D., and Adler, R., Photoreceptor survival-promoting activity in interophotoreceptor matrix preparations: characterization and partial purification, Exp. Eye Res., 50, 79, 1990.

11.   Dorey, C.K., Wu, G., Ebenstein, D., Garsd, A., and Weiter, J.J., Cell loss in the aging retina. Relationship to lipofuscin accumulation and macular degeneration, Invest. Ophthalmol. Vis. Sci., 30, 1691, 1989.

12.   Wing, G.L., Blanchard, G.C. and Weiter, J., The topography and age relationship of lipofuscin concentration in the retinal pigment epithelium. <u>Invest. Ophthalmol. Vis. Sci.</u>, 17, 601, 1978.

13.   Kolb, H. and Gouras, P., Electron Microscopic observations of human retinitis pigmentosa, dominantly inherited. <u>Invest. Ophthalmol. Vis. Sci.</u>, 13, 487, 1974.

SECTION IV

HUMAN RETINAL DEGENERATIONS

Inherited retinal degenerations have traditionally been studied best in animal models because of the ready availability of tissues of defined age and genetic background. Rodents, dogs, and cats with inherited degenerative disorders are used to define the mechanisms of inherited retinal diseases, and these sources of tissues for experimental studies will continue to be extremely important. However, any findings made on experimental animal tissues and animal models of inherited retinal diseases must ultimately be compared with those of human disorders. Therefore, it is of continuing importance to study disorders in human patients and human tissues whenever possible.

The chapters in this section describe new information derived through a variety of technologies that can be applied to patients or human donors with degenerative retinal disorders. Among the subjects presented are gene mapping studies of a large autosomal dominant pedigree, studies of the prevalence of altered refractive properties of the eye in a series of juvenile retinal disorders, pigmentary and histopathological studies of tissues from retinitis pigmentosa patients, and electrophysiological studies of individuals with various forms of metabolic disease. Collectively, these studies encompass virtually all of the contemporary experimental and diagnostic procedures that can be applied to the characterization of degenerative retinal disorders in man.

HISTOPATHOLOGY AND IMMUNOCYTOCHEMISTRY OF HUMAN RETINAL DYSTROPHIES

Ann H. Milam,[1] Steven J. Fliesler,[2]
Michael H. Chaitin,[3] and Samuel G. Jacobson[3]

[1]Department of Ophthalmology and RP Histopathology Laboratory,
University of Washington, Seattle, WA 98195
[2]Bethesda Eye Institute, St. Louis University, St. Louis, MO 63110
[3]Bascom Palmer Eye Institute, University of Miami, Miami, FL 33101

"Retinitis pigmentosa" (RP) comprises a group of inherited human retinal degenerations in which there is progressive loss of photoreceptor and retinal pigment epithelium (RPE) function.[1,2,3] Detailed histopathology studies of RP retinal photoreceptors and RPE are relatively few, due to scarcity of well preserved donor retinas from patients with retained vision. Since the gene defect is not yet known for most forms of human RP,[4] it is also desirable to study these valuable donor retinas by immunocytochemistry to determine if photoreceptor and RPE specific proteins are present with normal distribution. Such immunocytochemistry has been difficult to perform, since many donor retinas have been stored in fixatives containing glutaraldehyde (~2%), which reduces or abolishes tissue antigenicity and increases autofluorescence.

Increasing numbers of well preserved RP donor retinas are now available for study, due in part to the active donor program of the US National RP Foundation. We have found that antigenicity is restored and autofluorescence is diminished in glutaraldehyde-fixed retinas after treatment with sodium borohydride.[5,6] Immunocytochemical results from three RP retinas are presented here, with emphasis on one retina processed by this method.

I. CASE HISTORIES

A. DONOR # 184.

The patient was a 76 year old man who had night blindness since childhood and was diagnosed as having RP as a young adult.[6] His best corrected visual acuity OD (the eye studied here) was 20/25- after cataract surgery. Each fundus had an annular ring of bone spicule pigmentation. The 73 year old sister of the donor also had night blindness from childhood and was diagnosed as having RP at age 50. Her central vision is now 20/60 OD with a cataract and 20/50 OS uncorrected one year after cataract surgery. Each fundus showed attenuated retinal vessels and an annulus of depigmentation and bone spicule pigment in the midperipheral retina.

The parents of the donor did not have RP and the sister has no children. The donor had six children; none has RP nor do any of their children. Based on family history, the most likely diagnosis of the donor and his sister is multiplex RP. The donor had no history of ingestion of retinotoxic drugs and died of pneumonia on 1-28-89. The right eye was placed in fixative 3.5 hours *post mortem.*

B. DONOR #114

Initial observations on this patient's retina were reported previously by Fliesler *et al.*[7,8] The donor was a 39 year old man with X-linked (XL) RP. Seven years *ante mortem,* there was severely impaired visual acuity (6/120), and kinetic perimetry showed only a central island and small islands in the peripheral field. Each fundus showed an annular ring of bone spicule pigmentation from the pericentral to the peripheral retina. The patient's

history included carcinoma of the lung and chemotherapy three months prior to death. The patient died on 2-6-87 and the left eye was placed in fixative 6 hours *post mortem.*
C. DONOR # 215.

This 46 year old man was the brother of donor #114 and was also diagnosed as having RP. His fundi closely resembled his brother's, with classic bone spicule pigmentation, pale optic discs and attenuated retinal vessels. His medical history included malignant lymphoma and chemotherapy until one week before death. He died on 12-12-89 and the right eye was placed in fixative 60 min *post mortem.*

II. METHODS

The globe from donor #184 was stored in 2.5% glutaraldehyde and 1% paraformaldehyde in 0.1M phosphate buffer, pH 7.2 at room temperature for ~one month. Eyes from donors #114 and #215 were fixed initially in 2% paraformaldehyde and 2% glutaraldehyde in the same buffer for ~15 hours at 4° C, followed by storage in buffered 2% paraformaldehyde for 4 months (#215); retina #114 was stored in the same fixative, samples were processed initially after several weeks and subsequently after ~3.5 years. Some retinal samples were embedded in epoxy resin for conventional 1μm and 100 nm sections. Other samples were treated for recovery of antigenicity:[5,6] 4% sucrose in 0.13M phosphate buffer ("rinse buffer") at 20° C, 1 hr; 1% sodium borohydride in rinse buffer, 1 hr on shaker table; rinse buffer, 2-5 hr until bubbling ceased; 30% sucrose in phosphate buffer overnight at 4° C for 12 μm cryostat sections or embedment in LR-White resin.

For indirect immunofluorescence, cryostat sections were incubated overnight in primary antibodies against one of the following proteins: rod opsin (N or C terminius, F_1-F_2 loop),[9] blue cone opsin,[10] red/green cone opsin,[10] rod transducin α,[11] rod transducin βγ,[12] cone transducin α,[11] phosducin,[13] arrestin,[14] rod phosphodiesterase (α, β and γ subunits),[15] interphotoreceptor retinoid binding protein (IRBP),[16] cellular retinaldehyde binding protein,[16] cellular retinoic acid binding protein,[17] glial fibrillary acidic protein,[18] and rds protein ("peripherin").[19] The primary antibodies were prepared in rabbits or mice and the secondary antibodies were fluorescein isothiocyanate (FITC) labeled goat anti-rabbit or goat anti-mouse IgG, respectively. One μm LR-white sections were processed for light microscopy by immunogold-silver intensification.[20] Some cryostat sections were treated with FITC labeled peanut agglutinin lectin (PNA) for demonstration of cone sheaths.[21]

For each case of RP, an age and *post mortem* matched normal human retina was processed identically as a control.

III. OBSERVATIONS

A. DONOR #184. The detailed histopathology of this retina was presented previously.[6] The macula showed well preserved photoreceptors that were reduced in number by ~50%; the outer segments were reduced in length by ~30%. This correlated functionally with the patient's preserved central vision (20/25- after cataract surgery). Photoreceptors were present in the parafovea and far periphery but were very sparse in the region of bone spicule pigmentation. An unusual feature of this retina was organization of most remaining extramacular photoreceptors into rosettes and tubules instead of of a true photoreceptor layer (Figure 1). The rosettes were not associated with RPE cells but their lumina contained scattered macrophages, each engorged with lipofuscin and phagocytosed outer segment material at various stages of digestion.

This retina had been stored in 2.5% glutaraldehyde, which abolished antigenicity and led to very high immunofluorescence. Treatment with sodium borohydride restored antigenicity and reduced autofluorescence to an acceptably low level.

Immunocytochemistry revealed that most of the photoreceptors were cones with short outer segments. All cone outer segments and somata were reactive with anti-cone transducin α (Figure 2). Only a few cone outer segments were positive for red/green cone opsin, while the majority and longer cone outer segments were positive for blue cone opsin (Figure 3A). The lumina of the rosettes were stained with FITC-PNA and immunoreactive for IRBP (Figure 3B), which is characteristic of the interphotoreceptor matrix (IPM) in normal human retinas.

Few rod photoreceptors were retained; their outer segments were short or absent. These cells were reactive for each rod marker, including anti-rod opsin, -arrestin, -rod transducin α, transducin βγ, -rod PDE, and -phosducin, the latter of which reacts with both rods and cones in normal human retinas. Rods showed immunoreactivity for each marker throughout the outer segment and cytoplasm of the inner segment and soma but not nucleus. Finally, the tiny rod outer segments were reactive with anti-rds protein, as is also found in normal human retinas.[19]

High autofluorescence of the macrophage inclusions prohibited identification of specific cytoplasmic immunolabeling of these cells. The binding protein for cellular retinaldehyde had normal distribution in the cytoplasm of remaining RPE and hypertrophied Müller cells (Figure 4). Cellular retinoic acid binding protein showed normal distribution in Müller cells, which were also positive for glial fibrillary acidic protein, as noted previously in reactive Müller cells of rat retinas following photoreceptor death.[18]

B. Donor #114. As reported previously,[7,8] this retina showed marked loss of macular photoreceptors, which were reduced to a single layer of cone inner segments. The mid peripheral region of bone spicule pigmentation lacked photoreceptors, corresponding functionally to the ring scotoma. The far peripheral retina contained short rods and cones, which probably accounted for the small functional domains detected clinically. The far periphery of this retina showed normal immunoreactivity with anti-rod opsin, -IRBP,[7,8] -phosducin, -arrestin, and -cellular retinaldehyde binding protein and staining with FITC-PNA.

C. Donor #215. The histopathology of this retina closely resembled that of #114. Photoreceptors in the macula were reduced to a single layer of cone inner segments that lacked outer segments. The region of bone spicule pigmentation contained no photoreceptors and the far periphery contained decreased numbers of rods and cones with short outer segments. Some cones showed extreme densification of the cytoplasm.

The macula showed normal reactivity with the battery of antibodies tested except with anti-IRBP, which was completely negative. Maculas treated with FITC-PNA showed a thin layer of reactivity over the monolayer of cone inner segments. The far peripheral retina had normal reactivity with PNA and anti-IRBP, both of which showed normal localization in the IPM. Cones were readily found whose outer segments were reactive with anti-red/green cone opsin; however, no cone outer segments were labeled with the anti-blue cone opsin used in this study.

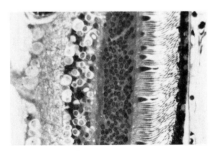 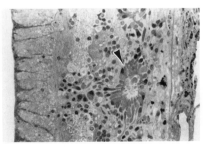

Figure 1. Parafoveas (1 μm epoxy sections, Richardson's stain). A. Control retina. Note continuous layer of RPE and normal thickness of rod and cone layer. ×75. B. Retina #184. Note marked loss of RPE and a photoreceptor rosette (➤) within the retina. ×75.

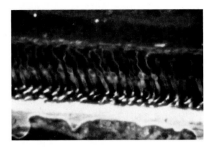
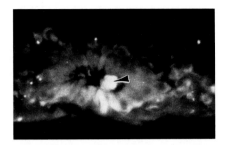

Figure 2. Immunofluorescence of cryostat sections. A. Normal human retina shows immunoreactivity for cone transducin α in all cone outer and inner segments and somata. X 90. B. Retina #184 shows immunoreactivity for cone transducin α in virtually all photoreceptors that comprise the rosettes. ◄, autofluorescent macrophage. ×250.

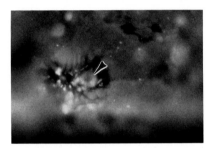
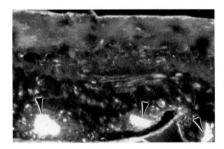

Figure 3. Immunolabeling of retina #184. A. Most of the cone outer segments are reactive with anti-blue cone opsin.   , autofluorescent macrophage. ×250. B. Rosette lumina are immunoreactive for IRBP (➤). ×100.

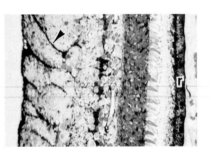
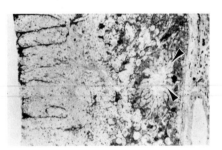

Figure 4. Immunogold labeling of 1 μm LR-white sections with anti-cellular retinaldehyde binding protein (CRALBP). A. Normal human retina. Dense labeling is restricted to the cytoplasm of RPE (r) and Müller cells (➤). ×75. B. Retina #184. Although the photoreceptors in the rosette are unlabeled (➤), the Müller fibers are strongly positive for CRALBP. Note lack of RPE cells in this region. ×75.

IV. DISCUSSION

This study demonstrates recovery of antigenicity in a glutaraldehyde-fixed RP donor retina (#184) by treatment with sodium borohydride. Sodium borohydride is thought to partially reverse deleterious effects of glutaraldehyde on tissue antigenicity by reduction of Schiff base double bonds to single bonds, allowing some restoration of antigen tertiary structure.[5] This recovery method should allow productive study of RP retinas stored in relatively high concentrations of glutaraldehyde (~2%), which to date have not been useful for immunocytochemistry. Donor retinas #114 and #215 had been fixed initially with glutaraldehyde-paraformaldehyde but stored in paraformaldehyde, which facilitated immunocytochemical studies.

An unusual feature of donor retina #184 was the organization of the remaining photoreceptors into prominent rosettes comprised primarily of cones immunoreactive with anti-blue but not -red/green cone opsin. Rosettes are not a recognized histopathologic feature of RP and are usually congenital; we cannot assess if the rosettes in this retina were congenital or represented a reactive change, perhaps secondary to profound loss of photoreceptors. Retention of viable cones and rods in these rosettes which are removed from RPE cells is provocative, in that the RPE is thought to subserve a variety of functions essential for photoreceptor viability. Macrophages in the rosette lumina are performing at least one RPE function, that of phagocytosis of outer segment tips. Assuming that these rosette outer segments contain functional visual pigments, this suggests that certain other RPE functions such as vitamin A delivery and metabolism, including isomerization, must be performed by alternate cells. Since cellular retinaldehyde binding protein is found in Müller fibers that surround the rosettes, it appears possible that Müller cells may subserve some aspects of vitamin A delivery to these photoreceptors, mediated possibly by IRBP in the rosette lumina.

In contrast to the observation that retina #184 contained primarily cones reactive with anti-blue cone opsin, several reports document preferential loss of blue sensitivity in RP.[22] Because of the recently described retinal degeneration that includes blue cone hypersensitivity, clinical testing of the affected sister of donor #184 was performed.[6] The sister had diminished rod and cone function. Results of psychophysical testing were consistent with a diagnosis of RP and not the enhanced S cone syndrome.[6,23,24]

Correlated with their severe loss of vision, the retinas of the two brothers with XL RP showed severe loss of photoreceptors, with retention of a single layer of cone inner segments but no rods centrally and decreased rods and cones with short outer segments in the far peripheral retinas. Immunocytochemistry of the macula from Donor #215 was normal, except for absence of IRBP reactivity. The region of the mid peripheral retina that lacked photoreceptors also lacked IRBP immunoreactivity. Normal IRBP reactivity in the far peripheral region of the same retina correlates with previous studies showing that IRBP is secreted predominantly by rod photoreceptors,[25, 26] which were present only in the far periphery. This result also corroborates previous reports of IRBP reactivity in RP retinas that still contain photoreceptors (autosomal dominant RP,[27] XL and autosomal recessive RP[28]).

Failure to identify blue cones immunocytochemically in retina #215 correlated with previous reports[22] that short wavelength (blue) sensitivity may be preferentially diminished in RP. It is not known if diminished blue cone sensitivity in RP reflects a specific loss of blue cones or simply death of all cone types which functionally would be most apparent for blue cones, the minority population.[10]

Immunocytochemistry of RP retinas using antibodies specific for rods, cones and Müller cells is useful for identification of these cell types, all of which have abnormal morphology. Virtually all antibodies tested produced immunostaining of the appropriate cell type or compartment, with the exception of anti-blue cone opsin and anti-IRBP in the macula of retina #215. Neither protein is likely to be a causal defect in this X-linked disease, since the genes for both blue cone opsin and IRBP are found on autosomal chromosomes 7 and 10, respectively.[29,30] When accompanied by age and *post mortem* matched human retinas as controls, positive immunoreactivity for the antigens tested here corroborates recent reports that the genes for four of these proteins, cellular retinaldehyde binding protein,[31] arrestin, IRBP and cone transducin α,[32] do not correspond to known loci for any form of RP.

V. ACKNOWLEDGEMENTS

This research was supported by The Louis Berkowitz Family Foundation, The National Retinitis Pigmentosa Foundation, Inc., The Chatlos Foundation, Inc., and NIH Research Grants EY0-1311, -1730 (AHM), -6045 (SJF), -6590 (MHC), -5627 (SGJ) and -2180 (MHC and SGJ), unrestricted departmental grants from Research to Prevent Blindness, Inc. (RPB), and by The Washington and Northern Idaho Lions' Sight Conservation Foundation. AHM is a Senior Scholar of RPB. The authors thank I. Klock, J. Chang, D. Possin, B. Clifton, R. Jones and C. Stephens for technical assistance. Special thanks go to J. Hennessey of the RP Foundation and to the scientists who generously provided antibodies used in this study.

VI. REFERENCES

1. Newsome, D.A., Retinitis pigmentosa, Usher's syndrome, and other pigmentary retinopathies, in *Retinal Dystrophies and Degenerations,*. Newsome, D. A., Editor, Raven Press, New York, 161, 1988.

2. Heckenlively, J.R., *Retinitis Pigmentosa*. J.B. Lippincott, Philadelphia, 1988.

3. Pagon, R.A., Retinitis pigmentosa. *Surv. Ophthalmol.,* 33, 137, 1988.

4. Dryja, T.P., McGee, T.L, Reichel, E., Hahn, L.B., Cowley, G.S., Yandell, D.W., Sandberg, M.A., and Berson, E.L., A point mutation of the rhodopsin gene in one form of retinitis pigmentosa. *Nature*, 343, 364, 1990.

5. Eldred, W.D., Zucker, G., Karten, H.J., and Yazulla, S., Comparison of fixation and penetration enhancement techniques for use in ultrastructural immunocytochemistry. *J. Histochem. Cytochem.,* 31, 285, 1983.

6. Milam, A.H. and Jacobson, S.G., Photoreceptor rosettes with blue cone opsin immunoreactivity in retinitis pigmentosa. *Ophthalmology,* in press, 1990.

7. Fliesler, S.J., Chaitin, M.H., and Jacobson, S.G., X-linked retinitis pigmentosa (XLRP): light and electron microscopic analysis. *Abst. Int. Cong. Eye Res.,* 45, 1988.

8. Fliesler, S.J., Chaitin, M.H., and Jacobson, S.G., X-linked retinitis pigmentosa (XLRP): histopathological and immunocytochemical analyses of a donor eye. *Invest. Ophthalmol. Vis. Sci. Supp.,* 30, 306, 1989.

9. Molday, R.S., Monoclonal antibodies to rhodopsin and other proteins of rod outer segments. In *Progress in Retinal Research,* Vol. 8, Osborne, N.N., and Chader, G. J., Editors, Pergamon Press, Oxford, 1988, Chap 8.

10. Lerea, C.L., Bunt-Milam, A.H., and Hurley, J.B., Alpha transducin is present in blue-, green- and red-sensitive cone photoreceptors in the human retina. *Neuron,* 3, 367, 1989.

11. Lerea, C.L., Somers, D.E., Hurley, J.B., Klock, I.B., and Bunt-Milam, A.H., Identification of specific transducin α subunits in retinal rod and cone photoreceptors. *Science,* 234, 77, 1986.

12. Navon, S.E., Lee, R.H., Lolley, R.N., and Fung, B. K.-K., Immunological determination of transducin content in retinas exhibiting inherited degeneration. *Exp. Eye Res.,* 44, 115, 1987.

13. Lee, R., Whelan, J., Lolley, R., and McGinnis, J., The photoreceptor-specific 33 kDa phosphoprotein of mammalian retina: generation of monospecific antibodies and localization by immunocytochemistry. *Exp. Eye Res.,* 46, 829, 1988.

14. Kamada, Y., Shichi, H., and Das, N.D., Localization and properties of an immunoreactive protein in bovine ciliary body similar to retinal S antigen. *Curr. Eye Res.,* 4, 207, 1985.

15. Lee, R.H., Navon, S.E., Brown, B.M., Fung, B.K.-K, and Lolley, R.N., Characterization of a phosphodiesterase-immunoreactive polypeptide from rod photoreceptors of developing *rd* mouse retinas. *Invest. Ophthalmol. Vis. Sci.,* 29, 1021, 1988.

16. Bunt-Milam, A.H. and Saari, J.C., Immunocytochemical localization of two retinoid binding proteins in vertebrate retinas. *J. Cell Biol.,* 97, 703, 1983.

17. Milam, A.H., DeLeeuw, A.M., Gaur, V.P., and Saari, J.C., Immunolocalization of cellular retinoic acid binding protein to Müller cells and/or a subpopulation of GABA-positive amacrine cells in retinas of different species. *J. Comp. Neurol.,* 296, 123, 1990.

18. Eisenfeld, A.J., Bunt-Milam, A.H., and Sarthy, P.V., Müller cell expression of glial fibrillary acidic protein after genetic and experimental photoreceptor degeneration in the rat retina. *Invest. Ophthalmol. Vis. Sci.,* 25, 1321, 1984.

19. Connell, G., Boscom, R., McInnes, R., and Molday, R.S., Photoreceptor cell peripherin is the defective protein responsible for retinal degeneration slow (rds). *Invest. Ophthalmol. Vis. Sci.,* 31, Abst. #1514, 1990.

20. Carter-Dawson, L. and Burroughs, M., Differential distribution of interphotoreceptor retinoid-binding protein (IRBP) around retinal rod and cone photoreceptors. *Curr. Eye Res.,* 8, 1331, 1989.

21. Blanks, J.D. and Johnson, L.V., Specific binding of peanut lectin to a class of retinal photoreceptor cells. A species comparison. *Invest. Ophthalmol. Vis. Sci.,* 25, 546, 1984.

22. Greenstein, V.C., Hood, D.C., Ritch, R., Steinberger, D., and Carr, R.E., S (blue) cone pathway vulnerability in retinitis pigmentosa, diabetes and glaucoma. *Invest. Ophthalmol. Vis. Sci.,* 30, 1732, 1989.

23. Jacobson, S.G., Marmor, M.F., Kemp, C.M., and Knighton, R.W., SWS (blue) cone hypersensitivity in a newly identified retinal degeneration. *Invest. Ophthalmol. Vis. Sci.,* 31, 827, 1990.

24. Marmor, M.F., Jacobson, S.G., Foerster, M.H., Kellner, U., and Weleber, R.G., Diagnostic clinical findings of a new syndrome with night blindness, maculopathy and enhanced S cone sensitivity. *Amer. J. Ophthalmol.,* 110, 124, 1990.

25. van Veen, T., Kitial, A., Shinohara, T., Barrett, D.J., Wiggert, B., Chader, G. J., and Nickerson, J.M., Retinal photoreceptor neurons and pinealocytes accumulate mRNA for interphotoreceptor retinoid-binding protein (IRBP). *FEBS Lett.,* 208, 133, 1986.

26. Hollyfield, J.G., Fliesler, S.J., Rayborn, M.E., Fong, S.-L., Landers, R.A., and Bridges, C.D.B., Synthesis and secretion of interstitial retinol-binding protein by the human retina. *Invest. Ophthalmol. Vis. Sci.,* 26, 58, 1985.

27. LaVail, M.M., Yasumura, D., and Hollyfield, J.G., The interphotoreceptor matrix in retinitis pigmentosa: preliminary observations from a family with an autosomal dominant form of disease. In *Retinal Degeneration: Experimental and Clinical Studies,* LaVail, M.M., Hollyfield, J.G., and Anderson, R.E., Editors, Alan R. Liss, Inc., New York, 51, 1985.

28. Schmidt, S.Y., Heth, C.A., Edwards, R.B., Brandt, J.T., Adler, A.J., Spiegel, A., Shichi, H., and Berson, E.L., Identification of proteins in retinas and IPM from eyes with retinitis pigmentosa. *Invest. Ophthalmol. Vis. Sci.,* 29, 1585, 1988.

29. Nathans, J., Thomas, D., and Hogness, D. S., Molecular genetics of human color vision: the genes encoding blue, green, and red pigments. *Science,* 232, 193, 1986.

30. Liou, G.I., Li, Y., Wang, C., Fong, L.-L., Bhattacharya, F.S. and Bridges, C.D.B., Bgl II RFLP recognized by a human IRBP cDNA localized to chromosome 10. *Nucleic Acids Res.,* 15, 3196, 1987.

31. Cotran, P.R., Ringens, P.J., Crabb, J.W., Berson, E.L., and Dryja, T.P., Analysis of the DNA of patients with retinitis pigmentosa with a cellular retinaldehyde binding protein cDNA. *Exp. Eye Res.,* 51, 15, 1990.

32. Ringens, P.J., Fang, M., Shinohara, T., Bridges, C.D., Lerea, C.L., Berson, E.L., and Dryja, T.P., Analysis of genes coding for S-antigen, interstitial retinol binding protein, and the alpha-subunit of cone transducin in patients with retinitis pigmentosa. *Invest. Ophthalmol. Vis. Sci.* 31, 1421, 1990.

PROGRESS IN THE LOCALISATION OF A LATE ONSET ADRP GENE

Peter McWilliam, Siobhan A. Jordan, Paul Kenna,
Marian M. Humphries, Rajendra Kumar-Singh, Elizabeth Sharp,
and Peter Humphries

Department of Genetics, Trinity College, Dublin 2, Ireland

I. Introduction

Retinitis pigmentosa (RP) describes a group of clinically and genetically heterogenous inherited retinopathies. Clinicial features include reduced night and peripheral vision, retinal pigment epithelium degeneration, retinal vessel attenuation and optic disk pallor.[1] RP can be genetically divided on the basis of mode of inheritance into X-linked, autosomal recessive and autosomal dominant forms.

We have previously reported a linkage in a large dominant Irish pedigree (TCDM1) to the polymorphic DNA marker D3S47 on the long arm of chromosome 3.[2] This marker maps close to the gene for rhodopsin, the pigment of the rod photoreceptors. Subsequently it was shown that a point mutation in this gene was responsible for a proportion (15/150) of ADRP cases.[3]

In a second Irish pedigree (TCDG1) we have shown that the disease gene is not segregating with this chromosome 3 locus,[4] confirming the presence of genetic heterogeneity in ADRP. Consequently, we have started a comprehensive linkage study designed to locate the site of the gene involved in this family.

It has recently been reported that CA repeats, present in 50-100,000 copies in the human genome, are frequently polymorphic.[5] These polymorphisms have the significant advantage over conventional RFLP's in that their average PIC value is greater than 0.5. Since they are assayed by the technique of PCR they are rapid and convenient to use as well as being highly informative. In addition, it has been shown that various repeat units associated with the poly A tract at the 3' end of Alu sequences can be polymorphic.[6] Oligodeoxynucleotide primer sequences spanning many of these simple sequence repeats have now been published. Here we report a preliminary study where ten of these 'microsatellite' repeats have been typed in TCDG1. Exclusion data representing about 300cM is presented.

II. MATERIALS AND METHODS

TCDG1
All individuals in the pedigree were assessed with corrected visual acuity and ERG using a modification of Arden's protocol[7] and direct and indirect ophthalmoscopy. Selected individuals had standard dark adaptometry and two colour dark adaptometry.[8]

PCR
Standard PCR reactions were carried out essentially as described by Weber and May[5] except that a 32-P dCTP was used. *Taq* D1\1A polymerase was obtained from Promega and used according to their specifications.

Data Analysis
Computations were performed using the data management package LINKSYS[9] in conjunction with the program LIPED.[10]

III. RESULTS AND DISCUSSION

The structure of TCDG1 is shown in Figure 1. The type of RP in this pedigree differs from that in TCDM1 by its later age of onset (mid-thirties, as opposed to early childhood) and the pattern of dark adaptometry. In TCDG1 there was greater elevation of rod threshold compared to cone, uniformly throughout the retina, whereas in TCDG1 there was simultaneous elevation of rod and cone thresholds in a regionalised pattern.

Figure 1:   TCDG1

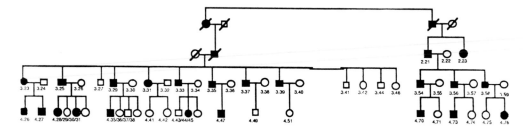

The calculated segregation ratio (0.51) in the pedigree did not differ significantly from that expected for a dominant gene, suggesting full penetrance. A number of cases of male to male transmission rule out the presence of an X-linked dominant gene. The pedigree shown in Figure 1 consists of two branches. While the right half has three generations, the left half only has two. This latter feature reduces the number of potentially informative meioses (24) and means that the use of highly informative markers is important in carrying out a linkage study in this family.

Table 1 lists the microsatellite markers used in this study. All of the markers are highly variable, showing between six and ten alleles. The PIC values vary from 0.46 to 0.81 with an average value of 0.66.

TABLE 1

Locus	PIC	Number of alleles	Reference
Amy2B	0.63	6	Dracopoli and Meisler (1990)[11]
D1S103	0.78	11	Weber *et al.* (1990a)[12]
ApoA2	0.65	6	Weber and May (1989)[5]
SST	0.46	6	Weber and May (1989)[5]
D3S61	0.78	8	Kumar-Singh *et al.* (1990)[13]
D14S42	0.65	10	Jordan *et al.* (1990a)[14]
TCRD	0.74	6	Jordan *et al.* (1990b)[15]
D16S261	0.66	6	Weber *et al.* (1990b)[16]
D17S250	0.81	10	Weber *et al.* (1990c)[17]
HMG14	0.50	6	Petersen *et al.* (1990)[18]

Table 2 shows the two point Lod scores obtained between RP and the various markers. No positive Lod scores are observed and all markers give significant exclusion. The probes exclude, at a Lod score of below -2, from between recombination fractions of 0.07 to 0.24. Assuming a recombination fraction of 0.1 to be roughly equivalent to 10 cM, this data excludes the disease-causing gene from approximately 300 cM or just under 10% of the genome. As further markers are typed, multipoint analysis can be used to exclude regions between loosely linked markers.

The last year has seen the development of many polymorphic markers based on simple sequence repeats. Such repeats can be selected easily by probing genomic libraries with the relevant repeat unit.[5] However, inspection of a sequence data base shows the presence of many repeats associated with Alu sequences and genes. Since an accurate map position for the repeats is often known, it is frequently possible to target specific regions, for example near candidate genes. This feature, coupled with the high degree of polymorphism and ease of use, makes these markers ideal for extended linkage studies and the localisation of disease genes.

TABLE 2
Two Point Lod Scores for Microsatellites in TCDG1

Probe	Chromosome	Recombination Fraction				
		0.05	0.10	0.15	0.20	0.25
Amy2B	1	-8.24	-4.77	-2.94	1.80	1.05
D1S103	1	-4.80	-2.91	-1.90	-1.25	-0.81
ApoA2	1	-11.62	-7.00	-4.53	-2.94	-1.86
SST	3	-5.82	-3.11	-1.97	-1.50	-6.80
D3S621	3	-4.92	-2.78	-1.66	-0.96	-0.51
D14S42	14	-10.33	-6.26	-4.07	-2.67	-1.70
TCRD	14	-6.54	-3.67	-2.19	-1.29	-0.72
D16S261	16	-2.81	-1.40	-0.76	-0.43	-0.27
D17S250	17	-2.86	-1.19	-0.42	-0.03	0.14
HGM14	21	-5.15	-2.41	-1.07	-0.33	0.08

Acknowledgements: This work has been supported by grants from the National RP Foundation of America, the George Gund Foundation, RP Ireland-Fighting Blindness and the British Retinitis Pigmentosa Society.

References

1. Hekenlively JR (1988). "Retinitis Pigmentosa," pp. 125-149, Lippincott, Philadelphia.
2. McWilliam P, Farrar GJ, Kenna P, Bradley D, Humphries MM, Sharp EM, McConnell DJ, Lawler M, Shiels D, Ryan C, Stevens K, Daiger S and Humphries P. (1989). Autosomal dominant retinitis pigmentosa (ADRP): Localisation of an ADRP gene to the long arm of chromosome 3. Genomics 5: 619-622.
3. Dryja TD, McGee TL, Reichel E, Hohn LB, Cowley GS, Yandell DN, Sandberg MA and Berson EL. (1990). A point mutation of the rhodopsin gene in one form of retinitis pigmentosa. Nature 343: 364-366.
4. Farrar GJ, McWilliam P, Bradley DG, Kenna P, Lawler M, Sharp EM, Humphries MM, Eiberg H, Conneally PM, Trofatter JA and Humphries P.

(1990). Autosomal dominant retinitis pigmentosa: Linkage to rhodopsin and evidence for genetic heterogeneity. Genomics 8: 35-40.

5. Weber JL and May PE. (1989). Abundant class of human polymorphisms which can be typed using the polymerase chain reaction. Am. J. Hum. Genet. 44: 388-396.

6. Economou EP, Bergen AW, Warren AC and Antonarakis SE. (1990). The polydeoxyadenylate tract of Alu repetitive elements is polymorphic in the human genome. Proc. Natl. Acad. Sci. 87: 2951-2954.

7. Arden GB, Carter RM, Hogg CR *et al.* (1981). A modified ERG technique and the results obtained in X-linked retinitis pigmentosa. Br. J. Ophthalmol. 67: 419-430.

8. Massof RW and Finkelstein D. (1981). Two forms of autosomal dominant primary retinitis pigmentosa. Doc. Ophthalmol. 51: 289-346.

9. Attwood J and Bryant S. (1988). A computer program to make analysis with LIPED and LINKAGE easier to perform and less prone to input errors. Ann. Hum. Genet. 52: 259.

10. Ott J. (1974). Estimation of the recombination fraction in human pedigrees: Efficient computation of the liklihood for human linkage studies. Amer. J. Hum. Genet. 26: 588-597.

11. Dracopoli NC and Meisler MH. (1990). Mapping the human Amylase gene cluster on the proximal short arm of chromosome 1 using a highly informative (CA)n repeat. Genomics 7:97-102.

12. Weber JL, Kwitek AE and May PE. (1990a). Dinucleotide repeat polymorphism at the D1S103 locus. Nucl. Acids Res. 18: 2199.

13. Kumar-Singh R, Bradley DG, Farrar GJ, Lawler M, Jordan SA and Humphries P. (1990). Autosomal dominant retinitis pigmentosa: A new multi-allelic marker (D3S621) genetically linked to the disease locus (RP4). Hum. Genet. in press.

14. Jordan SA, McWilliam P, O'Briain S and Humphries P (1990a). Dinucleotide repeat polymorphism at the D14S42 locus. Nucl. Acids Res, in press.

15. Jordan SA, McWilliam P, O'Briain S and Humphries P (1 990b). Dinucleotide repeat polymorphism at the TCRD locus. Nucl. Acids Res, submitted.

16. Weber JL, Kwitek AE and May PE. (1990b). Dinucleotide repeat polymorphisms at the D16S260, D16S261, D16S265, D16S266 and D16S267 loci. Nucl. Acids Res. 18: 4034.

17. Weber JL, Kwitek AE, May PE, Wallace MR, Collins FS and Ledbetter DH (1990c). Dinucleotide repeat polymorphisms at the D17S250 and D17S261 loci. Nucl. Acids Res. 18: 4640.

18. Petersen MB, Economou EP, Slaughenhaupt SA, Chakravarti A and Antonarakis SE (1990). Linkage analysis of the human HMG14 gene on chromosome 21 using a GT dinucleotide repeat as a polymorphic marker. Genomics 7: 136-138.

LINKAGE STUDIES AND RHODOPSIN MUTATION DETECTION IN AUTOSOMAL DOMINANT RETINITIS PIGMENTOSA: AN UPDATE

S.S. Bhattacharya, R. Bashir, J. Keen, D. Lester,
B. Lauffart, M. Jay,* A.C. Bird,* C.F. Inglehearn

University of Newcastle upon Tyne,
Department of Human Genetics, 19 Claremont Place,
Newcastle upon Tyne, NE2 4AA

*Institute of Ophthalmology, Moorfields Eye Hospital,
City Road, London

The term retinitis pigmentosa (RP) was first coined in the middle of the last century to describe a symptom associated with a variety of eye defects. Viral, toxic or ischaemic damage to the retina all can cause the death of photoreceptor cells, leading to pigmentary patches on the fundus. However, by far the most common cause of RP is the complex range of inherited eye defects, sometimes referred to as primary RP, with symptoms which include night blindness, narrowing of peripheral vision and retinal pigmentary patches, often leading to complete blindness.[1] Within this category, there is substantial variation in age of onset, mode of inheritance and clinical manifestations of the disease. RP families can be classified into X-linked, autosomal dominant and autosomal recessive categories, with further clinical heterogeneity even within these groups.[2] In the autosomal dominant class, patients have been classified clinically as type I and type II, based on age of onset,[3] which roughly corresponds to the categories D (diffuse) and R (regional) type, respectively, on the basis of functional loss of photoreceptors in the retina.[4] The autosomal recessive class includes cases where RP is found with other clinical defects, such as Usher's syndrome (RP and deafness). Also, many cases of RP are sporadic and therefore unclassifiable by these criteria.[5]

Reverse genetics seeks to identify unrelated genetic variants that coinherit with the defect, and so locate the causative genetic lesion.[6] By locating and identifying genes implicated in ADRP, researchers can begin to study exactly how the defect progresses and so can begin to look for ways of treating RP. In the short term, identification of the gene in one form of RP allows informed counselling in some families and is also a useful clue as to other candidate genes.

This approach has recently lead to considerable advance in the understanding of one of the categories of RP, namely autosomal dominant RP (ADRP). In 1989, McWilliam and colleagues reported a lod score of 14.7 with no recombination between marker C17 on chromosome 3q (D3S47) in a single large Irish D type family.[7] Our own laboratory demonstrated genetic heterogeneity by excluding linkage at this locus in a single large British R type family.[8] Reports from our own and other laboratories subsequently revealed three further C17 unlinked type II / R type families, one further D type family with a lod score of 5.5 and no recombination with C17, and one R type / type II family with linkage to C17 with a lod score of 4.78 at a recombination fraction of 0.08.[9,10,11,12]

The rod photopigment rhodopsin maps to 3q21-24,[13] close to locus D3S47, and was therefore a strong candidate for the ADRP gene in C17 linked families. Dryja et al. (1990) sequenced rhodopsin in 20 ADRP patients and found a point mutation in codon 23 (CCC-CAC, proline to histidine) in six of them.[14] By allele specific oligonucleotide hybridization (ASO), they demonstrated that this mutation was present in 17 of 148 ADRP patients, that is, in approximately 12%. However, results from our panel of ADRP families, together with those of two other European laboratories, demonstrate the absence of this mutation in 91 European families.[15] Subsequently, Dryja's laboratory reported three other mutations involving codons 347 and 58.[16] Almost 6% of patients on their genetic register had the codon 347 mutation.

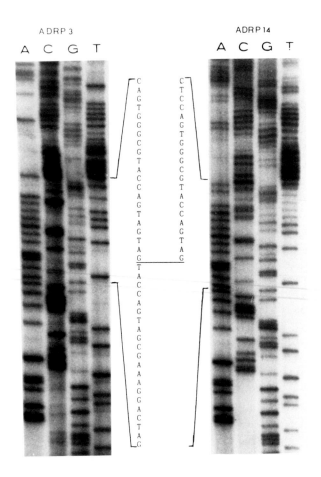

Figure 1. Rhodopsin exon 4 sequences from two C17 linked ADRP families, ADRP3 and ADRP14. Sequence was obtained as described elsewhere.[17] Briefly, a kinase end labelled internal primer was used to prime a sequenase (T7 DNA polymerase: USB) sequencing reaction on double stranded PCR amplified exon 4 template. The sequence in ADRP3 corresponds to the known human rhodopsin sequence. In the ADRP14 sequence, from a point a little above half way up, all bands are seen as a double image, since the three basepair deletion in half the amplified molecules frameshifts one half of the image relative to the other.

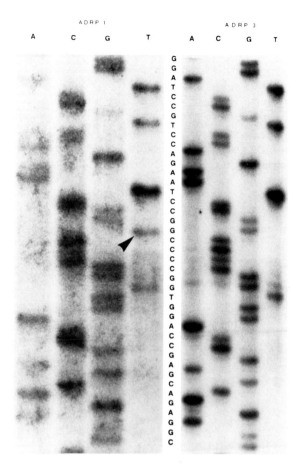

Figure 2. Rhodopsin exon 5 sequences from ADRP1 and ADRP3. In ADRP3 the sequence matches perfectly with the known sequence of human rhodopsin, while in ADRP14, an extra band (arrowed) clearly shows in the T track, corresponding to a CCG-CTG mutation in codon 347.

Our own laboratory works on a panel of 31 unrelated British ADRP families. These families have been examined by our clinical colleagues at Moorfields Eye Hospital, London. Direct genomic sequencing of the exons of the rhodopsin gene in one of our two C17 linked D-type families, ADRP14, showed a 3 base pair (bp) deletion (Figure 1) in one of them.[17] Codons 255 and 256 code for isoleucine residues, and lie within the sequence TCATCATCAT. Exactly which 3bp within this run is deleted is impossible to tell, but it has no consequence to the resultant mutation, since the translational reading frame of the protein is unaltered. However, in another C17 linked family, ADRP3, we have sequenced the entire coding sequence and found no mutations.

The process of genomic sequencing is time consuming, and we therefore felt it impractical to set about sequencing all of the remaining 29 families on our ADRP register. First we tested for the mutations already described. This revealed one family, ADRP1, which had the codon 347 (CCG-CTG) mutation first described by

Dryja and colleagues (Figure 2). We then used the mutations in ADRP14 and ADRP1 as controls, and found that it was possible to detect not only the small deletion but also the single base mismatch as mobility shifted heteroduplex bands on high resolution hydrolink polyacrylamide gels.[18] These are shown in Figures 3 and 4, respectively.

We then undertook to screen each exon of rhodopsin in this way in the remaining families, as a means of pinpointing mutations in the rhodopsin gene. To date, we have identified three mobility shifts, one in exon 4 and two in exon 3, each of which is present in all affected family members and absent in normals. In addition, we have located a deletion in exon 1 in an isolated patient from another family. One of the mobility shifts in exon 3 was present in two of our panel of 31 families, while the other, clearly a different shift and therefore almost certainly a different mutation, was in only one family. The exon 4 shift was also present in a single family. Sequence analysis of these mutations is currently being undertaken.

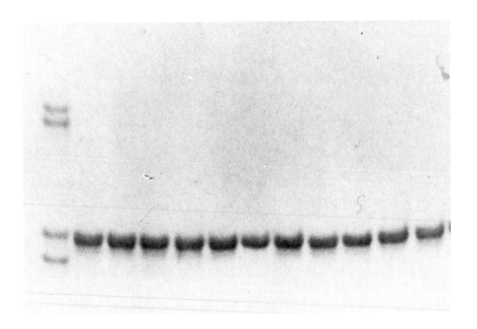

Figure 3. PCR of a 100bp section of rhodopsin exon 4 in a member of ADRP14 (to the left) and in 11 unaffected control DNAs, using primers ACAGAAGGCAGAGAAGGAGG and GAAGATGTAGAATGCCACGC. Amplified product was resolved on a 10% polyacrylamide gel. Since the primers used span the deletion in ADRP14, four bands can be seen in this individual. The lower two represent the 100bp product and the 3bp deleted 97bp product. The two bands above are heteroduplexes, composed of deleted plus strand with normal minus strand and deleted minus strand with normal plus strand.

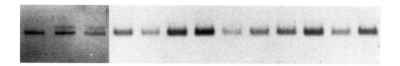

<u>Figure 4</u>. PCR of a 211bp fragment containing all of rhodopsin exon 5, from a normal and two affected individuals from ADRP1 (left), then from two affecteds from each of 5 other ADRP families in our panel (right). PCR was performed using primers AGTTCCAAGCACACTGTGGG and GGATGGGAGACGCCTATAGT, and products were resolved on a 10% hydrolink polyacrylamide gel (Hoefer UK). In the two ADRP1 affecteds, a heteroduplex band can be seen running above the main band.

In summary, we have identified the probable causative genetic lesion in 7 of our panel of 31 ADRP families, in coding sequences of the rhodopsin gene. This represents approximately 22% of the sample, and in all but one case these families have been diagnosed as having D-type ADRP. (The remaining case is awaiting confirmation of clinical status.) In contrast, as discussed previously, two of our R-type families show significant exclusion with probe C17, making it unlikely that they are caused by mutations in the rhodopsin gene. It is interesting to note that the estimated proportion of R-type to D-type in ADRP is about 4 to 1,[19] which corresponds to the frequency with which we have identified rhodopsin mutations in our families. However, we do not yet know whether the heteroduplex mobility shift technique detects all possible mutations. Further, in one case we have identified a D-type linked ADRP family for which genomic sequencing of the entire coding sequence has revealed no mutation. Also, Ollsen and coworkers have described an R-type family with significant linkage to C17 but at a recombination fraction of 0.08. Thus, ADRP can clearly result from mutations in the rhodopsin gene, and must also have a locus or loci elsewhere in the genome. However, it remains a possibility that there is another ADRP gene in the vicinity of the D3S47 locus, and that a range of phenotypes can result from mutations in these genes.

Figure 5 shows the rhodopsin mutations to date for which exact locations are known. Mutations do not appear to be confined to any one domain, but occur in the cytoplasmic, intradiscal and transmembrane regions of the protein. Neither do they occur within known functional motifs. It is therefore difficult to say exactly how a defect in rhodopsin could give rise to the pattern of loss of function and photoreceptor cell death associated with the later stages of ADRP. However, the fact that it does constitutes a significant clue as to other genes which may be implicated in other forms of RP. Clearly, any gene in the phototransduction cascade can now be tested as a candidate in RP families.

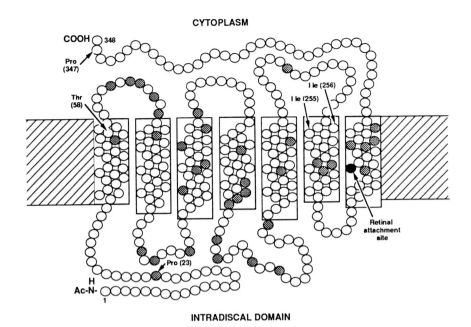

<u>Figure 5.</u>

Our own results revealed six different RP mutations in seven ADRP families. This contrasts with the results of Dryja and coworkers, who found that the codon 23 proline to histidine mutation accounted for 17 of 148 patients. However, haplotype analysis of genetic markers in the rhodopsin vicinity suggested that these patients may have a common ancestor. Further, this mutation appears to be specific to the North American population, while our finding of the codon 347 CCG-CTG mutation in ADRP1 suggests that this may have a more world-wide distribution. It appears increasingly unlikely, therefore, that any one mutation will account for a large fraction of ADRP families, as was the case for Cystic Fibrosis.[20] This might be expected for a dominant condition, where selection against carriers must have been significant historically and would therefore prevent a rhodopsin mutation rising to a high frequency in the human population. In cases where a mutation is found in more than one family, this may represent a mutation hotspot, or could prove to be some form of founder effect, as appears to be the case for the codon 23 mutation.

In the short term, it is now possible to offer informed counselling and carrier diagnosis to many of the ADRP families on our panel. That each has a different mutation makes diagnosis more difficult for a routine diagnostic laboratory. However, the mismatch detection technique described is so simple and rapid that it provides a viable means by which the problem could be approached. In addition, the finding of one RP gene must surely speed up the search for other causative genes.

ACKNOWLEDGEMENTS

We gratefully acknowledge the generous support provided by the National Retinitis Pigmentosa Foundation Fighting Blindness USA, George Gund Foundation, and the Wellcome Trust for funding this research. Thanks also go to Professor Calbert Phillips, Mr. Tony Moore, and Professor Barry Jay for clinical details and help with collecting the families, and to Pauline Battista for typing.

REFERENCES

1. Botermans CH: (1972). Primary pigmentary retinal degeneration and its association with neurological diseases. In Handbook of Clinical Neurology 13 (eds Vinken PJ an Bruyn GW). 148-379.

2. Kaplan J, Bonneau D, Frezal J, Munnich A, Dufier JL: (1990). Clinical and genetic heterogeneity in retinitis pigmentosa. Human Genet 85: 635-642.

3. Massof RW, and Finkelstein D: (1981). Two forms of autosomal dominant retinitis pigmentosa. Doc Ophthalmol 51: 289-346.

4. Lyness AL, Ernst W, Quinlan MP, Clover GM, Arden GB, Carter RM, Bird AC, Parker JA: (1985). A clinical, psychophysical and electroretinographic survey of patients with autosomal dominant retinitis pigmentosa. Brit J Ophthalmol 69: 326-339.

5. Jay M: (1982). Figures and fantasies: the frequencies of the different genetic forms of retinitis pigmentosa. Birth Defects orig art series 18: 167-173.

6. Botstein D, White RL, Skolnick M, Davis RW: (1980). Construction of a genetic linkage map using restriction fragment length polymorphisms. Am J Hum Genet 32: 314-31.

7. McWilliam P, Farrar GJ, Kenna P, Bradley DG, Humphries MM, Sharp EM, McConnell DJ, Lawler M, Sheils D, Ryan C, Stevens K, Daiger SP and Humphries P: (1989). Autosomal dominant retinitis pigmentsoa (ADRP): localisation of an ADRP gene to the long arm of chromosome 3. Genomics 5: 619-622.

8. Inglehearn CF, Jay M, Lester DH, Bashir R, Jay B, Bird AC, Wright AF, Evans HJ, Papiha 55 and Bhattacharya SS: (1990). No evidence for linkage between late onset autosomal dominant Retinitis Pigmentosa and Chromosome 3 locus D3547 (C17). Evidence for genetic heterogeneity. Genomics 6: 168-173.

9. Lester DH, Inglehearn CF, Bashir R, Ackford H, Esakowitz L, Jay M, Bird AC, Wright AF and Bhattacharya SS: (1990). Linkage to D3547 (C19) in one large family and exclusion in another: confirmation of genetic heterogeneity. Am J Hum Genet 47: 536-541.

10. Farrar GJ, McWilliam P, Bradley DG, Kenna P, Lawler M, Sharp EM, Humphries MM, Eiberg H, Conneally PM, Trofatter JA, Humphries P: (1990). Autosomal Dominant Retinitis Pigmentosa: Linkage to rhodopsin and evidence for genetic heterogeneity. Genomics 8: 35-40.

11.   Blanton SH, Cottingham AW, Giesenschlag N, Heckenlively JR, Humphries P and Daiger SP: (1990). Further evidence of exclusion of linkage between type II Autosomal Dominant Retinitis Pigmentosa (ADRP) and D3S47 on 3q. Genomics 8: 179-181.

12.   Olsson JE, Samanns C, Jimenez J, Pongratz J, Chand A, Watty A, Seuchter SA, Denton M and Gal A: (1990). Gene of Type II autosomal dominant retinitis pigmentosa maps on the long arm of chromosome 3. Am J Med Genet 35: 595-599.

13.   Nathans J, Piantanida TP, Eddy RL, Shaws TB and Hogness DS: (1986). Molecular genetics of inherited variation in human colour vision. Science 232: 203-210.

14.   Dryja TP, McGee TL, Reichel E, Hahn LB, Cowley GS, Yandell DW, Sandberg MA and Berson EL: (1990). A point mutation of the rhodopsin gene in one form of retinitis pigmentosa. Nature 343: 364-366.

15.   Farrar GJ, Kenna P, Redmond R, McWilliam P, Bradley DG, Humphries MM, Sharp EM, Inglehearn CF, Bashir R, Jay M, Watty A, Ludwig M, Schinzel A, Sammans AC, Gal A, Bhattacharya 55, Humphries P: (1990). Autosomal dominant retinitis pigmentosa: Absence of the rhodopsin codon 23 Proline-Histidine substitution in pedigrees of European origin. Am J Hum Genet 47: 941-945.

16.   Dryja TP, McGee TL, Hahn LB, Cowley GS, Olsson JE, Reichel E, Sandberg MA, Berson EL: (1990). Mutations within the rhodopsin gene in patients with autosomal dominant retinitis pigmentosa. New Engl J Med 323: 1302-1307.

17.   Inglehearn CF, Bashir R, Lester DH, Jay M, Bird AC, Bhattacharya SS: (1991). A three basepair deletion in the rhodopsin gene in a family with autosomal dominant retinitis pigmentosa. Am J Hum Genet 48: 26-30.

18.   Keen J, Lester DH, Inglehearn CF, Curtis A, Bhattacharya SS: (1991). Rapid detection of single base mismatches as heteroduplexes on hydrolink gels. Trends Genet. January issue.

19.   Farber MD, Fishman GA and Weiss RW: (1985). Autosomal dominantly inherited retinitis pigmentosa: visual acuity loss by subtype. Arch Ophthalmol 103: 524-528.

20.   Kerem B-S, Rommens JM, Buchanan JA, Markiewicz D, Cox TK, Chakravarti A, Buchwald M, Tsui L-C: (1989). Identification of the cystic fibrosis gene: Genetic analysis. Science 245: 1073-1080.

AMETROPIA IN RETINAL DISORDERS

Alan M. Laties, M.D.
Richard A. Stone, M.D.

Scheie Eye Institute
University of Pennsylvania School of Medicine

The discovery that visual manipulations such as lid suture, goggle application or dark rearing alter refractive states in young animals provides a new insight into ocular development, revealing that the retina takes part in the postnatal regulation of eye growth.[1] From experiments in monkey and chick and from clinical observations in children with conditions such as congenital ptosis,[2] it is now clear that normal ocular development depends on the quality of the retinal image in early life. Thus, in addition to transmitting visual information to the central nervous system, the retina also influences eye growth and refraction by participating in a feedback pathway presently just beginning to be characterized.[3] Supporting this conclusion are observations that intravitreal administration of retinal cell toxins also alters subsequent eye growth,[4] which suggests that accurate regulation of postnatal eye growth requires a functionally intact retina as well as a clear image. In the same way accurate performance of the retina's growth modulating role may fail in primary retinal disorders, and a high prevalence of refractive errors may represent a necessary consequence of particular retinal disturbances in the young.

To illustrate present evidence that juvenile retinal disorders may associate with altered refractive status, we briefly review salient aspects of four conditions. In each, normal refractive development fails in a way that may be characteristic of the retinal disorder. On this basis, the possibility exists that the present broad categories used to denote the phenotypic expression of hereditary retinal disorders might be refined through an improved ascertainment of refractive status. It also is possible that in instances where the retinal cell pathology is relatively specific and the refractive error is distinctive, appropriate studies might provide insight into the manner by which the retina participates in the regulation of refractive status. In order to realize either possibility, however, future clinical reports will require collection of more comprehensive data on the components of ocular refraction such as corneal curvature and axial length than are currently available.

DISTRIBUTION OF REFRACTIONS

As general background, the net refractive power of an eye is largely based on four components--radius of corneal curvature, lens power, anterior chamber depth and axial length--each of which is normally distributed. Sorsby and others have asserted that an as yet unexplained harmonization takes place by which compensatory changes of individual optical elements achieve the balance necessary for a good focus at distance.[5] In this regard, the population distribution of refractions generally shows a mid-zone excess at or near emmetropia. For instance, the Pullman Washington survey of children ages 5-17 found refractions clustered at 0.74 ± 0.90 diopters (S.D.);[6] these results differ little from 1033 young British men examined for army service in which 75% had refractions between 0 and +1.9 diopters.[5] When compared to a Gaussian distribution, two other aspects of the population distribution of refractive errors are remarkable: modest degrees of hyperopia and myopia are below expectation while the prevalence of high degrees of error, especially myopic error, exceeds expectation. The existence of an uncommon but distinct condition, pathological myopia, only partly explains the prominent myopic tail.

LEBER'S CONGENITAL AMAUROSIS

Clinically, Leber's Congenital Amaurosis presents as congenital blindness with nystagmus, sluggish pupillary reflexes and an electroretinogram that is unrecordable or nearly so under scotopic or photopic illumination. Signs of retinal degeneration on ophthalmoscopy, often subtle at first, include pigment mottling or irregularity, narrowed arterioles, and profound optic disc pallor. Leber's Congenital Amaurosis is currently classified as uncomplicated or complicated, depending on the absence or presence of defined disorders that include peroxisomal deficiency, ceroid lipofuscinosis and several syndromes yet to be categorized biochemically.[7,8] An early hyperopia that persists into adulthood is the rule for uncomplicated and probably so for complicated Leber's Congenital Amaurosis as well. The hyperopia is frequently of large extent; refractive errors usually range between +4 and +9.5 diopters.[9,10]

A component analysis of hyperopia in Leber's Congenital Amaurosis is not possible for lack of essential information. Direct measurements of corneal curvature, lens power and anterior chamber depth are not available; axial length measurements by ultrasound are few. The available ultrasound data do indicate that these eyes have abnormally short axial lengths, a finding compatible with Leber's original observation and subsequent clinical assertions that these eyes frequently remain small through life.[9]

Supporting the human data is a pilot survey of eye growth in the RCS rat, a species with an early onset retinal degeneration. Uehara et al. have recently measured axial and equatorial eye lengths in both pigmented and albino RCS rats at maturity, finding in both instances that the globes of the early retinal dystrophy rats were significantly smaller than those of congenic controls with normal retinas.[11]

RETINITIS PIGMENTOSA

Under the impact of molecular genetics, the presently accepted classification of retinitis pigmentosa (RP) by inheritance pattern is undergoing a substantial refinement; the classical inheritance grouped categories of retinitis pigmentosa are proving inadequate.[12,13] Undoubtedly in future years, RP will be characterized in a far more specific manner. Already we know for some patients with dominant retinitis pigmentosa of a gene locus at 3q and of several seemingly independent mutations within the rhodopsin gene in this region.[13,14,15] These co-segregate with retinitis pigmentosa in families, and therefore, it is presumed that each mutation is associated with the phenotypic expression of the disorder.   Phenotypic differences for each mutant locus are currently being sought. [15]

It has long been known that the prevalence of refractive errors in retinitis pigmentosa departs considerably from the general norm. Assessment of the type, degree and course of refractive errors in the same patients might well prove useful in subclassifying retinitis pigmentosa.   Usher's report that 18 of 48 patients with retinitis pigmentosa were myopic was but the first of many.[16] For example, Raski (1938) found myopia in 46% of his retinitis pigmentosa patients compared to a 12% prevalence among 12,000 general patients in the same eye clinic.[17]   So striking was this coincidence, Raski speculated about a significant connection, perhaps etiologic, between the myopia and retinitis pigmentosa.   Francois and Verriest first detected differential distributions of refractive errors according to inheritance type, reporting a particularly high prevalence of myopia in x-linked cases.[18] Sieving and Fishman also noted a high frequency of myopia in x-linked patients adding that it was often of substantial degree and monotonic distribution.[19] Subsequently, Berson et al. emphasized the high fre-quency of astigmatism in x-linked patients with a vertical axis for the minus cylinder.[20]

Measurements of the components of refraction in retinitis pigmen-tosa are lacking and consequently the associated myopia cannot be characterized as refractive or axial.   Such an evaluation could prove useful in several respects.   First, if different gene loci in individual types of RP prove to have differential effects on anterior segment refractive power versus axial length, then the clinical classification of retinitis pigmentosa patients could be improved.   Second, association of known genetic retinal defects with altered eye form and optics could provide valuable insights into the retinal mechanisms influencing post-natal ocular growth.

CONGENITAL STATIONARY NIGHT BLINDNESS

Among ophthalmic conditions Congenital Stationary Night Blindness is unusual in several respects, not least of all its being well de-scribed by its name.   Night blindness dominates the clinical picture. Within narrow limits it is stationary and thought to be present at birth.   Importantly, it is not a single entity but instead a symptom complex representative of several highly distinctive disorders. Autosomal dominant, autosomal recessive and x-linked modes of inheri-tance have been recognized.   For complete diagnosis, fundus reflect-ometry and electroretinography should complement measurement of dark adaptation and spectral sensitivity.[21,22]

Congenital Stationary Night Blindness predominantly affects rods; diminished or extinguished rod function is revealed by dark adaptometry and electroretinography.   Because visual acuity usually measures in the 6/9 - 6/30 range, cone function is also affected to some extent. Despite the patient's inability to see in the dark, all genetic types

show normal rhodopsin bleaching and regeneration on fundus reflect-
ometry. Fundus albipunctatus, sometimes included in the classification
of Congenital Stationary Night Blindness, represents an exception to
this statement. Since rhodopsin kinetics are normal in the presence of
faulty dark adaptation and electrical signals, a defect in signal origin
or neurotransmission of rod impulses has been suggested. (for a detailed
review, see Sharp et al.)[22]

While neither the distribution nor extent of refractive errors are
remarkable in autosomal dominant disease, myopia is conspicuous in x-
linked and recessive Congenital Stationary Night Blindness. In fact,
the frequency is so high that myopia is commonly described as part of a
syndrome in classifications and in article titles. For example, Merin
et al. titled their report "Syndrome of Congenital High Myopia with
Nyctalopia."[23] Based on 32 eyes from 25 different families, the average
myopia was 8 diopters. The frequent description of myopic changes in
the fundus speaks for an axial elongation, but confirmatory ultrasound
measurements are lacking.

Miyake further subclassified Congenital Stationary Night Blindness
into complete and incomplete types.[24] His incomplete type differs from
classical x-linked Congenital Stationary Night Blindness in two respects. First, there is a small but definite rod component to the dark
adaptation curve. Second, cone and rod electroretinographic responses
are each present but compromised, as opposed to preservation of the
photopic cone electroretinogram and complete absence of the scotopic rod
B-wave in the complete type. In his report, all twenty patients classified as incomplete were male and had pedigrees typical of x-linked
inheritance. They may represent a special population. Miyake's
complete type seems identical to previously described cases of x-linked
or recessive Congenital Stationary Night Blindness with myopia. The
mean of myopic error of -7.9 diopters in these patients corresponds
precisely to what has previously been recorded by others.[23] In contrast, patients with the incomplete type apparently experience a broad
distribution of refractive errors rather than any specific error. The
mean refractive error for 36 eyes in this group was -0.8 diopters, but
the large standard deviation (± 5.4 diopters) indicates a wider than
normal scatter of individual refractions.

In x-linked and recessive Congenital Stationary Night Blindness,
astigmatism also appears common. Merin et al. state that "most cases"
have it while Hill et al. recorded cylindrical errors in 14 of 16
eyes.[23,25] No particular axis is favored. Although much has yet to be
done to achieve a satisfactory classification for the different types of
Congenital Stationary Night Blindness, Miyake's work has led to the
complete form with myopia being designated by a subscript 1. Recently
geneticists have established a linkage to Xp 11.3 for this form.[26,27]

CONGENITAL ACHROMATOPSIA

Congenital achromatopsia represents a failure of cone development
such that color vision is either absent or grossly defective.[28] Pathological examinations have been performed in only a few eyes; in the
main, they have demonstrated cones of abnormal morphology and reduced

number. Autosomal recessive and x-linked forms are recognized.[29] In both, patients generally present with nystagmus, reduced visual acuity and photophobia. Squint is also common. Regarding refraction, several features are noteworthy. If calculated as spherical equivalents, there is a wide spread of refractions with no central tendency.[30,31,32] For instance, in a recent survey of 16 congenital achromats,[31] 8 were hyperopic, 2 plano and 6 myopic, with a range in refraction from +7.75 to -11.75 diopters. More striking is the prevalence and quality of astigmatism in achromatopsia. Of 32 eyes in the Haegerstrom-Portnoy et al. survey, 28 required a cylindrical correction of -1 diopter or more, with 24 of the 28 eyes having the minus axis near the 180 degree meridian. Partly because of the nystagmus, no published data on axial length or the optical powers of the cornea and lens are available to permit an analysis of the sources of these refractive errors.

CONCLUSION

In each of the four hereditary retinal disorders just reviewed the normal fine control over ocular refraction fails. Regulatory failure can manifest itself as a high prevalence of hyperopia or myopia with or without accompanying astigmatism or as a general loss of regulatory precision as evidenced by a wide range of refractions without the sharp mid-zone cluster seen in normal populations. In several of the conditions cited, the nature of the refractive error is distinctive. Unfortunately, a full analysis of the source of refractive error cannot be undertaken in these conditions for lack of essential measurements on the components of refraction that are readily measured in the clinic by keratometry and ultrasonography. Such measurements of the individual components of the eye's refractive power would allow comparisons to values in the normal population. By way of example, Sorsby divided refractive errors into two main types: correlational and component.[5] In correlational errors, the individual elements of refraction measure within normal variation, but there is failure of the mechanism that harmonizes them. In contrast, component errors result from an extreme value of one component, most often axial length, whose refractive effects overwhelm any possible compensation by other components such as lens and/or cornea. To the degree that refractive errors reflect deficiencies in retinal performance, more precise delineation of the state of the eye's refractive components in juvenile retinal disorders might reveal alterations characteristic of each. Improved definition of refractive errors and corresponding measurements of eye size and shape might also prove a useful adjunct in the search now underway for phenotypic differences among patients with grouped conditions, such as dominant retinitis pigmentosa, where individual and distinctive mutations at differing loci within a single gene, for instance rhodopsin, can be responsible for the retinal pathology.[15]

In addition to providing a more rigorous description for clinical phenotypes, careful longitudinal and cross-sectional component analysis in refractive development of patients with hereditary retinal disorders might also provide critical insights into the mechanisms controlling refraction. Occurring as they do, sometimes early or sometimes late and affecting rods and/or cones to a varied degree, careful scrutiny of the eye growth effects of individual retinal disorders might well reveal important clues to the retinal mechanisms that participate in the postnatal regulation of eye growth.

REFERENCES

1. Raviola, E. and Wiesel T.N., An animal model of myopia. New Eng. J. Med., 312, 1609-1615, 1985.
2. Hoyt, C.S., Stone, R.D., Fromer, C. and Billson, F.A., Monocular axial myopia associated with neonatal eyelid closure in human infants. Am. J. Ophthalmol., 91, 197, 1981.
3. Wallman, J. Emmetropization and myopia: results from experimental studies, in Researches into Refractive Anomalies, Flom, M. and Grosvenor, T., Butterworth, in press.
4. Wildsoet, C.F. and Pettigrew, J.D., Kainic acid-induced eye enlargement in chickens: differential effects on anterior and posterior segments Invest. Ophthalmol. & Vis. Sci., 29, 311, 1988.
5. Sorsby, A., Modern Ophthalmology, vol. 3, 2nd ed., J.D. Lippincott Co., Philadelphia, 1972, chap. 2.
6. Young, F.A., Beattie, R.J., Newby, F.J. and Swindel, M.T., The Pullman study--a visual survey of Pullman school children, Am. J. Optom. and Arch. Am. Acad. Optom. 31(3), 111 and 31(4), 192, 1954.
7. Dagi, L.R., Leys, M.J., Hansen, R.M. and Fulton, A.B., Hyperopia in complicated Leber's congenital amaurosis, Arch. Ophthalmol., 108, 709, 1990.
8. Karel, I., Clinical picture of congenital diffuse tapetoretinal degeneration in 42 cases, Acta Univ. Carol. Med., 15, 259, 1969.
9. Foxman, S.G., Wirtschafter, J.D. and Letson, R.D., Leber's congenital amaurosis and high hyperopia: a discrete entity. Acta XXIV International Congress of Ophthalmology, pp. 55-58, 1983.
10. Wagner, R.S., Caputo, A.R., Nelson, L.B. and Zanoni, D., High hyperopia in Leber's congenital amaurosis, Arch. Ophthalmol., 103, 1507, 1985.
11. Uehara, F., Yasumura, D. and LaVail, M.M., personal communication, 1990.
12. Bhattacharya, S.S., Wright, A.F., Clayton, J.F., et al., Close genetic linkage between X-linked retinitis pigmentosa and a restriction fragment length polymorphism identified by recombinant DNA probe L1.28, Nature, 309, 253, 1984.
13. McWilliam, P., Farrar, G.J., Kenna, P., Bradley, D.G., Humphries, M.M., Sharp, E.M, McConnell, D.J., Lawler, M., Sheils, D., Ryan, C., Stevens, K., Daiger, S.P. and Humphries, P., Autosomal dominant retinitis pigmentosa (ADRP): localization of an ADRP gene to the long arm of chromosome 3, Genomics, 5, 619, 1989.
14. Dryja, T.P., McGee, T.L., Reichel, E., Hahn, L.B., Cowley, G.S., Yandell, D.W., Sandberg, M.A. and Berson, E.L., A point mutation of the rhodopsin gene in one form of retinitis pigmentosa, Nature, 343, 364, 1990.

15. Dryja, T.P., McGee, T.L., Hahn, L.B., Cowley, G.S., Olsson, J.E., Reichel, E., Sandberg, M.A. and Berson, E.L., Mutations within the rhodopsin gene in patients with autosomal dominant retinitis pigmentosa, New Eng. J. Med., 323, 1302, 1990.
16. Usher, C.H., The Bowman lecture: VI. On a few hereditary eye affections, in Trans. Ophthalmol. Soc. U.K., 55, 164, 1935.
17. Raski, K. Über die refraktion der patienten mit pigmentdegeneration der netzhaut, Acta Ophthalmolgica Kbh., 16, 295, 1938.
18. François, J. and Verriest, G., Etude biometrique de la retinopathie pigmentaire, Ann. d'Oculistique, 195, 937, 1962.
19. Sieving, P.A. and Fishman, G.A., Refractive errors of retinitis pigmentosa patients, Br. J. Ophthalmol., 62, 163, 1978.
20. Berson, E.L., Rosner, B. and Simonoff, B.A., Risk factors for genetic typing and detection in retinitis pigmentosa, Am. J. Ophthalmol., 89, 763, 1980.
21. Carr, R.E., Ripps, H., Siegel, I.M. and Weale, R.A., Rhodopsin and the electrical activity of the retina in congenital night blindness, Invest. Ophthalmol. Vis. Sci., 5, 497, 1966.
22. Sharp, D.M., Arden, G.B., Kemp, C.M., Hogg, C.R. and Bird, A.C, Mechanisms and sites of loss of scotopic sensitivity: a clinical analysis of congenital stationary night blindness, Clin. Vision Sci., 5, 217, 1990.
23. Merin, S., Rowe, H., Auerbach, E. and Landau, J., Syndrome of congenital high myopia with nyctalopia, Am. J. Ophthalmol., 70, 541, 1970.
24. Miyake, Y., Yagasaki, K., Horiguchi, M., Kawase, Y. and Kanda, T., Congenital stationary night blindness with negative electroretinogram. A new classification, Arch. Ophthalmol., 104, 1013, 1986.
25. Hill, D.A., Arbel, K.F. and Berson, E., Cone electroretinograms in congenital nyctalopia with myopia, Am. J. Ophthalmol., 78, 127, 1974.
26. Musarella, M.A., Weleber, R.G., Murphey, W.H., Young, R.S.L., Anson-Cartwright, L., Mets, M., Kraft, S.P., Polemeno, R., Litt, M. and Worton, R.G., Assignment of the gene for complete X-linked congenital stationary night blindness (CSNB1) to Xp11.3, Genomics 5, 727, 1989.
27. Orth, U., Schinzel, A., Mächler, M. and Gal, A., X-chromosomal erbliche Nachtblindheit: Erkennen von Überträgerinnen durch Segregationsanalyse mit gekoppelten DNA-Markern, Klin. Mbl. Augenheilk., 196, 269, 1990.
28. Pokorny, J., Smith, V.C., Verriest, G. and Pinckers, A.J., Eds. Congenital and Acquired Color Vision Defects, Grune & Stratton, New York, 1979, 232.
29. Pokorny, J., Smith, V.C., Pinckers, A.J. and Cosijnsen, M., Classification of complete and incomplete autosomal recessive achromatopsia, Graefe's Arch. clin. exp. Ophthal., 219, 121, 1982.
30. Auerbach, E. and Merin, S., Achromatopsia with amblyopia. A clinical and electroretinographical study of 39 cases, Documenta Ophth., 37, 79, 1974.

31. Haegerstrom-Portnoy, G., Friedman, N., Adams, A.J., Schenck, M. and Hewlett, S., Vision of rod monochromats, <u>Invest. Ophthalmol. Vis. Sci.</u>(suppl.), 29, 74, 1988.

32. Evans, N.M., Fielder, A.R. and Mayer, D.L., Ametropia in congenital cone deficiency--achromatopsia: a defect of emmetropisation?, <u>Clin. Vision Sci.</u> 4, 129, 1989.

X-LINKED RETINITIS PIGMENTOSA:
ROD AND CONE ERG ABNORMALITIES IN HETEROZYGOTES

Samuel G. Jacobson, Katsuya Yagasaki and William J. Feuer

Department of Ophthalmology, University of Miami School of Medicine,
Bascom Palmer Eye Institute, Miami, Florida

Heterozygotes (carriers) of X-linked retinitis pigmentosa (XLRP) can show a tapetal-like reflex and/or retinal regions with pigmentary degeneration on ophthalmoscopic examination, and visual dysfunction by electroretinographic (ERG) and psychophysical testing.[1-7] In order to quantify and extend certain observations made in previous ERG studies of XLRP heterozygotes, we measured 12 parameters from the ERGs of both eyes of 22 XLRP heterozygotes and made statistical comparisons with results from 22 female control subjects.

We determined which rod and cone ERG amplitude, timing and sensitivity parameters were abnormal. Then, we investigated if there were any patterns to the rod and cone dysfunction by testing for correlations between parameters. Finally, the data from this study are drawn together with those in earlier work to provide guidelines for the minimum ERG evaluation of the heterozygous state of XLRP.

SUBJECTS AND METHODS

The XLRP heterozygotes (n=22; ages 18-71 years; mean age 40.3 years) in this study were from 16 different families. The criteria for selection of the heterozygotes and the results of their clinical examinations (including visual acuities, refractive errors and fundus findings) have been published.[7] There were 22 female control subjects (ages 16-64; mean age 39.5 years). Informed consent was obtained from the subjects in the study after full explanation of the procedures involved.

Electroretinography was performed with techniques already described and waveforms were measured conventionally.[7] The Naka-Rushton equation $[V = Vmax \cdot I^n/(I^n + K^n)]$ was applied to the measured amplitudes from the rod and cone flicker intensity series.[4,8-10] In the equation, V is rod b-wave or cone flicker peak-to-peak amplitude; Vmax, the amplitude at response saturation; I, the stimulus intensity; K, intensity at 1/2 Vmax; and n, the exponent responsible for the slope of the function.

The following 12 ERG parameters (numbered as in Tables 1 and 2) were used in the data analyses: b-wave amplitude [1] and implicit time [2] of the suprathreshold rod response to the 'dim blue' flash of a scotopically-matched pair of stimuli; Vmax [3] and log K [4] from the rod b-wave intensity response function; peak-to-peak amplitude [5] and timing [6] of a suprathreshold white light flicker response; Vmax [7] and log K [8] from the cone flicker intensity response function; amplitude [9] and timing [10] of the response to single white flashes at a suprathreshold intensity in the light-adapted state; and the amplitude [11] and implicit time [12] of the dark-adapted cone response, the digitally-subtracted result of the two waveforms from the scotopically-matched stimuli.[11]

Statistical analyses of the ERG data are in Tables 1 and 2. Table 1: Two sample t-tests were used to make intergroup comparisons of heterozygotes and controls for the 12 ERG parameters. For each parameter, the eye with the result tending more toward the 'abnormal' or more indicative of 'disease' was chosen for analysis [i.e. lower value for amplitude (parameter nos. 1,3,5,7,9,11), slower timing (nos. 2,6,10,12), and larger log K (nos. 4,8)] in both heterozygote and normal groups.[7] Table 2: Non-parametric correlations, Kendall's Tau-b (T_b), were used to investigate relationships between parameters in controls and heterozygotes and were evaluated separately in right and left eyes and with data from both eyes combined. As the results of all three analyses were very similar with respect to both correlation coefficients and significance levels, only the combined right eye - left eye data are presented. [12] To see if the change in pairs of parameters from the less to the more 'affected' eyes of heterozygotes tended to be in the same direction as across the group, we determined the slope of the vector connecting the two eyes of each person in the two parameter space for each pair of ERG measurements. These slopes were weighted by the length of this vector:[13]

$$\sqrt{(P_{1RE} - P_{1LE})^2 + (P_{2RE} - P_{2LE})^2} ,$$

where P_x is the value of parameter no. x; RE and LE are right and left eyes respectively. Two eyes with large interocular differences in both parameters would therefore be weighted more heavily than two eyes with similar values in one or both parameters. The Wilcoxon signed rank test was used to determine whether these slopes were significantly different from zero.

RESULTS

In Table 1, the t-tests compare the means of each ERG parameter value in the heterozygote and the control groups. All rod and cone amplitude parameters were significantly lower and all cone timing parameters significantly 'delayed' in heterozygotes compared to controls. The rod b-wave implicit time and log K for rod and cone ERGs were not significantly different in the two groups.[7]

Table 2 presents the results of investigation into correlations between rod and cone ERG parameters. In heterozygotes, the Kendall's (T_b) correlation coefficients show moderately strong, highly significant correlations between the rod and cone amplitude parameters. Pearson correlation coefficients (not shown) for these relationships were typically about 0.6. These parameters were similarly correlated in controls. Also significantly correlated, albeit more weakly, were log rod amplitude with measures of light-adapted cone timing in heterozygotes only, and rod sensitivity with cone sensitivity (i.e. log K parameters) in both heterozygotes and controls.

TABLE 1
Rod and Cone ERG Parameters in XLRP Heterozygotes
versus Normal Subjects

Parameter No.	Minimum or Maximum Value[a]		
	Normals mean (s.d.)	Heterozygotes mean (s.d.)	p-value
Rod			
1 Amplitude[b]	291.9 (52.4)	195.2 (85.8)	<0.001
2 Implicit Time[c]	76.3 (4.6)	80.1 (9.4)	0.1
3 Vmax[b]	360.0 (63.1)	242.4 (97.6)	<0.001
4 Log K	-2.287 0.167	-2.367 0.317	ns
Cone Flicker			
5 Amplitude	94.5 (27.8)	62.4 (28.7)	0.001
6 Timing	27.0 (1.0)	32.0 (4.1)	<0.001
7 Vmax	149.7 (38.4)	99.6 (48.6)	<0.001
8 Log K	-1.188 (0.268)	-1.101 (0.391)	ns
Cone, single flash, light-adapted			
9 Amplitude	73.3 (21.5)	54.8 (28.2)	0.019
10 Implicit time	27.1 (0.9)	29.9 (2.5)	<0.001
Cone, single flash, dark-adapted			
11 Amplitude	160.6 (48.5)	90.9 (62.4)	<0.001
12 Implicit time	45.9 (2.4)	48.5 (3.8)	0.013

s.d.=standard deviation
ns=not significant
[a], minimum amplitude parameters, maximum timing parameters, and higher intensity value for log K (highest intensity=0)
[b], amplitude parameters are in microvolts
[c], timing parameters are in milliseconds

TABLE 2
Correlation of Rod and Cone ERG Parameters

Parameter Nos.	Normals		Heterozygotes	
	Non-parametric correlations[a]		Non-parametric correlations[a]	Weighted Wilcoxon Signed Rank
Rod vs. cone amplitudes				
1 vs. 5	.57 (<.001)		.46 (<.001)	<.0001
1 vs. 9	.35 (<.001)		.50 (<.001)	.002
1 vs. 11	.23 (.016)		.49 (<.001)	.031
Rod amplitude[b] vs. cone timing				
1 vs. 6	-.08 (ns)		-.31 (.001)	.006
1 vs. 10	-.17 (.07)		-.34 (<.001)	ns
1 vs. 12	.14 (.10)		-.15 (.09)	ns
Rod vs. cone sensitivity (log K)				
4 vs. 8	.30 (.002)		.33 (<.001)	ns

[a], values shown are T_b (p-value)
[b], in log units
ns=not significant

Figure 1 shows graphs of the relationships in heterozygotes (squares) and controls (small circles) between: A) rod amplitude and dark-adapted cone amplitude (nos. 1 vs 11); B) rod amplitude and cone flicker amplitude (nos. 1 vs 5); and C) log rod amplitude and cone flicker timing (nos. 1 vs 6). Both eyes of each heterozygote are plotted and connected by lines; both eyes of controls are also plotted. As is evident from these graphs, the rod and both cone amplitude parameters were positively correlated in controls and heterozygotes while only in heterozygotes was cone timing inversely proportional to log rod b-wave amplitude.

The presence or absence of a tapetal-like reflex in heterozygotes has been used to subdivide XLRP families for molecular biology studies.[14] We enquired if there were any obvious differences in ERG relationships between heterozygotes with a tapetal-like reflex or from a family with tapetal-like reflexes (n = 10) and those without (n = 12). The graphs in Figure 1 show no obvious differences between the two groups; intergroup comparisons of minimum/maximum values confirmed that there were no significant differences.

DISCUSSION

Rod and cone ERG amplitude parameters were significantly lower and cone timing was delayed in heterozygotes compared with control subjects; these results are in agreement with those from earlier studies.[3-7] Although isolated ERG amplitude and timing abnormalities have been reported, more often previous studies have found combinations of parameter values to be abnormal in heterozygotes. The statistical analyses of our data from individual eyes revealed that there is a strong positive correlation of rod and cone ERG amplitude parameters in heterozygotes, like that in controls. This implies a parallel loss of rod and cone photoreceptor-mediated function in eyes of XLRP heterozygotes. What exactly this means at the cellular level becomes, of course, speculative. Arden et al[4] suggested that reduced rod Vmax without change in log K predicts a loss of rod function in relatively large patches of retina. Accepting this hypothesis as tenable and adding our data on cone parameters and the relationship of rod to cone ERG amplitude data, it might be predicted that both rod and cone function in large patches of retina would be seriously impaired, if not lost. Supporting this prediction are psychophysical evidence in some heterozygotes[15,16] and the finding of patches of retina with both rod and cone degeneration, as well as normal retinal areas, in a morphological study of an XLRP heterozygote.[17]

The negative correlation of log rod amplitude to cone flicker timing found in heterozygotes in this study is also evident when the tabulated data of earlier ERG studies are analyzed as in Table 2 of the present study [reference 3: (right eyes), T_b = -0.28, p-value = .043; reference 5, T_b = -0.52, p-value < .001]. This same relationship was explored in RP patients and a hypothesis involving impaired rod-cone interaction was advanced to explain at least some of the apparent dependency of cone timing on rod amplitude.[11]

It is recognized that accurate genetic diagnosis in RP is important for counselling of families as well as for genetic research. Despite the increasing importance of molecular genetics techniques, there can be little argument that ophthalmoscopy and/or the ERG are

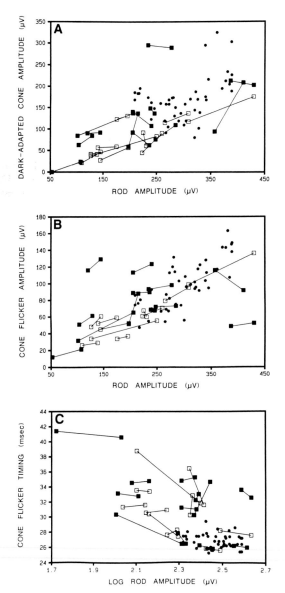

Figure 1 - Relationships between rod b-wave amplitude and cone ERG parameters in heterozygotes (unfilled squares, families with tapetal-like reflex; filled squares, no tapetal-like reflexes) and control subjects (circles). Lines connect data from the two eyes of each heterozygote.

currently the simplest methods for determining or confirming the heterozygous state of XLRP. Based on the results of this study and others in the literature, some guidelines can be offered for the minimum ERG examination and analysis in women being investigated for the heterozgous state of XLRP.

Given only one ERG test to do, it should be the cone flicker ERG performed in both eyes with white light at a single intensity that would evoke a response in normals with amplitudes of at least 40-50μV. The most important measurement to make therefrom would be timing. The facts to support this recommendation are as follows: 1) cone flicker timing is the most frequent or at least one of the most frequent ERG abnormalities in heterozygotes; 2) the other common abnormality, rod and/or cone amplitude reduction, is reflected in the delays of cone flicker timing; 3) normal amplitude ranges of rod, cone or mixed ERGs are wide and any laboratory establishing these norms would need many more control subjects (over a large age range[18]) than with cone flicker timing, the normal range of which is usually quite limited; 4) although both eyes of heterozygotes generally showed delayed timing to cone flicker in our previous work,[7] bilateral recordings would detect the minority of carriers who could show normal timing in one eye but an abnormally delayed signal in the other eye.

ACKNOWLEDGMENTS

This investigation was supported in part by the National Retinitis Pigmentosa Foundation, Inc. (Baltimore, MD), The Chatlos Foundation, Inc. (Longwood, FL), and Public Health Service Research Grant EY05627 (to SGJ). Dr. Yagasaki is now with the Department of Ophthalmology, Nagoya University School of Medicine, Japan.

REFERENCES

1. Krill AE, Observations of carriers of X-chromosomal-linked chorioretinal degenerations: Do they support the "inactivation hypothesis"? Am. J. Ophthalmol. 64,1029,1967.

2. Bird AC, X-linked retinitis pigmentosa. Br. J. Ophthalmol. 59,177,1975.

3. Berson EL, Rosen JB, Simonoff EA, Electroretinographic testing as an aid in detection of carriers of X-chromosome-linked retinitis pigmentosa, Am. J. Ophthalmol.87,460,1979.

4. Arden GB, Carter RM, Hogg CR, et al., A modified ERG technique and the results obtained in X-linked retinitis pigmentosa, Br. J. Ophthalmol. 67,419,1983.

5. Fishman GA, Weinberg AB, McMahon TT, X-linked recessive retinitis pigmentosa : Clinical characteristics of carriers, Arch. Ophthalmol. 104,1329,1986.

6. Peachey NS, Fishman GA, Derlacki DJ, Alexander KR, Rod and cone dysfunction in carriers of X-linked retinitis pigmentosa, Ophthalmology 95,677,1988.

7. Jacobson SG, Yagasaki K, Feuer WJ, Román AJ, Interocular asymmetry of visual function in heterozygotes of X-linked retinitis pigmentosa, Exp. Eye Research 48,679,1989.

8. Yagasaki K, Jacobson SG, Apáthy PP, et al., Rod and cone psychophysics and electroretinography: methods for comparison in retinal degenerations, Doc. Ophthalmol. 69,119,1988.

9. Naka KI, Rushton WAH: S-potentials from colour units in the retina of fish (Cyprinidae), J. Physiol. 185,536,1966.

10. Massof RW, Wu L, Finkelstein D, et al., Properties of electroretinographic intensity-response function in retinitis pigmentosa, Doc. Ophthalmol. 57,279,1984.

11. Birch DG, Sandberg MA, Dependence of cone b-wave implicit time on rod amplitude in retinitis pigmentosa, Vision Res. 27,1105,1987.

12. Ederer F, Shall we count numbers of eyes or numbers of subjects? Arch. Ophthalmol. 89,1,1973.

13. Morrison DF, Multivariate Statistical Methods, McGraw-Hill, New York, 1967,44.

14. Nussbaum RL, Lewis RA, Lesko JG, et al., Mapping X-linked ophthalmic diseases: II. Linkage relationship of X-linked retinitis pigmentosa to X chromosomal short arm markers, Hum. Genet. 70,45,1985.

15. Jacobson SG, Voigt W, Parel JM, et al., Automated light- and dark-adapted perimetry for evaluating retinitis pigmentosa, Ophthalmology 93,1604,1986.

16. Jacobson SG, Chiu MT, Yagasaki K, et al., Cone and rod dysfunction in carriers of X-linked retinitis pigmentosa, Invest. Ophthalmol. Vis. Sci. Suppl. 28,112,1987.

17. Szamier RB, Berson EL, Retinal histopathology of a carrier of X-chromosome-linked retinitis pigmentosa, Ophthalmol. 92,271,1985.

18. Weleber RG, The effect of age on human cone and rod ganzfeld electroretinograms, Invest. Ophthalmol. Vis. Sci. 20,392,1981.

EARLY ELECTROPHYSIOLOGICAL
FINDINGS IN CASES WITH METABOLIC DISEASES

Lillemor Wachtmeister
Department of Ophthalmology
Karolinska Institute/St. Erik's Eye Hospital
Stockholm, Sweden

ABSTRACT

The early ophthalmological and electrophysiological findings in some rare cases with metabolic diseases are presented.

In the cases of 5-oxoprolinuria, an "inborn error of metabolism," both the a- and b-wave amplitudes of the electroretinogram (ERG) were diminished and the amplitudes of the individual oscillatory potentials (OPs) either decreased or abolished, indicating an early disturbed rod pigment synthesis and photoreceptor function. In the patient with juvenile neuronal ceroid lipofuscinosis (JNCL), a "non-ganglioside storage disease," the amplitude of the b-wave was significantly reduced and the OPs all abolished. Thus, in the early course of JNCL the primary damage seems to be located in the inner part of the retina. In a case with long standing malabsorption of vitamin A causing a disturbed metabolism of rhodopsin and iodopsin, the summed amplitude of the OPs was lower during the initial phase of very low retinol level (0.21 μmol) and elevated rod as well as cone visual sensory thresholds. Hence, in this case with reversible and comparatively early form of vitamin A hypovitaminosis, the first measurable electrophysiological manifestation indicates a disturbed interaction of rod and cone activity.

In conclusion, the present report shows the usefulness of electrophysiological examination in cases with metabolic retinal diseases. Although there were minimal, if any, funduscopic changes, the ERG was pathological. The most sensitive test was the measurement of the OPs, indicating a disturbed function in the inner part of the retina and interaction between rod and cone activity.

I. INTRODUCTION

In many forms of retinal degeneration there is an underlying metabolic defect. Most cases are associated with a systemic disease, as there is a general metabolic disturbance affecting other parts of the body as well. Many of these metabolic degenerative retinal diseases are hereditary. Some are exceedingly rare and often inherited in a recessive mode. Others are acquired ones, secondary to i.e. malnutrition and seldom seen nowadays.

In many types of metabolic retinal dystrophy the fundus appearance may be non-specific. Very few cases have been examined (morphologically as well as functionally) in the early course of the disease and in most cases the exact cellular lesion is therefore unknown. The present report describes three rare metabolic types of retinal degenerations during a relatively early part of the disease. Although there were very few clinical ophthalmological findings, they all showed a disturbed retinal electrophysiological function which indicated the part of the retina that was primarily lesioned. The complete findings of these cases have been published elsewhere.[1,2,3,4,5]

II. CASE REPORTS

A. 5-OXOPROLINURIA (HEREDITARY GLUTATHIONE SYNTHETASE DEFICIENCY)

5-Oxoprolinuria, an inborn error of metabolism, is a rare hereditary autosomal recessive disease. The metabolic lesion is located at the glutathione synthesis step of the Γ-glutamyl cycle.[6] Markedly decreased concentrations of sulfhydryl containing glutathione and very low glutathione synthetase activity are found intracellularly. Lack of glutathione has been suggested to result in oxidative damage in specific regions of the brain. We studied two sisters with glutathione synthesis deficiency and found primary lesions also in the (neuro) retina, another part of the brain.[3,4]

The two sisters (J.G., 10 years and H.G., 7 years) have no other siblings. There was no known consanguinity. Funduscopy of both sisters showed very slightly disturbed foveal reflexes which were more ovale in shape than normal. The younger girl showed slight retinal peripapillary atrophy and delicate granular hyper-pigmentations in the peripheral parts of both fundi. Dark adaptation curves measured with a Goldmann Weekers adaptometer revealed slight but clearly reproducible elevations (½-1 log unit) of the threshold after thirty minutes of dark adaptation compared to normals in the same age group. Visual acuity, perimetry and colour sense were normal in both girls.

Routine single flash electroretinograms (ERG) were repeatedly pathological in both patients. The a- and b-wave amplitudes were diminished (Figure 1A) and the amplitudes of the oscillatory potentials (OPs) decreased or abolished (Figure 1B). This indicates a more generally disturbed electrophysiological function both in the outer layer of the retina, representing the a-wave, and the inner portion, reflected by the b-wave and the OPs.[7,8]

Sulfhydryl groups have been shown to be involved in the synthesis and bleaching of rhodopsin and have been suggested to be associated with visual excitation and phototransduction.[9] Therefore, these findings of an elevated threshold of the rod part of the adaptometric curve may indicate disturbed rod pigment (rhodopsin) synthesis and photoreceptor function, possibly caused by abnormal levels of sulfhydryl compounds.

Visual evoked cortical potentials (VECP) in response to checkerboard stimulation were normal in both sisters in the early course of the disease. The electroretinograms were also used to study the effects of longterm therapy with antioxidants (Thiola[R] - mercapto propionyl glycine and/or Vitamin E). However, no appreciable effect was observed either ophthalmologically or electrophysiologically.

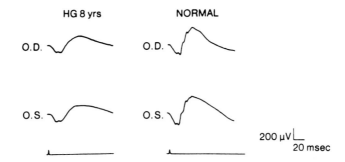

FIGURE 1A

Electroretinograms (ERGs) of both eyes of H.G. with 5-oxoprolinuria at the age of eight years recorded with a long time constant (= 1 sec) after ten minutes' dark adaptation at an interval of one min in response to full field flashes of maximal intensity (16) from a Grass photostimulator placed 75 cm from the eyes. For comparison, ERGs recorded from a person of the same age and normal eyes are shown to the right. The amplitudes of both the a- and b-waves were decreased about 40% in the patient with glutathione synthetase deficiency compared to the normal of the same age. OD = right eye, OS = left eye.

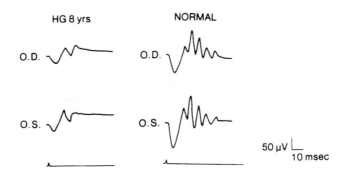

FIGURE 1B

ERGs recorded from the same patient as in Figure 1A with a short time constant (= 15 msec) in dark adaptation at an interval of 15 sec. The same photostimulator as in Figure 1A but placed 20 cm in front of the eyes. For comparison, ERGs recorded from a person of the same age with normal eyes are shown to the right. The amplitude of the second OP is substantially diminished and the latter abolished in the patient with glutathione synthetase deficiency. OD = right eye, OS = left eye.

B. JUVENILE NEURONAL CEROID LIPOFUSCINOSIS (JNCL)

Neuronal ceroid lipofuscinosis, a cerebroretinal degeneration inherited in a recessive autosomal mode, is the most common type of the so-called "nonganglioside" storage disease. It has been reported to have a deficiency of the selenium containing enzyme glutathione peroxidase[10,11] and thus a defective utilization of glutathione in the perioxidase reaction. Defective peroxidation has been postulated to cause free radical accumulation, damage to polyunsaturated fatty acids and subsequent formation of ceroid lipofuscin.[12] It is manifested by visual and intellectual deterioration, seizures and usually death before the age of 18 years.[13] An early case of JNCL is reported and, although there were very few clinical signs of retinal abnormalities, the ERGs were abnormal.[1,2]

The patient, 5½ years old, is the sister of a 10 year old boy who has JNCL. Both parents are in good health and non-consanguinous. Both fundi demonstrated minimal changes in the macula in the form of absent foveal reflexes and discrete yellow-white disclike oedema in both maculae. Her dark adaptation curve showed about 1 log unit increase of the threshold after 30 minutes compared to normals in the same age group. Her vision was 20/40 (Snellens E, 5 m) in both eyes. Binocular colour vision testing with pseudoisochromatic plates (Ishihara and Boström-Kugelberg) showed that she correctly named the colours. Peripheral visual fields tested in a Goldmann perimeter was normal in her right eye but difficult to evaluate in her left eye due to variable cooperation.

The ERGs of both eyes showed a significantly decreased amplitude of the b-wave and a slightly but not significantly reduced a-wave (Figure 2A). The OPs were all abolished (Figure 2B). Flicker ERG (30 Hz) showed low but distinct amplitudes. These findings suggest that the photoreceptors still seem to function in the early course of the disease, as the a-wave reflecting the activity of the photoreceptors in the outer retinal layer did not show any significant change. The primary damage seems to be located in the inner part of the retina, where the OPs and the b-wave have their origins.[7,8] This is in accordance with biochemical and morphological findings in canine NCL,[14] in which an early accumulation of lipofuscin in the ganglion cells and the cells of the inner nuclear layer of the retina has been described.

Visual evoked responses were of normal amplitudes and latencies bilaterally.

A treatment with selenium and Vitamin E seemed temporarily to improve visual function but no significant change of the ERG was found.

C. VITAMIN A DEFICIENCY

Vitamin A is an essential part of the photosensitive pigment of the rods and cones (rhodopsin and iodopsin). If the Vitamin A supply decreases, the cone pigments may capture all they require, while the rods will suffer from deficit. The first measurable clinical manifestation of Vitamin A hypovitaminosis is night blindness. In very severe Vitamin A deficiency irreversible degeneration of the retina and blindness occurs. We describe a case of long-standing malabsorption of Vitamin A causing a reversible and comparatively early form of hemeralopia.[5] The first measurable electrophysiological manifestation was a decreased summed amplitude of the OPs of the ERG, indicating a disturbed interaction between rod and cone activity.

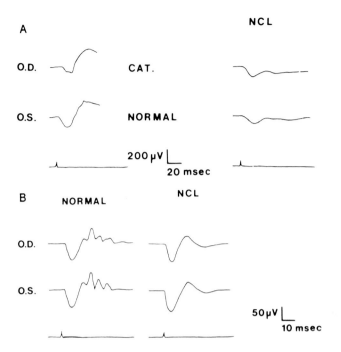

FIGURE 2A

On the right, ERGs of the patient with JNCL are depicted. The same recording conditions as in Figure 1A were used. For comparison, ERGs recorded from a patient of the same age with a cataract of the right eye and a normal left eye are shown on the left.

FIGURE 2B

On the right, ERGs recorded from the patient with JNCL are depicted. The same recording conditions as in Figure 1B were used. For comparison, ERGs recorded from a person of the same age but with normal eyes are shown on the left.

The patient is a 52-year old woman suffering from severe malabsorption of fat soluble vitamins after an intestinal by-pass operation due to morbid obesity. Six years later she was admitted to the hospital because of a six-month history of reduced vision, especially at night. Serum retinol was severely decreased (0.21 μmol/l).

Fundus examination revealed normal findings for her age. Dark adaptation curves measured in a Goldmann Weekers adaptometer after preadaptation to light using a standard technique showed a severely affected night vision (Figure 3). The cone sensitivity was reduced by about one log unit compared to normal. Rod vision was depressed to a greater extent and the threshold elevated above the normal by two and a half log units. Colour vision tested with pseudoisochromatic plates (Boström II and Boström-Kugelberg) showed a red-green defect. Her visual acuity was slightly decreased in both eyes (0.7 c.c./0.9 c.c.). Goldmann perimetry was normal.

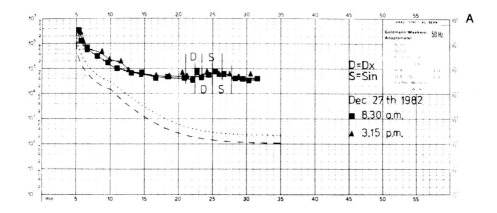

FIGURE 3

Dark adaptation curves of the patient with Vitamin A deficiency measured on the same day (December 27th, 1982) before (8.30 a.m.) and after (3.15 p.m.) injection of 300 000 IU vitamin A oleate for an oleate absorption test performed at 9.30 a.m. The dashed and stippled curves describe the mean and the upper limit of the normal range (+2.5) for a person of the same age group.

The ERG recorded before the therapy started showed normal amplitude and time characteristics of the major components (a- and b-waves) (Figure 4A left column). However, the summed amplitude of the OPs was subnormal (28-32%) (Figure 4A right column). Treatment with Vitamin A (i.m. injections and orally) increased the serum retinol level. Even though the retinol had not reached normal levels (0.52) and the cone and rod visual thresholds were elevated about 1 log unit, the characteristics of the OPs had normalized (Figure 4B right column).

These observations suggest that a disturbed interaction between rod and cone activity is a relatively early sign of retinal dysfunction in Vitamin A hypovitaminosis, as the OPs have been shown to represent both scotopic and photopic systems and reflect neuronal activity in the inner part of the retina.[15,16] Furthermore, the OPs seem to be the most sensitive of the components of the ERG to indicate electrophysiological malfunction of the retina in cases of Vitamin A deficiency.

III. DISCUSSION AND CONCLUSIONS

It is interesting to note that, in the three different types of retinal metabolic diseases with very sparse if any funduscopic findings, the ERG was pathological in three separate ways, which indicated where in the retinal neuronal pathway the lesions were located. The ERGs of the two sisters with 5-oxoprolinuria and well compensated acidosis showed decreased amplitudes of the a-wave as well as the b-wave and the OPs. These findings indicate strongly that the primary lesion is located

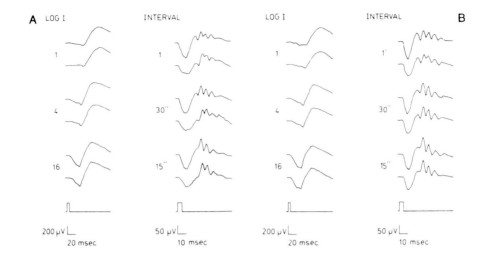

FIGURE 4A

Electroretinograms of the patient with vitamin A hypovitaminosis before therapy started. The ERGs were evoked by single white flashes in dark adaptation. In the left columns recordings with a long time constant (T = 1 sec) and in response to flashes of different intensities are shown. In the right column recordings with a short time constant (T = 15 msec) in response to flashes of maximum intensity (16) elicited at different interstimulus intervals are depicted.

FIGURE 4B

Electroretinograms from the same patient recorded during vitamin A therapy, but during a recurrence of hypovitaminosis. Same recording conditions as in Figure 4A.

in the photoreceptors, which in turn will affect the response of the second and third order neurons in the retinal pathway. Thus, the reduction of the amplitudes of the b-wave and OPs seems to be a consequence of a disturbed photoreceptor function in this disease. These observations are new and may aid in the identification of the more exact underlying mechanism of dysfunction of the photoreceptors and also may be a better tailored cure for this disease in the future.

In the case of JNCL, there was a significantly diminished b-wave and abolished OPs, but the a-wave was not significantly changed. This observation helped to identify the level of primary damage to the inner part of the retina also in human NCL. To the author's knowledge, this has not been known previously.

In the case of Vitamin A deficiency, the major components were unchanged, whereas the summed amplitude of the OPs was reduced when both the rod and cone visual thresholds were elevated and the colour vision defective. Thus, the OPs proved to be a useful tool to identify an early imbalance between the finely tuned interaction between scotopic and photopic systems in the inner part of the retina.

Secondly, the present findings are also in accordance with previous suggestions that the OPs seem to have separate origins compared to the major components, a- and b-waves.[7,8]

In conclusion, the present report shows the advantage of electrophysiological testing in cases with metabolic retinal diseases. Although there were minor, if any, ophthalmoscopic changes, the ERG was abnormal, and in different ways. The most sensitive test was the measurement of the OPs, indicating a disturbed function in the inner part of the retina and interaction between rod and cone activity.

IV. REFERENCES

1. Wachtmeister, L., Early clinical and electrophysiological diagnosis of neuronal ceroid lipofuscinosis. A case report. Ceroid-lipofuscinosis (Batten's disease) - Armstrong, D., Koppang, N. and Rider, J.A., Eds., Elsevier Biomedical Press, Amsterdam 1982, 95.
2. Wachtmeister, L., Clinical and electrophysiological findings in an early case of juvenile neuronal ceroid lipofuscinosis treated with selenium. In Docum. Ophthal. Proc. Series Vol 31 Niemeyer G. and Huber, Ch. Eds, Dr. W. Junk Publishers, The Hague, 1982, 209.
3. Wachtmeister, L. and Larsson, A., Ophthalmological findings in two sisters with hereditary glutathione synthetase deficiency (5-oxoprolinuria). Proceedings of the VIIth Congress of the European Society of Ophthalmology, Helsinki, 1985, 259.
4. Larsson, A., Wachtmeister, L., von Wendt, L., Andersson, R., Hagenfeldt, L. and Herrin, K.M., Psychometric and therapeutic investigation in two sisters with hereditary glutathione synthetase deficiency (5-oxoprolinuria), Neuropediatrics 16, 131, 1985.
5. Wachtmeister L., Björkhem, I., Diczfalusy, U. and Emami, A., Attempts to define the minimal serum level of Vitamin A required for normal visual function in a patient with severe fat malabsorption. Acta Ophthalmol. (Copenh) 66, 341, 1988.
6. Wellner, V.P., Sekura R., Meister, A. and Larsson, A., Glutathione synthetase deficiency, an inborn error of metabolism involving the Γ-glutamyl cycle in patients with 5-oxoprolinuria (pyroglutamic aciduria), Proc. Natl. Acad. Sci USA 71, 2505, 1974.
7. Wachtmeister, L. and Dowling, J., The oscillatory potentials of the mudpuppy retina. Invest. Ophthalmol. Vis Sci 17, 1176, 1978.
8. Heynen, H., Wachtmeister, L. and van Norren, D., Origin of the oscillatory potentials in the primate retina. Vision Res. 25, 1365, 1985.
9. Wald, G., and Brown P.K., The role of sulfhydryl groups in the bleaching and synthesis of rhodopsin. J. Gen. Physiol. 35, 797, 1952.
10. Jensen, E.G., Shukla, V.K.S., Gissel-Nielsen, G. and Clausen, J., Biochemical abnormalities in Batten's syndrome. Scand. J. Clin. Lab. Invest. 38, 309, 1978.
11. Jensen, G. and Clausen, J., Glutathione peroxidase in leucocytes, erythrocytes and serum in patients with juvenile type of neuronal ceroid lipofuscinosis.

Ceroid Lipofuscinosis (Batten's disease). Armstrong, D., Koppang, N. and Rider, J.A., Eds. Elsvier Biomedical Press, Amsterdam 1982, 301.

12. Zeman, W., Donahue, S., Dyken, P. and Green, J., The neuronal ceroid lipofuscinosis (Batten-Vogt syndrome). Handbook of Clinical Neurology. Leucodystrophies and Poliodystrophies. Vinken, P.J. and Bruyn, G.W., Eds. North Holland Publishing Co. Vol. 10, 1970, 617.

13. Zeman, W. and Dyken, P., Neuronal ceroid lipofuscinosis (Batten's disease): Relationship to amaurotic family idiocy. Pediatrics. 44, 570, 1969.

14. Armstrong, D., Neville, H., Koppang, N., and Wehling, D., Morphological and biochemical abnormalities in a model of retinal degeneration: Canine ceroid lipofuscinosis. Int. Symp. of the Neurochemistry in Retina), Athens, Greece, Aug. 28th-Sept 1st, 1979.

15. Wachtmeister, L., Incremental thresholds of the oscillatory potentials of the human electroretinogram in response to coloured light. Acta Ophthalmol. (Copenh) 52, 378, 1974.

16. Wachtmeister, L., Luminosity functions of the oscillatory potentials of the human electroretinogram. Acta Ophthalmol. (Copenh.) 52, 353, 1974.

17. Stodtmeister, R., The spectral sensitivity functions of human ERG wavelets. Ophthalmic Res. 5, 21, 1973.

CONE-ROD DEGENERATIONS

Bettina Sadowski and Eberhart Zrenner

University Eye Hospital, Department of Pathophysiology of Vision and Neuro-
Ophthalmology, Tuebingen, FRG.

KEY WORDS

Color vision, cone dystrophy, cone-rod dystrophy, dark adaptation, dazzle
sensitivity, electrooculogram, electrophysiology, electroretinogram, inheritance,
mesoptometry, pattern electroretinogram, perimetry, psychophysics.

I. INTRODUCTION

Cone degenerations and cone-rod degenerations in man have not drawn a lot of
attention in recent years, compared with rod and rod-cone degenerations. This is
puzzling, since a large number of new findings have emerged in molecular biology and
in animal studies that clearly indicate that degeneration mechanisms in cones may be
quite different from those in rods, e.g. as far as the fatty acid metabolism is concerned [1]
or the interstitial retinol-binding protein (IRBP) [2, 3, 4] or the interphotoreceptor matrix
(IPM) [5].

The first step for a reasonable study in humans is to have an ophthalmologically
well investigated, large group of patients suffering from cone degenerations [6].
Considering the comparatively rare occurrence of isolated cone degenerations, this seems
like a major obstacle. Investigations in large families with this disease are even more
rare [7], but are very helpful concerning investigations of the inheritance pattern. The
present paper is concerned with data of 40 patients with cone and cone-rod degeneration,
investigated within the last 5 years. Psychophysical and electrophysiological results are
presented and compared to each other, shedding new light on this group of diseases.
Several points need clarification beforehand: by definition patients with cone
degeneration have a normal rod electroretinogram, at least initially [8, 9]. Additionally
according to Krill's [10] observations, patients with primary cone degeneration may - with
increasing age - show rod involvement, the photopic part, however, being always more
affected than the scotopic one [7, 11, 12, 13]. Therefore, the disease of the patients with
primary cone degeneration described here shall be called: "cone-rod degeneration".
Unfortunately there exists no universally accepted classification of progressive cone and
cone-rod degenerations, although attempts to obtain such a classification have been
made [6, 11, 14, 15]. Krill et al. [6] distinguished central from diffuse cone dystrophy; other
attempts at classification are based on ERG findings [15], inheritance patterns [10] or
ophthalmoscopic findings [16]. Because of this lack of an universal classification scheme,
the reader shall not be surprised that all patients presented here were put into a single
group. Considering the quite variable expression of this disease it seems unhelpful to rely
on clinical phenotype and on functional parameters alone for subclassification. It is our

intention, however, to use this patient group in order to arrive at a new classification in coming years, based on molecular genetic parameters and / or biochemical findings.

II. METHODS

Each patient, transferred to us as a suspect of cone-rod degeneration, underwent a careful general ophthalmological investigation. The history of the patient was recorded with special attention to onset and progression of the disease, the history of the family with special attention to inheritance patterns. The typical symptoms of cone-rod degenerations were recorded (visual acuity, color vision and dazzle sensitivity) in respect to onset and progression. Refraction was determined either with correction glasses and / or with a Canon refractometer. Ophthalmoscopy and fundus photography was performed after dilating pupils with Mydriaticum Roche.

A. DARK ADAPTATION:

Testing was performed with a Tübingen perimeter; a test stimulus of 104 min was presented for 500 ms at a temporal retinal eccentricity of 20°. After dilatation ("Mydriaticum Roche") and light adaptation (850 cd·m^{-2}) for 10 minutes the test light was increased in steps of 0.1 log units from subthreshold values while monocular foveal fixation was maintained by means of a red mark in the center of the Ganzfeld globe. The patient was asked to respond by pressing a button as soon as he saw the test light. After 30 minutes a curve consisting of two parts separated by the rod-cone break was obtained (Figure 1).

For a detailed description see also Alexander and Fishman [17], Kohen et al. [18], Lorenz and Zrenner [19], Schneider and Zrenner [20], Zrenner [21], Zrenner et al. [22].

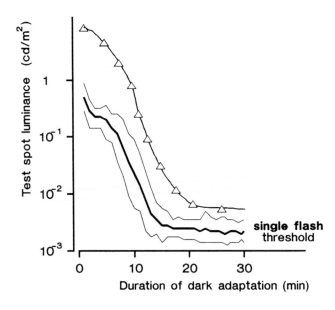

Fig. 1: Dark adaptation (lower curve) and cone flicker threshold during dark adaptation (upper curve (mean and +/- 2 SD). The duration of dark adaptation (min.) is plotted against the test spot luminance (cd m^{-2}) necessary for threshold detection (log units). The test spot has a diameter of 104´. Before starting measurements the retina is bleached for 10 minutes (850 cd m^{-2}). Symbols (△, ○) indicate an example of a patient with cone-rod dystrophy (see text).

B. MESOPTOMETRY:

After calibration of the instrument (Mesoptometer II, Oculus, Dutenhofen) and adaptation of the patient to 0.1 cd·m^{-2} for 5 minutes, a Landolt ring was presented to the patient with decreasing contrast (1:23 to 1:1.14). The threshold was found when three different out of four possible positions of the Landolt ring were recognized correctly within 5 seconds. The same procedure was performed for a background of 0.032 cd·m^{-2}.

Subsequently, in presence of a dazzling light the patient fixated in between two fixation points while trying to recognize Landolt rings in 5 different positions from 12 h to 6 h over 3 h. A detailed description was given by Aulhorn and Harms [23].

C. THE ELECTROOCULOGRAM (EOG):

The pupils were dilated with "Mydriaticum Roche". After 30 minutes of dark adaptation gold cup electrodes were placed at the nasal and temporal canthi of both eyes and the patient was grounded with an ear clip electrode. He fixated two red fixation lights ten times alternatively every 2nd minute for ten minutes. The fixation lights had a distance of 30 degrees visual angle. After light adaptation (150 cd·m^{-2}) to a homogeneously illuminated Ganzfeld bowl for 4 minutes a recording was made in the light adapted state and repeated subsequently 4 times every two minutes. The amplitudes obtained during each recording period were averaged. The ratio between the maximum amplitude during the light adapted state and the amplitude recorded during the preceding dark phase results in a light/dark ratio. The range +/- 2 SD of our normal population is 1.36 to 1.86. For details see Zrenner [24].

D. THE GANZFELD ELECTRORETINOGRAM (ERG):

Pupils were dilated ("Mydriaticum Roche") and the patient was dark adaptated for 30 minutes. After local anesthesia ("Conjuncain^R-EDO^R sine", Dr. Mann Pharma) Henkes contact lens electrodes were placed on the cornea using "Methocel Dispersa" as contact medium. Reference gold cup electrodes were placed at the temples. The patient was grounded via an ear clip electrode and placed in front of a Nicolet Ganzfeld bowl in supine position. Recordings were made with the Nicolet compact four computer.

ERGs were performed according to the ISCEV/NRPF standard [25]:

1) The rod response was elicited in the dark adapted eye by a white flash of 3.9 mcd·s·m^{-2}. The flash was repeated 6 times every 0.5 seconds. The responses were amplified, bandpass filtered (1 to 250 Hz), averaged and stored on floppy discs.

2) The maximal response was recorded under identical conditions with a white flash of 2500 mcd·s·m^{-2} and an interstimulus interval of 5 seconds.

3) Oscillatory potentials were recorded similarly to the maximal response, however with a band pass filter of 100 to 250 Hz and an interstimulus interval of 10 seconds. Subsequently the photopic recordings started after light adaptation of 10 minutes (32 cd · m^{-2}).

4) Immediately after the beginning of light adaptation a 30 Hz flicker response was evoked (2000 mcd·s·m^{-2}); after 10 minutes the recording was repeated.

5) The white flash cone response was elicited by flashes of 2500 mcd·s·m^{-2} presented at an interstimulus interval of 0.6 seconds.

E. THE PATTERN ERG (PERG):

For registration of the PERG we used gold foil electrodes which were attached to the lower lid of the non-dilated eyes. Anaesthesia was not obligatory, but was found to be helpful in some patients ("Conjuncain^R EDO^R sine", Dr. Mann Pharma). The patient's refraction was corrected optimally. Vertical white and black sinusoidal bars with a contrast of 97 % served as stimuli, presented at a temporal frequency of 8 Hz in 5 different frequencies: 0.22, 0.45, 0.9, 1.8, 2.7 cycles per degree. The monitor subserved a visual angle of 12.6 x 15.5 deg. The distance between the patient's eyes and the monitor was 1.25 m. The resulting potentials were amplified, averaged and the second harmonic component was calculated by Fourier analysis. The method was described in detail by Hess et al. [26], Marx and Zrenner [27], Zrenner [28].

III. RESULTS:
CLINICAL OBSERVATIONS

As shown in Table 1, the distribution of sexes was approximately equal in this patient group. The average age at the time of investigation was near 28 years, with a wide span, the youngest patient being 5 years old, the oldest being 61 years old. The onset, as reported by the patient, was in average 20 years +/- 10 years. The 40 patients came from altogether 36 families; within the patient group there are 4 families with 2 members. All patients reported progression of their symptoms. An autosomal dominant inheritance pattern could be established in 32 % of the patients, an autosomal recessive one in 8 %; due to small family size, simplex or multiplex pattern in 60 % of the patients, a clear inheritance pattern could not be established.

Visual acuity varied considerably; two thirds of the patients had a visual acuity below 0.5, a fifth of the patients had a visual acuity between 0.5 and 0.8, one eighth of the patients had a visual acuity better than 0.8. Myopia was found in 74 % of the cases, hyperopia in 19 % and emmetropia in 7 % of the patients. A pathological glare sensitivity was found in 63 % of the patients, while it was normal in 28 %. In 9 % glare sensitivity could not be determined, because the test pattern could not be seen.

TABLE 1

General Ophthalmological Findings in Patients with Cone-Rod Dystrophy

Number of patients	40	♂ = 52 %	♀ = 48 %
Average age	28 years +/- 23 years		
Onset	20 years +/- 10 years		
Progression	yes		
Inheritance	autosomal dominant = 32 %	autosomal recessiv = 8 %	unknown = 60 %
Visual acuity	< 0,5 = 67 %	0,5 - 0,8 = 20 %	> 0,8 = 13 %
Refraction	myopia = 74 % in 35 % larger -3,0	hyperopia = 19 %	emme-tropia = 7 %
Glare sensitivity	pathological = 63 %	normal = 28 %	unknown = 9 %

The ophthalmoscopic findings are summarized in Table 2. Fundus pictures in primary cone degeneration were found to be quite variable, even within the same family and within patients in the same age group. In approximately a quarter of the patients the optic nerve or at least a section of the optic nerve head showed a slight pallor. The macula varied from normal (17 %) to bull's eye shaped or even large lesions in the retinal pigment epithelium. The pigment epithelium of the retinal periphery was involved in 30 % of the patients. A small number of patients showed narrow retinal vessels.

TABLE 2

Fundus Findings in Patients with Cone-Rod Dystrophy

Optic Nerve	pale	26 %	normal	74 %
Macula	pigment alterations	83 %	normal	17 %
Periphery	involved	30 %	normal	70 %
Retinal vessels	narrow	6 %	normal	94 %

FUNCTIONAL TESTS

A. DAZZLE SENSITIVITY:

In Figure 2 visual acuity is plotted against luminance of a white area of 8.2 x 8.2 degree on top of which black Landolt figures were presented. In the normal population (grey area) visual acuity increases up to a luminance of the test field of approximately 1 000 cd·m^{-2}; it stays constant with further increase of luminance or only slightly decreases. In patients with cone-rod dystrophy the maximum visual acuity (given in %) was reached already at lower luminance levels and fell off considerably, when the luminance of the testfield was further increased, which correlates nicely with the high dazzle sensitivity of these patients [29].

B. VISUAL FIELDS:

As determined by Octopus perimetry (program 21 or 31), visual fields were normal in 46 eyes of 23 patients. At first this seems surprising; however considering that the Octopus Perimeter has a very low background luminance, the rod system determines the threshold and due to the relatively large raster, the physiological rod scotoma is missed. If determined by means of other perimeters (Tübinger Automatic Perimeter etc.) with higher background luminance or with red test flashes usually a central scotoma emerges. Half of the pathological visual fields revealed a central scotoma, 13 % a ring scotoma and 32 % a concentric constriction of the visual field, despite a normal rod electroretinogram.

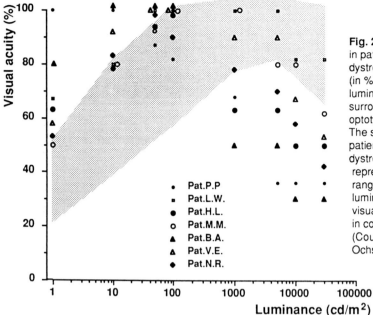

Fig. 2: Glare sensitivity in patients with cone-rod dystrophy. Visual acuity (in %) is plotted against luminance (cd/m2) of the surround on which the optotype is presented. The symbols indicate the patients with cone-rod dystrophy; the grey zone represents the normal range (+/- 2 SD). At high luminance the patients´ visual acuity decreases in comparison to normals. (Courtesy of Dr. Heike Ochsner.)

Legend within figure:

- Pat.P.P
- Pat.L.W.
- Pat.H.L.
- Pat.M.M.
- Pat.B.A.
- Pat.V.E.
- Pat.N.R.

Y-axis: Visual acuity (%)

X-axis: Luminance (cd/m²)

C. COLOR VISION:

Color vision of these patients was determined by the Farnsworth-Munsell 100-Hue test (n = 37) and evaluated according to Kitahara [30]. Normal total error scores were found in approximately one fifth (n = 7) of the patients. Most of the patients revealed a tritan pattern (n = 8), an erratic pattern (n = 7) or a scotopic pattern (n = 11) indicating that the discrimination of the colored cups is mainly governed by rods. A small fraction of patients showed protan (n = 3) or deutan (n = 1) defects.

Interestingly, color vision and visual acuity is not necessarily deteriorating in parallel. Usually only with visual acuity deteriorating below approximately 0.5, the total error score in the Farnsworth-Munsell 100-Hue test reaches very pathological values.

D. DARK ADAPTATION:

Final dark adaptation threshold was normal in 6 of 16 investigated patients. An increased cone threshold was found in 4 patients (see Figure 1), the rod threshold was never found to be elevated. The function as a whole was elevated in 4 patients.

E. ELECTRORETINOGRAM:

As shown in Figure 3 (panel a and b), the b-wave in response to a white test flash of 3,9 mcd·s·m-2 after 30 minutes of dark adaptation showed amplitudes and implicit times within the normal range +/- 1 Standard Deviation (SD) indicated by grey zones. When a strong test flash was used (2.5 cd·s·m-2) the amplitude reached pathological values and prolonged implicit times were seen (Figure 3, panel c and d), indicating some rod involvement at higher light intensities. The cone b-wave, recorded with white flashes in presence of a background of approximately 32 cd·m-2 revealed amplitude values of approximately half the normal size and quite prolonged implicit times as shown in Figure 4 (panel a and b).

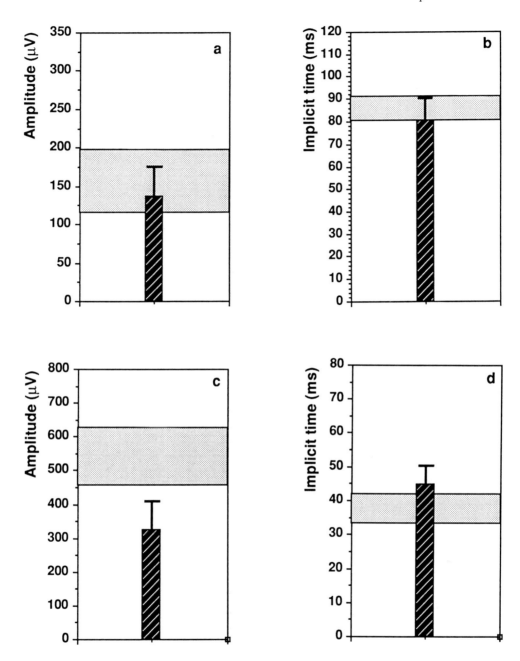

Fig. 3: Amplitude (μV) and implicit time (ms) of rod b-wave (according to the ISCEV-Standard) in the ERG of patients with cone-rod dystrophy. The normal range is indicated by a horizontal bar (+/- 1 SD). Data in panel a and b were obtained in response to a weak flash (3.9 mcd s m^{-2}), those in panel c and d in response to a strong flash (2.5 cd s m^{-2}).

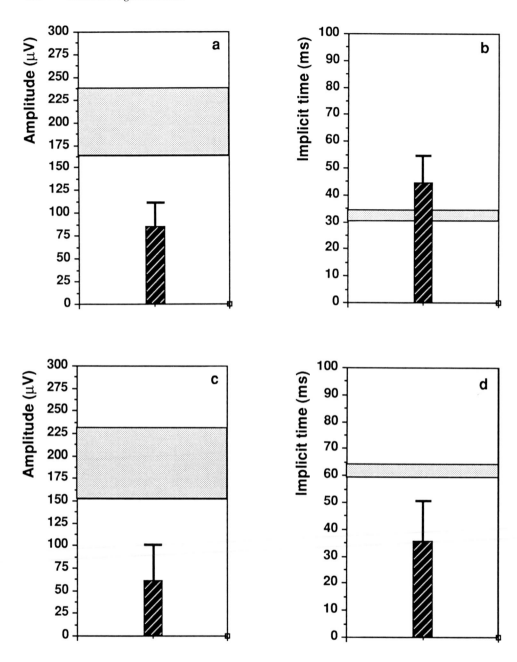

Fig. 4: Amplitude (μV) and implicit time (ms) of cone b-wave (according to the ISCEV-Standard) in the ERG of patients with cone-rod dystrophy. The normal range is indicated by a horizontal bar (+/- 1 SD). Data in panel a and b were obtained in response to a white flash in presence of a background of approximately 32 cd m-2, those in panel c and d in responseto a 30 cycles per second white flash.

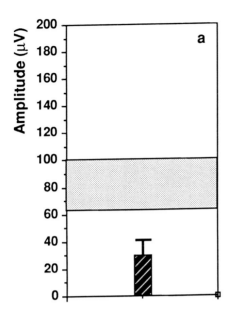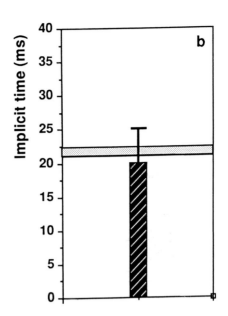

Fig. 5: Amplitude (μV) and implicit time (ms) of oscillatory potentials (according to the ISCEV-Standard) in the ERG of patients with cone-rod dystrophy. The normal range is indicated by a horizontal bar (+/- 1 SD).

Flicker responses (Figure 4, panel c and d) in response to a 30 cycles per sec white flash light were approximately half the normal range in the group as a whole and showed a phase shift.

Surprisingly, also the oscillatory potentials were affected. As shown in Figure 5 (panel a and b) the amplitudes reached only half the normal values, while latencies were within the normal range.

F. PATTERN ELECTRORETINOGRAM (PERG):

The pattern electroretinogram was recorded in response to sinusoidal gratings of increasing spatial frequency. The normal range is shown in Figure 8 (triangles and hatched area). In all the 9 patients which underwent pattern electroretinography, the amplitudes of the second harmonic response of the pattern electroretinogram were reduced.

G. ELECTROOCULOGRAM (EOG):

The electrooculogram was recorded in the conventional way. After 30 min of dark adaptation a standing potential was recorded (for a 30° eye movement). The subsequent illumination in a Ganzfeld globe (150 cd·m^{-2}) resulted in a light rise of the standing potential, usually observed during the eighth minute after switching on the Ganzfeld. The results are shown in Figure 7, ranked according to the size of the light/dark ratio. Surprisingly, despite normal rod electroretinograms, the electrooculogram in more than half of the patients was below normal. No supernormal electrooculograms were found. Only two values of the light/dark ratio of the patients' eyes were above the normal mean.

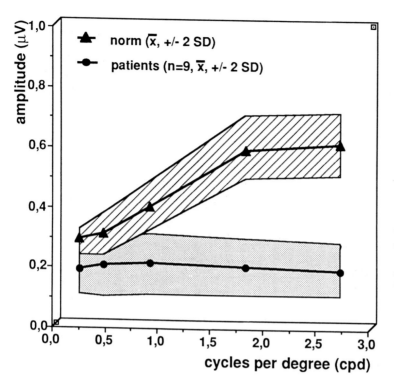

Fig. 6: Pattern ERG of 9 patients suffering from cone-rod dystrophy; mean and +/- 1 SD of the amplitude (µV) of the second harmonic plotted against spatial frequency (cpd). The norm is represented by triangles (mean) and hatched area (+/- 1 SD). In patients with cone-rod dystrophy (points (mean) and grey zone (+/- 1 SD) the second harmonic is heavily reduced.

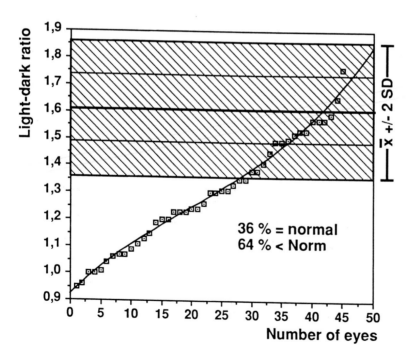

Fig. 7: EOGs in patients with cone-rod dystrophy. EOG values of individual eyes (open square) are ranked.

IV. DISCUSSION

The typical patient with cone-rod degeneration notices problems with visual acuity below age 30, complains about progression of the symptoms, suffers from myopia and very often reveals an autosomal dominant inheritance pattern. Most authors also find that the disease starts in the first two or three decades of life [6, 8, 16], but according to Krill and Deutman [7] the disease can begin at any age. Progression of the disease differentiates between stationary cone dysfunctions and progressive cone dystrophies or degenerations [7, 13]. All our patients showed progression of their symptoms, which puts them into the cone-rod degeneration or dystrophy group. Krill [10], Krill et al. [6] and Weleber and Eisner [13] found a correlation between age of onset and speed of progression: they pointed out that the progression advances more rapidly in patients with onset at early age of life. The observation time of 5 years in our patients is not long enough to draw a similar conclusion.

An autosomal dominant inheritance is the most common pattern in cone-rod dystrophy as also found by Krill and Deutman [7] and Krill et al. [19]. The small families and the low occurrence of this disease have resulted in the assumption that spontaneous mutations occur rather often in these patients according to Jimenez et al. [8] and Krill [10]. Krill et al. [6] observed even more commonly sporadic cases than familial ones. However, due to the variable penetrance and difficulties in tracking exactly the family tree, a dominant pattern cannot always be established, even if present.

Besides decreased visual acuity the main symptom is a pathological dazzle sensitivity. Many authors pointed out that patients with cone-rod dystrophy suffer from photophobia [8, 9, 15, 16, 31], which is a subjective sign and therefore difficult to establish [6]. The method of determining visual acuity at different levels of adaptation demonstrated here is a good indicator for measuring dazzle sensitivity. Patients with cone-rod dystrophy are even dazzled at low luminance levels.

The fundus can be highly variable [14], from normal [32] to bull's eye and extensive lesions in the retinal pigment epithelium, rendering the ophthalmological picture as unsuited for classification, since the complete range of variations can occur in single families. To our opinion changes in the ophthalmological picture are not very helpful for diagnosing cone-rod dystrophy in the initial stages of this disease; they seem to depend rather on age of onset and on progression of the disease [7, 31] and most often pathologic electrophysiological and psychophysical findings preceed fundus alterations [14, 31]. In the majority of our patients the fundus was normal or near normal, often with mild pigment alterations; Weleber and Eisner [13] have made similar observations. The most typical fundus finding in patients with cone-rod dystrophy in literature, however, is the bull's eye [6]. To our opinion the bull's eye lesion is a very late sign in cone-rod dystrophy and certainly not an obligatory sign. A very detailed description of fundus changes in patients with cone-rod dystrophy can be found in Krill [10], Krill et al. [6] and Weleber and Eisner [13]. Fishman [16] observed a correlation between fundus findings and electrophysiological results. He found out that patients with a lesion clinically localized in the fovea and patients with peripheral pigmentary changes show an affection of the scotopic part in psychophysical (elevated rod threshold in the dark adaptation curve) and electrophysiological (reduced scotopic amplitude in the ERG) tests. Patients with bull's eye lesions or atrophic foveal lesion show a normal photopic and scotopic ERG.

Since color vision is a function that heavily involves cones, it is obvious that we expect a disturbed color vision in patients with cone-rod dystrophy, as also found by most authors [7, 8, 9, 11, 13, 14, 15, 16]. According to Köllner's rule [33] the blue cone system and its interaction with longer wavelength sensitive cones is affected in the majority of patients. If visual acuity drops below 0.5, severe color vision disturbances are seen [6]. Marked color vision disturbances rarely preced the loss of visual acuity in cone-rod dystrophies.

Although the rod b-wave is normal, some b-wave pathology can be found with strong test lights in the dark adapted eye. In parallel to increased photophobia, rod b-waves become smaller with high test light intensities; either rods cannot handle the high incidence of light quanta or a regulation involving rod-cone interaction comes into effect. Cone b-waves and flicker amplitudes always are reduced (by definition) and surprisingly, the oscillatory potentials are reduced as well, again pointing to additional defects in the rod pathway. The fact that oscillatory potentials are reduced in amplitude does not suggest that the disease process affects the inner retina, since the implicit times of the oscillatory potentials are normal.

The pattern electroretinogram shows decreased amplitudes, marking the loss of physiological functions in the central retina.

The alterations in visual fields indicate that a loss of cones can occur either from the center towards the periphery or from the periphery towards the center. Surprisingly rarely are all cones affected simultaneously, as far as they determine the increment threshold in perimetric tests. It seems also very surprising, that the electrooculogram shows a reduced light/dark ratio in a rather large number of these patients, since the electrooculogram is driven mainly by rods it represents mainly the large areas of the peripheral retina. Apparently, in many patients the interaction between retinal pigment epithelium and photoreceptors is affected early in the course of the disease. This leads us to the tentative assumption that the primary defect might be found in the retinal pigment epithelium cells, at least in a large subpopulation of patients with cone-rod degeneration. The disease process then would most probably affect a mechanism that is involved in normal cone regeneration but not necessarily to the same degree in rod regeneration. Rods seem only affected, if the primary disease process in the pigment epithelium leads progressively to a considerable general disturbance or death of retinal pigment epithelium cells. Based on the observations in the visual field testing, we do not assume that the process affects rods and cones equally at the posterior pole, at least in a large proportion of our patients. On the other hand, we cannot assume that our patient population is genetically uniform. We might rather deal with several defects, also those involved directly in the functional maintenance of rods, that are directly responsible for rod dysfunction.

REFERENCES

1. Birkle D.L., Bazan N.G.: The arachidonic acid cascade and phospholipid and docosahexaenoic acid metabolism in the retina, in Progress in Retinal Research, Vol. 5, Osborne N., Chader G., Eds., Pergamon Press, Oxford, 1986, 309.

2. Bok D.: Structure and function of the retinal pigment epithelium - receptor complex, in Retinal Diseases, Tso, M.O.M., Eds., J.B. Lippincott Company, Philadelphia, 1988, 3.

3. Gonzalez-Fernandez F., Fong S.-L., Liou G.I., Bridges C.D.B.: Interstitial retinol-binding protein (IRBP) in the RCS rat: effect of dark-rearing. Invest. Ophthalmol. Vis. Sci., 26, 1381, 1985.

4. Veen T. van, Ekstrom P., Wiggert B., Lee L., Hirose Y., Sanyal S., Chader G.J.: A developmental study of interphotoreceptor retinoid-binding protein (IRBP) in single and double homozygous rd and rds mutant mouse retinae. Exp. Eye Res., 47, 291, 1988.

5. Schmidt S.Y., Heth C.A., Edwards R.B., Brandt J.T., Adler A.J., Spiegel A. Shichi H., Berson E.L.: Identification of proteins in retinas and IPM from eyes with retinitis pigmentosa. Invest. Ophthalmol. Vis. Sci., 29, 1585, 1988.

6. Krill A.E., Deutman A.F., Fishman M.: The cone degenerations. Doc. Ophthalmol., 35, 1, 1973.

7. Krill A.E., Deutman A.F.: Dominant macular degenerations. The cone dystrophies. Am. J. Ophthalmol., 73, 3, 352, 1972.

8. Jiménez-Sierra J.M., Ogden T.E., Van Boemel G.B.: Inherited retinal diseases. The C.V. Mosby Company, St. Louis, 1989, 166.

9. Ripps H., Noble K.G., Greenstein V.C., Siegel I.M., Carr R.E.: Progressive cone dystrophy. Ophthalmol., 94, 11, 1987.

10. Krill A.E.: Hereditary retinal and choroidal diseases, Vol. 2, Harper & Row Publishers, Inc., Hagerstown, 1977, 421.

11. Berson E.L., Gouras P., Gunkel R.D.: Progressive cone degeneration, dominantly inherited. Arch. Ophthalmol., 80, 77, 1968.

12. Lith G.H.M. van: Electroophthalmology II. Indications and interpretation. Doc. Ophthalmol. Proc. Ser., 3, 257, 1973.

13. Weleber R.G., Eisner A.: Cone degeneration ("Bull's-eye dystrophies") and color vision defects, in Retinal Dystrophies and Degenerations, Newsome D.A., Eds., Raven Press, New York, 1988, 233.

14. Berson E.L., Gouras P., Gunkel R.D.: Progressive cone-rod degeneration. Arch. Ophthalmol., 80, 68, 1968.

15. Goodman G., Ripps H., Siegel I.M.: Cone dysfunction syndromes, Arch. Ophthalmol., 70, 214, 1963.

16. Fishman G.A.: Electroretinography and inherited macular dystrophies. Retina, 5, 172, 1985.

17. Alexander K.R., Fishman G.A: Rod-cone interaction in flicker perimetry. Br. J. Ophthalmol., 68, 303, 1984.

18. Kohen L., Zrenner E., Schneider T.: Der Einfluß von Theophyllin und Coffein auf die sensorische Netzhautfunktion des Menschen. Fortschr. Ophthalmol., 83, 338, 1986.

19. Lorenz B., Zrenner E.: Retinal Dysfunction in hereditary myopia associated with choroidal degeneration. Is there a correlation to the degree of myopia? in Advances in Biosciences 62, Research in Retinitis Pigmentosa, Zrenner E., Krastel H., Goebel H.-H., Eds., Pergamon Press, Oxford, New York, 1987, 137.

20. Schneider T., Zrenner E.: Rod-cone interaction in patients with fundus flavimaculatus. Br. J. Ophthalmol., 71, 10, 762, 1987.

21. Zrenner E.: Neue differentialdiagnostische Möglichkeiten in der Sinnesphysiologie, in Neuerungen in der ophthalmologischen Diagnostik und Therapie, Lund O.-E., Waubke T.N., Eds., Enke, Stuttgart, 1988, 154.

22. Zrenner E., Kohen L., Krastel H.: Einschränkungen der Netzhautfunktion bei Konduktorinnen der Chorioideremie. Fortschr. Ophthalmol., 83, 602, 1986.

23. Aulhorn E., Harms H.: Das Mesoptometer, ein Gerät zur Prüfung von Dämmerungssehen und Blendungsempfindlichkeit. Ber. Dt. Ophthalmol. Ges., 66, 425, 1965.

24. Zrenner E.: Grundlagen elektrophysiologischer Untersuchungen in der Augenheilkunde. in Degenerative Erkrankungen des Auges, Lund O.-E., Waubke T. N., Eds., Enke, Stuttgart, 1983, 129.

25. Marmor M.F., Arden G.B., Nilsson S.E., Zrenner E.: At last . A standard electroretinography protocol. Standard for clinical electroretinography. Arch. Ophthalmol., 107, 813, 1989.

26. Hess R.F., Baker C.L., Zrenner E., Schwarzer J.: Differences between electroretinograms of cat and primate. J. Neurophysiol., 56, 747, 1986.

27. Marx R., Zrenner E.: Sensitivity distribution in the central and midperipheral visual field determined by pattern electroretinography and harmonic analysis. Doc. Ophthalmol., 73, 347, 1990.

28. Zrenner E.: The physiological basis of the pattern electroretinogram, in Progress in Retinal Research, Osborne N., Chader J., Eds., Pergamon Press, Oxford, 9, 1989, 427.

29. Ochsner H.B.: Beziehung zwischen Sehschärfe und Testfeldleuchtdichte bei blendungsempfindlichen Patienten mit Neuritis nervi optici, Rethinopathia diabetica und Glaukom, <u>Diss.</u>, Ludwigs-Maximilians-Univ., Munich, 1989.

30. Kitahara K.: An analysis of the Farnsworth-Munsell 100-Hue test. <u>Doc. Ophthalmol. Proc. Series</u>, 39, 233, 1984.

31. Sloan L.L., Brown D.J.: Progressive retinal degeneration with selective involvement of the cone mechanism. <u>Am. J. Ophthalmol.</u>, 54, 629, 1962.

32. Deutmann A.F.: <u>The hereditary dystrophies of the posterior pole of the eye</u>, Van Gorcum & Comp., Assen, 1971, 181.

33. Koellner H.: <u>Die Störungen des Farbensinns,</u> Karger, Berlin, 1912.

ACKNOWLEDGEMENT

We are indebted to the Max-Planck Society for the support of this study, Heike Ochsner for permitting to quote the graph on dazzle sensitivity. The study was supported by the German Research Council Grant Zr. 1/7-1.

PIGMENTARY PATTERNS IN RETINITIS PIGMENTOSA

N.Orzalesi, A.Porta, G.Staurenghi, C.Pierrottet
Department of Ophthalmology
University of Milan
San Paolo Hospital
Milan (Italy)

RP patients may be conventionally divided into Cone-Rod (CR) or Rod-Cone (RC) subtypes according to cone and rod erg responses examined separately (1)(2).

Patients with advanced disease (unrecordable erg, a visual field of less than 10 degrees and dark adaptation test results showing severe night blindness) may be difficult to classify into either of these subtypes, at least with the routine work-up as performed in the majority of RP centers.

The aim of our study was to determine whether there was any association between 9 specific pigmentary patterns of the fundus and RC or CR subtypes: if this were the case, pigmentary patterns could be added to other indirect (non-erg) criteria for the diagnosis of CR or RC RP, particularly in advanced forms and in the case of an inadequate electrophysiological work-up.

PATIENTS AND METHODS

The patients involved in the present study attended the Lombardy RP Referral Center (Milan) during the first 18 months of its activity. During this period more than 300 patients were examined according to the protocol prepared by Heckenlively (3) (table 1).

TABLE 1: RP DIAGNOSTIC PROTOCOL

- ocular and medical history
- family history with pedigree
- best corrected visual acuity
- colour vision testing
- goldmann kinetic perimetry
- dark adaptation test
- biomicroscopy
- applanation tonometry
- scotopic and photopic erg
- fundus photographs
- fluorescein angiography
- audiogram
- blood tests
- medical,pediatric,otola-
  ryngologic,neurologic
  consultation

The protocol was completed in 171 subjects   listed in table 2.

TABLE 2

171 pts (96 m./75 f.)   mean age 37.37 yrs.
                                ranging 0.33 - 83

141 PRIMARY FORMS   30 SECONDARY FORMS
      only ocular)   (RP syndromes)
- 112 autosomic recessive   - 7 Usher I
- 13 autosomic dominant   - 8 Usher II
- 7 x-linked recessive   - 9 L.M.B.B.
- 10 still to define   - 2 Alstrom
                               - 1 Saldino-Mainzer
                               - 3 unknown

In order to divide RP patients into CR and RC subtypes, we used the "direct" erg criteria whenever possible and, in cases where the erg was unrecordable, "indirect" criteria based on ocular history and psychophysical testing (3) (table 3,4,5).

TABLE 3: CR TYPE INCLUSION CRITERIA

- Direct criteria:
* Cone-erg more severely affected than rod-erg with both cone and rod-erg abnormal;
- Indirect criteria:
* Final Rod Threshold elevation of 2.00 Log Units or less;
* Visual field ring scotomata between 5-30 degrees with concentric (onion like) rings in later stages;
* History of no or late onset night blindness (>20);

TABLE 4: RC TYPE INCLUSION CRITERIA

- Direct criteria:
* Rod-erg more severely affected than cone-erg with both cone and rod-erg abnormal;
- Indirect criteria:
* History of early onset night blindness (<20);
* Final Rod Threshold elevation of 3.50 Log Units or greater;
* Visual field larger jumps in sensitivity among isopters as well as ring scotomata between 30-50 degrees.

TABLE 5: EXCLUSION CRITERIA

1) Congenital RP: LCA (Leber Congenital Amaurosis) where the erg performed within the first year of life is extinguished and a typical erg pattern cannot be distinguished (4);
2) Secondary forms: with other organic or sistemic involvement;
3) Nonspecific forms in which, in the absence of a recordable erg, indirect criteria did not allow a distinction to be made between cone and rod involvement;
4) Incomplete fundus documentation.

115 patients were considered eligible for the study and divided into CR and RC groups with (erg+) and without (erg-) recordable erg (table 6).

TABLE 6

	CR RP			RC RP		
	tot	erg+	erg-	tot	erg+	erg-
	5 7	25	32	58	18	40
mean age	43.98	41.13	46.16	39.70	39.83	39.64
onset of symptoms	22.46	24.05	21.24	11.56	14.47	10.26
onset of night blind.	25.31	24.60	25.86	12.44	14.65	11.45
duration(presumed)	20.88	15.91	24.71	29.42	25.12	31.35
RE visual acuity	0.41	0.54	0.32	0.47	0.55	0.43
LE visual acuity	0.42	0.57	0.30	0.57	0.87	0.44
RE visual field (*)	2.86	3.96	2.01	2.08	2.00	2.12
LE visual field (*)	2.63	3.70	1.80	2.14	2.08	2.17
aut. recessive pts.	52	22	30	43	14	29
aut. dominant pts.	3	2	1	10	3	7
X-l. recessive pts.	2	1	1	1	-	1
still to be defined	-	-	-	4	1	3

(*) note: reported in units representing ranges of size with IV-4 Goldmann isopter (1 = field < 5 degrees; 2 = field 5-15 degrees; 3 = field 16-30 degrees; 4 = field 31-50 degrees; 5 = field > 50 degrees), measured from fixation to the edge of the field in each quadrant and averaged.

The following well-established pigmentary patterns were considered:
1) bull's eye: complete ring-like perifoveal EPR window defect on fluorescein angiography (figure 1);

2) macular window RPE defects;

3) macular hypofluorescence: decreased fluorescence in the macula as compared to the surrounding areas; perifoveal capillary net undetectable;

4) macular atrophy: areolar atrophy of RPE and choriocapillaris in the macula;

5) pericentral RPE atrophy (regional atrophy): patches of RPE loss along the major vascular arcades (figure 2);

6) diffuse retinal atrophy: loss of RPE and choriocapillaris spread throughout the fundus;

7) salt and pepper appearance: a diffuse scattering of pigment in a salt and pepper distribution;

8) bone spicules: pigment dispersion adhering to the arteriolar vessels (figure 3);

9) sine pigmento: little or no pigment deposition.

The data were analyzed with the Chi-square test of independence with Yates' correction and, in the case of stratification, by means of the Fisher's exact test.

RESULTS

Contingency tables, comparing the prevalence of each pigmentary pattern in both CR and RC subtypes are shown below.

(note: (+) = with the pigmentary pattern; (-) = without the pigmentary pattern)

TABLE 7

BULL'S-EYE

total of patients	+	-	T
CR	13	44	57
RC	13	45	58
T	26	89	115

patients with recordable ERG	+	-	T
CR	7	18	25
RC	4	14	18
T	11	32	43

.01037	CHI-SQUARE	.12536
.9189	SIGNIFICANCE	.7233

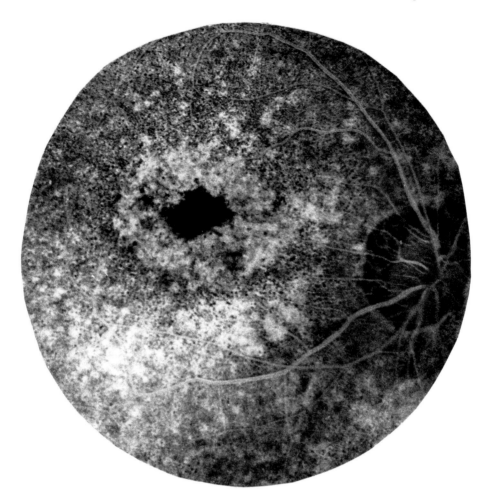

Figure 1: bull's eye

TABLE 8

MACULAR WINDOW RPE DEFECTS

total of patients				patients with recordable ERG			
	+	-	T		+	-	T
CR	1 3	4 4	5 7	CR	4	2 1	2 5
RC	7	5 1	5 8	RC	3	1 5	1 8
T	2 0	9 5	1 1 5	T	7	3 6	43

2.80788	CHI-SQUARE	.01307
.0938	SIGNIFICANCE	.9090

TABLE 9

MACULAR HYPOFLUORESCENCE

total of patients				patients with recordable ERG		
	+	−	T		+	−	T
CR	1 2	4 5	5 7	CR	6	1 9	2 5
RC	1 6	4 2	5 8	RC	4	1 4	1 8
T	2 8	8 7	1 1 5	T	1 0	3 3	4 3

.29391   CHI-SQUARE   .00442
.5877   SIGNIFICANCE   .9474

TABLE 10

MACULAR ATROPHY

total of patients				patients with recordable ERG		
	+	−	T		+	−	T
CR	1 6	4 1	5 7	CR	7	1 8	2 5
RC	1 3	4 5	5 8	RC	4	1 4	1 8
T	2 9	8 6	1 1 5	T	1 1	3 2	4 3

.23244   CHI-SQUARE   .12536
.6299   SIGNIFICANCE   .7233

TABLE 11

PERICENTRAL RPE ATROPHY

total of patients				patients with recordable ERG		
	+	−	T		+	−	T
CR	2 5	3 2	5 7	CR	1 1	1 4	2 5
RC	1 7	4 1	5 8	RC	4	1 4	1 8
T	4 2	7 3	1 1 5	T	1 5	2 8	43

1.78923	CHI-SQUARE	1.90974
.1810	SIGNIFICANCE	.1670

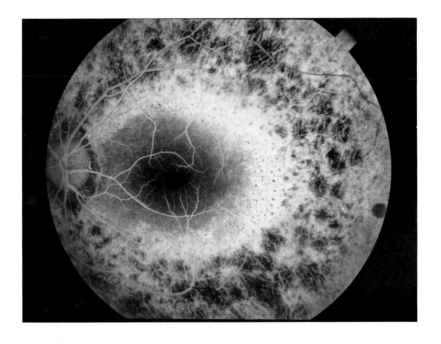

Figure 2: pericentral rpe atrophy

TABLE 12

DIFFUSE ATROPHY

total of patients				patients with recordable ERG		
	+	−	T		+	−	T
CR	1 4	4 3	5 7	CR	3	2 2	2 5
RC	1 8	4 0	5 8	RC	6	1 2	1 8
T	3 2	8 3	1 1 5	T	9	3 4	4 3

1.01279	CHI-SQUARE	3.10525
.3142	SIGNIFICANCE	.0780

TABLE 13

SALT-PEPPER APPEARANCE

total of patients				patients with recordable ERG		
	+	−	T		+	−	T
CR	2 6	3 1	5 7	CR	1 4	1 1	2 5
RC	3 0	2 8	5 8	RC	1 1	7	1 8
T	5 6	5 9	1 1 5	T	2 5	1 8	4 3

.87158	CHI-SQUARE	.22881
.3505	SIGNIFICANCE	.6324

TABLE 14

BONE SPICULE

total of patients

	+	-	T
ŒR	4 3	1 4	5 7
RC	5 1	7	5 8
T	9 4	2 1	1 1 5

patients with recordable ERG

	+	-	T
ŒR	1 6	9	2 5
RC	1 7	1	1 8
T	3 3	1 0	43

5.20847	CHI-SQUARE	4.51282
.0125	SIGNIFICANCE	.0132

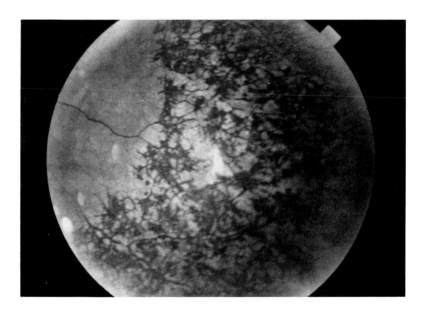

Figure 3: bone spicule

TABLE 15

SINE PIGMENTO

total of patients					patients with recordable ERG			

	+	-	T
CR	1 1	4 6	5 7
RC	4	5 4	5 8
T	1 5	1 0 0	1 1 5

	+	-	T
CR	6	1 9	2 5
RC	1	1 7	1 8
T	7	3 6	4 3

3.35069	CHI-SQUARE	2.44081
.0672	SIGNIFICANCE	.1182

DISCUSSION

The most frequent pigmentary pattern found in the 115 patients was bone spicule (81.7% of all subjects and 75% of patients with recordable ERG) (table 14).
Given the .01 result of the Chi-Square test, this pattern may be considered positively associated with the RC subtype both in cases with recordable and unrecordable erg. However the association is probably slight and the predictive value (i.e. the ratio between the actual number of RC patients with bone spicule and the total number of patients with bone spicule) is .54, which is equivalent to say that for every 2 patients with bone spicules, 1 must be an RC RP patient.
The presumed duration of the disease (from the onset of first symptoms to the moment of our visit) is longer in the RC group than in the CR group (29.42 yrs. vs 20.88 yrs) and this could have been a confounder, as increased frequency of bone-spicules in RC could be due only to the duration of the disease. However, stratification by age indicates that in all strata bone spicule were significantly more frequent in RC than in CR (Fisher exact test).
Next in frequency were salt and pepper pattern (48.7%) (table 13), pericentral RPE atrophy (36.5%) (table 11) and diffuse retinal atrophy (27,8%) (table 12) none of which significantly correlated with either the CR or RC subtypes.

Fundus patterns relating to macular aspects were present in about one fouth of our cases: macular atrophy (25%) (table 10), macular hypofluorescence (24.3%) (table 9) and bull's eye which appears to be equally distributed between CR and RC subtypes, both in the erg recordable groups and in the totality of cases (22.5%) (table 7).

Macular window defects (table 8) and sine pigmento (table 15) were slightly more frequent in CR, without attaining the level of significance.

Our data suggest that morphological fundus changes can hardly be used for differentiating RC and CR involvement in RP.

Only bone spicules are significantly related to the RC subtype while, surprisingly enough, macular changes, in particular bull's eye, seem not associated with CR.

The great limitation of this kind of study is the limited number of subject it involves, and the number decreases dramatically in the meticulous but necessary effort to increase homogeneity of subtypes and significance of the differences between them (in our case the initial number of 300 patients had to be reduced to 115 eligible cases).

We have little doubt that, with larger numbers, other associations could have been demonstrated, and that more sophisticated statistical analyses (including multivariate analysis of the duration of disease, pattern of inheritance, association of fundus changes, etc.) could have been performed.

Finally we may express some doubt as to the clinical relevance of CR and RC subtyping, as the majority of fundus changes that we have considered are common to both.

REFERENCES

1) Krill AE: Rod-cone dystrophies. In Krill AE,   Archer DB (eds): Krill's Hereditary Retinal and Choroidal Diseases pp 479-644. Harper & Row, Hagerstown, 1977
2) Berson EL, Gouras P, Gunkel RD. Progressive cone-rod degeneration. Arch Ophthalmol 80:68-76,1968
3) Heckenlively,JR, Retinitis Pigmentosa, Lippincott, Philadelphia, 1988
4) Foxman SG, Heckenlively JR, Bateman JB, Wirtschafter JD. Classification of congenital and early onset RP. Arch of Ophthalmol 103:1502-6,1985

ACKNOWLEDGMENTS

We are indebted to Italian Retinitis Pigmentosa Association of Milan for supply and management of patients examined in the present study.

SECTION V

MOLECULAR BIOLOGY OF RETINAL DEGENERATIONS

A precise definition of the genetic basis for inherited retinal diseases will ultimately come from studies of the molecular biology of both human and animal tissues. Indeed, during the last two years, extraordinary strides have been made in this area, both to map several forms of inherited retinal disease in the human genome and to identify the specific mutations in retinal specific genes.

The chapters presented in this section deal with the molecular biological studies of retinal diseases. Two chapters on the *rd* mouse precisely identify the site of the mutation, as well as the point mutation responsible for this defect in the beta subunit of cyclic GMP phosphodiesterase. The chapter on the *rds* mouse identifies the defective gene product in this mutation as the minor outer segment specific protein, peripherin. Several papers describe transgenic mouse studies using constructs with photoreceptor specific gene promoters coupled to reporter genes. An interesting paper describes the role of viruses in retinal degenerative processes. The authors of the last chapter were asked by the editors to speculate on the possible mechanism(s) of retinal degeneration that results from point mutations in rhodopsin. Collectively, the chapters presented in this section provide a comprehensive overview of the molecular biological studies that are being applied to understanding inherited retinal diseases.

THE MOLECULAR BIOLOGY OF RETINAL DEGENERATIONS

PERSPECTIVES AND NEW DIRECTIONS

Wolfgang Baehr and Muayyad R. Al-Ubaidi

Cullen Eye Institute, Department of Ophthalmology, Baylor College of Medicine, Houston, TX 77030

In recent years, a variety of molecular biological techniques have enhanced our understanding of retinal degenerations in human and animal models. Three methods, however, stand out as being particularly useful for the molecular characterization of genes: first, the polymerase chain reaction (PCR), which allows rapid in-vitro amplification of a gene of interest and subsequent analysis by direct sequencing or cloning. PCR has led to the identification of several point mutations in the opsin gene which may be causative for some forms of human autosomal dominant retinitis pigmentosa (ADRP). Second, subtraction cloning, which allows enrichment of specific DNA probes not easily obtainable by other procedures, and subsequent isolation of candidate genes for a particular retinal degeneration; and third, transgenic mouse technology, which allows incorporation of a particular gene or gene construct into the genome of a mouse, a powerful method for monitoring the consequence of gene expression in a living animal. In the following paragraphs, the three methods will be summarized and their major achievements in the molecular biology of retinal degenerations will be briefly highlighted.

I. THE POLYMERASE CHAIN REACTION (PCR)

The principle of PCR is to amplify target DNA <u>in-vitro</u> by repetitive primer annealing and extension[1]. After each primer extension, the produced double stranded DNA is denatured and primers are reannealed. With each cycle, the DNA product dou-

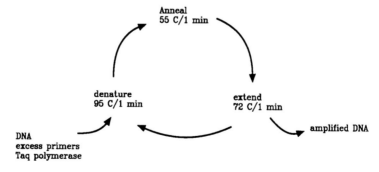

Figure 1. Schematic diagram of the polymerase chain reaction. After 20 cycles, amplification of target DNA is 2^{20} or over 1-million-fold

bles and eventually increases millionfold (Figure 1). PCR became an automated procedure only two years ago with the introduction of Taq polymerase[2] (designated "Molecule of the year" by <u>Science</u> 1989), a heat resistent DNA polymerase isolated from <u>Thermus aquaticus</u>, a microorganism found in Yellowstone hot springs. The reaction depends on the specificity of the oligonucleotide primers used, and the fidelity of incorporation of nucleotides by the DNA polymerase. Taq polymerase incorporates up to 150 nucleotides/ sec/ mole depending on the DNA template, and the misincorporation rate is as low as 2×10^{-4}/cycle[2].

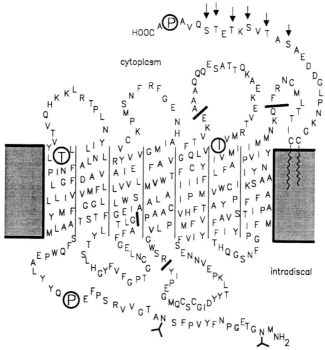

Figure 2. Human opsin and mutations identified in patients affected with Autosomal Dominant Retinitis Pigmentosa (ADRP). Mutated residues are circled. A Y attached to an Asn (N) depicts a glycosylation site, vertical arrows point to phosphorylation sites near the C-terminus. Bars indicate the positions of introns within the gene.

By amplifying exon 1 of the human opsin gene, Ted Dryja and Eliot Berson and their collaborators[3] at Harvard Medical School detected a Pro to His mutation at codon 23 (P23H) in 17 of 148 unrelated patients affected with ADRP. No mutation was found in over 100 randomly selected, unaffected patients. One family of British ancestry showed cosegregation of the point mutation with the disease, indicating that the P23H mutation of opsin may be causative for the form of autosomal dominant retinitis pigmentosa found in this family. Shortly after this discovery, several other point mutations and a microdeletion were identified in various exons of the opsin gene. Ted Dryja and his collegues[4] described a T58R (Thr to Arg transversion at position 58 in exon 1), and a P347I (Pro to Ile at position 347 in exon 5) mutation (Dr. Jane E. Olsson, this session), and additionally Shomi Bhattacharya and his collaborators identified a deletion of a codon for Ile (position 255 or 256 in exon 4, figure 2) (Dr. Shomi S. Bhattacharya, this session). Pro(23), but not Thr(58), I(255 or 256), and Pro(347), is conserved in vertebrate and invertebrate opsins, and related G protein receptors[5].

II. SUBTRACTION CLONING

The principle of subtraction cloning (Figure 3) is to "subtract" cDNA of tissue B (not containing the probe of interest, e.g. degenerated retina lacking photoreceptors) from cDNA of tissue A (containing the probe of interest, e.g. intact retina)[6]. This procedure enriches for a specific cDNA which may be contained in tissue A in very small amounts. For subtraction cloning, a large amount of cDNA (micrograms) of tissue A is first produced by reverse transcription. Then, double stranded cDNA of tissue B which contains many of the transcripts of tissue A, but not the target mRNA, is isolated from a cDNA library. The two cDNA pools are combined in a carefully balanced ratio, denatured ("melted"), annealed to each other under specific conditions (phenol emulsion), and the single stranded cDNA which does not have a complement in tissue B is isolated. Isolation of the cDNA is classically achieved by hydroxylapatite chromatography which separates

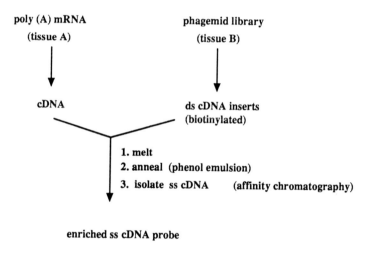

Figure 3. Schematic procedure for subtraction cloning. Subtraction of tissue B from tissue A yields a bank of single stranded (ss) candidate cDNAs which can be analyzed further.

double stranded and single stranded DNA. More efficiently, the DNA to be subtracted may be labeled by biotinylation, and any DNA that binds to the biotinylated probes may be removed by affinity chromatography on Streptavidine Sepharose. The enriched single stranded DNA may be used for screening a library of tissue A which will provide a bank of candidate clones. Screening of the bank of clones by secondary procedures the strategy of which depends on the system used, will finally yield a few candidates to be analyzed further. Such a procedure has been especially successful in the identification of the gene causative for the rds (retinal degeneration slow) mutation[7], and the rd mutation in mouse[8,9]. The rds gene product was later identified to be identical to peripherin, an intrinsic membrane protein of unknown function found in rod disk membranes (Dr. Robert S. Molday, this session). One of the final candidate cDNAs for the rd mutation was found to encode the beta subunit of cGMP phosphodiesterase[7,8] (Dr. Cathy Bowes, this session).

III. TRANSGENIC MOUSE TECHNOLOGY

Several methods have been devised to introduce foreign DNA into both somatic and germ cells of animals. The most important accomplishment for germ-line transformation was the development of techniques for removing embryos, culturing them in vitro, and reimplanting them in foster mothers where they proceed through the normal embryogenic developmental pathways[10]. The first transgenic mice were produced by microinjecting the monkey virus SV40 DNA into the blastocoel cavity of early embryos[11]. Subsequently, the majority of transgenic mice have been produced by microinjecting recombinant DNA directly into pronuclei of fertilized eggs[10].

To direct expression of a gene to photoreceptors of transgenic mice, a gene construct consisting of a structural gene and upstream sequences which regulate its expression must be generated by molecular cloning. We have utilized regulatory sequences of two photoreceptor genes that are well characterized: human interphotoreceptor retinoid-binding protein (IRBP)[12,13] and mouse rhodopsin[14,15]. Both antigens are abundantly expressed in rod photoreceptors, and to a much lesser extent in pinealocytes, which are considered rudimentary photoreceptors. The human IRBP-gene spans more than 11 kb and is interrupted by three introns, all of which are positioned near the 3' end of the coding sequence. The major transcription start site is located at an adenine 119 bp upstream of ATG. Minor sites were located within 18 bp upstream and downstream of this site. No CCAAT or TATA boxes can be identified upstream of the transcription start. The mouse opsin gene spans less than 5 kb and is split into five exons and four introns, an organization characteristic of other mammalian opsin genes. Transcription of the mouse opsin gene starts at an adenine 93 bp upstream of ATG. In contrast to the IRBP gene, the transcription starting point of the mouse opsin gene is preceded by both a TATAA and CAAT box at conventional distances.

The first construct (Fig. 4A) that has been successfully used to target gene expression to the retina[13] consists of a 1.3 kb fragment designated as IRBP promoter and a bacterial gene encoding chloramphenicol acetyl transferase (CAT). Microinjection of this construct yielded six transgenic families, all of which expressed the bacterial CAT gene, concomitant with endogeneous IRBP, predominantly in the retina and to a lesser extent in the pineal gland. Other tissues did not express detectable levels of the transgene product. These results established that a 1.3 kb fragment from the 5' end of the human IRBP gene directs expression of a transgene to a visual subdivision of the central nervous system.

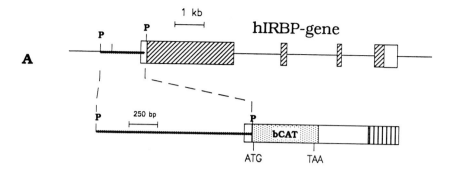

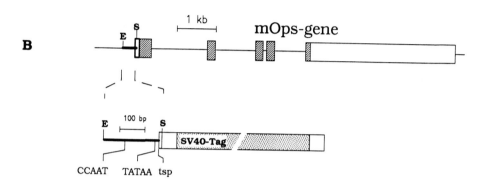

Figure 4. Map of the hIRBP-CAT and MoT1 constructs used for microinjection. A, schematic representation of the human IRBP gene and the bCAT /hIRBP promoter construct. Hatched boxes, coding sequences of exons. White boxes, untranslated regions. The promoter fragment used in the construct is flanked by two PvuII (P) sites. bCAT, bacterial chloramphenicol transferase gene. B, schematic representation of the mouse opsin gene. The promoter is flanked by an EcoR1 (E) and a SacI (S) site. SV40-Tag, the gene encoding SV40 large T-antigen.

The second construct (Fig. 4B) is a fusion gene consisting of 250 bp mouse opsin promoter sequence and Simian Virus 40 (SV40) large T-antigen (SV40-Tag)[16]. SV40 T-antigen was chosen as an antigen for its capability to induce a variety of tumors, thus generating heritable abnormalities[17]. The construct, MoT1, was microinjected into one day old FVB/N mouse embryos. Three transgenic lines were established by mating the founder mice to normal C57BL/6 mice. Early expression (3 days) of the transgene was detected in the retina by PCR with Tag specific primers. The heterozygous offspring of one family showed normal ERG response, while the homozygous offspring showed a negative ERG response and absence of photoreceptor cells as seen by light microscopy. Negative ERG responses were recorded for both heterozygous and homozygous offspring of the second family. Light microscopic analysis of the developing retina in the heterozygous offspring of the second family showed normal progression of the retina until day 10. From day 10 on, differences between normal and transgenic retinas appear. Rod outer segments never develop properly, as judged by the thickness of the photoreceptor layer. At day 21, the outer nuclear layer has degenerated to a single layer of nuclei. The origin of the remaining nuclei is as yet undetermined.

IV. PERSPECTIVES

The techniques briefly highlighted in this introduction will continue to provide ever increasing information about genes, point mutations, and the consequences of their expression in human individuals and in animal models. Generation of subtraction libraries enriched in cDNAs of a specific cell type will continue to be a valuble tool for characterizing hitherto unknown genes. Owing to the polymerase chain reaction and direct gene sequencing, the identification of point mutations in genes encoding photoreceptor proteins has been remarkably fast. In less than one year, four mutations have been characterized in the human opsin gene alone. Undoubtedly, mutations in other genes will be discovered in the near future thereby further enhancing our understanding of retinal degenerations. Finally, the expression of foreign antigens and mutated genes in transgenic mice has given us a powerful tool to follow the consequences of their expression in a living animal.

REFERENCES

1. Saiki, R.K., Scharf, S., Faloona, F., Mullis, K.B., Horn, G.T., Erlich, H.A. and Arnheim, N. Enzymatic amplification of beta-globin genomic sequences and restriction site analysis for diagnosis of sickle cell anemia, Science, 230, 1350, 1985.

2. Saiki, R.K., Gelfand, D.H., Stoffel, S., Scharf, S.J., Higuchi, R., Horn, G.T., Mullis, K.B. and Erlich, H.A. Primer-directed enzymatic amplification of DNA with a thermostable DNA polymerase, Science, 239, 487, 1988.

3. Dryja, T.P., McGee, T.L., Reichel, E., Hahn, L.B., Cowley, G.S., Yandell, D.W., Sandberg, M.A. and Berson, E.L. A point mutation of the rhodopsin gene in one form of retinitis pigmentosa, Nature, 343, 364, 1990.

4. Dryja, T.P., McGee, T.L., Reichel, E., Hahn, L.B., Cowley, G.S., Yandell, D.W., Sandberg, M.A. and Berson, E.L. Point mutation of the human rhodopsin gene in patients with autosomal dominant retinitis pigmentosa, Inv. Ophthal. Vis. Sci., 31, 309, 1990.

5. Applebury, M.L. and Hargrave, P.A. Molecular Biology of Visual Pigments, Vision Res., 26, 1881, 1986.

6. Travis, G.H. and Sutcliffe, J.G. Phenol emulsion-enhanced DNA-driven subtractive cDNA cloning: Isolation of low-abundance monkey cortex-specific mRNAs, Proc. Natl. Acad. Sci. U.S.A., 85, 1696, 1988.

7. Travis, G.H., Brennan, M.B., Danielson, P.E., Kozak, C.A. and Sutcliffe, J.G. Identi-

fication of a photoreceptor-specific mRNA encoded by the gene responsible for retinal degeneration slow (rds), <u>Nature</u>, 338, 70, 1989.

8. Bowes, C., Danciger, M., Kozak, C.A. and Farber, D.B. Isolation of a candidate cDNA for the gene causing retinal degeneration in the rd mouse, <u>Proc. Natl. Acad. Sci. U.S.A.</u>, 86, 9722, 1990.

9. Bowes, C., Li, T., Danciger, M., Baxter, L.C., Applebury, M.L. and Farber, D.B. Retinal degeneration in the rd mouse is caused by a defect in the beta subunit of rod cGMP phosphodiesterase, <u>Nature</u>, 347, 677, 1990.

10. Palmiter, R.D. and Brinster, R.L. Germline transformation of mice, <u>Ann. Rev. Gen.</u>, 20, 465, 1986.

11. Small, J.A., Blair, D.G., Showalter, S.D. and scangos, G.A. Analysis of a transgenic mouse containing simian virus 40 and v-myc sequences, <u>Mol. Cell. Biol.</u>, 5, 642, 1985.

12. Liou, G.I., Ma, D.P., Yang, Y.W., Geng, L., Zhu, C. and Baehr, W. Human interstitial retinoid-binding protein: Gene structure and primary sequence, <u>J. Biol. Chem.</u>, 264, 8200, 1989.

13. Liou, G.I., Geng, L., Al-Ubaidi, M.R., Matragoon, S., Hanten, G., Baehr, W. and Overbeek, P.A. Tissue-specific expression in transgenic mice directed by the 5'-flanking sequences of the human gene encoding interphotoreceptor retinoid-binding protein, <u>J. Biol. Chem.</u>, 265, 8373, 1990.

14. Baehr, W., Pittler, S.J., Champagne, M.S. and Al-Ubaidi, M.R. The mouse opsin gene: Molecular basis of multiple transcripts determined by the polymerase chain reaction (PCR), <u>Inv. Ophthal. Vis. Sci.</u>, 1990.

15. Al-Ubaidi, M.R., Pittler, S.J., Champagne, M.S., Triantafyllos, J.T., McGinnis, J.F. and Baehr, W. Mouse opsin: Gene structure and molecular basis of multiple transcripts, <u>J. Biol. Chem.</u>, 265,1990.

16. Al-Ubaidi, M.R., Overbeek, P.A., Naash, M.I. and Baehr, W. Expression of a viral oncogene in the retina of transgenic mice, <u>Inv. Ophthal. Vis. Sci.</u>, 31, 298, 1990.

17. Overbeek, P.A., Chepelinsky, A.B., Khillan, J.S., Piatigorsky, J. and Westphal, H. Lens-specific expression and developmental regulation of the bacterial chloramphenicol acetyltransferase gene driven by the murine alphaA-crystallin promoter in transgenic mice, <u>Proc. Natl. Acad. Sci. U.S.A.</u>, 82, 7815, 1985.

STUDIES ON THE GENE DEFECT OF THE *rd* MOUSE

Debora B. Farber, Michael Danciger and Cathy Bowes

Jules Stein Eye Institute, UCLA School of Medicine,
Los Angeles, California 90024-7008, USA.

For many years we have been working on the inherited retinal degeneration affecting the *rd* mouse. Biochemical defects were described as early as 1974, implicating elevated levels of cGMP[1] resulting from deficient cGMP-phosphodiesterase (cGMP-PDE) activity[2] as the possible cause of photoreceptor cell death. Later on, a lack of phosphorylation of rhodopsin was also found to occur in the *rd* retina when *in vitro* experiments were performed.[3] The phosphorylation defect, though, seems to be secondary to the deficiency in cGMP-PDE activity and is associated with increased activity of protein phosphatase 2A, which is the enzyme that removes phosphate from phosphorylated rhodopsin.[4] Thus, the phosphorylation reaction may proceed normally in the *rd* retina but the accelerated activity of the phosphatase prevents the detection of the phosphorylated visual pigment. What causes increased phosphatase 2A activity is still not known, but it does not look like there is an abnormality in the enzyme's molecule, since by chromatographic methods we have been able to demonstrate that the enzymes from normal and *rd* retinas are comparable.[4] However, the elevated levels of cGMP in the *rd* retina may stimulate phosphatase 2A activity and prevent the detection of phosphorylated rhodopsin, as has been shown to occur in isolated rod outer segments of rat retina.[5] This, therefore, would be a consequence of the deficient activity of cGMP-PDE.

cGMP-PDE is a key enzyme in the phototransduction process of rod photoreceptors. Its activation by light is mediated by components of the visual cell which include rhodopsin, transducin (a heterotrimeric protein composed of α, β and γ subunits) and GTP. Rhodopsin kinase, arrestin (also called 48 kDa protein or S-antigen) and ATP are involved in the deactivation of cGMP-PDE (for a review, see [6]). The enzyme is composed of two large subunits with catalytic activity (α and β, molecular weights 88,000 and 84,000, respectively) and two identical small inhibitory subunits (γ, molecular weight 11,000).[7,8] Evidently, the abnormal functioning of cGMP-PDE in the *rd* retina could result from lesions in the structure or function of any of the activators/deactivators of the enzyme or from the absence or defective composition of any of its α, β or γ subunits.

Our previous investigations indicated that the mRNAs as well as the proteins from the *rd* retina corresponding to opsin, α, β and γ transducin, arrestin and the γ subunit of cGMP-PDE are comparable to those from control retina in terms of size,[9] amount and onset of expression.[10] Gene mapping studies confirmed that none of these proteins (with the exception of transducin γ which has not been investigated as yet), was the primary site of the *rd* disease since no one maps to mouse chromosome 5,[11-15, 16] the location that had been assigned by linkage analysis to the *rd* gene.[17] Furthermore, cGMP-PDE is synthesized normally in the *rd* retina.[18] However, the enzyme is always present at lower levels in *rd* retina than in control retina, suggesting that either the *rd* cGMP-PDE has a change in its amino acid composition or structure which makes it more unstable, or that increased proteolytic activity in the *rd* photoreceptors may result in its faster degradation.[18] Preliminary experiments investigating the activity of several proteases in *rd* and control retinas showed comparable results with the

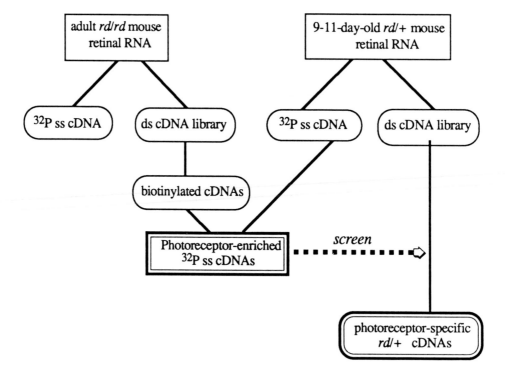

Figure. 1. Outline of the steps followed for the isolation of normal mouse (*rd/+*) photoreceptor-specific clones.

normal and affected tissues.[19] As we will describe in the next paragraphs, we know by now that the abnormality resides in one of the subunits of the rod-specific cGMP-PDE.

The approach that allowed us to identify and isolate the retinal component responsible for the degeneration of the *rd* mouse photoreceptors made use of basic molecular biological techniques. We based our strategy on the assumption that the mRNA encoded by the *rd* gene would be expressed differently in affected and normal visual cells, and on the fact that the adult *rd* retina is devoid of photoreceptor cells and their specific mRNAs. The first step of our procedure was to prepare a radiolabeled probe consisting of photoreceptor-enriched cDNAs. This probe was obtained by subtractive cloning.[20] An outline of the steps and different cDNAs used is shown in Figure 1. A large excess of adult *rd/rd* cDNAs was biotinylated and hybridized to a pool of radiolabeled, single stranded cDNAs from 9-11-day-old normal *rd/+* mouse retina (this mouse age was chosen for all experiments to ensure the greatest amount of age-matched retinal tissue before complete degeneration of the *rd/rd* photoreceptors). Theoretically, all the cDNAs of the adult *rd/rd* retina will hybridize the cDNAs from the inner retinal layers of normal retina, leaving radiolabeled, single stranded *rd/+* photoreceptor cDNAs unhybridized. These were separated on a streptavidin-Sepharose column from the excess biotinylated, *rd/rd* driver DNA and the non-photoreceptor *rd/rd* • *rd/+* cDNA hybrids. This probe was then used to screen a 9-11-day-old normal *rd/+* retinal cDNA library for homologous sequences and the positive clones were re-screened with adult *rd/rd* single-stranded cDNAs to confirm their photoreceptor-specific nature.

The selection of a candidate cDNA for the *rd* gene from the set of 400 photoreceptor-specific clones obtained was carried out by means of differential screening with probes consisting of 9-11-day-old *rd/+* and *rd/rd* mouse single-stranded retinal cDNAs.[20] Of the 3 clones that hybridized differently with the two probes, only one clone, zr.408, hybridized more faintly on Northern blots to 9-11-day-old *rd/rd* RNA than to the age-matched normal RNA. zr.408 then became the focus of our studies. Several properties of this cDNA made it a strong candidate for the *rd* gene:

1) In all Northern blots that we analyzed (which contained samples of *+/+*, *rd/+*, and *rd/rd* retinal RNAs from mice at various postnatal ages) zr.408 hybridized to a slightly larger, less abundant transcript, in the developing *rd/rd* retina compared with the normal *rd/+* and *+/+* retinas. RNA samples of *rd/rd* mice which had lost all of their photoreceptor cells (30-days-old or older) did not hybridize with zr.408. The size difference in the mRNA could be the result of alternative splicing, of the presence of different poly-adenylation sites or it could stem from a structural alteration in the corresponding gene of the *rd/rd* mouse. Quantification of the mRNA

hybridized by zr.408 in slot blots containing retinal RNA samples from developing *rd/rd* and *rd/+* animals showed that at postnatal day 1 the expression of the putative *rd* cDNA is already abnormal in *rd/rd* retina.[20] This occurs before the cGMP levels become elevated in the *rd* photoreceptor cells and, therefore, constitutes the earliest molecular lesion demonstrated to date in the *rd* mouse disease.

2) In Southern blots of normal (+/+) and *rd/rd* mouse genomic DNAs, zr.408 detected restriction fragment length polymorphisms (RFLPs). This suggests a structural difference between the +/+ and *rd/rd* gene sequences at sites homologous to zr.408. That such a difference is real was confirmed by the pattern of hybridization of zr.408 with the *rd/+* mouse DNA, which showed both the +/+ and *rd/rd* mouse DNA polymorphisms at about half the intensity observed for each in the DNAs from the homozygous mice.[20]

3) Chromosomal mapping of zr.408 using Southern blot hybridization to DNA from 14 hamster-mouse somatic cell hybrids showed no discordancies for the localization of this cDNA on mouse chromosome 5, whereas several discordancies were observed for the assignment of zr.408 to any other mouse chromosome.[20]

4) In a three-point intersubspecific backcross study we showed that zr.408 hybridizes to mouse DNA sequences that lie between the genes encoding α-fetoprotein (*Afp*) and β-glucuronidase (*Gus*). The position of the gene corresponding to zr.408 relative to *Afp* and *Gus* was comparable to the position of the *rd* gene in standard mouse gene maps.[21]

5) In an interspecific backcross study, using *rd/rd* mice made congenic for the normal allele of *rd*, derived from the wild mouse *Mus spretus*, we showed that the zr.408 co-segregates with the phenotypic expression of the *rd* disease, retinal degeneration.[21]

The results described above are consistent with our characterization of zr.408 as the normal product of the *rd* locus. In the following paragraphs we will summarize the work that we carried out next in order to identify the protein encoded by the *rd* gene.

Based on the biochemical evidence obtained in the previous years of study of the *rd* mouse, our initial attention was directed to the α and β subunits of rod-specific cGMP-PDE (we had already cloned and sequenced the γ subunit of the enzyme present in *rd* retina[22] and found that it is identical to that in the rods of normal mouse retina[23]). A collaboration was established with Dr. Meredithe Applebury who provided us with the cDNAs for the bovine cGMP-PDE α and β subunits. A strong hybridization of zr.408 with cGMP-PDEβ cDNA indicated that our candidate cDNA had homologous sequences with the cDNA encoding this subunit of the enzyme. We then proceeded to use zr.408 and the bovine probes to screen normal mouse (+/+) retinal cDNA libraries. None of the isolated clones were full-length;

Mouse PDE β-cDNA

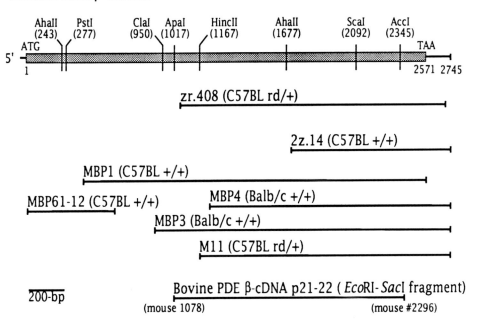

Figure 2. Restriction map of the mouse photoreceptor cGMP-PDE β-subunit cDNA. Depicted in the diagram are the relative sizes and positions of the various cDNA clones (including zr. 408) used to determine the full-length sequence of the cGMP-PDE β cDNA. Some of these clones were also used as probes in Northerns and Southerns. The filled box indicates the open reading frame.

thus, we needed to use the polymerase chain reaction to obtain fragments which together would span the complete mRNA sequence (Figure 2).

The nucleotide sequence of the mouse cGMP-PDEβ cDNA is shown in figure 3. It has 82% identity with the bovine transcript; zr.408 is a truncated clone which corresponds to two-thirds of the total sequence (from base 1,114 through base 2,706). There is only one nucleotide changed in the zr.408 sequence, which may be due to a polymorphic difference in the mouse strains that were used for the preparation of the libraries, confirming the

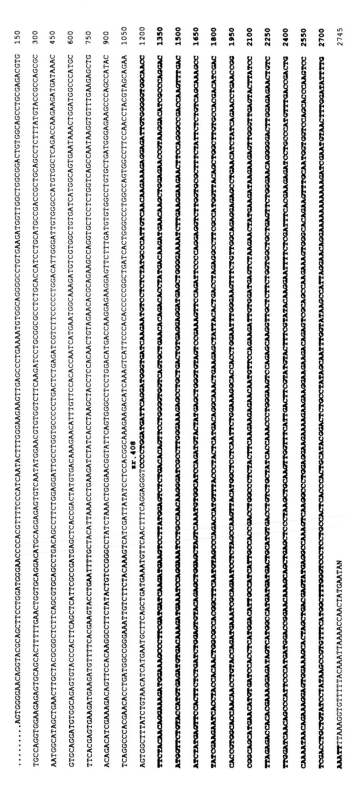

Figure 3. Nucleotide sequence of mouse cGMP-PDE β subunit cDNA. The sequence of zr.408 is depicted by the bold portion of the sequence.

```
1     - - - S G E Q V R S F L D G N P T F S H Q Y F G K K L S P E N V A G A C E D G W L A D C G S L R D V
51    C Q V E E S A A L F E L V Q D M Q E S V N M E R V V F K I L R R L C T I L H A D R C S L F M Y R Q R
101   N G I A E L A T R L F S V Q P D S L L E D C L V P P D S E I V F P L D I G I V G H V A Q T K K M I N
151   V Q D V A E C T H F S S F A D E L T D Y V T K N I C S T P I M N G K D V V A V I M A V N K L D G P C
201   F T S E D E D V F T K Y L N F A T L N L K I Y H L S Y L H N C E T R R S Q V L L W S A N K V F E E L
251   T D I E R Q F H K A F Y T V R A Y L N C E R Y S V G L L D M T K E K E F F D V W P V L M G E A Q P Y
301   S G P R T P D G R E I V F Y K V I D Y I L H G K E D I K V I P T P P A D H W A L A S G L P T Y V A E
351   S G F I C N I M N A S A D E M F N F Q E G P L D D S G W V I K N V L S M P I V N K K E E I V G V A T
401   F Y N R K D G K P F D D Q D E V L M E S L T Q F L G W S V L N T D T Y D K M N K L E N R K D I A Q D
451   M V L Y H V R C D K D E I Q E I L P T R D R L G K E P A D C E E D E L G K I L K E E L P G P T K F D
501   I Y E F H F S D L E C T E L E L V K C G I Q M Y Y E L G V V R K F Q I P Q E V L V R F L F S V S K A
551   Y R R I T Y H N W R H G F N V A Q T M F T L L M T G K L K S Y Y T D L E A F A M V T A G L C H D I D
601   H R G T N N L Y Q M K S Q N P L A K L H G S S I L E R H H L E F G K F L L A E E S L N I Y Q N L N R
651   R Q H E H V I H L M D I A I I A T D L A L Y F K K R T M F Q K I V D E S K N Y E D K K S W V E Y L S
701   L E T T R K E I V M A M M M T A C D L S A I T K P W E V Q S K V A L L V A A E F W E Q G D L E R T V
751   L D Q Q P I P M M D R N K A A E L P K L Q V G F I D F V C T F V Y K E F S R F H E E I L P M F D R L
801   Q N N R K E W K A L A D E Y E A K V K A L E E E K K K E E D R V A A K K V G T E V C N G G P A P K S
851   S T C C I L
```

Figure 4. Deduced amino acid sequence of mouse cGMP-PDE β subunit.

nature of our candidate *rd* cDNA.[24] Figure 4 shows the deduced amino acid sequence of cGMP-PDE β-subunit. At the amino acid level, the percent identity between mouse and bovine cGMP-PDEβ subunits is 93.1%, indicating that this protein has been very well conserved through evolution.

In order to further confirm that zr.408 is a part of the cGMP-PDEβ gene, we compared the pattern of hybridization of genomic DNA from *rd/rd*, *rd/+* and normal murine tissues with several murine and bovine cGMP-PDEβ cDNA probes along with zr.408. All probes detected RFLPs that distinguished the *rd* and wild-type genotypes; in addition, the patterns of hybridization of zr.408 and a mouse cGMP-PDEβ probe to murine poly(A)$^+$ RNAs from normal, *rd/rd* and *rd/+* retinas were identical.[24]

The observations summarized in the paragraphs above support the conclusion that cGMP-PDEβ is encoded by the normal counterpart of the *rd* gene. Definitive proof of this will come from our ongoing transgenic studies in which we are attempting to place a functional copy of the cGMP-PDEβ gene in the photoreceptor cells of *rd* mice. We hope that the transgene will achieve correction of the disease phenotype.

ACKNOWLEDGEMENTS

We wish to thank Dr. John Flannery for his continued participation in discussion of these studies. We also acknowledge the technical assistance of Ana Lia Rapoport and Vincent Guerena. This work was supported by National Institutes of Health grants EY02651 and EY08285 (D.B.F.) and Core grant EY00331; a Center grant from the National Retinitis Pigmentosa Foundation; and a grant from the George Gund Foundation. DBF is the recipient of a Research to Prevent Blindness Senior Scientific Investigators Award.

REFERENCES

1. Farber, D. B. and Lolley, R. N., Cyclic guanosine monophosphate: Elevations in degenerating photoreceptor cells of the C3H mouse retina, *Science*, **186**, 449, 1974.

2. Farber, D. B and Lolley, R. N., Enzymatic basis for cyclic GMP accumulation in degenerative photoreceptor cells of mouse retina, *J. Cyclic Nucleotide Res.*, **2**, 139, 1976.

3. Shuster, T. A. and Farber, D. B., Rhodopsin phosphorylation in developing normal and degenerative mouse retinas, *Invest. Ophthalmol. Vis. Sci.*, **27**, 264, 1986.

4. Palczewski, K., Farber, D. B. and Hargrave, P.A., Elevated level of protein phosphatase 2A activity in retinas of *rd* mice, *Exp. Eye Res.*, 1991, in press.

5. Shuster, T. A. and Farber, D. B., Phosphorylation in sealed rod outer segments: the effects of cyclic nucleotides, *Biochemistry*, **23**, 515, 1984.

6. Farber, D. B. and Shuster, T. A., Cyclic nucleotides in retinal function and degeneration. In *The Retina: A model for cell biology studies,*, Part 1, Adler,R. and Farber, D.B., Academic Press, Orlando, FL, 1986, 239.

7. Baehr, W., Devlin, M. J., Applebury, M. L., Isolation and characterization of cGMP phosphodiesterase from bovine rod outer segments, *J. Biol. Chem.*, **254**, 11669, 1979.

8. Fung, B, K, -K., Young, J. H., Yamane, H. K., Griswold-Prenner, I., Subunit stoichiometry of retinal rod cGMP phosphodiesterase, *Biochemistry*, **29**, 2657, 1990.

9. Bowes, C. and Farber, D. B., mRNAs coding for proteins of the cGMP cascade in the degenerative retina of the *rd* mouse, *Exp. Eye Res.*, **45**, 467, 1987.

10. Bowes, C., van Veen, T. and Farber, D. B., Opsin, G-protein and 48-kDa protein in normal and *rd* mouse retinas: developmental expression of mRNAs and proteins and light/dark cycling of mRNAs, *Exp. Eye Res.*, **47**, 369, 1988.

11. Danciger, M., Kozak, C. A. and Farber, D. B., The gene for the α-subunit of retinal rod transducin is on mouse chromosome 9, *Genomics,* **4**, 215, 1989a.

12. Danciger, M., Tuteja, N., Kozak, C. A. and Farber, D.B., The gene for the γ-subunit of retinal cGMP-phosphodiesterase is on mouse chromosome 11, *Exp. Eye Res.*, **48**, 303, 1989b.

13. Danciger, M., Kozak, C. A., Tsuda, M., Shinohara, T. and Farber, D. B., The gene for retinal S-antigen (48-kDa protein) maps to the centromeric portion of mouse chromosome 1 near *Idh-1, Genomics,* **5**, 378, 1989c.

14. Danciger, M., Farber, D. B., Peyser, M. and Kozak, C. A., Mapping of the gene for the β-subunit of retinal transducin (*Gnb-1*) to distal mouse chromosome 4 and demonstration of additional homologous sequences on chromosomes 5 and 8, *Genomics,* **6**, 428, 1990a.

15. Danciger, M., Kozak, C. A,, Li, T., Applebury, M. L., Farber, D. B., Genetic mapping demonstrates that the α-subunit of retinal cGMP-phosphodiesterase is not the site of the *rd* mutation, *Exp. Eye Res.*, **51**, 185, 1990b.

16. Elliott, R. W., Sparkes, R. S., Mohandas, T., Grant, S. G. and McGinnis, J. F., Localization of the rhodopsin gene to the distal half of mouse chromosome 6, *Genomics,* **6**, 635, 1990.

17. Sidman, R. L. and Green, M. C., Retinal degeneration in the mouse; location of the *rd* locus in linkage group XVII, *J. Hered.*, **56**, 23, 1965.

18. Farber, D. B., Park, S. and Yamashita, C., Cyclic GMP-phosphodiesterase of *rd* retina: biosynthesis and content, *Exp. Eye Res.*, **46**, 363, 1988.

19. Farber, D. B., unpublished data, 1990.

20. Bowes, C., Danciger, M., Kozak, C. A. and Farber, D. B., Isolation of a candidate cDNA for a gene causing retinal degeneration in *rd* mouse. Proc. Natl. Acad. Sci., U.S.A., **86**, 9722, 1989.

21. Danciger, M., Bowes, C., Kozak, C.A., LaVail, M.M. and Farber, D. B., Fine mapping of a putative *rd* cDNA and its cosegregation with *rd* expression, *Invest. Ophthalmol. Vis. Sci.,* **31**, 1427, 1990c.

22. Tuteja, N., Tuteja, R. and Farber, D. B., Cloning and sequencing of the γ-subunit of retinal cyclic GMP-phosphodiesterase from *rd* mouse, *Exp. Eye Res.*, **48**, 863, 1989.

23. Tuteja, N. and Farber, D. B., γ-subunit of mouse retinal cyclic GMP-phosphodiesterase: cDNA and corresponding amino acid sequences, *FEBS Letters,* **232**, 182, 1988.

24. Bowes, C., Li, T., Danciger, M., Baxter, L. C., Applebury, M. L. and Farber, D. B., Retinal degeneration in the *rd* mouse is caused by a defect in the β–subunit of rod cGMP-phosphodiesterase, *Nature,* **347,** 677, 1990.

IDENTIFICATION OF THE PRECISE MOLECULAR DEFECT RESPONSIBLE FOR BLINDNESS IN THE MOUSE RETINAL DEGENERATION MUTANT, *rd*

Steven J. Pittler and Wolfgang Baehr

Department of Ophthalmology, Cullen Eye Institute, Baylor College of Medicine, Houston, Texas 77030

I. SUMMARY

An autosomal recessively inherited retinal degeneration, *rd*, was described in the mouse almost forty years ago. Histopathologically, the mutant mice display a complete loss of rod photoreceptor cells by postnatal day (pn) 20. The earliest detectable abnormality, however, is a marked elevation of retina cGMP levels beginning at pn 6. Biochemical studies suggested a defect may reside in one of the subunits of the rod cGMP phosphodiesterase (cGMP PDE). More recently the mouse cGMP PDE β-subunit gene was mapped near the *rd* locus on chromosome 5. It was also suggested that the β-subunit transcript was abnormal in size and abundance. In order to compare the sequences of the rod cGMP phosphodiesterase β-subunit in normal and *rd* mouse, we characterized cDNA clones from a normal mouse retina library and reverse transcription-PCR amplified products of pn 9-11 *rd* retina RNA. Six sequence differences were found including one leading to a nonsense mutation in the PDE β-subunit mRNA of the *rd* mouse. The stop codon truncates the normal gene product predicting a peptide of ~30 kD that does not contain the presumed catalytic domain. We suggest that the apparent alterations in size and abundance of the β-subunit transcript are not the primary cause of the *rd* disorder. Rather, the truncation of the β-subunit caused by a premature stop codon is responsible for the retinal degeneration and subsequent blindness that occurs in the *rd* mouse, thereby establishing the identity of the *rd* locus as the gene encoding the rod cGMP phosphodiesterase β-subunit. In this chapter we review the history of the *rd* mouse from its discovery to our finding of the specific molecular defect.

II. RESULTS AND DISCUSSION

A. HISTORY OF THE MOUSE RETINAL DEGENERATION MUTANT, *rd*

Retinal degeneration was first noted in the mouse with the now extinct mutant rodless (*r*) described in 1924[1]. In 1951 another mouse mutant, termed *rd*, was found almost simultaneously in wild populations throughout Europe[2-4], and in inbred laboratory strains[5]. The morphological characteristics of these mice were strikingly similar, suggesting that *r* and *rd* were allelic. Retinas of *rd* mice appear to develop normally until pn 9-10 when the rod photoreceptors begin to degenerate[6]. By pn 20 rod photoreceptor cells are absent, yet cones and other retinal cells remain intact[7]. The *rd* locus was initially shown to be linked to the β-glucuronidase gene[8], in linkage group XVII[9] which is now known to be mouse chromosome 5. Later it was shown that *rd* is very tightly linked to the pigmentation mutant gene, *le*, and this easily distinguished marker was useful for genetic studies[10].

Several studies were performed during the early 70's to provide clues to the biochemical nature of the defect[11]. Finally, in 1974 cGMP levels in the *rd* retina were found to be considerably higher than normal prior to any signs of morphological degeneration[12]. It was later shown that cGMP PDE activity was deficient in the developing *rd* retina[13], suggesting a defect in the enzyme itself or in some regulatory component. Monoclonal antibodies specific to cGMP PDE were used to show the apparent absence of immunoreactive material in pre-degenerative *rd* retinas[14]. Using polyclonal antibodies it was later shown that the γ-subunit and at least one large subunit of the cGMP PDE are present at low levels, but a normal subunit complex is not formed[15]. This was the first study to provide direct biochemical evidence that the defect may reside within a subunit of the rod cGMP phosphodiesterase. It was later suggested that a defect in the rod cGMP phosphodiesterase β-subunit gene is responsible for the retinal degeneration, based on chromosome localization, RFLP detection, altered transcription levels, and a slight difference in the migration of the β-subunit mRNA in formaldehyde-agarose gels[16-18]. We show that the mouse cGMP PDE β-subunit gene is indeed identical to the *rd* locus by identifying a nonsense codon that truncates the normal gene product.

B. MOUSE ROD PHOTORECEPTOR cGMP PHOSPHODIESTERASES

Rod photoreceptor cGMP phosphodiesterase (PDE) is a three subunit enzyme that functions as a signal amplifier in phototransduction (reviewed in[19,20]). Rod PDE consists of three subunits[21], termed α, β, γ , with SDS-PAGE mobilities of 88K (α), 84K (β), and 13K (γ). Comparison of the predicted amino acid sequences from mouse PDE α and β-subunit cDNAs[22] (Figure 1) revealed a high overall homology (72%) and a very high sequence similarity (90%) of the putative catalytic domain. The regions that are the least well conserved in the mouse α and β-subunits are at the N-terminus (first 100 residues) and at the C-terminus (last 30 residues). The domain with the greatest sequence similarity is located near the C-terminus, consisting of approximately 300 amino acids. This region is also conserved between several eukaryotic cyclic nucleotide phosphodiesterases[23-26] and is thought to contain at least part of the active site of the enzyme. The open reading frame of the mouse β-subunit cDNA sequence predicts an 856 residue polypeptide (Figure 2), three amino acids longer than bovine β[27]. The sequence similarity to its bovine counterpart is very high (93%). The mouse α-subunit contains 859 residues, the same number found in bovine and human α-subunits[28,29]. Mouse[30], human[31], and bovine[32] γ-subunits are highly conserved 87 residue polypeptides containing a region highly enriched in basic residues.

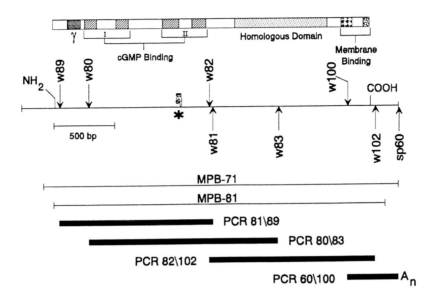

Figure 1 Schematic of PCR Generated and cDNA Clones from *rd* and Normal Mouse Retina RNA

At the top is a representation of functional domains within the cGMP PDE β-subunit. A region near the N-terminus (marked γ) may be involved in the interaction with the PDE γ-subunit. Two domains (marked I and II) that contain consensus sequence motifs for cyclic nucleotide binding[33] are shown. The presumed catalytic domain that is homologous to several eukaryotic cyclic nucleotide phosphodiesterases[23-26] is located near the C-terminus. At the C-terminus is a Caax box signalling posttranslational modification involving isoprenylation, proteolysis, and carboxymethylation[34]. Near the C-terminus is a short stretch of charged residues that may, in conjunction with the Caax processing, be involved in membrane binding as shown for p21^{ras} [35]. Primers used to amplify cDNA (W80-W102 and SP60) are shown. Primer sp60 amplifies from the poly A tail designated A$_n$. The asterisk and pointing icon mark the site of the nonsense mutation in the *rd* cDNA. Two full length cDNAs, MPB-71 and MPB-81 are represented as single lines. Filled rectangles represent the amplified PCR products from *rd* and normal cDNA.

C. ALTERNATIVE SPLICING OF THE MOUSE ROD cGMP PDE β-SUBUNIT GENE

Surprisingly, during our analysis of β-subunit cDNAs[22], two clones were identified containing a 10 bp insertion. The insertion caused a shift in the reading frame introducing a stop codon 16 codons after the insertion point, generating a truncated β subunit (termed β'). The existence of an mRNA in the mouse retina RNA population with the 10 bp insertion was verified by PCR amplification. Thus, the predicted β' polypeptide has a C-terminus different from β, is 55 residues shorter lacking a Caax motif[36], but does contain most of the catalytic domain. The β' transcript was shown to arise via alternative use of an acceptor splice site[22], demonstrating the first phototransduction gene that may produce more than one gene product.

Mouse cGMP PDE β-Subunit cDNA Sequence

```
GCATTAGCAAAGTTCACAGGACGCTCTCGCCTGTTCCCTGCAACATCTCTGGTGCTAGCT60
AAGGGTCTCCTATGATGTAGGGGGCACAGCAGCAGGAACACCATGAGCCTCAGTGAGGAA120
                 *                                M  S  L  S  E  E

CAGGTACGCAGCTTCCTGGATGGGAACCCCACGTTTGCCCATCAATACTTTGGGAAGAAG180
 Q  V  R  S  F  L  D  G  N  P  T  F  A  H  Q  Y  F  G  K  K

      C
TTGAGCCCTGAAAATGTGGCAGGGGCCTGTGAAGATGGTTGGCTGGCGGACTGTGGCAGC240
 L  S  P  E  N  V  A  G  A  C  E  D  G  W  L  A  D  C  G  S

CTGCGAGAGCTGTGCCAGGTGGAAGAGAGTGCAGCACTTTTTGAACTGGTGCAGGACATG300
 L  R  E  L  C  Q  V  E  E  S  A  A  L  F  E  L  V  Q  D  M

CAGGAGAGTGTCAATATGGAACGTGTGGTCTTCAAGATCCTGCGGCGCCTCTGCACCATC360
 Q  E  S  V  N  M  E  R  V  V  F  K  I  L  R  R  L  C  T  I

CTGCATGCCGACCGCTGCAGCCTCTTTATGTACCGCCAGCGCAATGGCATAGCTGAACTT420
 L  H  A  D  R  C  S  L  F  M  Y  R  Q  R  N  G  I  A  E  L

      A
GCTACGCGGCTCTTCAGCGTGCAGCCTGACAGCCTTCTGGAGGATTGCCTGGTGCCCCCT480
 A  T  R  L  F  S  V  Q  P  D  S  L  L  E  D  C  L  V  P  P

GACTCTGAGATCGTCTTCCCCCTGGACATTGGGATTGTGGGCCATGTGGCTCAGACCAAG540
 D  S  E  I  V  F  P  L  D  I  G  I  V  G  H  V  A  Q  T  K

AAGATGATAAACGTGCAGGATGTGGCAGAGTGTCCCCACTTCAGCTCATTCGCCGATGAG600
 K  M  I  N  V  Q  D  V  A  E  C  P  H  F  S  S  F  A  D  E

CTCACCGACTATGTGACAAAGAACATTTTGTCCACACCAATCATGAATGGCAAAGATGTC660
 L  T  D  Y  V  T  K  N  I  L  S  T  P  I  M  N  G  K  D  V

GTGGCTGTGATCATGGCAGTGAATAAACTGGATGGCCCATGCTTCACGAGTGAAGATGAA720
 V  A  V  I  M  A  V  N  K  L  D  G  P  C  F  T  S  E  D  E

GATGTTTTCACGAAGTACCTGAATTTTGCTACATTAAACCTGAAGATCTATCACCTAAGC780
 D  V  F  T  K  Y  L  N  F  A  T  L  N  L  K  I  Y  H  L  S

TACCTCCACAACTGTGAGACACGCAGAGGCCAGGTGCTCCTCTGGTCAGCCAATAAGGTG840
 Y  L  H  N  C  E  T  R  R  G  Q  V  L  L  W  S  A  N  K  V

TTTGAAGAGCTGACAGACATCGAAAGACAGTTCCACAAGGCCTTCTATACTGTCCGGGCC900
 F  E  E  L  T  D  I  E  R  Q  F  H  K  A  F  Y  T  V  R  A

TATCTAAACTGCGAACGGTATTCAGTGGGCCTCCTGGACATGACCAAGGAGAAGGAGTTC960
 Y  L  N  C  E  R  Y  S  V  G  L  L  D  M  T  K  E  K  E  F

TTTGATGTGTGGCCTGTGCTGATGGGAGAAGCCCAGCCATACTCAGGCCCACGAACACCT1020
 F  D  V  W  P  V  L  M  G  E  A  Q  P  Y  S  G  P  R  T  P
```

```
GATGGCCGGGAAATTGTCTTCTACAAAGTCATCGATTATATCCTCCACGGCAAAGAAGAC1080
 D  G  R  E  I  V  F  Y  K  V  I  D  Y  I  L  H  G  K  E  D

ATCAAAGTCATTCCCACACCCCCGGCTGATCACTGGGCCCTGGCCAGTGGCCTTCCAACC1140
 I  K  V  I  P  T  P  P  A  D  H  W  A  L  A  S  G  L  P  T

    A
TACGTAGCAGAAAGTGGCTTTATCTGTAACATCATGAATGCTTCAGCTGATGAAATGTTC1200
 Y  V  A  E  S  G  F  I  C  N  I  M  N  A  S  A  D  E  M  F
 *
                                                      T
AACTTTCAGGAGGGGCCCCTGGATGATTCAGGATGGGTGATCAAGAATGTCCTCTCTATG1260
 N  F  Q  E  G  P  L  D  D  S  G  W  V  I  K  N  V  L  S  M

CCCATTGTCAACAAGAAAGAGGAGATTGTGGGGGTGGCAACCTTCTACAACAGGAAAGAT1320
 P  I  V  N  K  K  E  E  I  V  G  V  A  T  F  Y  N  R  K  D

GGAAAGCCCTTCGATGATCAAGATGAAGTCCTTATGGAGTCTCTGACACAGTTCCTGGGG1380
 G  K  P  F  D  D  Q  D  E  V  L  M  E  S  L  T  Q  F  L  G

TGGTCAGTGCTGAACACAGACACCTATGACAAGATGAACAAGCTGGAGAACCGTAAGGAC1440
 W  S  V  L  N  T  D  T  Y  D  K  M  N  K  L  E  N  R  K  D

ATCGCCCAGGACATGGTTCTGTACCATGTGAGATGTGACAAAGATGAAATCCAGGAAATC1500
 I  A  Q  D  M  V  L  Y  H  V  R  C  D  K  D  E  I  Q  E  I

CTGCCAACAAGGGATCGCCTTGGGAAAGAGCCTGCTGACTGTGAGGAGGATGAGCTGGGG1560
 L  P  T  R  D  R  L  G  K  E  P  A  D  C  E  E  D  E  L  G

AAAATCTTGAAGGAAGAACTTCCAGGGCCGACCAAGTTTGACATCTATGAGTTCCACTTC1620
 K  I  L  K  E  E  L  P  G  P  T  K  F  D  I  Y  E  F  H  F

TCTGATCTGGAGTGTACAGAGCTGGAGCTAGTCAAATGTGGCATCCAGATGTACTATGAG1680
 S  D  L  E  C  T  E  L  E  L  V  K  C  G  I  Q  M  Y  Y  E

CTGGGTGTAGTCCGAAAGTTCCAGATTCCCCAGGAGGTCTTGGTGCGCTTTCTATTCTCT1740
 L  G  V  V  R  K  F  Q  I  P  Q  E  V  L  V  R  F  L  F  S

GTCAGCAAAGCCTATCGAAGAATCACCTACCACAACTGGCGCCACGGCTTCAATGTAGCC1800
 V  S  K  A  Y  R  R  I  T  Y  H  N  W  R  H  G  F  N  V  A

CAGACCATGTTTACCCTACTCATGACAGGCAAACTGAAGAGCTATTACACTGACCTAGAG1860
 Q  T  M  F  T  L  L  M  T  G  K  L  K  S  Y  Y  T  D  L  E

GCCTTCGCCATGGTTACAGCTGGCTTGTGCCACGACATCGACCACCGTGGCACCAACAAC1920
 A  F  A  M  V  T  A  G  L  C  H  D  I  D  H  R  G  T  N  N

CTGTACCAAATGAAATCGCAGAATCCTCTAGCCAAGTTACATGGCTCCTCAATTCTGGAA1980
 L  Y  Q  M  K  S  Q  N  P  L  A  K  L  H  G  S  S  I  L  E

AGGCACCACCTGGAATTTGGGAAGTTTCTGTTGGCAGAGGAGAGCCTGAACATCTATCAG2040
 R  H  H  L  E  F  G  K  F  L  L  A  E  E  S  L  N  I  Y  Q

AACCTGAACCGGCGGCAGCATGAACATGTGATCCACCTCATGGACATTGCCATCATTGCC2100
 N  L  N  R  R  Q  H  E  H  V  I  H  L  M  D  I  A  I  I  A

ACCGACCTGGCCCTCTACTTCAAGAAGAGAACAATGTTCCAGAAGATTGTGGATGAGTCT2160
 T  D  L  A  L  Y  F  K  K  R  T  M  F  Q  K  I  V  D  E  S

AAGAACTATGAAGATAAGAAGAGTTGGGTTGAGTACTTATCCTTAGAGACCACACGAAAG2220
 K  N  Y  E  D  K  K  S  W  V  E  Y  L  S  L  E  T  T  R  K

GAGATAGTCATGGCCATGATGATGACTGCATGTGACCTGTCTGCTATCACCAAACCCTGG2280
 E  I  V  M  A  M  M  M  T  A  C  D  L  S  A  I  T  K  P  W
```

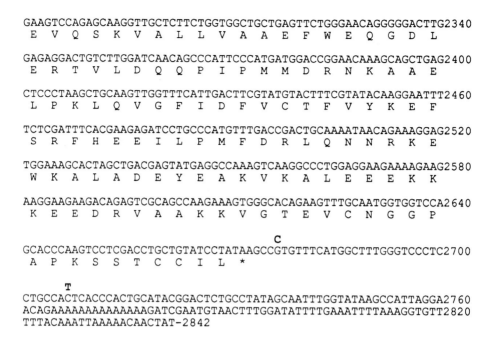

```
GAAGTCCAGAGCAAGGTTGCTCTTCTGGTGGCTGCTGAGTTCTGGGAACAGGGGGACTTG2340
 E   V   Q   S   K   V   A   L   L   V   A   A   E   F   W   E   Q   G   D   L

GAGAGGACTGTCTTGGATCAACAGCCCATTCCCATGATGGACCGGAACAAAGCAGCTGAG2400
 E   R   T   V   L   D   Q   Q   P   I   P   M   M   D   R   N   K   A   A   E

CTCCCTAAGCTGCAAGTTGGTTTCATTGACTTCGTATGTACTTTCGTATACAAGGAATTT2460
 L   P   K   L   Q   V   G   F   I   D   F   V   C   T   F   V   Y   K   E   F

TCTCGATTTCACGAAGAGATCCTGCCCATGTTTGACCGACTGCAAAATAACAGAAAGGAG2520
 S   R   F   H   E   E   I   L   P   M   F   D   R   L   Q   N   N   R   K   E

TGGAAAGCACTAGCTGACGAGTATGAGGCCAAAGTCAAGGCCCTGGAGGAAGAAAAGAAG2580
 W   K   A   L   A   D   E   Y   E   A   K   V   K   A   L   E   E   E   K   K

AAGGAAGAAGACAGAGTCGCAGCCAAGAAAGTGGGCACAGAAGTTTGCAATGGTGGTCCA2640
 K   E   E   D   R   V   A   A   K   K   V   G   T   E   V   C   N   G   G   P

                                   C
GCACCCAAGTCCTCGACCTGCTGTATCCTATAAGCCGTGTTTCATGGCTTTGGGTCCCTC2700
 A   P   K   S   S   T   C   C   I   L   *

     T
CTGCCACTCACCCACTGCATACGGACTCTGCCTATAGCAATTTGGTATAAGCCATTAGGA2760
ACAGAAAAAAAAAAAAAAAGATCGAATGTAACTTTGGATATTTTGAAATTTTAAAGGTGTT2820
TTTACAAATTAAAAACAACTAT-2842
```

Figure 2 Sequence of cGMP PDE β-Subunit cDNAs from Normal and *rd* Mouse

The complete sequence of a full length cGMP phosphodiesterase β-subunit cDNA (MPB-71) isolated from a normal mouse retina cDNA library is shown with the predicted protein sequence below. Asterisks denote stop codons that delimit the open reading frames for the predicted protein products. Nucleotide differences found in the *rd* mouse β-subunit sequence are shown in bold letters above the normal sequence. The only amino acid change produces an ochre mutation converting codon 347, tyrosine (TAC), to a stop codon (TAA).

D. THE GENE DEFECT RESPONSIBLE FOR RETINAL DEGENERATION IN THE *rd* MOUSE

Studies in the 70's from the laboratory of Richard Lolley[12,13] represented groundbreaking work that led to intense investigation of the role of cGMP in phototransduction, and implicated a defective cGMP PDE as the primary cause of retinal degeneration in the *rd* mouse. More recently the cGMP PDE β-subunit gene was mapped near the *rd* locus on mouse chromosome 5, and the α- and γ-subunit genes were shown to map to other chromosomes (see below). The *rd* mouse retina β-subunit mRNA was reported to differ in size by 300 bp compared to that of normal mouse retina[16]. We amplified by PCR overlapping segments of the protein coding region, and the entire 3' untranslated region, of *rd* and normal mouse retina poly A RNA and found no difference in the size of amplified products[37]. The suggested size difference may result from a gel anomaly caused by gross differences in the amount of β-subunit mRNA present in *rd* and normal retina samples. The difference in β-subunit mRNA levels was reported, and suggested to be the primary cause of the *rd* phenotype[16,17]. It was previously shown that cGMP PDE is present at very low levels and inactive in pn 9-11 pre-degenerative *rd* retinas, in contrast to the abundant, active enzyme present in pn 9-11 normal mouse retinas[14,15]. It is possible that the α-subunit transcript is also of low abundance, due to coordinate regulation of the genes which would explain the lower level of cGMP PDE identified in the *rd* mouse retina prior to morphological signs of degeneration.

We began characterization of the β-subunit mRNA in normal and *rd* mouse to identify any differences that may exist in the predicted protein sequences. Poly A RNA from pn 9-11 *rd* and normal adult retinas was used as a template for reverse transcription to produce cDNA. The cDNA products were amplified by PCR with primers that are specific to the β-subunit cDNA sequence and with a primer that amplifies from the poly A tail[38] (Figure 1). With the exception of 46 residues at the N-terminus the entire sequence of the protein coding region of the *rd* PDE β-subunit cDNA was determined. Comparison of the sequence to that of the normal β-subunit cDNA revealed six differences (Figure 2). Two of the differences occur in the 3' untranslated region, three are silent changes within the protein coding region, and one (C to A at nt 1143, Figure 2) introduces an ochre mutation that would truncate the normal expressed product to a ~30 kD peptide fragment. This mutation is consistent with a previous observation[15] that intact α- and β-subunits are required to produce a functional cGMP PDE holoenzyme.

E. CHROMOSOME LOCATION OF PHOTORECEPTOR cGMP PDE SUBUNIT GENES IN MAMMALS

One aspect of the candidate gene approach[29] to the study of hereditary retinal degeneration involves chromosome mapping of the suspect genes. All of the genes encoding rod and cone cGMP PDE subunits have been mapped in human, bovine and

Table 1
Chromosome Localization and Synteny of PDE Genes

	α	β	γ	Cone (α')
Mouse	18	5	11	(19)[a]
Human	5	4p	17	(10q)
Bovine	U22	U15	U21	U26

[a]The mouse and human cone cGMP PDE α' gene locations are predictions based on syntenic relationships conserved in these species.

mouse using somatic cell hybrid DNA and *in situ* hybridization technologies. We mapped the human α-subunit gene[29] to chromosome 5 (5q31.2-q34), and the human β-subunit gene to the short arm of chromosome 4[39] near the Huntington's chorea disease locus. The human γ-subunit gene maps to chromosome 17 (17q11.2-

21.1)[31,40] and mouse γ maps to chromosome 11[41]. Bovine rod PDE α, β, and γ genes, and the cone PDE α' gene map to linkage groups U22, U15, U21 and U26, respectively[42]. The mouse α-subunit gene maps to chromosome 18[43]. Based on synteny mouse and human cone PDE genes are expected to map to chromosomes 19, and 10, respectively. Chromosome assignments determined and predicted by synteny are shown in Table 1.

III. ACKNOWLEDGEMENTS

We gratefully acknowledge the determination and expert technical assistance of Ms. Andrea K. Lee. We thank Drs. Richard N. Lolley and Rehwa H. Lee for critical review of the manuscript, helpful discussion, and providing homozygous and heterozygous *rd* retinas. We also thank Dr. James F. McGinnis for homozygous pn 9-11 *rd* retina poly A RNA. Supported by an NIH/NEI EY06172 Neurobiology Fellowship, and the Knights Templar Eye Foundation, Inc. to S.J.P., and grants from NIH/NEI EY08123, the National Retinitis Pigmentosa Foundation, the Gund Foundation, and the Retina Research Foundation to W.B., WB is a recipient of a Jules and Doris Stein Research to Prevent Blindness Professorship.

IV. REFERENCES

1.   Keeler, C.E., The inheritance of a retinal abnormality in white mice, *Proc. Natl. Acad. Sci. U.S.A.*, 10, 329, 1924.

2.   Brückner, R., Spaltlampenmikroskopie und Ophthalmoskopie am Auge von Ratte und Maus, *Document. Ophthalmol.*, 5-6, 452, 1951.

3.   Sorsby, A., Koller, P.C., Attfield, M., Davey, J.B. and Lucas, D.R., Retinal dystrophy in the mouse: histological and genetic aspects, *J. Exp. Zool.*, 125, 171, 1954.

4.   Tansley, K., Hereditary degeneration of the mouse retina, *Brit. J. Ophthalmol.*, 35, 573, 1951.

5.   Dunn, T.B., The importance of differences in morphology of inbred strains, *J. Nat. Cancer Inst.*, 15, 573, 1954.

6.   Noell, W.K., Differentiation, metabolic organization, and viability of the visual cell, *A. M. A. Arch. Ophthalmol.*, 60, 702, 1958.

7.   Carter-Dawson D.L., LaVail, M. M., and Sidman, R. L., Differential effect of the *rd* mutation on rods and cones in the mouse retina. *Invest. Ophthalmol. Vis. Sci.*, 17, 489, 1978.

8.   Paigen, K. and Noell, W.K., Two linked genes showing a similar timing of expression in mice, *Nature*, 190, 148, 1961.

9.   Sidman, R.L. and Green, M.C., Retinal degeneration in the mouse: Location of the *rd* locus in linkage group XVII, *J. Heredity*, 56, 23, 1965.

10.   LaVail, M.M. and Sidman, R.L., C57BL/6J mice with inherited retinal degeneration, Arch. Ophthalmol., 91, 394, 1974.

11. Robb, R. M., Electron microscopic histochemical studies of cyclic 3', 5'-nucleotide phosphodiesterase in the developing retina of normal mice and mice with hereditary retinal degeneration, *Tr. Am. Ophth. Soc.*, LXXII, 650, 1974.

12. Farber, D.B. and Lolley, R.N., Cyclic guanosine monophosphate: elevation in degenerating photoreceptor cells of the C3H mouse retina, *Science*, 186, 449, 1974.

13. Farber, D.B. and Lolley, R.N., Enzymic basis for cyclic GMP accumulation in degenerative photorceptor cells of mouse retina, *J. Cycl. Nucleotide Res.*, 2, 139, 1976.

14. Lee, R.H., Lieberman, B.S., Hurwitz, R.L. and Lolley, R.N., Phosphodiesterase probes show distinct defects in rd mice and Irish setter dog disorders, *Invest. Ophthalmol. Vis. Sci.*, 26, 1569, 1985.

15. Lee, R.H., Navon, S.E., Brown, B.M., Fung, B.K.-K. and Lolley, R.N., Characterization of a phosphodiesterase-immunoreactive polypeptide from rod photoreceptors of developing *rd* mouse retinas, *Invest. Ophthalmol. Vis. Sci.*, 29, 1021, 1988.

16. Bowes, C., Danciger, M., Kozak, C.A. and Farber, D.B., Isolation of a candidate cDNA for the gene causing retinal degeneration in the *rd* mouse, *Proc. Natl. Acad. Sci. U.S.A.*, 86, 9722, 1989.

17. Bowes, C., Li, T., Danciger, M., Baxter, L.C., Applebury, M.L. and Farber, D.B., Retinal degeneration in the *rd* mouse is caused by a defect in the β subunit of rod cGMP phosphodiesterase, *Nature*, 347, 677, 1990.

18. Danciger, M., Bowes, C., Kozak, C.A., LaVail, M. M., and Farber, D.B., Fine mapping of a putative *rd* cDNA and its co-segregation with *rd* expression, *Invest. Ophthalmol. Vis. Sci.*, 51, 185, 1990.

19. Stryer, L., Molecular basis of visual excitation, Cold Spring Harbor Symp. Quant. Biol., LIII, 283, 1988.

20. Chabre, M. and Deterre, P., Molecular mechanism of visual transduction, *Eur. J. Biochem.*, 179, 255, 1989.

21. Baehr, W., Devlin, M.J. and Applebury, M.L., Isolation and characterization of cGMP phosphodiesterase from bovine rod outer segments, *J. Biol. Chem.*, 254, 11669, 1979.

22. Baehr, W., Champagne, M.S., Lee, A.K. and Pittler, S.J. Complete cDNA sequences of mouse rod photoreceptor cGMP phosphodiesterase α- and β-subunits, and identification of β', a putative β-subunit isozyme produced by alternative splicing of the β-subunit gene, *FEBS Lett.*, in press.,1991.

23. Beavo, J.A., Multiple isozymes of cyclic nucleotide phosphodiesterase, *Adv. Sec. Mess. Phosphopro. Res.*, 22, 1, 1988.

24. Charbonneau, H., Prusti, R.K., LeTrong, H., Sonnenburg, W.K., Mullaney, P.J., Walsh, K.A. and Beavo, J.A., Identification of a noncatalytic cGMP-binding domain conserved in both the cGMP-stimulated and photoreceptor cyclic nucleotide phosphodiesterases, *Proc. Natl. Acad. Sci., U.S.A.*, 87, 288, 1990.

25.   Gillespie, P.G. and Beavo, J.A. Characterization of a bovine cone photo-receptor phosphodiesterase purified by cyclic GMP-sepharose chromatography, *J. Biol. Chem.*, 263, 8133, 1988.

26.   Pittler, S.J. and Baehr, W., The molecular genetics of retinal photoreceptor proteins involved in cGMP metabolism, in *The Molecular Biology of the Retina: Basic and Clinically Relevant Studies*, Chader, G.J. and Farber, D.B. Eds., Wiley-Liss, Inc., New York, 1991, 33.

27.   Lipkin, V.M., Khramtsov, N.V., Vasilevskaya, I.A., Atabekova, N.V., Muradov, K.G., Gubanov, V.V., Li, T., Johnston, J.P., Volpp, K.J. and Applebury, M.L., β-Subunit of bovine rod photoreceptor cGMP phospho-diesterase. Comparison with the phosphodiesterase family, *J.Biol.Chem.*, 265, 12955, 1990.

28.   Ovchinnikov, Y.A., Gubanov, V.V., Khramtsov, N.V., Ischenko, K.A., Zagranichny, V.E., Muradov, K.G., Shuvaeva, T.M. and Lipkin, V.M., Cyclic GMP phosphodiesterase from bovine retina Amino acid sequence of the α-subunit and nucleotide sequence of the corresponding cDNA, *FEBS Lett.*, 223, 169, 1987.

29.   Pittler, S.J., Baehr, W., Wasmuth, J.J., McConnel, D.G., Champagne, M.S., VanTuinen, P., Ledbetter, D. and Davis, R.L., Molecular characterization of human and bovine rod photoreceptor cGMP phosphodiesterase α-subunit and chromosomal localization of the human gene, *Genomics*, 6, 272, 1990.

30.   Tuteja, N. and Farber, D.B., γ-subunit of mouse retinal cyclic GMP phosphodiesterase: cDNA and corresponding amino acid sequence, *FEBS Lett.*, 232, 182, 1988.

31.   Tuteja, N., Danciger, M., Klisak, I., Tuteja, R., Inana, G., Mohandas, T., Sparkes, R.S. and Farber, D.B., Isolation and characterization of cDNA encoding the γ-subunit of cGMP phosphodiesterase in human retina, *Gene*, 88, 227, 1990.

32.   Ovchinnikov, Y.A., Lipkin, V.M., Kumarev, V.P., Gubanov, V.V., Khramtsov, N.V., Akhmedov, N.B., Zagranichny, V.E. and Muradov, K.G., Cyclic GMP phosphodiesterase from cattle retina Amino acid sequence of the γ-subunit and nucleotide sequence of the corresponding cDNA, *FEBS Lett.*, 204, 288, 1986.

33.   Holbrook, S.R. and Kim, S.-H. Molecular model of the G protein α-subunit based on the crystal structure of the H*ras* protein, *Proc. Natl. Acad. Sci. U.S.A.*, 86, 1751, 1989.

34.   Maltese, W.A., Posttranslational modification of proteins by isoprenoids in mammalian cells, *FASEB J.*, 4, 3319, 1990.

35.   Hancock, J.F., Paterson, H. and Marshall, C.J., A polybasic domain or palmitoylation is required in addition to the CAAX motif to localize p21[ras] to the plasma membrane, *Cell*, 63, 133, 1990.

36.   Magee, T. and Hanley, M., Sticky fingers and CAAX boxes, *Nature*, 335, 114, 1988.

37.   Pittler, S. J. and Baehr, W., unpublished data, 1990.

38. Al-Ubaidi, M.R., Pittler, S.J., Champagne, M.S., Triantafyllos, J.T., McGinnis, J.F. and Baehr, W., Mouse opsin: Gene structure and molecular basis of multiple transcripts, *J. Biol. Chem.*, 265, 20563, 1990.

39. Plummer, S., Pittler, S. J., Baehr, W., and Wasmuth, J. J., unpublished data, 1990.

40. Ledbetter, D., Baehr, W., and Pittler, S. J., unpublished data, 1990.

41. Danciger, M., Tuteja, N., Kozak, C.A. and Farber, D.B., The gene for the γ-subunit of retinal cGMP phosphodiesterase is on mouse chromosome 11, *Exp. Eye Res.*, 48, 303, 1989.

42. Gallagher, D. S., Pittler, S. J., Baehr, W., and Womack, J. E., unpublished data, 1990.

43. Danciger, M., Kozak, C. A., Li, T., Applebury, M. L., and Farber, D. B., Genetic mapping demonstrates that the α-subunit of retinal cGMP-phosphodiesterase is not the site of the *rd* mutation, *Exp. Eye Res.*, 51, 185, 1990.

MOLECULAR STRUCTURE AND PROPERTIES OF PERIPHERIN/rds THE NORMAL PRODUCT OF THE GENE RESPONSIBLE FOR RETINAL DEGENERATION IN THE rds MOUSE

Greg Connell, Laurie L. Molday, Delyth Reid and Robert S. Molday
Department of Biochemistry
University of British Columbia
Vancouver, B.C. Canada, V6T 1W5

I. INTRODUCTION

Retinal degeneration in the *rds* (retinal degeneration slow) mutant mouse is characterized by a failure in the photoreceptor cells to develop outer segments and a slow progressive loss in photoreceptor cells such that few photoreceptor cells remain one year after birth.[1-4] The *rds* mutation has been localized to mouse chromosome 17 by Démant and coworkers,[5] and a candidate gene for the *rds* defect has been recently identified by Travis *et al.*[6] using differential and substractive screening procedures. In the latter study the normal *rds* gene was found to encode for a photoreceptor cell specific protein of 346 amino acids. The mutant *rds* gene contained an insertion of 10 kb of foreign DNA into an exon region of the normal gene. Thus, if translation of the mutant mRNA does occur in the *rds* mouse, an abnormal protein would be produced which would lack the C-terminal 87 amino acids present in the normal protein.[6]

In earlier studies outer segments of bovine rod photoreceptor cells have been shown to contain a membrane protein called peripherin.[7] Anti-peripherin monoclonal antibodies used with immunogold labeling techniques suggest that peripherin is preferentially localized along the rim and incisures of outer segment disks. Peripherin migrates with rhodopsin as a 35 kDa polypeptide on SDS-polyacrylamide gels run in the presence of a disulfide reducing agent. In the absence of a reducing agent, bovine peripherin preferentially migrates as a 66-68 kDa doublet. The cDNA for bovine peripherin recently has been cloned and sequenced by established recombinant DNA methods.[8] Sequence analysis indicates that the cDNA codes for a polypeptide chain of 346 amino acids containing three consensus sequences for N-linked glycosylation and four possible hydrophobic transmembrane domains. Comparison of the bovine peripherin sequence with the protein encoded by the normal mouse *rds* gene indicates that the two proteins are 92.5% identical.[9] On this basis, we consider peripherin and the normal *rds* protein as the same protein from different species. Accordingly, we will now refer to peripherin as peripherin/*rds*. Recently, the cDNA for the rat peripherin/*rds* protein has also been cloned, sequenced and reported to be highly homologous to the normal mouse peripherin/*rds* protein.[10]

In this paper we compare the primary structures of the bovine, mouse, and rat peripherin/*rds* proteins in relation to the proposed model for the organization of this protein in the outer segment disk membrane.[8] The purification, expression and partial characterization of peripherin/*rds* protein are also described as an initial step in defining its molecular structure and role in photoreceptor outer segment morphogenesis and cell function.

II. PRIMARY STRUCTURE OF BOVINE, MOUSE AND RAT PERIPHERIN/rds PROTEIN

The protein sequences for the peripherin/*rds* protein from bovine,[8] mouse[6] and rat[10] photoreceptor outer segments have been reported from cDNA cloning and sequence analysis (Figure 1). In the case of the bovine peripherin/*rds* protein, the N-terminal protein sequence of the purified protein has also been determined and shown to be identical to the N-terminal protein sequence derived from cDNA analysis except for the absence of the initiator methionine residue.[8] It is likely that the initiator methionine is also removed in the mature mouse and rat proteins.

```
BOVINE   ALLKVKFDQKKRVKLAQGLWLMNWFSVLAGIIIFGLGLFLKIELRKRSDV   50
MOUSE    ALLKVKFDQKKRVKLAQGLWLMNWLSVLAGIVLFSLGLFLKIELRKRSEV   50
RAT      ALLKVKFDQKKRVKLAQGLWLMNWLSVLAGIVLFSLGLFLKIELRKRSDV   50
         ************************.******..*.************.*

BOVINE   MNNSESHFVPNSLIGVGVLSCVFNSLAGKICYDALDPAKYAKWKPWLKPY   100
MOUSE    MNNSESHFVPNSLIGVGVLSCVFNSLAGKICYDALDPAKYAKWKPWLKPY   100
RAT      MDNSESHFVPNSLIGVGVLSCVFNSLAGKICYDALDPAKYAKWKPWLKLY   100
         *.*********************************************** *

BOVINE   LAVCVLFNVVLFLVALCCFLLRGSLESTLAHGLKNGMKFYRDTDTPGRCF   150
MOUSE    LAVCIFFNVILFLVALCCFLLRGSLESTLAYGLKNGMKYYRDTDTPGRCF   150
RAT      LAVCVFFNVILFLVALCCFLLRGSLESTLAYGLKNGMKYYRDTDTPGRCF   150
         ****..***.******************.*******.***********

BOVINE   MKKTIDMLQIEFKCCGNNGFRDWFEIQWISNRYLDFSSKEVKDRIKSNVD   200
MOUSE    MKKTIDMLQIEFKCCGNNGFRDWFEIQWISNRYLDFSSKEVKDRIKSNVD   200
RAT      MKKTIDMLQIEFKCCGNNGFRDWFEIQWISNRYLDFSSKEVKDRIKSNVD   200
         *************************************************

BOVINE   GRYLVDGVPFSCCNPNSPRPCIQYQLTNNSAHYSYDHQTEELNLWLRGCR   250
MOUSE    GRYLVDGVPFSCCNPSSPRPCIQYQLTNNSAHYSYDHQTEELNLWLRGCR   250
RAT      GRYLVDGVPFSCCNPSSPRPCIQYQLTNNSAHYSYDHQTEELNLWLRGCR   250
         **************.**********************************

BOVINE   AALLSYYSNLMNTTGAVTLLVWLFEVTITVGLRYLHTALEGMANPEDPEC   300
MOUSE    AALLNYYSSLMNSMGVVTLLVWLFEVSITAGLRYLHTALESVSNPEDPEC   300
RAT      AALLNYYSSLMNSMGVVTLLIWLFEVSITAGLRFLHTALESVSNPEDPEC   300
         ****.***.***.*.****.*****.**.***.******...*******

BOVINE   ESEGWLLEKSVPETWKAFLESVKKLGKGNQVEAEGEDAGQAPAAG   345
MOUSE    ESEGWLLEKSVPETWKAFLESFKKLGKSNQVEAEGADAGPAPEAG   345
RAT      ESEGWLLENSVSETWKAFLESFKKLGKSNQVEAEAADAGQAPEAG   345
         ********.**.*********.*****.******..***.**.**
```

Figure 1: Alignment of the protein sequences for bovine[8], mouse[6] and rat[10] peripherin/*rds* using the Clustal program of PC/Gene (IntelliGenetics, Mountain View, CA.). The (*) indicate that amino acids are perfectly conserved; the (.) indicate amino acids are well conserved. The initiator methionine is not included. Solid lines indicates putative membrane spanning domains.

Taking this into account, the peripherin/*rds* proteins for these three species consist of 345 amino acids and have a molecular weight of about 39 kDa. The alignment of the sequences for bovine, mouse and rat peripherin/*rds* is shown in Figure 1.

The primary structures for bovine, mouse and rat peripherin/*rds* show a high degree of homology. The bovine and mouse proteins are 92.5% identical; the bovine and rat proteins are 91.3% identical; and the mouse and rat proteins are 97.1% identical. Kyte-Doolittle hydropathy plots[11] are essentially identical and indicate the presence of four hydrophobic segments of 17 to 23 amino acids which are flanked by a positively-charged arginine or lysine residues on the C-terminal end.[8] These four segments are potential membrane spanning domains as indicated in the models illustrated in Figure 2. The view that peripherin/*rds* is an integral membrane protein is supported by experimental studies indicating that detergents are required to solubilize peripherin from the membrane.[7] Another common feature is the presence of 13 conserved cysteine residues, 6 of which are found in pairs. According to the proposed model, two of these cysteine pairs and three single cysteine residues are present in the disk lumen or intradiskal space. Since the reducing potential in the disk lumen, like the extracellular compartment, is expected to be low relative to the cytoplasmic compartment, it is possible that some or all of these cysteine residues may form intrachain and/or interchain disulfide bonds. Interchain disulfide bonding has been proposed to explain the observation that peripherin/*rds* preferentially migrates as a dimer on SDS-polyacrylamide gels in the absence of a disulfide reducing agent.[7]

Bovine and mouse peripherin/*rds* proteins contain three consensus sequences for N-linked glycosylation (-N-X-S- or -N-X-T-), whereas the rat protein contains only two. Bovine peripherin/*rds* has potential N-linked glycosylation sites at asparagines N_{52}, N_{228}, and N_{262}; mouse peripherin/*rds* has potential sites at asparagines N_{52}, N_{228} and N_{214}; and rat peripherin/*rds* has potential sites at asparagines N_{214} and N_{228}. In the model depicted in Figure 2, these sites are all localized within the intradisk or lumen compartment where, as in the case of rhodopsin, one would expect oligosaccharide chains on glycoproteins to reside. The presence of N-linked glycosylation of bovine peripherin/*rds* has been confirmed by enzymatic removal of the oligosaccharide chains with either Endo H or N-Glycanase F.[8] Although the exact site is not known, conservation of the consensus sequence at asparagine N_{228} suggests that this is a likely site for N-linked glycosylation of peripherin/*rds*.

The model shown in Figure 2 suggests that peripherin/*rds* contains one relatively small intradiskal hydrophilic loop of 21 amino acids (K_{41}-N_{61}) and one large hydrophilic loop of 142 amino acids (R_{122}-T_{263}). The large loop, if globular in conformation, may be expected to extend over 20 Å (2 nm) from the phospholipid bilayer of the disk membrane. The function of these highly conserved domains is not known, but one can speculate that the large segment may be involved in protein-protein interactions which may help to stabilize the highly curved disk structure. Protein segments exposed on the cytoplasmic side consist of a short, conserved, positively charged N-terminal region of 17 amino acids (A_1-Q_{17}), a short conserved loop of 22 amino acids (K_{79}-Y_{100}), and a highly charged C-terminal segment of 63 amino acids (R_{283}-G_{345}). The C-terminal region, which is not as well conserved as the rest of the protein, is a highly antigenic domain. Immunocytochemical labeling studies using monoclonal antibodies clearly indicates that the C-terminal segment is exposed on the cytoplasmic surface of disk membranes.[7,8] The four hydrophobic putative transmembrane domains are suggested to be α-helical in conformation on the basis of analogy with other known eukaryotic membrane proteins.

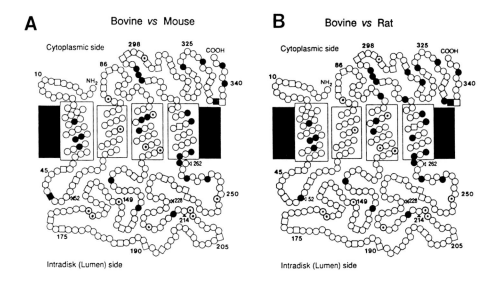

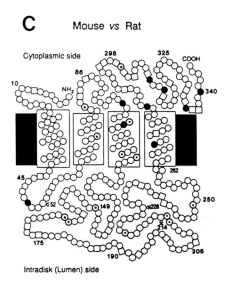

Figure 2: A model for the structural organization of peripherin/*rds* within the disk membrane[8] showing the location of amino acid differences. The negatively (hexagons) and positively charged (squares) amino acids are indicated. **A.** Bovine sequence is indicated by open symbols; mouse sequence differences are shown by filled symbols; possible N-linked glycosylation sites for bovine peripherin/*rds* are given by open triangles and for mouse peripherin/*rds* by closed triangles. **B.** Bovine sequence is indicated by open symbols; rat sequence differences are shown by filled symbols; possible N-linked glycosylation sites for the bovine protein are given by open triangles and for the rat protein by the closed triangles. **C.** Mouse sequence is indicated by open symbols; rat sequence differences are shown by filled symbols; possible N-linked glycosylation sites for the mouse protein are shown by the open triangles and for the rat protein by the closed triangles. Cysteine residues are indicated (⊙).

III. MONOCLONAL ANTIBODIES TO PERIPHERIN/rds

Monoclonal antibodies are valuable probes to study the structure and function of proteins. Previously, two monoclonal antibodies (Mabs) have been produced against peripherin/*rds* by the immunization of mice with either purified bovine rod outer segments (Mab 2B6) or rat retinal extracts (Mab 3B6).[7] Both these Mabs have been shown to label the peripherin/*rds* protein from bovine outer segment membranes on Western blots.

Since the sequences of bovine, mouse and rat peripherin/*rds* are published, it is now possible to determine the binding sites or epitopes by studying the crossreactivity of Mab 2B6 and Mab 3B6 to peripherin/*rds* from these mammalian species. As shown with Western blots in   Figure 3, the anti-rat antibody Mab 3B6 labeled rat peripherin/*rds* most intensely, but it also intensely labeled the bovine protein as previously shown.[7] In contrast, the mouse peripherin/*rds* protein was not labeled. The anti-bovine Mab 2B6 antibody showed a different pattern of crossreactivity. This antibody labeled bovine peripherin/*rds*, but not the rat or mouse protein (Figure 3). The crossreactivity of these antibodies to human peripherin/*rds* protein was also studied. Mab 3B6 showed some crossreactivity to human peripherin/*rds* protein. No crossreactivity of Mab 2B6 was detected with the

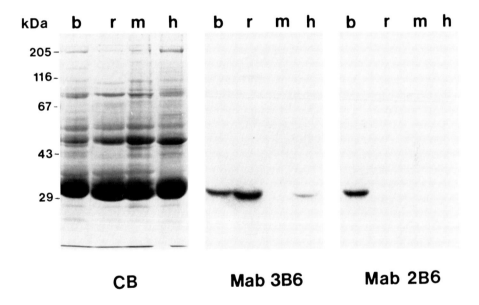

Figure 3: Immunocrossreactivity of monoclonal antibodies Mab 3B6 and Mab 2B6 to purified   outer segments of bovine (b), rat (r), mouse (m) and human (h) photoreceptor cells. SDS polyacrylamide gels were either stained with Coomassie Blue (CB) or transferred to Immobilon membranes and labeled with Mab 3B6 or Mab 2B6 and ^{125}I-goat anti-mouse Ig for autoradiography.

human protein. Immunoscreening of a λgt-11 expression library has indicated that both Mab 2B6 and Mab 3B6 bind to an epitope within the C-terminal 35 amino acids (V_{311}-G_{345}) of the bovine protein.[8] Comparison of this C-terminal 35 amino acid sequence of bovine, mouse and rat (Figure 1) indicates that the proline at position 340 (P_{340}) in mouse peripherin/*rds* is the only amino acid within this region which is unique to the mouse sequence, i.e. not found in either the rat or bovine C-terminal sequences. On this basis one would predict that the glutamine at position 340 (Q_{340}) is required for Mab 3B6 binding such that substitution with a proline, as found in the mouse sequence, would abolish binding. This change and changes in alanine and glutamic acid at position 336 and/or position 343 probably contribute to the inability of Mab 2B6 to bind rat and mouse peripherin/*rds*. In recent studies, we have shown that a synthetic peptide made to the C-terminal 14 amino acids of bovine peripherin/*rds* binds to both the Mab 3B6 and Mab 2B6 antibodies (Illing and Molday, unpublished observations). The sequence of the human peripherin/*rds* protein is not available at the present time, but one can expect that there are amino acid changes within the C-terminal 14 amino acids such as to affect the binding of Mab 2B6 and to a lesser extent Mab 3B6.

IV. IMMUNOAFFINITY PURIFICATION OF PERIPHERIN/rds

Purification of the peripherin/*rds* protein is an important step for analysis of its molecular structure and function. Since peripherin/*rds*, like rhodopsin, is a membrane glycoprotein having a subunit molecular weight of 39 kDa, it is necessary to develop specific methods to separate and purify peripherin/*rds* from rhodopsin and other membrane-associated proteins of outer segments. Immunoaffinity chromatography is a particularly valuble method for this purpose. Recently, we

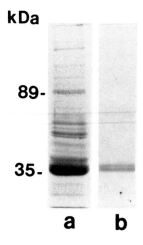

Figure 4: Immunoaffinity purification of peripherin/*rds* from bovine rod outer segments. Coomassie blue stained SDS-polyacrylamide gels of bovine rod outer segments (a) and purified peripherin/*rds* (b). CHAPS solubilized rod outer segments were passed through a Mab 2B6 antibody - Sepharose column and the peripherin/*rds* was eluted with 0.05 M formic acid in CHAPS detergent.

have covalently linked monoclonal antibody Mab 2B6 to Sepharose 2B by the CNBr procedure [11], and we have used this matrix to isolate peripherin/*rds* from bovine ROS membranes solubilized in either CHAPS or Triton X-100 detergents. Under these conditions peripherin/*rds* can be selectively bound to this immunoaffinity column and eluted at low pH. As shown in Figure 4, the purified peripherin/*rds* protein migrates as a doublet of apparent molecular weight of 34-36 kDa on SDS-polyacrylamide gels run in the presence of a disulfide reducing agent. Western blotting indicates that the purified peripherin/*rds* protein is essentially free of rhodopsin. It is unclear why bovine peripherin migrates as a doublet in reduced and nonreduced state.[7] It is possible that the doublet represents a single peripherin polypeptide with different forms of posttranslational modifications such as glycosylation. Alternatively, there may be two closely related forms of bovine peripherin which are associated with one another under nondenaturing conditions. Further studies are now in progress to resolve this question.

V. EXPRESSION OF PERIPHERIN/rds IN MONKEY KIDNEY (COS) CELLS

In order to obtain further insight into the molecular structure and properties of peripherin/*rds* protein, the bovine protein was expressed in the monkey kidney COS-1 cell line. This was carried out by first constructing the full length coding region for bovine peripherin from clones λ.11,λ.17 and λ.18 and from a synthetic oligonucleotide containing the six N-terminal amino acids not present in the cDNA clones.[8] The synthetic oligonucleotide was designed to also contain a Kozak consensus sequence for the efficient initiation of translation and a BamH1 cloning site. This DNA construct was cloned into the expression vector pAX111, generously provided by Drs. R. Kay and R.K. Humphries of the Terry Fox Laboratories, Vancouver, B.C., and used to transfect monkey kidney COS-1 cells. Expression of peripherin/*rds* in COS-1 cells was confirmed by both immunofluorescence and Western blot analysis. As shown in Figure 5, COS-1 cell-expressed peripherin/*rds* migrated as two closely spaced bands on SDS gels run in the presence of a disulfide reducing agent. In the absence of the reducing agent, the expressed peripherin/*rds* protein, like the native outer segment protein, migrated as a dimer. This suggests that the dimer of peripherin is composed of two identical polypeptide chains linked by interchain disulfide bonds. The possibility that some heterodimer formation occurs in rod outer segments, however, cannot be excluded. It is of interest to note that peripherin/*rds* protein in rod outer segment appears to be more abundant when SDS-gel electrophoresis is carried out in the absence of a reducing agent. This appears to be an artifact which arises from the differential efficiency of transfer of reduced and unreduced peripherin/*rds* to Immobilon membranes. Since peripherin/*rds* comigrates with rhodopsin under reducing conditions, more abundant rhodopsin appears to saturate the binding sites on the Immobilon transfer membrane limiting the binding of peripherin/*rds*. Under nonreducing conditions, peripherin/*rds* migrates as a dimer and accordingly, is separated from most of the rhodopsin. Under these conditions peripherin/*rds* can readily bind to the Immobilon membrane.

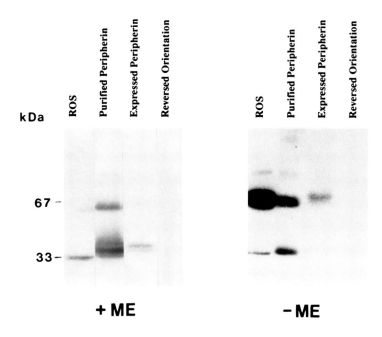

Figure 5: Western blots of bovine rod outer segments (ROS), purified peripherin/*rds*, and postnuclear homogenate of COS-1 cells transfected with the pAX 111 vector containing the peripherin/*rds* coding sequence in the correct or reversed orientation. Western blots were labeled with Mab 2B6 monoclonal antibody and ^{125}I-goat anti-mouse Ig for autoradiography. SDS polyacrylamide gel electrophoresis was run in the presence (+ ME) and absence (- ME) of the disulfide reducing agent, 2-mercaptoethanol.

VI. LOCALIZATION OF PERIPHERIN/rds IN ROD OUTER SEGMENTS

Immunocytochemical labeling studies using Mab 2B6 and Mab 3B6 have shown that peripherin/*rds* is predominantly localized within the outer segments of photoreceptor cells. Post-embedding immunogold labeling studies indicated that the peripherin/*rds* protein is distributed around the periphery of bovine and rat rod outer segments in the region where the disks come in close contact with the plasma membrane.[7] The resolution of this technique, however, is not sufficient to determine whether peripherin/*rds* is present along the rims of the disks or on the plasma membranes. This was resolved by carrying out pre-embedding immunogold labeling studies of hypotonically lysed rod outer segments[8] and isolated disks.[7] Results of these studies using both Mab 2B6 and Mab 3B6 indicate that peripherin/*rds* is preferentially localized along the rim region and incisures of the disks. Recently, Travis *et al.*[13] have generated a polyclonal antiserum against a synthetic peptide corresponding to a segment near the C-terminus of the mouse peripherin/*rds* protein. Their immunofluorescence studies have shown that mouse peripherin/*rds* protein is also predominantly distributed in the outer segments. Post-embedding immunogold labeling studies, however, suggested that peripherin/*rds* in mouse outer segments is uniformly distributed throughout the outer segment. This would further suggest that the peripherin/*rds* protein is present in the lamellar region of the disks. The basis for the difference in distribution observed for bovine and rat rod outer segments using monoclonal antibodies and mouse rod outer segments using polyclonal antipeptide antiserum is not clear at the present time.

VII. CONCLUSIONS

Initial studies of Travis et al.[6] on the identification of the gene responsible for retinal degeneration in the *rds* mouse have led to the identification of peripherin (now referred to as peripherin/*rds*) as the normal product for this gene.[9] Sequence analyses and biochemical studies indicate that it is a transmembrane glycoprotein of 345 amino acids having four potential transmembrane spanning regions and three consensus sequences for N-linked glycosylation. The sequences for bovine, mouse and rat peripherin/*rds* protein are highly conserved as indicated by alignments in Figure 1. The sequences of the human[14] and cat[15] peripherin/*rds* proteins have been recently obtained, and it is likely that the sequences of these proteins will be closely related to those of bovine, mouse, and rat. A computer search of protein

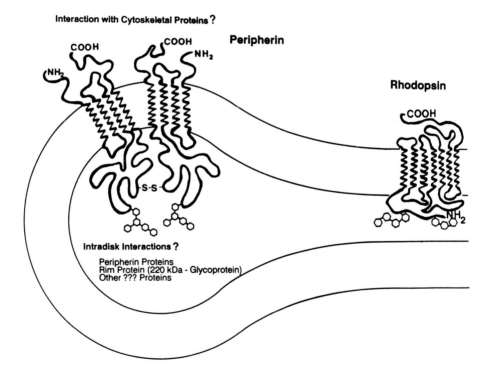

Figure 6: Schematic diagram showing the organization of peripherin/*rds* and rhodopsin within the disk membrane based on sequence and monoclonal antibody labeling studies.

data bases have failed to show any obvious relationship of peripherin/*rds* to other proteins of known function. This and the phenotype of the *rds* mutation suggest that peripherin/*rds* has a specific role in photoreceptor outer segment morphogenesis. Possible function of peripherin/*rds* is not known at the present time. On the basis of studies which localize peripherin/*rds* to the rim regions of disks, one may speculate that this protein is involved in forming and maintaining the highly curved rim region of the disk through protein-protein interactions within the intradiskal space (Figure 6). Alternatively, the cytoplasmic surface may serve to anchor fibrous proteins which have been observed to link the rim region of the disks to adjacent disks and to the plasma membrane.[16]   Further studies are needed to define the role of peripherin/*rds* in normal photoreceptor cell structure and function and in understanding why mutation in the rds gene prevents outer segment morphogenesis and results in the slow degeneration of the photoreceptor cells.

Acknowledgements: We wish to thank Drs. Robert Kay and Keith Humphries of the Terry Fox Laboratories in Vancouver, B.C. for their generous gift of the pAX 111 expression vector.   These studies were supported by grants from the RP Eye Research Foundation of Canada and the Medical Research Council of Canada.

REFERENCES

1.   Van Nie, R., Ivanyi, D. & Demant, P., A new H-2 linked mutation, *rds*, causing retinal degeneration in the mouse, *Tissue Antigens* 12, 106, 1978.

2.   Sanyal, S. & Jansen, H.G., Absence of receptor outer segments in the retina of *rds* mutant mice, *Neurosci. Lett.* 21, 23, 1981.

3.   Cohen, A.I., Some cytological and initial biochemical observations on photoreceptors in retinas of *rds* mice, *Invest. Ophthalmol. Vis. Sci.*, 24, 832, 1983.

4.   Jansen, H.G. & Sanyal, S., Development and degeneration of retina in *rds* mutant mice: Electron microscopy, *J. Comp. Neurol.*, 224, 71, 1984.

5.   Demant, P., Ivanyi, D. & Van Nie, R., The map position of the rds gene on the 17th chromosome of the mouse, *Tissue Antigens*, 13, 53, 1979.

6.   Travis, G.H., Brennan, M.B., Danielson, P.E., Kozak, C.   & Sutcliffe, J.G. Identification of a photoreceptor-specific mRNA encoded by the gene responsible for retinal degeneration slow (*rds*), *Nature*, 338, 70, 1989.

7.   Molday, R.S., Hicks, D. & Molday, L., Peripherin. A Rim-specific membrane protein of rod outer segment discs. *Invest. Ophthalmol. Vis. Sci.,*   28, 50, 1986.

8. Connell, G. & Molday, R.S., Molecular cloning, primary structure, and orientation of the vertebrate photoreceptor cell protein peripherin in the rod outer segment disk membrane, *Biochemistry,* 29, 4691, 1990.

9. Connell, G., Bascom, R., McInnes, R. and Molday, R.S., Photoreceptor cell peripherin is the defective protein responsible for retinal degeneration slow (*rds*), *Invest. Ophthalmol. Vis. Sci.*, 31, 309, Abst #1514, 1990.

10. Begy, C. and Bridges, C.D., Nucleotide and predicted protein sequence of rat retinal degeneration slow (*rds*), *Nucl. Acid Res.*, 18, 3058, 1990.

11. Kyte, J. and Doolittle, R.F., A simple method for displaying the hydrophobic character of a protein, *J. Mol. Biol.*, 157, 105, 1982.

12. Cuatrecasas, P., Protein purification by affinity chromatography, *J. Biol. Chem.*, 245, 3059, 1970.

13. Travis, G. H. , Sutcliffe, J.G. and Bok, D. Characterization of the mouse retinal degeneration slow (*rds*) gene product, *Proc. Intern. Soc. Eye Res.*, Vol VI., 213, Abst. #756, 1990.

14. Dryja, T.P., Grondin, V.J., Ringens, P., Cotran, P., Berson, E.L. and Travis, G., Isolation of human retinal cDNA fragments homologous to the murine *rds* gene transcript, *Invest. Ophthal. Vis. Sci.* 30, 43, Abst #1., 1989.

15. Snyder, S.K., Curtis, R., Narfstrom, K., Gorin, M.B., RT/PCR analysis of the orthologous rds transcript in two feline models of hereditary retinal disease, *Invest. Ophthal. Vis. Sci.* 31, 311, Abst #1524, 1990.

16. Roof, D. and Heuser, J.E. Surfaces of rod photoreceptor disk membranes: Integral membrane components, *J. Cell Biol.* 95, 487, 1982.

TISSUE-SPECIFIC EXPRESSION OF IRBP GENE IN TRANSGENIC MICE:
THE DEVELOPMENT OF A POSSIBLE ROUTE TO STUDY RETINAL DEGENERATIONS

Gregory I. Liou[*], L. Geng[+] and Suraporn Matragoon[*]
Cullen Eye Institute, Baylor College of Medicine,
Houston, Texas 77030, USA

I. INTRODUCTION

Interphotoreceptor retinoid-binding protein (IRBP) is a fatty acid-conjugated[1,2] glycoprotein expressed in vertebrate retinal photoreceptors.[1,2] IRBP is also expressed in pinealocytes, although at relatively lower levels.[3] In the retina, IRBP is secreted into the interphotoreceptor matrix where it binds visual retinoids, and thus has been suggested to participate in the visual process as a carrier for visual retinoids.[4,5] This important role has recently been demonstrated by in vitro evidence in amphibian eyes which shows that IRBP supports the delivery of all-trans-retinol to the retinal pigment epithelium (RPE),[6] as well as promotes rhodopsin regeneration.[7]

IRBP may also play important roles in the normal development of the retina. In the developing mouse retina, IRBP is expressed when inner segments of the photoreceptors start to differentiate.[8] How IRBP is involved in this process is unclear. Expression of IRBP is greatly reduced in one case of retinitis pigmentosa,[9] and in a number of animal models for hereditary retinal degeneration (rd), such as rd mice (which also show impaired secretion of IRBP),[10] and in early development of Abyssinian cats with a recessively inherited rd.[11] In all of these diseases, photoreceptors within the retina degenerate, although at variable rates. Recently, mutations in genes that cause some of these degenerations have been found, these include: a mutation in the rod opsin gene in one form of autosomal dominant retinitis pigmentosa;[12] in the gene coding for rod disc peripherin in retinal degeneration slow (rds) mouse;[13] and in the gene coding for the ß subunit of rod phosphodiesterase in rd mouse.[14] Whether or not IRBP gene is directly related to any form of photoreceptor degeneration as yet unidentified, it should be interesting to know how IRBP is related to the process of photoreceptor degeneration in these diseases.

Because of the physiological roles in the normal tissue and the special features in the diseased tissue, the expression of the gene coding for IRBP as well as those coding for other retinal proteins involved in vitamin A metabolism, phototransduction (such as human opsin gene and mouse rd gene) and the structure of the photoreceptors (such as mouse rds gene) should be examined and used as "candidate genes" for

[*] Current address: Department of Ophthalmology, Medical College of Georgia, Augusta, GA 30912-3400

[+] Current address: Department of Rheumatology, Hospital for Sick Children, Toronto, Ontario, Canada M5G 1X8 studies of the hereditary retinal degenerations. We recently reported the use of gene transfer experiments in mice to identify a transcriptional regulatory region of the human IRBP gene.[15] This region has been shown to regulate the expression of IRBP in a tissue-specific manner. We describe here the identification of this tissue-specific promoter and how it may provide a valuable tool for transgenic studies of retina development and degeneration.

II. HUMAN IRBP GENE STRUCTURE AND PRIMARY SEQUENCE

The structure of the human IRBP gene and its 5'-flanking region, IRBP-S3, was reported previously.[15,16] The gene spans about 12 kilobases and is interrupted by three introns, all of which are positioned near the 3'-end of the coding sequence. The coding region of 3741 bases contains four homologous segments of about 900 bases each with sequence similarity between them being as high as 60%. This interesting feature suggests that the human gene is generated by quadruplication of an ancestral gene. The deduced amino acid sequence predicted a signal peptide of 17 amino acids and a mature protein of 1230 residues. Two putative N-linked glycosylation sites are located in highly conserved domains in the center of the first and second segment of IRBP. A region containing 41 amino acids at the C-terminal end of the 3rd segments of IRBP has 15 matching amino acids with an intradiscal loop of rhodopsin. The significance of this interesting feature is unknown.

III. THE REGULATION OF HUMAN IRBP GENE

A. CONSTRUCTION OF THE IRBP-CAT FUSION GENE

Because IRBP is expressed in a tissue-specific manner, we predict the promoter of its gene confers tissue specificity, and is located, like most of the other genes, at the 5'-flanking region.[17] As observed for many other eucaryotic genes, the 5'-flanking fragment of human IRBP gene lacks TATA and CAAT boxes within conventional distances upstream of the transcription start site, and the putative promoter region appears to be GC-rich. To identify sequences in the IRBP-S3 that regulate transcription and confer tissue specificity, we fused a 1329-bp PvuII fragment overlapping the transcription start site to the coding sequences of the bacterial chloramphenicol acetyltransferase (CAT) gene (Figure 1),[18] and this was used to generate transgenic mice.

B. GENERATION OF TRANSGENIC MICE

Transgenic mice were generated by microinjection of the fusion gene into one-cell stage FVB/N embryos.[19] Six independent transgenic founder (F_0) animals, five females and one male, were identified by Southern hybridization. Two of the F_0 mice transmitted the IRBP-CAT sequences to approximately 50% of their offspring. The remaining four F_0 mice had lower transmission rates (14 to 35%), suggesting that these mice were mosaic. The copy numbers of the integrated DNA ranged from 3 to about 100 in the F_1 mice (Table 1).

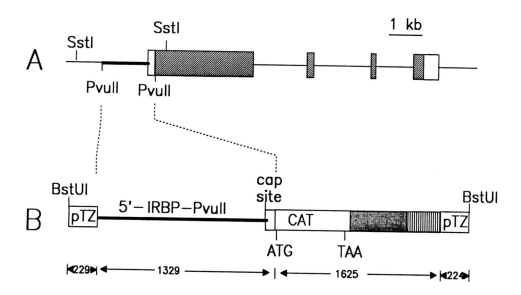

Figure 1. Human IRBP gene and construction of the IRBP-CAT fusion gene.
A, the distribution of exons (boxes), introns (lines), and flanking regions of the human IRBP gene.[16] The hatched boxes represent the protein coding regions. **B,** IRBP-CAT fusion gene. A 1329-bp PvuII fragment containing IRBP sequences from −1311 to +19 bp was fused with HindIII linkers[20] to the 5' end of a CAT gene in the promoterless CAT plasmid pTZCAT.[20] The CAT gene (1625 bp) consists of the CAT coding and noncoding sequences, an SV40 fragment containing the small t-antigen intron (stippled box), and a SV 40 fragment containing the early region polyadenylation site (box with vertical lines).[18] The 3407-bp BstUI restriction fragment was used for microinjections.

Table I
The copy number, transmission rate, and CAT activity
in the transgenic mouse families

Family	Copy number	Transmission		CAT activity			
		Per-Cent	Number screened	Neuro-retina	PECS	Pineal	Cere-brum
				milliunits/mg protein			
101	30	53	19	1350	33	NT	0.2
102	3	35	17	4	0.3	NT	<0.01
103	20	53	53	674	25	NT	0.04
104	5	22	9	700	17	75	<0.01
105	100	22	32	200	93	14	NT
106	30	14	37	933	14	103	<0.01

Copy numbers in F_1 animals were determined by dot blot hybridization to ^{32}P-labeled IRBP-CAT construct and scintillation counting of positive dots. Copy number per haploid genome was estimated by comparison to standards containing known amounts of IRBP-CAT DNA mixed with nontransgenic mouse DNA. Percent transmission was determined by screening the offspring of F_0 x wild type matings by means of dot blot and/or Southern hybridizations to tail DNA. CAT activities were assayed as described,[20] except that the incubation time was 30 min and the amount of soluble protein per assay was adjusted to ensure a linear range of acetylation (40% or lower). Radioactive spots were excised and counted. One unit of CAT activity was defined as the amount of enzymatic activity catalyzing acetylation of 1 μmol of chloramphenicol/min at 37° C. PECS, retinal pigment epithelium acompanied by choroid and sclera. NT, not tested.

C. EXPRESSION OF CAT GENE IN TRANSGENIC MICE

1.   Tissue-Specificity of CAT Expression in Transgenic Mice

F_1 mice from all six families were screened to determine the tissue specificity of the IRBP-CAT gene expression and one of them representing all families is shown in Figure 2. Retinas were separated into two components, the neuro-retina and the RPE accompanied by choroid-sclera (PECS). The RPE cells and photoreceptor outer segments interdigitate rendering their quantitative separation difficult.[21] In all six families, high levels of CAT activity were present in neuro-retina, PECS, and the pineal gland. CAT activity was not detected in other tissues. These results indicate that the human IRBP promoter functions appropriately in transgenic mice and directs gene expression specifically to the mouse tissues that contain endogenous IRBP.

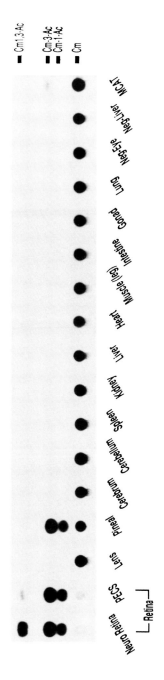

Figure 2. CAT activities. Various tissues of F1 mice were assayed as described earlier.[20] Assay conditions for the retinal tissues are nonlinear. Five µg of soluble protein were used in each assay, except for pineal, for which only 1.5 µg of protein was available. The unacetylated (Cm), monoacetylated (Cm-1-Ac and Cm-3-Ac), and diacetylated (Cm-1,3-Ac) forms of chloramphenicol are shown. PECS, retinal pigment epithelium accompanied by choroid and sclera. MCAT, an extract of cultured embryonic chick primary myoblasts transfected with a CAT gene promoted by a chicken skeletal muscle actin gene promoter.[15]

2.   Quantitation of CAT Expression

The relative levels of CAT activity in various tissues were determined on one F_1 mouse in each family (Table 1). The neuro-retinas showed the highest[1] levels of CAT activity in all six families. CAT activities measured in the pineal glands of the three families tested were around 10% of the activities in the neuro-retinas. CAT activities in the cerebral cortexes were near background levels.

IRBP-CAT expression in the pineal gland is not surprising. It is generally accepted that a major population of mammalian pinealocytes evolved from pineal photoreceptor cells, which are photosensitive in lower vertebrates.[3] During evolution, these pineal photoreceptor cells appear to have been progressively transformed into endocrine secretory cells. However, mammalian pinealocytes and retinal photoreceptors still share a number of[3] common proteins, such as IRBP, arrestin, rhodopsin kinase, and opsin.[3] It is thought that in higher vertebrates the pineal gland may play a role in the regulation of circadian rhythms.

3.   Determination of CAT-Expressing Cells in the Retina

a.   Northern Analysis

The presence of CAT activity in the PECS was unexpected, since the endogenous IRBP gene is expressed specifically in the photoreceptor cells of the neuro-retina.[2] To determine whether the IRBP-CAT gene is transcribed in both neuro-retina and retinal PECS, poly (A$^+$) RNAs were isolated from these tissues of an F_1 mouse of family 101 and analyzed by Northern hybridization (Figure 3A). Transcripts encoding IRBP (5.7 kb),[5] and the CAT transgene (1.9 kb) were detected exclusively in the neuro-retina. The CAT activity detected in the PECS may therefore be the consequence of[1] normal phagocytosis of photoreceptor outer segments by the RPE cells.[21] Alternatively, the CAT activity in the PECS may be attributed to incomplete separation of PECS from photoreceptor outer segments which may contain significant amounts of CAT enzyme.

b.   Cellular Localization of IRBP-lacZ Expression in Transgenic Mice

To determine whether human IRBP promoter is active specifically in the photoreceptors within the neuro-retina, the same 1.3 kb PvuII fragment fused to lacZ gene was used to generate five families of transgenic mice. Three families showed photoreceptor-specific[23] expression of ß-galactosidase activity (data not shown).[23] These studies using transgenic mice demonstrate that a 1.3 kb fragment from the 5' end of the human IRBP gene is sufficient to promote photoreceptor-specific gene expression in vivo.

4.   Effect of Transgene Expression on Endogenous IRBP Expression

To determine whether the integration of the IRBP-CAT construct altered the endogenous IRBP transcription, retinal poly (A$^+$) RNAs from F_1 mice of families 101 and 105 were analyzed. The endogenous 5.7 kb IRBP mRNA was present at similar levels in transgenic and non-transgenic mice as judged[20] by comparison with the expression of the ß-actin gene (Figure 3B),[20] clearly indicating normal expression of endogenous IRBP in transgenic mice.

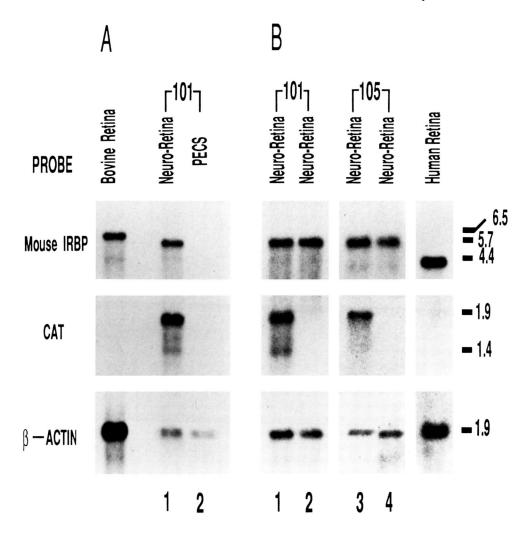

Figure 3. Northern analysis of poly(A$^+$) RNAs. RNA samples of 2μg were separated on formaldehyde denaturing gels and then blotted to Zeta-Probe. Hybridization probes are indicated on the left: Mouse IRBP, a 722-bp mouse IRBP cDNA, corresponding to human IRBP cDNA positions 3089 to 3810;[16] CAT, the IRBP-CAT construct; and ß-actin, the chicken cytoplasmic ß-actin cDNA.[20] **A,** neuro-retina (lane 1) and PECS (lane 2) poly(A$^+$) RNAs from a transgenic F$_1$ mouse of family 101. **B,** neuro-retina poly(A$^+$) RNAs from transgenic families 101 and 105; lanes 1 and 3, transgenic mice; lanes 2 and 4, nontransgenic littermates. The sizes of the hybridizing transcripts (in kilobases) were estimated by comparison to an RNA ladder [Bethesda Research Laboratory].

IV. TRANSGENIC MICE AS PROBES INTO RETINA DEGENERATION

Transgenic mice may provide new insights into mammalian development mechanisms by involving either change or inactivation of pre-existing genes.[24] IRBP may be used as a candidate gene to study the effect of its mutation or absence to the development of the mouse retina. For example, the expression of antisense IRBP RNA in the photoreceptors may form RNA-RNA hybrids and thereby impair IRBP gene expression by stoichiometric nature of the inhibition.[25] Alternatively, the inclusion of ribozymes in antisense molecules could not only form RNA-RNA hybrids, but also catalytically cleave a phosphodiester bond in the IRBP RNA strand and thereby could process a large number of IRBP mRNA.[26] Finally, it is possible to study the function of IRBP gene in the mouse by establishing a null allele in the germ line through the application of homologous recombination (gene targeting) in embryonic stem cells.[27]

The development and degeneration of mammalian photoreceptors may also be studied in transgenic mice by involving the selective destruction of photoreceptors as a means to address their functional necessity and interrelations with other developing cells. For example, engineered diphtheria toxin A gene with confined toxicity may be used with IRBP promoter to specifically ablate developing photoreceptors.[24] Future development in the research of retinal degeneration awaits for the result of current experiments using these strategies.

V. CONCLUSION

The goal of our research is to study how retinal degenerations may be related to IRBP gene expression. As a first step toward this goal, we have used the gene transfer experiments in mice to identify a transcriptional regulatory region of the human IRBP gene, and have established that a 1.3 kb fragment from the 5' end of the human IRBP gene is sufficient to direct transgene expression to the retinal photoreceptors. Future experiments may include genetic ablation of IRBP in transgenic mice to address the function of IRBP, and genetic ablation of developing photoreceptors to address their relations with other developing cells.

VI. ACKNOWLEDGEMENTS

This study was supported by NIH National Eye Institute Grant EY-03829, a grant from the RP Foundation Fighting Blindness, and an unrestricted grant to the Department of Ophthalmology from Research to Prevent Blindness, Inc.

VII. REFERENCES

1. Bazan, N. G., Reddy, T. S., Redmond, T. M., Wiggert, B. and Chader, G. J., Endogenous fatty acids are covalently and noncovalently bound to interphotoreceptor retinoid-binding protein in the monkey retina, J. Biol. Chem., 260, 13677, 1985.

2. van Veen, T., Katial, A., Shinohara, T., Barret, D. J., Wiggert, B., Chader, G. J. and Nickerson, J. M., Retinal photoreceptor neurons and pinealocytes accumulate mRNA for interphotoreceptor retinoid-binding protein (IRBP), FEBS Lett., 208, 133, 1986.

3. Bridges, C. D. B., Landers, R. A., Fong, S.-L. and Liou, G. I., Interstitial retinol-binding protein (IRBP) in rat and bovine pineal organs: Evolutionary vestige or functional molecule?, in Pineal and Retinal Relationships, O'Brien, P. J. and Klein, D. C., Eds., Academic Press, New York, 1986, 383.

4. Chader, G. J., Interphotoreceptor retinoid-binding protein (IRBP): A model protein for molecular biological and clinically relevant studies, Invest. Ophthalmol. Vis. Sci., 30, 7, 1989.

5. Liou, G. I., Geng, L. and Baehr, W., Interphotoreceptor reinoid-binding protein: Biochemistry and molecular biology, in The Molecular Biology of the Retina: Basic and Clinically Relevant Studies, Chader, G. J. and Farber, D., Eds., Alan R. Liss, New York, 1990, in press.

6. Okajima, T-I., L., Pepperberg, D.R., Ripps, H., Wiggert, B. and Chader, G. J., Interphotoreceptor retinoid-binding protein: Role in delivery of retinol to the pigment epithelium, Exp. Eye Res., 49, 629, 1989.

7. Okajima, T-I. L., Pepperberg, D. R., Ripps, H., Wiggert, B. and Chader, G. J., Interphotoreceptor retinoid-binding protein promotes rhodopsin regeneration in toad photoreceptors. Proc. Natl. Acad. Sci. USA, 87, 6907, 1990.

8. Carter-Dawson, L., Alvarez, R. A., Fong, S.-L., Liou, G. I., Sperling, H. G. and Bridges, C. D. B., Rhodopsin, 11-cis vitamin A, and interstitial retinol-binding protein (IRBP) during retinal development in normal and rd mutant mice, Dev. Biol., 116, 431, 1986.

9. Rodrigues, M. M., Wiggert, B., Hackett, J., Lee, L., Fletcher, R. T. and Chader, G. J., Dominantly inherited retinitis pigmentosa: Ultrastructure and biochemical analysis, Ophthalmology, 92, 1165, 1985.

10. van Veen, T., Ekstrom, P., Wiggert, B., Lee, L., Hirose, &., Sanyal, S. and Chader, G. J., A developmental study of interphotoreceptor retinoid-binding protein (IRBP) in single and double homozygous rd and rds mutant mouse retinae, Exp. Eye Res., 47, 291, 1988.

11. Narfstrom, K. and Nilsson, S. E. G., Hereditary retinal degeneration in the Abyssinian cat: An update on laboratory findings, presented at Symposium on retinal degenerations, Stockholm, Sweden, July 24 - 27, 1990.

12. Dryja, T. P., McGee, T. L., Reichel, E., Hahn, L. B., Cowley, G. S., Yandell, D. W., Sandberg, M. A. and Berson, E. L., A point mutation of the rhodopsin gene in one form of retinitis pigmentosa, Nature, 343, 364, 1990.

13. Connell, G., Boscom, R., McInnes, R. and Molday, R. S., Photoreceptor cell peripherin is the defective protein responsible for retinal degeneration slow (rds), Invest. Ophthalmol. Vis. Sci., 31 (suppl), 309, 1990.

14. Bowes, C., Li, T., Danciger, M., Baxter, L. C., Applebury, M. L. and Farber, D. B., Retinal degeneration in the rd mouse is caused by a defect in the ß subunit of rod cGMP-phosphodiesterase, Nature, 347, 677, 1990.

15. Liou, G. I., Geng, L., Al-Ubaidi, M. R., Matragoon, S., Hanten, G., Baehr, W. and Overbeek, P. A., Tissue-specific expression in transgenic mice directed by the 5'-flanking sequences of the human gene encoding interphotoreceptor retinoid-binding protein, J. Biol. Chem., 265, 8373, 1990.

16. Liou, G. I., Ma, D. P., Yang, Y.W., Geng, L., Zhu, C. and Baehr, W., Human intersitital retinoid-binding protein-gene structure and primary sequence, J. Biol. Chem., 264, 8200, 1989.

17. Smale, S. T. and Baltimore, D., The initiator as a transcription control element, Cell, 57, 103, 1989.

18. Gorman, C. M., Merlino, G. T., Willingham, M. C., Pastan, I. and Howard, B. H., The rous sarcoma virus long terminal repeat is a strong promoter when introduced into a variety of eukaryotic cells by DNA-mediated transfection, Proc. Natl. Acad. Sci. USA, 79, 6777, 1982.

19. Overbeek, P. A., Lai, S. P., van Quill, K. R. and Westphal, H., Tissue-specific expression in transgenic mice of a fused gene containing RSV terminal sequences, Science, 231, 1574, 1986.

20. Grichnik, J. M., Bergsma, D. J. and Schwartz, R. J., Tissue restricted and stage specific transcription is maintained within 411 nucleotides flanking the 5' end of the chacken a-skeletal actin gene, Nucleic Acid Res., 14, 1683, 1986.

21. Bok, D., Retinal photoreceptor-pigment epithelium interactions, Invest. Ophthalmol. Vis. Sci., 26, 1659, 1985.

22. Takahashi, J.S. and Zatz, M., Regulation of circadian rhythmicity, Science, 217, 1104, 1982.

23. Overbeek, P.A. and Yokoyama, T., personal communication, 1990.

24. Hanahan, D., Transgenic mice as probes into complex systems, Science, 246, 1265, 1989.

25. Weintraub, H. M., Antisense RNA and DNA, Scientific American, 262, 40, 1990.

26. Sarver, N., Cantin, E. M., Chang, P. S., Zaia, J. A., Ladne, P. A., Stephens, D. A. and Rossi, J. J., Ribozymes as potential anti-HIV-1 therapeutic agents, Science, 247, 1222, 1990.

27. DeChiara, T.M., Efstratiadis, A. and Robertson, E.J., A growth-deficiency phenotype in heterozygous mice carrying an insulin-like growth factor II gene disrupted by targeting, Nature, 345, 78, 1990.

IRBP GENE EXPRESSION IN THE DYSTROPHIC RETINA OF THE MUTANT *rds* MOUSE

Neeraj Agarwal, Izhak Nir, and David S. Papermaster
Department of Pathology,
University of Texas Health Science Center at San Antonio,
San Antonio, Texas 78284

I. ABSTRACT

The genetic defect in the *rds* mouse was recently localized to the peripherin gene. Although this mutation may explain the morphogenesis defect, i.e. the failure to form outer segments, the reasons for subsequent cell death are not clear. Previously, we demonstrated that the capability to synthesize opsin, an outer segment integral membrane protein, is not compromised by the mutation, although retinal opsin content is considerably reduced as a consequence of continued phagocytic destruction of abortive outer segment membranes by the pigment epithelium. We have now studied a secreted protein that is also synthesized by the rod: interstitial retinol binding protein (IRBP). This protein has recently been linked to photoreceptor cell death in several animal models of retinal dystrophy. Substantial levels of IRBP mRNA, IRBP synthesis and content were observed by 1 month of age, at a time coincident with pronounced photoreceptor death. IRBP was localized by immunocytochemistry in the interphotoreceptor matrix, as expected. As a result of these observations, we propose that cell death is probably not due to the inability of the abnormal photoreceptors to produce or secrete IRBP.

II. INTRODUCTION

In the *rds* mouse, photoreceptor outer segments do not develop normally during photoreceptor morphogenesis.[1] The abnormal photoreceptors die at a slow rate, as determined by the reduction in outer nuclear layer width or cell count, until photoreceptor nuclei largely disappear by one year.[2] Recently the *rds* gene was identified by Travis et al.[3] and the gene product was found by Connell et al.[4] to be peripherin. Peripherin may have a structural function in the stabilization of the outer segment disc rim or the binding of the disc rim to cytoskeletal elements.[5] The complete absence of peripherin in the homozygote or its partial absence in the heterozygote might explain the failure of *rds* rods and cones to form or maintain a normal outer segment. Why the *rds* mutation and its attendant defect in morphogenesis leads to photoreceptor cell death is not self evident, however.

We have now investigated the gene expression of interphotoreceptor retinol binding protein (IRBP) in the *rds* retina.   IRBP is synthesized in the rod inner segments and secreted into the interphotoreceptor space where it mediates the transport of retinol between the pigment epithelium (PE) and the photoreceptor cells.[6,7,8,9]   A role for IRBP in photoreceptor cell death has been proposed in various retinal dystrophies.   Gonzalez-Fernandez et al.[10] correlated reduced levels of IRBP with photoreceptor cell death in the RCS rat.   These authors suggested that, since IRBP is capable of binding α-tocopherol, it might function as an anti-oxidant.   Thus, loss of IRBP could enhance photoreceptor membrane degradation.   Reduced levels of IRBP in the interphotoreceptor space were also implicated in the photoreceptor death of the Abyssinian cat.[11]   These authors proposed that IRBP may also function as a buffer system for free retinoids, thus protecting membranes from their toxic effects.   We therefore explored whether changes in IRBP gene expression developed in the course of photoreceptor death in *rds* mouse retinas.   IRBP mRNA levels, its synthetic rate, content and ultrastructural localization were investigated in young mice, shortly after the photoreceptors would mature in normal mice, and at later phases of the retinal degeneration.

III.   MATERIALS AND METHODS

Animals: BALB/c mice were obtained from Jackson Laboratories (Bar Harbor, Maine).   Mutant 020/A *rds/rds* mice were obtained from Dr. Janet Blanks, University of Southern California, Los Angeles, from a colony that originated in the Netherlands and was distributed by Dr. Sanyal.   The animals were bred locally for four years and maintained under a 12h/12h dark/light cycle with exposure to low (3-5 foot candles) light levels.   The handling of the mice was in accordance with ARVO resolution on the use of animals in research and NIH and AAALAC guidelines.   Mice at various ages were sacrificed 1-2 h after the onset of light by exposure to CO_2.

Northern Blot Analysis: IRBP mRNA levels were studied as previously described.[12]   Briefly, RNA was extracted with guanidinium isothiocyanate and isolated on a CsCl gradient as described by Chirgwin et al.[13]   Purified total retinal RNA was separated by electrophoresis as described by Lehrach et al.[14] and transferred to a Nytran nylon membrane (S. & S. Inc.).   The blot was then subjected to hybridization with [^{32}P]-oligolabeled human IRBP cDNA (H.4 clone), or a β-actin genomic DNA probe as controls, using the procedure described by Maniatis et al.[15]   The IRBP probe was kindly provided by Dr. Gregory Liou of Baylor College of Medicine, Houston, TX, and the β-actin genomic DNA probe by Dr. U. Nudel of the Weizman Institute, Rheovot, Israel.[12]

In Vitro Protein Synthesis: Six to eight retinas were incubated in methionine-free medium containing 10 μCi/ml of [^{35}S]-methionine (NEN) for a period of 2 hours at 37°C with shaking, following the method of St. Jules and O'Brien[16] and as described in detail previously.[17]   Briefly, after incubation, the retinas were homogenized, solubilized and electrophoresed on a 10% SDS polyacrylamide gel.[18]   The gel was then stained with Coomassie blue, dried and autoradiographed. In a separate experiment, after incubation was completed, the incubation medium was collected, proteins were precipitated by addition of an equal volume of acetone and the precipitates were dried, solubilized and electrophoresed. No labeled proteins were detected in the medium after this short period of incorporation (data not shown).

Immunoblotting: Immunoblotting was conducted by a modification of the procedure of Towbin et al.[19] as described by Deretic and Hamm[20] using rabbit anti-bovine IRBP antibody followed by a peroxidase detection sequence. The antibody was also provided by Dr. Liou. To avoid IRBP losses during isolation of retinas, quantitative estimates of IRBP levels in *rds* eyes as compared with normal BALB/c eyes were obtained by sonication of whole eyes, solubilization, removal of the lens, electrophoresis and densitometric analysis of the immunoblots as described by Agarwal et al.[12]

Post Embedding Immunocytochemical Procedures: Dark- or light-adapted mice were sacrificed by CO_2 exposure. Following enucleation, the anterior eye cup and the lens were removed, and the posterior eye cup was fixed in the dark or in the light with 4% formaldehyde and 1% glutaraldehyde (in 0.1M phosphate buffer pH 7.0), for 1 hour at room temperature. Small tissue strips were then dehydrated and embedded in LR Gold (Polysciences) at 4°C as described by Nir et al.[17] IRBP was localized with a rabbit anti-bovine IRBP at 100 μg/ml, followed by biotinyl sheep anti-rabbit Fab dimer and a streptavidin gold 5 nm conjugate (Janssen). Labeling was also carried out with rabbit anti-monkey IRBP 50 μg/ml, followed by goat anti-rabbit IgG and a rabbit anti-goat 5nm gold conjugate (Janssen). The anti-monkey IRBP antibodies were kindly provided by Dr. B. Wiggert at NEI, Bethesda MD.[21] The sections were stained with uranyl acetate and lead citrate before viewing under the electron microscope.

IV. RESULTS

IRBP mRNA Levels: Retinas from *rds* mice, 11d to 365d old, were studied. A representative northern blot is shown in Figure 1. The *rds* retina mRNA in the northern blot was compared with 11 and 30d old BALB/c retina, bovine retina and mouse liver. A 5.8 Kb transcript was found in the BALB/c and *rds* retina. The IRBP cDNA did not hybridize with the liver RNA but did hybridize to an IRBP transcript in bovine retina of a slightly larger size. In the *rds* retinas, the IRBP transcript was found in all ages except at 365d old, which is in accordance with the almost complete photoreceptor cell loss at this age.[2] Densitometric quantitation of IRBP band density, followed by correction for loss of photoreceptors as the mice age, demonstrated that nearly normal levels of transcription of the IRBP gene occurred in both 11 and 30 d old *rds* mice when compared to BALB/c controls (data not shown).

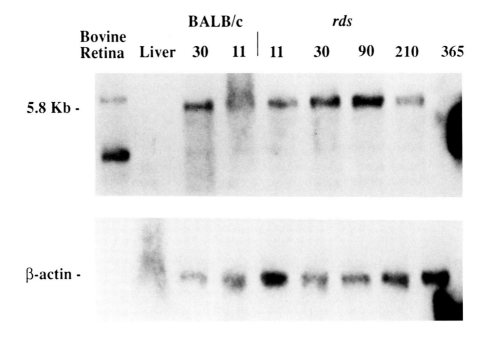

Figure 1. IRBP mRNA. Northern blot analysis of IRBP mRNA in 11 and 30d old BALB/c retinas and 11d to 365d *rds* retinas. Total retinal RNA (5mg/lane) was probed with human (H.4) ^{32}P-oligolabeled IRBP cDNA. A 5.8 Kb transcript was observed for BALB/c and *rds* mice total retinal RNA. A β-actin transcript served as an internal control for the loading of total RNA in each lane. The artifact on the right of the figure was generated by high levels of binding of the probes to an RNA standard ladder (lane not shown).

IRBP Synthesis: Newly synthesized IRBP was measured by the incorporation of [^{35}S]-methionine in retinas from *rds* mice of various ages, 30d to 11m old, and the newly synthesized IRBP was compared to retinas of 30d old BALB/c mice. The results of a representative experiment are depicted in Figure 2. A radiolabeled IRBP band was seen in 30d old *rds* retinas. It was greatly reduced by 90d and thereafter.

IRBP Content: The persistence of IRBP in the *rds* retina at various ages was determined by antibody binding on immunoblots of solubilized retinas. The results, as depicted in Figure 3, show that IRBP can be clearly detected in *rds* retinas up to 28d. There is a noticeable reduction in the band density thereafter but IRBP still persists in older retinas. Since the different lanes were loaded with equal amounts of retinal tissue, the major reduction in IRBP at 90d and 210d reflects, in part, photoreceptor cell loss. This result was explored more fully by determining the quantity of IRBP in solubilized eyes to eliminate the possible loss of IRBP during retinal isolation (Figure 4).

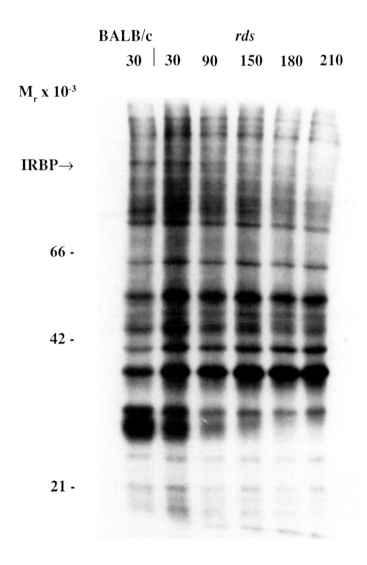

Figure 2. Biosynthesis of IRBP *in vitro*. Incorporation of [^{35}S]-methionine into newly synthesized IRBP in BALB/c and *rds* retinas at various ages. The retinal proteins were run on a 10% SDS-PAGE and the gels were autoradiographed. The [^{35}S]-methionine-labeled IRBP band is indicated by the arrow.

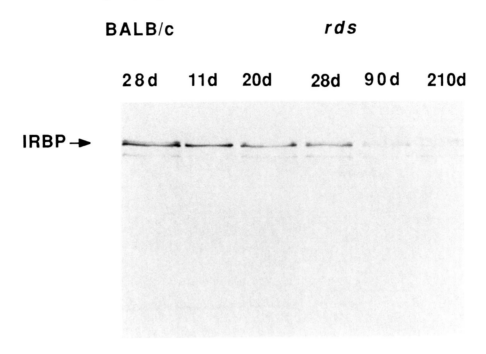

Figure 3. Immunoblot analysis of the IRBP in *rds* and BALB/c mice. A 10% SDS gel was electrophoretically blotted onto a PVDF Immobilon membrane (Millipore). The IRBP was detected with rabbit anti-bovine IRBP and peroxidase-conjugated anti-rabbit IgG. The IRBP band is indicated by the arrow. The other faint band is caused by non-specific binding. Substantial levels of IRBP are seen in *rds* retinas up to 28d. At 90d and 210d, IRBP levels are greatly reduced but still noticeable. Since the different lanes were loaded with equal amounts of retina tissue, the reduced levels at 90d and 210d are partly due to photoreceptor cell loss. The steady state levels of IRBP were quantitatively estimated in 33d old *rds* eyes and compared with 41d old BALB/c eyes (Figure 4). The lanes were loaded with varying amounts of solubilized eye tissue (minus the lens) in order to avoid overloading of the gel, as described in the legend of Figure 4. Densitometric analysis of the immunoblot revealed that the IRBP content in the *rds* eye is reduced by 70% in comparison with the IRBP content in BALB/c eye. Since 43% of the photoreceptors are lost by this age, the reduction in IRBP content is due, to a considerable extent, to rod cell death.

Localization of IRBP in both young and old rds retinas: In 3 month old retinas, IRBP was clearly detected in the interphotoreceptor space and the Golgi region (Figures 5 and 6). In 9 month old retinas, IRBP in the interphotoreceptor space was still evident (Figure 7), although it was often reduced in comparison to the density observed in younger retinas. It is noteworthy that Golgi labeling in photoreceptors of old retinas (Figure 7) is as dense as that observed in young retinas (Figure 6). Since the number of photoreceptor cells is greatly reduced in the older retinas, the reduction in interphotoreceptor labeling might reflect reduction in IRBP production per retina rather than production per cell.

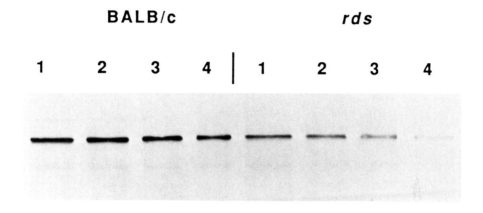

BALB/c　　　　　*rds*

1　　2　　3　　4　|　1　　2　　3　　4

Figure 4. Quantitation of IRBP content. Densitometric analysis of immunoblots from 41d old BALB/c and 33d old *rds* eyes. Decreasing amounts of BALB/c and *rds* eye tissues were loaded in the different lanes as follows: 1, 0.024; 2, 0.018; 3, 0.012; and 4, 0.006 eyes, respectively. Densitometric analysis revealed a linear relationship between the amount of tissue loaded and the measured band density. Comparison between the BALB/c and *rds* mice revealed that the *rds* IRBP content in the 33d old *rds* eye was reduced by 70% when calculated on a per retina basis.

V. DISCUSSION

IRBP mRNA transcripts persist in the *rds* retina at least to the age of 7m old. Hence, the early abnormalities in the formation of outer segment do not abolish the transcriptional activity of the IRBP gene. The reduction in the mRNA band density in the northern blot, as a function of age, correlates with the level of cell loss. IRBP synthesis was clearly detected in 1m old *rds* retinas. It was, however, greatly reduced by 3m and at later ages and also correlates with the level of cell loss. It should be noted, however, that detectable mRNA persists for longer periods than detectable IRBP synthesis. Also, immunochemistry, and particularly immunocytochemistry, revealed the presence of persisting IRBP at late stages of degeneration. Hence, the reduced synthesis may be a reflection of limited sensitivity of the detection technique. Quantitative analysis of IRBP content in 33d old *rds* retinas, as compared with 41d old BALB/c, showed a reduction of 70% in the *rds* retina as calculated per retina basis. Since cell loss in the *rds* retina of this age is about 45%,[22] it is apparent that the reduction is in large part due to cell loss. In a previous quantitative study, van

Veen et al.[23] calculated that the IRBP content in 30d old *rds* retinas is only slightly reduced in comparison to normal BALB/c retinas. The reasons for this discrepancy are not clear. Regardless, both studies clearly indicate the presence of considerable amounts of IRBP at a time when photoreceptors are degenerating at a rapid rate.

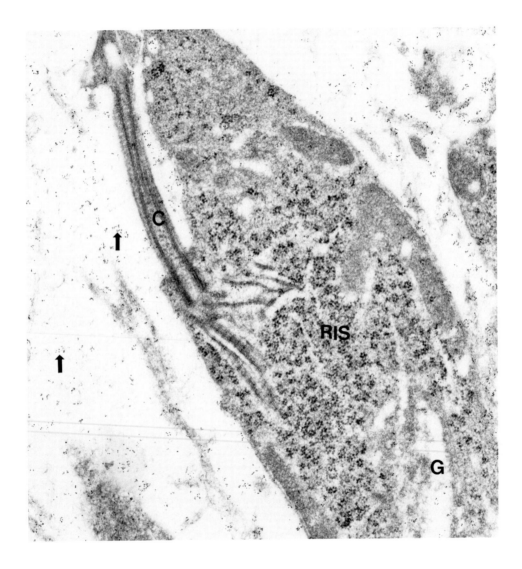

Figure 5. IRBP localization in the 3 month old *rds* mouse retina. Labeling with rabbit anti-bovine IRBP followed by biotinylated sheep anti-rabbit IgG and streptavidin gold (5nm). Substantial labeling is seen in the interphotoreceptor space (arrows). In *rds* photoreceptors, a cilium (C) is extended from the inner segment (IS) but an outer segment is not formed at the tip of the cilium.   ×37,000.

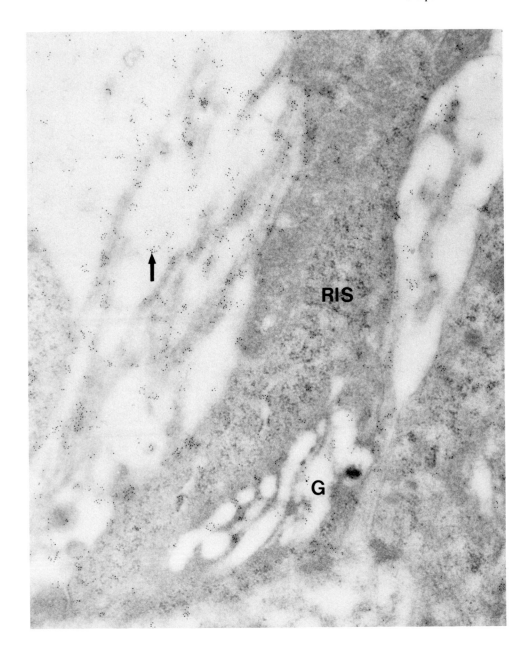

Figure 6.   Localization of IRBP in the Golgi of the 3 month old *rds* **mouse photoreceptor.** Labeling with rabbit anti-monkey IRBP followed by goat anti-rabbit IgG and rabbit anti-goat IgG - 5nm gold. Part of an inner segment (RIS) which contains a Golgi region (G) is seen. IRBP is localized in the Golgi region and in the interphotoreceptor space (arrow).   ×42,700.

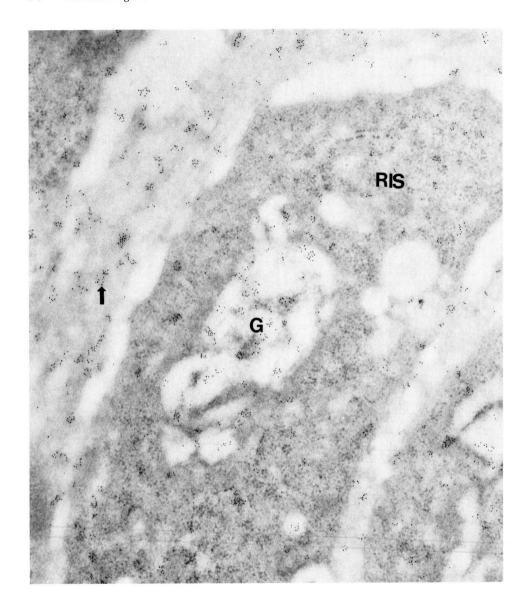

Figure 7. Persistence of IRBP in the Golgi of 9 month old *rds* mouse photoreceptor.
Labeling with IRBP as described in Figure 6. Part of an inner segment (RIS) with
a Golgi region (G) is seen. The Golgi region is clearly labeled. IRBP is also
localized in the interphotoreceptor space (arrow). The membranous structures which
are observed in the interphotoreceptor space (arrows) are either Müller cells or
pigment epithelium processes. ×42,700.

In a recent study, we established that opsin gene expression is little affected by the *rds* mutation, although the steady state opsin content in young *rds* retinas is low -- ca. 3% of normal. The opsin mRNA levels were 60-70% of normal, and opsin synthetic rates were comparable to normal retinas.[12] In older retinas, opsin mRNA persisted, but opsin synthesis fell below detection.[22] Thus, both IRBP and opsin appear to be expressed and synthesized by the subset of surviving *rds* photoreceptors at nearly normal levels and decline concordantly with the death of the photoreceptors.

The IRBP which is detected in the immunoblots was also localized by means of immunoelectron microscopy to the interphotoreceptor space in both young and old *rds* retinas. The persistence of IRBP in old *rds* retinas was also detected, with light microscopic immunocytochemistry, by van Veen et al.[23] These authors observed that at the later stages of degeneration the IRBP is sequestered intracellularly and suggested that secretion of IRBP might be affected in the *rds* retina, which in turn might be a factor in the less differentiated and/or degenerated state of the *rds* retina. In our present electron microscopic localization of IRBP, we were able to detect IRBP in both the Golgi and the interphotoreceptor space of young and old *rds* retinas. Reduced labeling of IRBP in the interphotoreceptor space was noted in older retinas, but this might reflect a reduction in the number of IRBP-secreting photoreceptor cells as the retinal degeneration progressed. The suggestion that changes in IRBP might be associated with photoreceptor cell death is of interest, since abnormalities in the IPM were reported in other retinal dystrophies such as the RCS rat.[24] It was subsequently proposed that IRBP may play a role in photoreceptor cell death in the RCS rat[10] and the Abyssinian cat.[11] In considering a role for reduced IRBP level in the *rds* retinal dystrophy, the kinetics of photoreceptor cell death should be evaluated. During the first month, between 11d and 30d, photoreceptor cell density was reduced by 41%, as compared with a 25% reduction in cell density in the next two months.[24] Nevertheless, IRBP mRNA, IRBP synthesis and IRBP content were higher in the period between 11d and 30d in comparison to the period between 30d and 90d. Hence, while 41% of photoreceptors were lost in the first month of degeneration, at the same time period IRBP content, mRNA, and synthesis were at their highest levels in the *rds* retina. Thus, at least the initial major photoreceptor cell loss is unlikely to be due to significant changes in IRBP gene expression.

Recently, Carter-Dawson and Burrough[25] reported that localization of IRBP, by immunoelectron microscopy, revealed that, by 18d, labeling density of IRBP in the apical PE region of the *rds* retina was low in comparison to normal. Whether the reduced labeling in the apical PE region was due to reduction in synthesis, to increased degradation, or to abnormal distribution of IRBP in the diseased retina was not clear. Although differences in IRBP distribution throughout the IPM were not apparent in the present study, a detailed quantitative analysis will have to be done in order to establish regional differences, especially since the distribution of IPM is affected by light in the normal rat.[26] In any case, even if such differences exist they should be evaluated in reference to our present biochemical and molecular observation that at an early stage of degeneration both IRBP content and synthesis might not be significantly affected. Hence, reduced labeling density of IRBP in the apical PE region might be a secondary result of the abnormal morphology of the *rds* retina. In the absence of outer segments, there is an abnormal increase in the volume of the interphotoreceptor space, which IRBP, even if synthesized and secreted normally, could fail to occupy. The apical PE region, being at the farthest distance from the site of synthesis, i.e. the inner segments, might result in a greater reduction in the IRBP labeling density simply because the enlarged IPM space in the *rds* retina cannot be fully occupied with IRBP. Alternatively, if IPM molecules move during the light cycle, the forces generating this movement may be altered by the structure of the *rds* photoreceptors and may be further perturbed by the cell loss that is characteristic of the later stages of the degeneration.

Acknowledgements: We wish to thank Dr. Barbara Schneider and Dusanka Deretic for helpful discussions, Dr. Z.D. Sharp for the β-actin probe, to Nancy Ransom for excellent E.M. immunocytochemistry and Tammy Lowe for preparing the manuscript. Supported in part by NIH (EY-6892).

REFERENCES

1. Sanyal, S. and Jansen, H.G. (1981). Absence of receptor outer segment in the retina of the *rds* mutant mouse. *Neuroscience Letters* 21:23-26.
2. Sanyal, S. and Hawkins, R.K. (1986). Development and degeneration of retina in *rds* mutant mice: Effects of light on the rate of degeneration in albino and pigmented homozygous and heterozygous mutant and normal mice. *Vision Research* 26:1177-1185.
3. Travis, G.H., Brennan, M.B., Danielson, P.E., Kozak, C.A. and Sutcliffe, J.G. (1989). Identification of a photoreceptor-specific mRNA encoded by the gene responsible for retinal degeneration slow (*rds*). *Nature* 338:70-73.
4. Connell, G., Boscom, R., McInnes, R., and Molday, R.S. (1990). Photoreceptor cell peripherin is the defective protein responsible for retinal degeneration slow (*rds*). *Invest. Ophthalmol. Vis. Sci.* (Suppl) 31:309.
5. Molday, R., Hicks, D., and Molday, L. (1987). Peripherin: A rim-specific membrane protein of rod outer segment discs. *Invest. Ophthalmol. Vis. Sci.* 28:50-61.
6. Adler, A.J. and Martin, K.J. (1982). Retinol-binding proteins in bovine interphotoreceptor matrix. *Biochem. Biophys. Res. Comm.* 108:1601-1608.
7. Bunt-Milam, A.H. and Saari, J.C. (1983). Immunocytochemical localization of two retinal binding proteins in vertebrate retina. *J. Cell Biol.* 97:703-712.
8. Chader, G.J., Wiggert, B., Lai, Y-L., Lee, L., and Fletcher, R. (1983). Interphotoreceptor retinoid binding protein: A possible role in retinoid transport to the retina. In *Progress in Retinal Research* (Eds. Osborn, N. and Chader, G.J.) Pergamon Press, Oxford. pp 162-189.

9. Fong, S-L., Liou, G.I., Landers, R.A., Alvarez, R.A., Gonzalez-Fernandez, F., Glazebrook, P.A., Lam, D.M.K., and Bridges C.D.B. (1984). Characterization, localization, and biosynthesis of an interstitial retinol binding protein in the human eye. *J. Neurochem.* 42:1667-1676.

10. Gonzalez-Fernandez, F., Landers, R.A., Glazebrook, P.A., Fong, S-L., Liou, G.I., Lam, D.M.K. and Bridges, C.D.B. (1984). An extracellular retinal-binding glycoprotein in the eyes of mutant rats with retinal dystrophy: Development, localization and biosynthesis. *J. Cell Biol.* 99:2092-2098.

11. Narfström, K., Nilsson, S.-E., Wiggert, B., Lee, L., Chader, G.J. and van Veen, T. (1989). Reduced level of interphotoreceptor retinoid-binding protein (IRBP): A possible cause for retinal degeneration in the Abyssinian cat. *Cell Tissue Res.* 257:631-639.

12. Agarwal, N., Nir, I. and Papermaster, D.S. (1990). Opsin synthesis and mRNA levels in dystrophic retinas devoid of outer segments in retinal degeneration slow (*rds*) mice. *J. Neuroscience* 10:3275-3285.

13. Chirgwin, J.M., Przybyla, A.E., MacDonald, R.J. and Rutter, W.J. (1979). Isolation of biologically active ribonucleic acid from sources enriched in ribonuclease. *Biochemistry* 18:5294-5299.

14. Lehrach, H., Diamond, D., Wozney, J.M. and Boedtker, H. (1977). RNA molecular weight determination by gel electrophoresis under denaturing condition: A critical reexamination. *Biochemistry* 16:4743-4751.

15. Maniatis, T., Fritsch, E.F., and Sambrook, J. (1982). In *Molecular Cloning: A Laboratory Manual.* Cold Spring Harbor Laboratory. p. 202.

16. St. Jules, R.S. and O'Brien, P.J. (1986). The acylation of rat rhodopsin *in vitro* and *in vivo*. *Exp. Eye Res.* 43:929-940.

17. Nir, I., Agarwal, N., Sagie, G. and Papermaster, D.S. (1989). Opsin distribution and synthesis in degenerating photoreceptors of *rd* mutant mice. *Exp. Eye Res.* 49:403-421.

18. Laemmli, U.K. (1970). Cleavage of structural proteins during the assembly of the head of bacteriophage T_4. *Nature* 227:680-685.

19. Towbin, H., Staehelin, T. and Gordon, J. (1979). Electrophoretic transfer of proteins from polyacrylamide gels to nitrocellular sheets: Procedure and some applications. *Proc. Natl. Acad. Sci.* 76:4350-4354.

20. Deretic, D. and Hamm, H.E. (1987). Topographic analysis of antigenic determinants recognized by monoclonal antibodies to the photoreceptor guanyl nucleotide binding protein, transducin. *J. Biol. Chem.* 262:10839-10847.

21. Wiggert, B., Lee, L., Rodrigues, M., Hess, H., Redmond, T.M., and Chader, G.J. (1986). Immunocytochemical distribution of retinoid binding proteins in selected species. *Invest. Ophthalmol. Vis. Sci.* 27:1041-1049.

22. Nir, I. Agarwal, N., and Papermaster, D.S. (1990). Opsin gene expression during early and late phases of retinal degeneration in *rds* mice. *Exp. Eye Res.* 51:257-267.

23. van Veen, T., Ekstrom, P., Wiggert, B., Hirose, Y., Sagal, S. and Chader, G.J. (1988). A developmental study of interphotoreceptor retinoid-binding protein (IRBP) in single and double homogeneous *rd* and *rds* mutant mouse retinae. *Exp. Eye Res.* 47:291-305.

24. LaVail, M.M., Pinto, L.H. and Yasumura, D. (1981). The interphotoreceptor matrix in rats with inherited retinal dystrophy. *Invest. Ophthalmol. Vis. Sci.* 21:658-668.

25. Carter-Dawson, L. and Burrough, M. (1989). Interphotoreceptor retinoid-binding protein (IRBP) in the postnatal development of *rds* mouse retina: EM immunocytochemical localization. *Exp. Eye Res.* 49:829-841.

26. Uehara, F., Matthes, M.T., Yasumura, D. and LaVail, M.M. (1990). Light-evoked changes in interphotoreceptor matrix. *Science* 248:1633-1636.

MOLECULAR MECHANISMS REGULATING CELLULAR AND SUBCELLULAR CONCENTRATIONS OF GENE PRODUCTS IN MOUSE VISUAL CELLS.

James F. McGinnis, Phillip L. Stepanik, Valentine Lerious, and James P. Whelan.
Dept of Anatomy & Cell Biology, Brain Research Institute and the Mental Retardation Research Center, University of California, Los Angeles, CA 90024

INTRODUCTION

The mechanisms underlying the regulation of the activity of genes which are important in the phototransduction process of vision and/or in the regulation of photoreceptor cell metabolism are significant neurobiological problems about which relatively little is known. We have been especially interested in studying the processes by which the concentrations of cell-specific gene products are regulated in mammalian photoreceptor cells. Toward this end, we have developed immunological and recombinant DNA probes and have used them to study the retinas of normal mice and of mice with hereditary retinal degeneration under different environmental lighting conditions. The application of these probes has resulted in two very interesting observations. First, the subcellular localization of some photoreceptor-specific proteins is transient and dependent on the lighting environment to which the animal is exposed. Second, the activities of the genes for some of these photoreceptor-specific proteins are noncoordinately regulated and show cyclic changes during the normal light/dark cycle.

The rapid light-dependent shift in subcellular localization of some proteins involved in phototransduction has a dramatic effect on their concentrations in the inner and outer segments of the rods and it therefore must have a corresponding effect on the rates of the reactions catalyzed by these proteins. Similarly, the cyclic changes in the concentration of specific mRNA's for these proteins will change the total cellular concentration of these proteins on a cyclic basis. These processes appear to be related to each other and to the development and maintenance of the differentiated status of the rod photoreceptor cells. Data supporting these conclusions will be presented along with an experimental model which summarizes and correlates these changes with other events occurring in photoreceptor cells.

METHODS

Animals: Albino Balb/cJ mice were bred and maintained in the animal vivarium at UCLA under a 12 hour light\dark cycle. Specific conditions were as described previously by Whelan & McGinnis, 1988[1]. All dissections of animals sacrificed in the dark were done with dim red light whereas normal room lighting was used for animals sacrificed from the light cycle. Polyclonal antisera were generously provided by Drs. Dale Gregerson (anti-rhodopsin and S-antigen) and Rehwa Lee (anti-phosducin and beta transducin).

Immunocytochemistry: Monospecific antisera were used for immunocytochemistry on formaldehyde-fixed mouse retinas employing the ABC avidin-biotin-peroxidase method (Vector Laboratories) with modifications, as described previously [1]. Six-micron thick, paraffin embedded sections were then treated in succession with 2% normal goat serum in Tris buffer, diluted primary serum, biotinylated goat anti-rabbit IgG, and the ABC complex. Specific binding was visualized with a solution of 0.05% diaminobenzidine and 0.01% hydrogen peroxide. Sections were washed, dehydrated and mounted before examination on a Nikon Microphot microscope.

RNA: Isolation of RNA was performed by the method of Chomzynski and Sacci[2] as described previously[3]. Both eyes from a single animal were put into one microfuge tube and total RNA extracted. Total RNA was quantitated spectrophotometrically at OD $_{260}$ and 10 ug from each sample was electrophoresed as described previously by Baehr et al[4], in a 1 % agarose gel containing formaldehyde and transferred to Nytran sheets by capillary action using the method of Thomas[5]. For slot blot analysis, 0.1, 0.3 and 1.0 ug of total RNA was applied to Nytran sheets using an S&S slot blot apparatus. Mouse cDNA's corresponding to opsin and S-antigen, cloned as previously described[6,7], were labelled with P^{32} by the random primer method[8]. The probes were hybridized to the filters in 50% formamide containing 1.5X SSC (0.225 M NaCl, 0.023 M Na citrate) at 42°C for 19 hours. The filters were washed three times in 2X, 0.5X, and 0.1X SSC, 1% SDS, at 55°C for 20 minutes and exposed to Kodak XAR5 film with an intensifier screen at -70°C for various times. The bands were quantitated by densitometry using a Bio-Rad Model 620 Video Densitometer in conjunction with Bio-Rad software on an IBM AT.

RESULTS AND DISCUSSION

We, like others, have felt that a first step in elucidating the underlying mechanisms involved in the formation and preservation of the functional status of the visual cells is to identify proteins and/or mRNA's which are unique to photoreceptor cells. Antibodies specific for three soluble proteins - phosducin (33k), B-transducin (37k), S-antigen (arrestin or 48k) and one membrane protein, rhodopsin - were obtained and used to investigate the cellular localization of these proteins in the retinas of mice which were either light-adapted or dark-adapted[1]. The results from one such experiment are shown in Figure 1 and demonstrate that the immunocytochemical localization of the soluble proteins is transient and dependent on the lighting environment to which the animal is exposed.

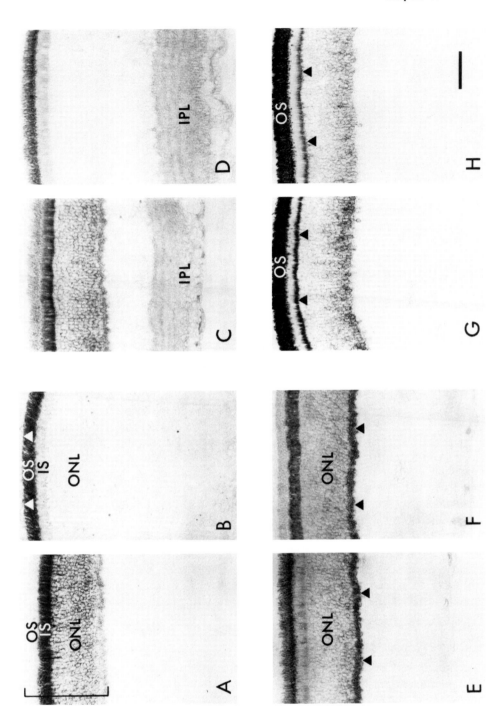

In light-adapted mice (A,C,E,G) phosducin (A) and beta transducin (C) were present mainly in the inner segments (IS) whereas 48k (E) was found almost exclusively in the rod outer segments (OS). When dark-adapted (B,D,F,H) animals were examined, the strongest stain for phosducin (B) and for beta-transducin (D) was found in the OS of the photoreceptors whereas the staining for 48k (F) had shifted to IS of these rod cells. The staining for the integral membrane protein rhodopsin does not shift with the lighting conditions (G and H, respectively).

The light-induced shift in immunocytochemical staining of these proteins may be due to (a) actual movement of the proteins between the IS and OS of the PR cell, (b) a "masking and unmasking" of antigenic sites on the proteins, or (c) a combination of both. Initial indirect evidence supporting intracellular protein movement was obtained by utilizing the rds (retinal degeneration slow) mouse mutant. The rds mutant mouse has PR cells that do not develop rod outer segments (Sanyal, et al[9]) but do have inner segments and detectable levels of proteins involved in the visual cascade (J. McGinnis, unpublished observations). We reasoned that if actual movement between IS and OS of the PR cell was occurring then the translocating proteins would have no OS into which they could shift in the rds mouse. As a result, we would expect immunocytochemical staining of the IS in both light and dark adapted animals. However, if the epitopes were being masked and unmasked, then the staining should appear and disappear in the IS of these mice in response to their exposure to light. We found that the IS of these mutant mice always stained positive for the presence of each of the proteins (33k, 37k and 48k) irrespective of their exposure to light (data not shown). These data suggest the mechanism for light-induced shifts in staining in the normal retina involves the actual movement of the proteins between the IS and OS.

To directly investigate the mechanism by which the shift in staining was occurring, the OS of the rod PR cells were isolated from light- and dark-adapted mice and their contents analyzed by Western transfer blots using a mixture of monospecific sera against S-antigen and beta transducin. The results (Figure #2) demonstrated that the OS isolated from light-adapted animals have a three-fold increase in 48 k protein as compared to OS from dark-adapted animals. Similarly, the data also show that the amount of beta transducin in the same light-adapted OS is about 2 times less than that found in dark-adapted retinas.

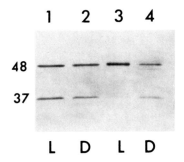

Figure 2. Western analysis of light (L) and dark (D)-adapted mouse retinal extracts. Samples of extracts isolated from whole retinas (5 micrograms) (lanes 1 and 2) or outer segments (3 micrograms) (lanes 3 and 4) were electrophoresed on an SDS polyacrylamide gel, transferred to nitrocellulose, and incubated with antisera that react with beta Transducin (37 kd) and S-antigen (48 kd). The bands were visualized by radiography and quantitated by densitometry. Reprinted with permission from Whelan & McGinnis, 1988; Copyright A. R. Liss, Inc.

These data are consistent with the shifts in staining shown in Figure 1 and demonstrate that beta Transducin and 48 kd are actually moving between the OS and the IS in response to light. The amounts of Tb and 48k in <u>total</u> retina preparations from light and dark-adapted animals were unchanged, suggesting that the differences in the Tb and 48k content of the OS were not due to changes in protein synthesis or degradation during light to dark shifts.

The intensity, duration and wavelength of the light which is required for this molecular movement has not yet been identified. Red light, which does not bleach rhodopsin, does not result in the light adapted response suggesting that rhodopsin is the light absorbing molecule which initiates this process. Developmentally, this mechanism is present as early as the staining can be detected and the outer segments are present. The <u>rd</u> mouse exhibits the ability to translocate these photoreceptor specific proteins up until the cells degenerate, suggesting that a defect in this process is not directly involved in the death of its rod cells (data not shown).

Time course studies were performed on eyes that were dissected from mice at various times after change from light to dark conditions. Figure 3 shows the results of such an analysis for anti-48 kd serum. As was shown in Figure 1F, 48 kd is localized to the IS after a two hour dark-adaptation (Fig. 3A). At 30 seconds after the animal is exposed to light (the shortest time tested), it is already apparent that relocalization of antigen is occurring (Fig. 3B). Accumulating 48 kd can be visualized at the proximal end of the OS, nearest to the connecting cilium. By two minutes after the animal has been exposed to light the staining has decreased markedly in the IS and the staining in the proximal end of the OS has increased (Fig. 3C). After ten minutes of light exposure, the immunoreactivity in the OS continues to increase and spread across the entire OS length while staining in the IS has been reduced to background levels (Fig. 3D). When examined after extended periods of light (Fig. 3E), the entire OS can be seen filled with reaction product.

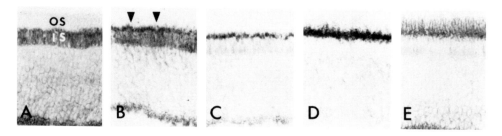

Figure 3. Time course analysis of 48 kd shifting in dark-adapted Balb/c mice moved into the light. In the dark-adapted animal, 48 kd is localized to the IS and the outer plexiform layer (A). Within thirty seconds after exposure to light (B), accumulating immunoreactivity can be seen in the proximal OS (arrowheads). At two minutes (C), staining in the IS has decreased to background levels and OS staining has increased. The anti-48 kd reaction product has begun to fill throughout the OS by 10 minutes of light exposure (D). When retinas from animals exposed to light for 240 minutes were examined, the reaction product was found throughout the OS (E). Magnification is × 490. Reprinted with permission from Whelan & McGinnis, 1988; Copyright A. R. Liss, Inc.

It is reasonable to expect that the directed movement of specific populations of protein molecules requires some mechanism which recognizes specific epitopes on the proteins. During transit from the inner to the outer segment, any site(s) that may be mechanistically involved might be masked or unmasked. Evidence in support of this was sought by observing the kinetics of movement of 48k during its transition from the rod inner segment to the outer segment using polyclonal and monoclonal antibodies which recognize discrete epitopes on 48k (data not shown). Except for differences in sensitivity, the monoclonal antibodies produced data indistinguishable from the polyclonal antisera suggesting that those specific epitopes were not masked during transit, at least during the time points tested.

We also observed that after a short period of time in the light, the inner segments again began to stain positive for 48k without any apparent diminution in the staining of the outer segments. This suggested that the new staining might reflect the presence of newly synthesized 48k which in turn might reflect an increase in the amount of specific mRNA for this protein. To test this, Northern and slot blot hybridization assays were developed to quantitate the amount of opsin and 48k mRNA's present in total RNA from mouse retinas. Data for the opsin mRNA assay are seen in Figure 4 and demonstrate that the signal (OD mm) is directly proportional to the amount of RNA applied. As an additional control, 1.0 ug of RNA from adult <u>rd</u> mice (photoreceptorless) did not produce a detectable signal under the same conditions. Therefore, the assay is linear and may be used to quantitate the amount of opsin mRNA present in each sample. Densitometric quantitation of Northern transfers gave essentially the same results as the slot blot assay. A similar slot blot assay was set up for 48k mRNA and essentially identical data obtained. Separate Nytran sheets were generated for use with opsin and 48k probes because stripping and reprobing the same sheet did not give quantitative data.

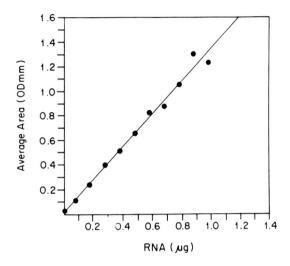

Figure 4. Linearity of slot blot hybridization assay for quantitating the amount of opsin mRNA present in total RNA from mouse eye, minus the lens. The densitometry signal (ODmm) is plotted vs the total micrograms of RNA applied to each slot.

To determine if there are any differences in the amounts of specific mRNA's for mouse opsin and 48k in light- and dark-adapted animals, mice were sacrificed at hourly intervals during the normal light-dark cycle to which they are routinely exposed and the mRNA's quantitated. Results from such an experiment are plotted in Figure 5 and indicate that 48k and opsin mRNA's both change in a cyclic manner during the light/dark cycle and that these changes are not coordinated. Opsin mRNA shows a 3-5 fold change with a sharp rise occurring during the middle of the dark cycle and a slower decline shortly after the lights come on. However, 48k mRNA changes by 5-8 fold with an increase shortly after the lights are turned on and a symmetrical decrease during the dark cycle. Northern analysis of the mRNA's present at selected times (maximas and minimas) showed no qualitative changes in either opsin or 48k mRNA's. Whenever the animals were in the dark, 48k was in the outer segments and 37k was in the inner segments. In the light the positions reversed.

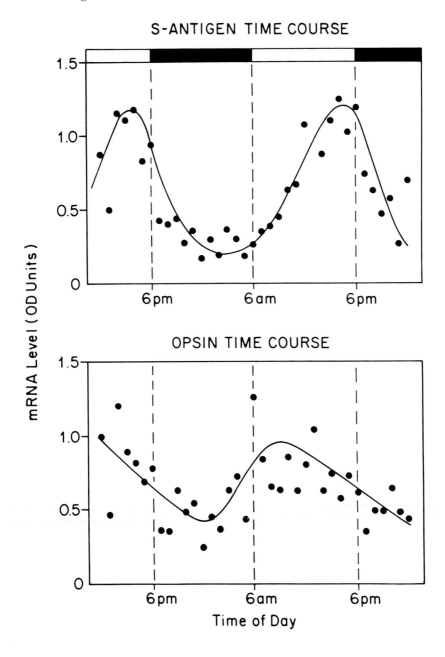

Figure 5. Cyclic, noncoordinated changes in the amounts of mRNA's for mouse opsin and S-antigen during the normal light dark cycles. Mice were sacrificed every hour for each of 36 hours and the amount of mRNA present at each time point was determined by slot blot hybridization assays using mouse cDNA's for opsin and S-antigen. See text for discussion.

To increase the amount of a mRNA, either the rate of synthesis must increase or the rate of degradation must decrease or a combination of both must occur. By analyzing the kinetics of the changes in the amounts of mRNA, it is possible to distinguish among these alternative mechanisms. The amount of mRNA present at any new steady state level is determined by the ratio of its rate of synthesis to its rate of degradation. However, the time course of approach from one steady state to a new steady state is determined solely by the rate of degradation.[10,11] Therefore, from the data for 48k in Figure 3, the fold change in mRNA may be calculated and the log of this value plotted for each time (t) against time t.

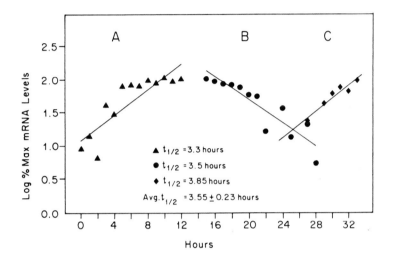

Figure 6. Kinetic analysis of the time course of change in the amount of S-antigen mRNA from one steady state level to another during the light/dark cycle. Data are from Figure 5 and are plotted as describe in the text. The lines are computer generated by linear regression analysis of the plotted points and indicate that the rate constant for degradation (the slope) of S-Antigen mRNA is essentially the same irrespective of whether the amount of mRNA is increasing or decreasing. Therefore, the quantitative changes observed in the amount of S-antigen mRNA are due to changes in the transcriptional activity of the gene for S-antigen with little or no changes in the rate of degradation of the mRNA.

From this data, the slope of the line is the rate constant of degradation and the half life of the mRNA can be determined. The results of such an analysis are shown in Figure 6 and demonstrate that the half life of the 48K mRNA is the same, about 3.5 hours, irrespective of whether the amount of mRNA is decreasing when the lights go off or increasing when the lights come on. Therefore, the changes in the amounts of S-antigen mRNA are due to changes in the transcriptional activity of its gene with no detectable changes in the stability of its mRNA. The changes in opsin mRNA are more complex and appear to be due to a combination of changes in both the rates of synthesis and degradation. A diagrammatic summary of our data, and that of others, concerning the differences observed in the mammalian retina during the light/dark cycle is presented in Figure 7.

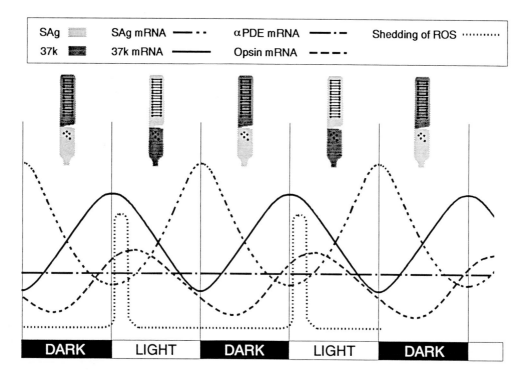

Figure 7. Schematic model representing the temporal changes during the light/dark cycle in: A) The subcellular localization of photoreceptor-specific proteins; B) The concentration of their specific mRNA's; and C) The shedding of the tips of the rod outer segments.

The light-dependent subcellular locations of 48k and beta-transducin are indicated within the drawings depicting the IS and the OS of the rod cells. During the light cycle S-antigen is in the OS and B-transducin is in the IS. Their positions rapidly reverse during the dark cycle. Alpha-transducin has been shown to move in the same direction as beta transducin.[12] These positional changes result in very large shifts in the subcellular concentration of these photoreceptor specific proteins and we think these translocations are functionally related to the mechanism of phototransduction.

When examined shortly after shifting from dark to light, reaction product is found closely associated with the proximal end of the OS, close to the connecting cilium (Fig. 3B). Even after extended periods of light, the strongest staining for 48 kd is still found in this region (Fig. 3E). The localization of phototransduction proteins to this region would agree with the demonstration that the majority of photoactivation (as measured by rhodopsin bleaching) is localized to the basal or proximal end of the outer segment during short light flashes.[13]

During the dark cycle the amount of opsin mRNA begins to increase until shortly after the lights come on, at which time, it decreases at a slower rate until the middle of the next dark cycle when it again increases. In contrast, S-antigen mRNA begins to increase as soon as the lights come on and continues until the lights go off. This cycle is repeated but unlike that for opsin mRNA, it is very symmetrical.

Because transducin moves, and in a direction opposite to 48k, our model predicts that the level of its mRNA would vary in a cyclic manner similar to that of 48k but out of phase by 12 hours. Therefore, when the lights go off and transducin moves to the outer segment, our model would predict that the transcriptional activity of its gene will increase until the lights come on and then subsequently decrease, coincident with transducin moving to the inner segment. The genes for other photoreceptor specific proteins which do not move may show cyclic variations in activity like the rhodopsin gene or they may simply remain at some developmentally determined steady state level. Monospecific antibodies against 23k, another photoreceptor specific protein,[6] demonstrate that it does not move in response to light/dark changes (Stepanik & McGinnis, unpublished observation). Analysis of its mRNA with a cDNA probe (Lerious & McGinnis, unpublished observation) shows no cyclic changes. The enzyme, cGMP PDE, has been reported not to move,[14] and the activity of its gene might also be constant as suggested in Figure 7.

The tips of the rod outer segments are shed synchronously when the lights come on in the morning.[15] This is indicated graphically in Figure 7. The 3-5 fold increase in the amount of rhodopsin mRNA preceding the shedding of the tips suggests that the cell is anticipating the shedding and has made new rhodopsin molecules for insertion into the newly synthesized discs at the base of the rod outer segment. Because the tips are shed in the light, they also contain 48k. Thus when 48k moves from the inner segment to the outer segment, the photoreceptor cell begins to make more 48k mRNA resulting in an increase in the total cellular content of 48k and renewed transient staining of the inner segment.

The absorption of a photon of light by rhodopsin results initially in the activation of alpha transducin molecules which in turn activate cyclic GMP phosphodiesterase molecules which catalyze the hydrolysis of cGMP resulting in the closure of the ion channels. This cycle continues, with signal amplifications of 10 to 100 fold at each step, until the cycle is broken when 48k binds to the activated rhodopsin and prevents it from further activating alpha-transducin. The light-dependent positional changes in these photoreceptor specific proteins are consistent with the increased utilization of the rods in dim light or darkness and decreased use in the light. In the dark, 48k is in the inner segment, transducin is in outer segment and the visual cycle remains active even with low levels of activated rhodopsin. In the light when rods are less active, 48k is in the outer segments, alpha- & beta-transducin are in the inner segments and the visual cycle in the rods is inhibited.

We have demonstrated that the movement of these photoreceptor specific proteins is light-dependent and not circadian. Our data are in agreement with that of Brann and Cohen[12] who showed the movement of alpha transducin to be in the same direction as we have found for beta transducin. However, they concluded that the movement was diurnal rather than light-dependent. Broekhuyse et al[16] demonstrated a light dependent shift of 48k as did Philip et al[14] in support of the directional shifts that we have found for 48 k and transducin. We have not determined the molecular mechanism(s) by which this movement occurs, but it may be similar to the actin- or microtubule-dependent, directed movement of proteins which occurs in axonal transport in other neuronal cell populations in the central nervous system.[16]

Similar cyclic changes in the retinal mRNAs have been observed by Bowes et al [17] during the light/dark cycle. In fish and toads, Korenblot & Fernald [19] have recently observed cyclic changes in opsin mRNA which were shown to be regulated by both circadian rhythm and light. We have demonstrated that the cyclic changes in the levels of mRNA for S-antigen are due to actual changes in the transcript-ional activity of its gene and suggest that the changes in mRNA levels for the other photoreceptor specific proteins are also due to effects on gene activity. These cyclic changes are initiated either by light, an internal circadian clock, or a combination of both. Experiments are currently underway to distinguish among these alternatives and to identify and characterize the molecular events associated with these changes and to correlate them with photoreceptor renewal and the phototransduction process of vision. Further, it remains to be shown if defects in these mechanisms may play a role in some forms of human diseases which result in blindness, whether inherited (such as retinitis pigmentosa), or the result of retinal light damage, or as occurs with the age related changes associated with macular degeneration.

ACKNOWLEDGEMENTS

We thank John Triantafyllos and Hratch Demerjian for their technical contributions to some of this work, Dale Gregerson for antibodies to opsin and S-antigen, and Rehwa Lee for antibodies to B-transducin and phosducin. Supported in part by funds from USPHS EY06030, EY06085 and EY06639.

REFERENCES

1.   Whelan JP, and McGinnis JF. Light-dependent subcellular movement of photoreceptor proteins. J. Neurosci. Res. 20: 263, 1988.

2.   Chomczynski, P and Sacchi, N. Single step method of RNA isolation by acid guanidinium thiocyanate- phenol-chloriform extraction. Anal. Biochem. 162, 156 1987.

3.   Baehr, W., J.T. Triantafyllos, D. Falk, K. Bugra, and J. F. McGinnis. Isolation and molecular analysis of the mouse opsin gene. FEBS Letters. 238, 253, 1988.

4.   Al-Abaidi, MR, Pittler, SJ, Champagne, NS, Triantafyllos, JT, McGinnis, JF & Baehr, W. Mouse opsin: Gene structure and molecular basis of multiple transcripts. J. Biol Chem. <u>265</u>, In Press, 1990.

5.   Thomas, PT. Hybridization of denatured RNA transferred or dotted to nitrocellulose paper. <u>Methods in Enzymology</u> <u>100</u>, 255, 1983.

6.   McGinnis, JF & Leveille, PJ. A biomolecular approach to the study of the expression of specific genes of the retina.   J. Neuroscience Research <u>16</u>, 157-165, 1986.

7.   Tsuda, MS, K. Bugra, J.P. Whelan, J.F. McGinnis and T. Shinohara. Cloning and sequence analysis of mouse retina S-antigen cDNA. Gene <u>73</u>: 11, 1988.

8.   Feinberg, AP, & Volelstein, B. A technique for radiolabeling DNA restriction endonuclease fragments to high specific activity.   Anal. Biochem. <u>132</u>, 6, 1983.

9.   Sanyal,S, De Ruiter A, Hawkins RK. Development and degeneration of retina in <u>rds</u> mutant mice: Light microscopy. J. Comp. Neurol. <u>194</u>, 193, 1980.

10. Berlin, CM, and Schimke, RT. Enzyme synthesis and degradation in animal tissues. Mol Pharmacol. <u>1</u>, 149, 1965.

11. Almagor, H., and Paigen, K. Chemical kinetics of induced gene expression: Activation of transcription by noncooperative binding of multiple regulatory molecules. Biochem. <u>27</u>, 2094, 1988.

12. Brann MR and Cohen LV. Diurnal expression of transducin mRNA and translocation of transducin in rods of rat retina. Science <u>235</u>: 585, 1987.

13. Makino CL, Howard LN, and Williams TP, Intracellular topography of rhodopsin bleaching. Science <u>238</u>: 1716, 1987.

14. Philip NJ, Chang W, and Long K. Light-stimulated movement in rod photoreceptor cells of the rat retina. FEBS <u>225</u>: 127, 1987.

15. LaVail, MM. Circadian nature of rod outer segment disc shedding in the rat. Inv. Ophth. Vis Sci. <u>19</u>: 407, 1980.

16. Broekhuyse RM, Tolhuizen EFJ, Janssen APM, and Wilkens HJ. Light-induced shift and binding of S-antigen in retinal rods. Current Eye Res. <u>4</u>: 613, 1985.

17.   Vale RD. Intracellular transport using microtubule-based motors. Ann. Rev. Cell Biol. 3: 347, 1987.

18.   Bowes, C, vanVeen, T, and Farber, DB. Opsin, G-protein and 48kDa protein in normal and rd mouse retinas: Developmental expression of mRNA's and proteins and light/dark cycling of mRNA's. Exp. Eye Res. 47, 369, 1988.

19.   Korenblot, JI, and Fernald, RD, Circadian rythm and light regulate opsin mRNA in rod photoreceptors. Nature 337, 454, 1989.

SPECULATIONS ON THE MOLECULAR BASIS OF
RETINAL DEGENERATION IN RETINITIS PIGMENTOSA

Paul A. Hargrave* and Paul J. O'Brien[‡]

*Department of Ophthalmology and Department of
Biochemistry and Molecular Biology,
University of Florida
Gainesville, Florida 32610
[†]Health Research Associates, Rockville, Maryland 20850

This work is supported in part by grants EY 06225 and EY 06226 from the National Eye Institute of the National Institutes of Health, and by an unrestricted departmental grant from Research to Prevent Blindness, Inc. P.A.H. is Francis N. Bullard Professor of Ophthalmology.

ABSTRACT

Mutations in the human rhodopsin gene have been reported to be the cause of some cases of autosomal dominant retinitis pigmentosa. From our current knowledge of rhodopsin structure and function relationships and with the aid of studies on animal models of retinal degeneration, we speculate on the molecular basis of the disease process. It is proposed that the reported mutations in rhodopsin may lead to a protein of altered structure that is incapable of normal folding, glycosylation and binding of retinal and is incapable of transport from the endoplasmic reticulum and expression of normal receptor function.

INTRODUCTION

Retinitis pigmentosa is a group of diseases characterized by night blindness and loss of midperipheral visual field. Progression of the disease may result in complete loss of photoreceptor cells in the retina. Retinitis pigmentosa is genetically heterogeneous and is caused by mutant alleles at a variety of loci within the human genome. Its incidence in the United States is 1 in 3,500 births, of which in Maine 43% of cases are autosomal dominant, with the remainder being autosomal recessive, X-linked, and isolated cases of undetermined origin.[1] Recently one form of autosomal dominant retinitis pigmentosa has been shown to be linked to point mutations in the rhodopsin gene.[1-3] It is not immediately clear how such a mutation might be responsible for the clinical picture observed to occur in this disease. In this article we consider in outline some things that are known about the biosynthesis, structure, function and turnover of rhodopsin and suggest how failures of various elements in these processes might lead to photoreceptor cell malfunction and death seen in retinal degenerative disease.

DISCUSSION

THERE ARE MANY STEPS IN WHICH MISTAKES COULD OCCUR IN THE SYNTHESIS AND
TRANSPORT OF RHODOPSIN

DNA in the rod cell nucleus encodes the primary structure of the
protein rhodopsin (Figure 1).   RNA for the protein sequence is transcribed and processed there and makes its way to the endoplasmic
reticulum.   There it is translated on membrane-bound ribosomes to
produce the nascent opsin polypeptide.   We envision that during this
translational process the opsin becomes acetylated at its amino-
terminus, glycosylated on two of its amino-terminal asparagine
residues, and folds appropriately so that it is inserted into the
membrane and forms the correct transmembrane elements.   During this
process a stabilizing disulfide bridge is formed between cysteines 110
and 187,[4] and the opsin three dimensional structure is produced that
will allow binding of 11-<u>cis</u> retinal and the formation of functionally
active rhodopsin.

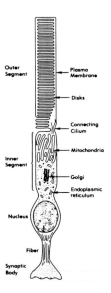

Figure 1.   Diagrammatic representation of a vertebrate photoreceptor.
This highly differentiated cell consists of outer and inner segments,
nucleus and synaptic body.   Rhodopsin molecules are synthesized in the
rough endoplasmic reticulum and transported through the cisternae of
the Golgi complex.   Transport vesicles then carry rhodopsin past the
packed mitochondria in the inner segment apex to the base of the
connecting cilium where they fuse with the plasma membrane.   Rhodopsin
is then transported by a poorly-understood mechanism to the point of
evagination of new plasma membrane folds at the base of the outer
segment.   These basal folds seal to form isolated discs enclosed within
the plasma membrane.   Ultimately, the oldest discs are shed as a packet
with plasma membrane at the tip of the outer segment.   The packet is
phagocytized by the pigment epithelial cell and digested by lysosomal
enzymes.

In order for a protein to proceed from the site of its synthesis on the endoplasmic reticulum (ER), a number of recognition and sorting events must take place. These events involve some recognition processes that are well known, such as signal sequences, and many that are not well understood at all. Immediately upon synthesis the opsin polypeptide must be inserted into the membrane of the ER. This is a process that, for many proteins, requires that the protein not be tightly folded. In some situations there are ATP-dependent "unfoldases", possibly heat-shock-like proteins, that maintain the nascent polypeptide in an unfolded state. In others there are proteins associated with ribosomes, known as "trigger factors", that appear to form 1:1 complexes cotranslationally with the nascent polypeptide. In some cases signal recognition particles, a complex of RNA and proteins, bind the nascent polypeptide as it is being elaborated and deliver it to the ER docking protein, permitting the signal sequence to interact with the signal sequence receptor. Regardless of the mechanism, the conformation of a nascent protein is critical for its delivery to the proper membrane.[5] Failure of a protein to acquire the appropriate conformation or insertion signal will cause it to accumulate at the site of synthesis.[6]

Almost immediately after the N-terminus of rhodopsin enters the lumen of the ER, two asparagine residues are glycosylated with a large oligosaccharide with the composition of $Glc_3Man_9GlcNAc_2$.[7] As the rhodopsin is completed and passes from the ER to the transitional elements, the three glucose (Glc) residues and one or two mannose (Man) residues are removed by specific enzymes. As transport continues, membrane vesicles containing rhodopsin bud from the transitional elements of the ER and fuse with the cis cisternae of the Golgi apparatus where another mannosidase removes up to three more mannose residues. The rhodopsin then proceeds to the medial Golgi cisternae by another vesicle budding and fusion. Here a transferase adds an N-acetylglucosamine (GlcNAc) and another mannosidase may remove one or two mannose residues. Another vesicle-mediated step sends the rhodopsin to the trans-Golgi cisternae where a transferase adds a galactose residue to some of the rhodopsin molecules.[8] Finally, after passing into the trans-Golgi network, rhodopsin is transported in vesicles to the base of the connecting cilium which, in frogs, is seen as the periciliary ridge complex.[9,10] The transport of proteins from the ER through the Golgi may be a bulk flow process down a pH gradient that represents a default pathway to send proteins to the cell surface. Nevertheless, each one of these specific enzyme-catalyzed reactions[7] could be influenced by an amino acid substitution.

A MUTANT RHODOPSIN MIGHT NOT INTERACT PROPERLY WITH THE SORTING MECHANISMS RESPONSIBLE FOR THE FORMATION OF DISC MEMBRANES.

Transport of rhodopsin from the periciliary ridge complex at the base of the connecting cilium to the plasma membrane of the rod outer segment (ROS) is poorly understood. What is impressive, however, is the sorting mechanism that allows discs to be formed from the plasma membrane resulting in two entirely different membranes, from the standpoint of protein composition.[11] This sorting mechanism probably involves cytoskeletal elements to which certain proteins are selectively bound. This can be inferred from the work of Vaughan and Fisher

(1989),[12] in which exposure of a rabbit retina to cytochalasin B, which inhibits actin functions, resulted in abnormal, overgrown basal ROS discs.   Once again, a mutation in rhodopsin could markedly influence its ability to bind to another protein at this step in the sorting process.   A genetic defect in the minor disc protein peripherin leads to cell death in the rds mutant mouse.[13]   This could also occur with a rhodopsin mutation.

MUTATIONS IN THE RHODOPSIN GENE MAY AFFECT RHODOPSIN'S ABILITY TO FORM A FUNCTIONAL PHOTORECEPTOR PROTEIN.

The first report of a point mutation in human rhodopsin linked to retinitis pigmentosa showed the change of proline 23 to histidine to be responsible for the phenotype.   At the present time, 17 unrelated patients have been shown to bear this mutation;[1,2]   Two additional sites of mutation have been reported; proline 347 to leucine or serine (10 patients), threonine 58 to arginine (1 patient; Figure 2),[3] and omission of isoleucine 255/256.[14]   The result of these mutations is progressive disease; photoreceptor cell deaths occur over a period of years.   One must conclude that if the defect in rhodopsin is the basic defect responsible for the disease symptoms, then we must seek to explain the disease processes as results emanating from the alterations in rhodopsin structure and function.

Other visual pigment gene defects lead to loss of visual function. The various human color vision deficiencies result from alterations in the genes for the red, green and blue visual pigment genes.[15]   These include gene deletions, gene fusions, and mutation in the regulatory elements controlling expression of these genes.   In one case of red cone visual pigment gene deficiency, a point mutation of cysteine 187 to arginine has been shown to be responsible.[16]   This mutation would make formation of the disulfide bridge impossible and lead to a protein of reduced structural stability.

Several of the ninaE _Drosophila_ mutants selected for visual deficiency have been shown to have mutations in their rhodopsin gene.[17] These defects have been shown to result from changes in the rhodopsin sequence of proline 120 to leucine (ninaE^{P318}), glycine 128 to arginine (ninaE^{332}) and tryptophan 289 to arginine (ninaE^{P334}) (Figure 2).   One suspects that in all of the above cases, the visual defect stems directly from a functional defect in rhodopsin.

HUMAN RHODOPSIN MUTANT PROLINE 23 TO HISTIDINE MUST BE FUNCTIONALLY IMPAIRED.

How does the mutation of human rhodopsin proline 23 in retinitis pigmentosa lead to photoreceptor cell degeneration?   Proline is structurally different from the other amino acids found in proteins; its α-amino group forms part of its cyclic side chain.   It can adopt a cis or trans configuration but cannot assume all the usual angles of rotation.   Proline is frequently found in bends and turns in proteins. In spite of the great diversity of amino-terminal sequences in opsins and in other G-protein-linked receptors, proline is frequently found in this part of the sequence.[2]   This suggests a structural role for proline 23 in rhodopsin and related receptors.   At the time of writing, the rhodopsin Pro 23-His mutant protein has not been expressed or its

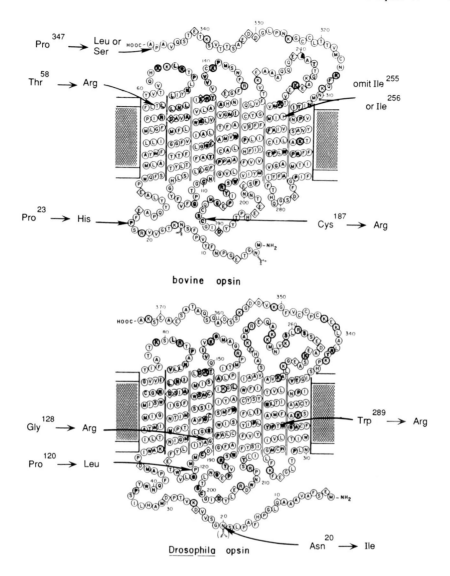

bovine opsin

Drosophila opsin

Figure 2. Sites of mutations in vertebrate and invertebrate opsins. Topographic models are shown for bovine opsin (which will be identical to that for human opsin) and <u>Drosophila</u> opsin (reproduced from ref. 17). Mutations in human opsin that result in retinitis pigmentosa are Pro[23]→His (refs. 1,2), Thr[58]→Arg (ref. 3), Pro[347]→Leu or Ser (ref. 3), and omission of Ile[225] or Ile[256] (ref. 14). Mutation of Cys[187]→Arg in the red cone visual pigment leads to loss of red cone visual function.[15] Mutations in <u>Drosophila</u> visual pigment that lead to photoreceptor cell degeneration include Pro[120]→Leu,Gly[128]→Arg,Trp[289]→Arg (ref. 18), and Asn[20]→Ile (ref. 19).

properties studied. However, <u>deletion mutants</u> of bovine rhodopsin have been prepared whose properties shed light on the role of this amino acid. Four deletion mutants in rhodopsin's amino terminal region are defective and all share similar defects.[20] Deletions were made of residues 7-10, 11-14, 18-20 or 21-29. The resultant mutant rhodopsin bound retinal only 10 to 20% that of wild type, was abnormally glycosylated, and had essentially lost its ability to activate transducin. Upon SDS gel electrophoresis there was an enhanced tendency to aggregate compared to wild type rhodopsin. This suggests that these alterations to the amino terminus of the protein lead to an opsin that does not glycosylate and fold properly, aggregates and is unable to proceed through the endoplasmic reticulum and Golgi vesicles properly and serve as an effective substrate for glycosyltransferases. Few of these opsin molecules appear to form the correct conformation that allows them to bind retinal to form a functionally competent rhodopsin. For those molecules that do bind retinal and respond to light, the metarhodopsin subsequently formed would probably be insufficiently stable to activate transducin.

MUTATIONS IN RHODOPSIN'S TRANSMEMBRANE SEGMENTS MAY DISRUPT PROTEIN PACKING.

Substitution of arginine for threonine 58 (Thr-58-Arg) has been reported to result from a gene defect responsible for retinitis pigmentosa.[3] Such a substitution would result in the sterically small uncharged amino acid side chain of threonine being replaced by the large positively-charged amino acid side chain of arginine. Position 58 in rhodopsin is located in the first transmembrane segment of the polypeptide chain (Figure 2), and is predicted to be located on the helix surface facing the interior of the protein.[21] Here it would be involved in specific interactions with other amino acid side chains and the substitution of a large charged amino acid side chain would be structurally disruptive. Such an altered protein could be unable to fold properly and bind retinal and would be unlikely to leave the endoplasmic reticulum.

Affected members of a family with autosomal dominant retinitis pigmentosa have been identified in which rhodopsin's isoleucine 255 (or 256) is omitted.[14] The site of this mutation, eliminating one of two sequential isoleucine residues, occurs within transmembrane helix 6 of the rhodopsin molecule (Figure 1). The effect of truncating this sequence $Val^{254}Ile^{255}Ile^{256}Met^{257}Val^{258}$ to $Val^{254}Ile^{255}Met^{256}Val^{257}$ will have the effect of replacing each of the following 20 amino acids in helix 6 with a different amino acid! This single amino acid omission is therefore equivalent to 20 sequential mutations. Tryptophan 265's bulky side chain would occupy the site for cysteine 264; proline 267, which introduces a 20° "kink" in the helix, would occupy the site of valine 266, and would be displaced vertically and shifted 100° with respect to its proper place in the helix. This will drastically disrupt the intricate side-chain packing so important in stabilizing the protein core structure. There is little doubt that such a protein would be unable to form a stable 7-helical bundle and bind retinal and would be unable to proceed from the endoplasmic reticulum.

HOW DOES A MUTATION IN RHODOPSIN'S CARBOXYL-TERMINUS RESULT IN RETINITIS PIGMENTOSA?

Rhodopsin's carboxyl-terminal amino acid is alanine-348. Mutations of the adjacent proline-347 to serine or leucine have been identified in autosomal dominant retinitis pigmentosa.[3] Proline-347 is invariant in each of the dozen vertebrate rhodopsins for which sequence information is available. Yet it is not immediately obvious how this amino acid in this penultimate position might be functionally important. It is difficult to imagine that a mutation in this near terminal position would impair rhodopsin's structural stability.

The carboxyl-terminal sequence of rhodopsin is a highly-accessible part of the molecule. The bond Gln^{344}-Val^{345} is exquisitely sensitive to proteolysis,[22] and Gln^{344} is easily modified by the high-molecular-weight enzyme transglutaminase.[23] Rhodopsin's carboxyl-terminal region is also readily accessible for antibody binding.[24] Rhodopsin kinase binds to photoactivated rhodopsin and phosphorylates serines and threonines in the adjacent sequence 334-343. In studies with model peptide substrates, rhodopsin kinase is able to phosphorylate peptides lacking Pro^{347} equally as well as those that contain it, thus suggesting that Pro^{347} is not important in the phosphorylation reaction. It could, however, be important in the binding of rhodopsin kinase to photoactivated rhodopsin. This is a critical first step preceding the phosphorylation reaction, and rhodopsin's carboxyl-terminal peptide 337-348 represents part of the binding site for rhodopsin kinase.[25]

It is intriguing to consider the possibility that the carboxyl-terminal sequence of rhodopsin contains information important for the vectorial transport of rhodopsin to its location in the outer segment. Some mechanisms must exist to assure rhodopsin's vectorial transport and it is reasonable to assume that this information is encoded in the protein structure.

There is precedent for such an argument. Amino-terminal hydrophobic signal sequences code for membrane insertion, and a carboxyl-terminal tetrapeptide sequence has been identified with retention of proteins within the endoplasmic reticulum. Proteins carrying the LysAspGluLeu sequence (KDEL in single letter code) at their carboxyl terminus are returned from post-Golgi compartments to the endoplasmic reticulum.[26] This KDEL sequence cannot be mutated or shifted from the carboxyl-terminus or the protein carrying this alteration will be secreted. Normally secreted proteins are retained in the endoplasmic reticulum or their secretion is greatly retarded when they carry the KDEL sequence.

Most vertebrate opsins carry a ValAlaProAla carboxyl-terminal sequence, and all vertebrate opsins to date have the Val and the Pro invariant. It is possible that the structural motif ValXxxProXxx is required at rhodopsin's carboxyl terminus in order for it to proceed normally from the endoplasmic reticulum to its cellular destination. The hypothesis that this region of the sequence is important in rhodopsin cellular transport could be tested by the use of site-specific mutants.

PROLINE CIS-TRANS ISOMERISM MAY AFFECT RHODOPSIN'S ABILITY TO FOLD
PROPERLY.

One can imagine cases in which a normal gene for rhodopsin is
present, but failure of another gene to function properly prevents the
functioning of rhodopsin. Such a situation exists with the ninaA
mutants in Drosophila. Flies mutant for the ninaA locus have a 10-
fold reduction in the levels of rhodopsin in their R1 to R6 photoreceptor cells. However, mutant flies have normal levels of expression of
the photoreceptor gene.[27] This suggests that some posttranslational
process may be defective. The ninaA gene has been found to encode a
protein homologous with the known protein, cyclophilin, that has been
shown to have a prolyl cis-trans isomerase activity.[28] This isomerase
activity may be necessary to achieve the proper folding of rhodopsin
and the absence of the isomerase could lead to an abnormally low level
of the properly folded and functionally active rhodopsin.

BINDING OF RETINAL MAY BE IMPORTANT FOR RHODOPSIN TRANSPORT.

Newly synthesized opsin accumulates in the rough ER of isolated
rat retinas incubated in the absence of any source of retinal.[29] In
contrast, when [^{3}H]-retinal was provided in the intact eye by intravitreal injection, the new opsin molecules acquired a retinal
chromophore while in the rough ER[30] and were rapidly translocated to
the rod outer segment.[31] The pigment epithelium provided retinal in
the latter two studies. It is not difficult to imagine that amino acid
substitution in the opsin polypeptide could modify its ability to form
a Schiff base with retinal, a process known to induce a conformational
change in the protein. Should this conformational change be essential
for a recognition event in intracellular transport, a reduction or
cessation of transport could occur. In the miniature poodle affected
with progressive rod-cone degeneration, there is a documented reduction
in intracellular transport of rhodopsin,[32] resulting in a reduced rate
of outer segment renewal.[33] Although the disorder appears to involve a
defect in polyunsaturated fatty acid metabolism,[34] a point mutation in
rhodopsin is not ruled out.

A RHODOPSIN MUTATION COULD COMPROMISE ITS INTERACTION WITH POST-
TRANSLATIONAL PROCESSING ENZYMES.

Many enzymes act sequentially on rhodopsin to produce its final
complement of oligosaccharides. Fliesler and Basinger (1985)[35] and
Fliesler, Rayborn and Hollyfield (1986)[36] have shown that tunicamycin
prevents addition of rhodopsin's oligosaccharides. This unglycosylated
rhodopsin can still be transported to the disc forming region but
normal disc membranes are not formed. Thus rhodopsin's oligosaccharides may be required for normal disc membrane morphogenesis.
[Although it is possible that other glycoproteins, such as peripherin[13]
could be responsible for disc morphogenesis.] When rhodopsin does not
become glycosylated there is progressive shortening of the outer
segments due to lack of outer segment membrane assembly which leads
eventually to photoreceptor cell death.[37] Since various amino acid
substitutions and deletions have been experimentally shown to result in
abnormal glycosylation of rhodopsin,[20] certain rhodopsin mutations
could clearly be implicated in photoreceptor cell degeneration.

Site-specific mutagenesis of <u>Drosophila</u> rhodopsin provides direct evidence for the importance of the glycosylation site. A germline transformed <u>Drosophila</u> mutant has been created in which the glycosylation site Asn[20] has been replaced with an isoleucine.[19] Extremely low opsin levels are detected in photoreceptors of this mutant. Rhabdomere organization is aberrant and undergoes age-dependent deterioration. Thus the Asn[20], and probably its glycosylation, plays a critical role in rhodopsin maturation and rhabdomere integrity.

WHY SHOULD A MUTATION IN THE RHODOPSIN GENE LEAD TO ROD CELL DEATH OBSERVED IN RETINITIS PIGMENTOSA?

We have considered a number of mutations and experimental systems in which alterations in rhodopsin structure lead to accumulation of rhodopsin in inner segment membranes or in the failure to form disc membranes. The rhodopsin mutations that have been found responsible for retinitis pigmentosa have been in patients with the autosomal dominant form of RP; i.e., the patient is heterozygous for the defective rhodopsin gene, carrying one copy of the authentic rhodopsin gene and one copy of the mutant gene for rhodopsin. In this case, normal and defective rhodopsin molecules could be produced in the rod cell endoplasmic reticulum in equal numbers of copies if the mutation does not affect translation rates or assembly. The normal rhodopsin molecules would proceed through the stages of the biosynthesis and intracellular transport normally, whereas the mutant rhodopsin molecules might be unable to proceed satisfactorily. They might fail to move from the endoplasmic reticulum to the Golgi apparatus. Evidence for this has been obtained by expression in COS cells of the gene for a rhodopsin with a deletion in the IV-V loop.[20] This mutant rhodopsin accumulates in the endoplasmic reticulum, failing to reach the plasma membrane in the manner of the wild type protein. A similar observation has been made for the <u>Drosophila</u> ninaA mutant, where rhodopsin is found in the endoplasmic reticulum but not in the rhabdom.[38] Such accumulation of protein must interfere with the normal processes of the rod cell and strain its ability to carry on its normal biosynthetic activities and continue to direct proteins efficiently to their destined location. Cellular energy in the form of ATP is expended to nonproductive purposes and a variety of basic cellular functions are undoubtedly compromised. The rate of renewal of outer segment components will be decreased due to the reduced amount of functional rhodopsin that is produced. This places the cellular components at greater risk to damage by oxidative processes. If cell membrane integrity were compromised by lowered availability of ATP to maintain ion gradients, or lipid peroxidation which led to increased membrane permeability, cell death could result. One can imagine that the environment and exposure to stress by individual cells may be different. This could be responsible in part for individual cellular variation in different parts of a retina and in different individuals with the same genetic trait.

CONCLUSION

There are numerous points in the synthesis, modification and transport of rhodopsin and in its physiological actions where an amino acid substitution or deletion could result in significant impairment of rhodopsin function and of normal cellular processes. Cumulatively these malfunctions could result in cell death. On the bright side, introduction of selected mutations into transgenic animals could mimic inherited diseases and produce model systems for the study of therapeutic approaches. Because of the high degree of differentiation of the photoreceptor, such transgenic models could yield profound insights into some of the more challenging cell biological questions surrounding intracellular transport, protein sorting and membrane biogenesis.

REFERENCES

1. Berson, E. L., Ocular findings in a form of retinitis pigmentosa with a rhodopsin gene defect, Trans. Am. Ophth. Soc., in press, 1990.
2. Dryja, T. P., McGee, T. L., Reichel, E., Hahn, L. B., Cowley, G. S., Yandell, D. W., Sandberg, M. A. and Berson, E. L., A point mutation of the rhodopsin gene in one form of retinitis pigmentosa, Nature, 343, 364, 1990.
3. Dryja, T. P., McGee, T. L., Hahn, L. B. Cowley, G. S., Olsson, J. E., Reichel, E., Sandberg, M. A. and Berson, E. L., Mutations within the rhodopsin gene in patients with autosomal dominant retinitis pigmentosa, N. Eng. J. Med., 323, 1302, 1990.
4. Karnik, S. S. and Khorana, H. G., Assembly of functional rhodopsin requires a disulfide bond between cysteine residues 110 and 187, J. Biol. Chem., 265, 17520, 1990.
5. Sabatini, D. D. and Adesnik, M. B., The biogenesis of membranes and organelles, in The Metabolic Basis of Inherited Disease, Vol. 1, 6th ed., Scrivner, C. R., Baudet, A. L., Sly, W. S., and Valle, D., Eds., McGraw-Hill, New York, 1989. 177.
6. Rose, J. K. and Doms, R. W., Regulation of protein export from the endoplasmic reticulum, Ann. Rev. Cell. Biol., 4, 257, 1988.
7. Kornfeld, R. and Kornfeld, S., Assembly of asparagine-linked oligosaccharides, Ann. Rev. Biochem., 54, 631, 1985.
8. Smith, S. B., St. Jules, R. S. and O'Brien, P. J., Transient hyperglycosylation of rhodopsin with galactose, Exp. Eye Res., submitted, 1990.
9. Papermaster, D. S., Schneider, B. G., and Besharse, J. C., Vesicular transport of newly synthesized opsin from the Golgi apparatus toward the rod outer segment, Invest. Ophthalmol. Vis. Sci., 26, 1386, 1985.
10. Defoe, D. M. and Besharse, J. C., Membrane assembly in retinal photoreceptors II. Immunocytochemical analysis of freeze fractured rod photoreceptor membranes using anti-opsin antibodies, J. Neurosci., 5, 1023, 1985.
11. Molday, R. S. and Molday, L. L., Differences in the protein composition of bovine retinal rod outer segment disk and plasma membranes isolated by a ricin-gold-dextran density perturbation method, J. Cell Biol., 105, 2589, 1987.
12. Vaughan, D. K. and Fisher, S. K., Cyotochalasin D disrupts outer segment disc morphogenesis in situ in rabbit retina, Invest. Ophthalmol. Vis. Sci., 30, 339, 1989.

13. Connell, G., Bascom, R., McInnes, R., and Molday, R. S., Photoreceptor cell peripherin is the defective protein responsible for retinal degeneration slow (rds), <u>Invest. Ophthalmol. Vis. Sci.</u>, 31 (Suppl.), 309, 1990.

14. Inglehearn, C. F., Bashir, R., Lester, D. H., Jay, M., Bird, A. C., and Bhattacharya, S. S., A 3-b.p. deletion in the rhodopsin gene in a family with autosomal dominant retinitis pigmentosa, <u>Am. J. Human Genetics</u>, 48, in press, 1991.

15. Nathans, J., Thomas, D. and Hogness, D. S., Molecular genetics of human color vision: The genes encoding blue, green, and red pigments, <u>Science</u>, 232, 193, 1986.

16. Nathans, J., Davenport, C. M., Maumenee, I. H., Lewis, R. A., Hejtmancik, J. F., Litt, M., Lovrien, E., Weleber, R., Bachynski, B., Zwas, F., Klingaman, R. and Fishman, G., Molecular genetics of human blue cone monochromacy, <u>Science</u>, 245, 831, 1989.

17. Falk, J. D. and Applebury, M. L., The molecular genetics of photoreceptor cells, <u>Prog. Ret. Res.</u>, 7, 89, 1988.

18. Washburn, T. and O'Tousa, J. E., Molecular defects in <u>Drosophila</u> rhodopsin mutants, <u>J. Biol. Chem.</u>, 264, 15464, 1989.

19. O'Tousa, J. E., Requirement of N-linked glycosylation site in <u>Drosophila</u> rhodopsin, submitted for publication, 1991.

20. Doi, T., Molday, R. S., and Khorana, H. G., The role of intradiscal domain in rhodopsin assembly and function, <u>Proc. Natl. Acad. Sci., USA</u>, 87, 4991, 1990.

21. Hargrave, P. A., McDowell, J. H., Feldmann, R. J., Atkinson, P. H., Rao, J. K. M. and Argos, P., Rhodopsin's protein and carbohydrate structure: Selected aspects, <u>Vis. Res.</u>, 24, 1487, 1984.

22. Kühn, H., Mommertz, O. and Hargrave, P. A., Light-dependent conformational change at rhodopsin's cytoplasmic surface detected by increased susceptibility to proteolysis, <u>Biochim. Biophys. Acta</u>, 679, 95, 1982.

23. McDowell, J. H., Ubel, A., Brown, R. A., and Hargrave, P. A., Transglutaminase modification of rhodopsin in retinal rod outer segment disk membranes, <u>Arch. Biochem. Biophys.</u>, 249, 506, 1986.

24. Molday, R. S., Monoclonal antibodies to rhodopsin and other proteins of rod outer segments, <u>Prog. Ret. Res.</u>, 8, 173, 1989.

25. Palczewski, K., Arendt, A., McDowell, J. H., and Hargrave, P. A., Substrate recognition determinants for rhodopsin kinase: Studies with synthetic peptides, polyanions, and polycations, <u>Biochemistry</u>, 28, 8764, 1989.

26. Pelham, H. R. B., Control of protein exit from the endoplasmic reticulum, <u>Annu. Rev. Cell. Biol.</u>, 5, 1, 1989.

27. Zuker, C. S., Mismer, D., Hardy, R. and Rubin, G. M., "Ectopic expression of a minor Drosophila opsin in the major photoreceptor cell class", <u>Cell</u>, 55, 475, 1988.

28. Shieh, B.-H., Stamnes, M. A., Seavello, S., Harris, G. L. and Zuker, C. S., <u>ninaA</u>, a gene required for visual transduction in <u>Drosophila</u> encodes a homolog of the cyclosporine A binding protein, <u>Nature</u>, 33, 67, 1989.

29. St. Jules, R. S. and O'Brien, P. J., The acylation of rat rhodopsin in vitro and in vivo, <u>Exp. Eye Res.</u>, 43, 929, 1986.

30. St. Jules, R. S., Wallingford, J. C., Smith, S. B., and O'Brien, P. J., Addition of the chromophore to rat rhodopsin is an early post-translational event, Exp. Eye Res., 48, 653, 1989.

31. St. Jules, R. S., Smith, S. B., and O'Brien, P. J., The localization and timing of post-translational modifications of rat rhodopsin, Exp. Eye Res., 51, 427, 1990.

32. Fahlman, C. S., O'Brien, P., and Aguirre, G., The kinetics of label incorporation into normal and progressive rod-cone degeneration (prcd) affected rods, Invest. Ophthalmol. Vis. Sci., 31 (Suppl.), 546, 1990.

33. Aguirre, G., Alligood, J., O'Brien, P., and Buyukmihci, N., Pathogenesis of progressive rod-cone degeneration in miniature poodles, Invest. Ophthalmol. Vis. Sci., 23, 610, 1982.

34. Wetzel, M. G., Fahlman, C. S., Maude, M. B., Alvarez, R. A., O'Brien, P. J., Acland, G. M., Aguirre, G. D., and Anderson, R. E., Fatty acid metabolism in normal miniature poodles and those affected with progressive rod-cone degeneration (prcd), in Inherited and Environmentally Induced Retinal Degenerations, LaVail, M. M., Anderson, R. E., and Hollyfield, J. G., Eds., Alan R. Liss, Inc., New York, 1989. 427.

35. Fliesler, S. J. and Basinger, S. F., Tunicamycin blocks the incorporation of opsin into retinal rod outer segment membranes, Proc. Natl. Acad. Sci., 82, 1116, 1985.

36. Fliesler, S. J., Rayborn, M. E., and Hollyfield, J. G., Membrane morphogenesis in retinal rod outer segments: Inhibition by tunicamycin, J. Cell Biol., 100, 574, 1986.

37. Fliesler, S. J., Rapp, L. M., and Hollyfield, J. G., Photoreceptor-specific degeneration caused by tunicamycin, Nature, 311, 575-577, 1984.

38. Colley, N., personal communication.

CAN VIRUSES TRIGGER RETINAL DEGENERATIVE PROCESSES

JOHN J. HOOKS, SUSAN ROBBINS, BARBARA WIGGERT,
GERALD J. CHADER AND BARBARA DETRICK[+]

Immunology & Virology Section, Laboratory of Immunology,
Laboratory of Retinal Cell & Molecular Biology, National Eye Institute,
and [+]Vaccine Research & Development Branch, Division of AIDS,
National Institute of Allergy & Infectious Diseases,
National Institutes of Health, Bethesda, Maryland

I. INTRODUCTION

The consequences of virus host interactions are numerous and varied. Some of the fascinating things that viruses can do include: infecting tissues without inducing inflammatory responses; replicating in cells throughout life without causing cell damage; replicating in cells causing tissue damage or interfering with developmental processes and then disappearing completely from the body; replicating and triggering immune-mediated diseases. Sometimes, in spite of causing no detectable damage, they interfere with differentiated ("luxury") functions. Dr. Cedric Mims has summarized these types of pathogenic relationships in the following way. "As long as there are diseases of unknown etiology there will be suggestions that viruses are responsible. Not because viruses are the last resort in the search for aetiological agents, but because of the unique and fascinating things that viruses can do."[1]

Degenerative and inflammatory diseases of the posterior pole of the eye are common causes of impaired vision and blindness throughout the world. Between 500,000 and 1,000,000 Americans suffer severe visual impairment from retinal and choroidal diseases. Retinal degenerative disorders consist of a diverse group of diseases frequently associated with a genetic predisposition; however, many cases are of unknown cause. Viral infections often precede acute multifocal placoid pigment epitheliopathy (APMPPE) and acute macular neuroretinopathy, and therefore are under suspicion as causative agents.[2,3] The purpose of this report is to review the ways by which viruses could induce retinal degenerative processes and to present data demonstrating that coronaviruses can induce an acute and long-lasting disease of the retina.

II. VIRUS - HOST INTERACTIONS

Interest in the ways in which viruses produce disease has been growing in parallel with our appreciation of the complexity of these pathogenic processes. Classically, these pathogenic processes have been subdivided into five general mechanisms: (1) direct lysis of cells, (2) transformation of cells, (3) altered specialized cellular function, (4) immunopathology and (5) autoimmunity.

These classical approaches have generated study of selected subtle and insidious virus-host interactions. Three of these approaches may provide insight into possible retinal degenerative diseases (Table 1). In the first virus-host interaction, the virus can induce the destruction of a specialized cell, such as a Müller cell or RPE cell. Once the destruction is complete, the virus is no longer available for detection. An example of this relationship is the picornavirus (EMC-) or reovirus-induced pancreatic beta cell destruction leading to loss of insulin and development of diabetes in the mouse.[4] In the second virus-host interaction, the virus can induce the loss of a cellular "luxury" function. An example of this relationship is the

TABLE 1. VIRUS HOST INTERACTIONS

TYPE	EXAMPLE
Destruction of specialized cells	Picornavirus (EMC) or Reovirus induced pancreatic beta cell destruction leading to loss of Insulin and development of diabetes.
Loss of cellular "luxury" function	Arenavirus (LCM) infect and stop pituitary cells from producing growth hormone, resulting in stunted growth (mice). LCM can stop pancreatic beta cell production of insulin.
Virus-induced immune mediated disease	Picornavirus (Theiler's Virus) can induce an immune destruction of CNS myelin - demyelination.

arenavirus (LCM) which infects and stops pituitary cells from producing growth hormone, resulting in stunted growth in mice.[5] In this instance, the virus does not kill the cell but rather just shuts off a specialized function. In the retina, one could expect extensive dysfunction if opsin or IRBP synthesis were curtailed or if ion transport or phagocytosis were inhibited. In the third virus-host interaction, the virus can induce an immune mediated disease. An example of this relationship is the picornavirus (Theiler's virus), which can induce an immune destruction of CNS myelin, resulting in a demyelination in mice which resembles multiple sclerosis in man.[6]

Not only can viruses induce insidious consequences, they may also act in a way that masks their true etiologic role, suggesting a genetic disease. This may be accomplished in at least two ways. First, some persistent virus infections cause diseases that follow genetic patterns. For example, scrapie virus infections in sheep follow patterns observed in autosomal recessive disease; similarly, Kuru in humans has a familial incidence. Second, the susceptibility to viral diseases can be determined genetically. Therefore, some of these diseases actually do appear to have a genetic basis. An example of this is Theiler's virus-induced, immune mediated demyelination.

III. CORONAVIRUS - INDUCED RETINAL DESTRUCTION

Fortified with the knowledge of the diverse capabilities of viruses, we have initiated studies to identify ways in which viruses can trigger retinal degenerations. Coronaviruses were selected as the first candidate virus. Coronaviruses are positive-sense, single-stranded RNA viruses which have long been known to cause a variety of diseases in man and animals.[7,8] Frequently, these viruses have been exploited as models to study the pathogenic processes involved in diseases of the nervous system.

Experimentally, the coronavirus (mouse hepatitis virus, strain JHM) was inoculated into adult BALB/C mice and the animals were evaluated for ocular disease.[9,10] We have found that murine coronavirus can induce ocular disease and this system can be used as a model for studying retinal degenerative diseases. This model has many unique features. The virus is capable of inducing an acute infection in the presence of mild inflammation. The initial retinal damage is followed by clearance of the virus within 7 days and progressive retinal destruction, even months after the virus is gone.

The typical pattern of events following intravitreal or anterior chamber inoculation of JHM is as follows. Multiple, focal lesions are evident as early as day 3, with subsequent involvement of the entire retina by day 10 to 15. The outstanding characteristics of the disease are initial multifocal changes in the ganglion cell, pigment epithelial cells, photoreceptor cells and Müller cells. Viral antigens were detected in all layers of the neural retina by day 3 to 6 but were absent after day 7. Infectious virus was detected at the time when viral antigens were observed. The drop in viral antigen expression was correlated with an elevation in virus specific antibody. Significant retinal abnormalities, notably photoreceptor degeneration, persisted through 8 weeks.

Coronavirus   Retinopathy

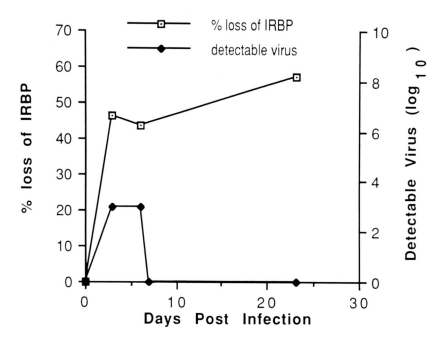

Figure 1. Reduction of IRBP concentration in retinas after intravitreal injection of JHM virus (1.5 X 10⁴ PFU). Retinas were harvested from uninjected, mock-injected and virus-injected mice on days 3, 6 and 23. Corneas were excised, the lenses removed, and the retinas tested for IRBP in a quantitative immuno-slot-blot assay. IRBP concentration was expressed as nanograms/milligram protein. Infectious virus was recovered from isolated retinas in a standard plaque assay. None of the mock-injected eyes yielded any infectious virus.

IV. CORONAVIRUS INFECTION ALTERS DISTRIBUTION AND AMOUNT OF IRBP

This coronavirus model illustrates the potential of an acute viral infection causing later degenerative changes in the retina. We wanted to determine if these persistent retinal alterations were associated with biochemical changes, particularly a change in an important "luxury" protein expressed by photoreceptor cells. In order to do this, we examined the effect of coronavirus infection (after intravitreal inoculation) on interphotoreceptor-retinoid binding protein (IRBP), the glycolipoprotein in the interphotoreceptor matrix thought to transport retinoids between the photoreceptor and the RPE.[11] Significant and expected changes in IRBP distribution accompanied virus-associated retinal pathology. We found that IRBP had diffused into the neural retina, away from the interphotoreceptor matrix region, by 3 days after inoculation. Moreover, the level of IRBP in isolated retinas, measured in an immuno-slot-blot assay, decreased significantly by day 3 and remained low through day 23 (Figure 1). These results demonstrate that the virus can induce biochemical changes in the retina which persist and progress long after the virus is detectable. These data suggest that retinal degenerations of "unknown" etiology could be caused by viral infections and that these processes can significantly alter both the concentration and localization of an important photoreceptor protein.

V. SUMMARY

In summary, these studies show that viruses are capable of entering the retina and replicating in selected retinal cells. The host responds with minimal immune reactivity within the retina, but of sufficient quantity to eliminate the virus. The selective nature of the coronavirus replication probably allows this clearance to take place without inflammatory disease. The fascinating part of this picture is what follows. Pathological alterations, both biochemical and morphological, persist in the retina for weeks and months after the virus is cleared. These studies provide evidence that viruses may indeed trigger retinal degenerative processes and provide a model for such studies in the human.

VI. REFERENCES

1.   Mims, C.A., Viral aetiology of diseases of obscure origin, *Brit. Med. Bull.* 41, 63, 1985.
2.   Annesley, W.H., Tomer, T.L. and Shields, J.A., Multifocal placoid pigment epitheliopathy, *Am. J. Ophthalmol.* 76, 511, 1973.
3.   Bos, P.J.M. and Deutman, A.F., Acute macular neuroretinopathy, *Am. J. Ophthalmol.* 80, 573, 1975.
4.   Rodrigues, M., von Wedel, R.S., Lampert, P.W. and Oldstone, M.B.A., Pituitary dwarfism in mice persistently infected with lymphocytic choriomeningitis virus, *Lab. Invest.*, 49, 48, 1983.
5.   Oldstone, M.B.A., Rodrigues, M.M., Daughaday, W.H. and Lampert, P.W., Viral perturbation of endocrine function to disordered cell function, disturbed homeostasis and disease. *Nature* (Lond) 307, 278, 1984.
6.   Rodrigues, M., Pierce, M.L. and Howie, E.A., Immune response gene products (Ia antigen) on glial and endothelial cells in virus-induced demyelination. *J. Immunol.* 138, 3438, 1987.
7.   Homes, K.V., Coronaviridae and their replication, in Fields Virology Vol 1, 2nd ed., Fields, B.N. and Knipe, D.M., Eds., Raven Press, New York, 1990, chap. 29.
8.   McIntosh, K.M., Coronaviruses, in Fields Virology Vol 1, 2nd ed., Fields, B.N. and Knipe, D.M., Eds., Raven Press, New York, 1990, chap. 30.
9.   Robbins, S.G., Hamel, C.P., Detrick, B. and Hooks, J.J., Murine coronavirus induces an acute and long-lasting disease of the retina, *Lab Invest.*, 62, 417, 1990.

10. Robbins, S.G., Detrick, B. and Hooks, J.J., Ocular tropisms of murine coronavirus (Strain JHM) following inoculation by various routes, *Invest. Ophthal. Vis. Sci.* (in press) 1991.

11. Chader, G.J., Interphotoreceptor retinol-binding protein (IRBP): a model protein for molecular biological and clinically relevant studies. *Invest. Ophthalmol. Vis. Sci.*, 30, 7, 1989.

INDEX

C

Calcium
   cyclic GMP-phosphodiesterase interaction,
      168—170
   interphotoreceptor matrix response, 231
Carbohydrate groups, in pigmented epithelium/
      rhodopsin-containing membrane interactions,
      203—215
   in disc membranes, 204—207
   galactosylated rhodopsin and, 207, 212
   neoglycoprotein effects, 208, 209
   phosphomannosyl receptors and, 209—211
   in rhodopsin liposomes, 204, 206, 208—213
Cardiolipins, 67
Carotenoid deprivation
   in *Drosophila*, 62, 64—67
   P-face particle response, 64
   rhabdomere response, 64—65, 68—69
   tunicamycin effects, 66—67
Cat, see Abyssinian cat
Cellular retinaldehyde binding protein, 111
Cellular retinoic acid binding protein, in retinitis
      pigmentosa, 363, 364, 366
Cerebral cortex, fatty acid content, 118—122
Cerebroside, 67
Cerebrum, interphotoreceptor retinoid-binding
      protein gene expression in, 483
Chloramphenical acetyl transferase gene, construc-
      tion of, 440—441, 480, 481
Cholesterol
   in light-damaged rod outer segments, 195, 196
   in retinitis pigmentosa, 131
   transport, 154
Chondroitin sulfate, see Proteoglycans, chondroitin
      sulfate
Chondroitin sulfate, rhodopsin-liposome binding
      effects, 211
Choriocapillaris, of diabetic rats, 243—253
   basal laminae thickening, 245, 246
   endoplasmic reticulum swelling, 245, 246
   ferritin binding, 247—249, 251
   intercapillary space changes, 245, 250
   luminal surface charge distribution, 243, 249, 251
Chromophore, photochemical damage, 183
Chromosome 10, cGMP-phosphodiesterase subunit
      genes, 462
Chromosome 17, *rds* defect locus, 467
Chromosome 18, cGMP-phosphodiesterase a-subunit
      gene, 462
Chromosome 19, cGMP-phosphodiesterase subunit
      genes, 462
Chylomicron, 152
Ciliary neuron trophic factor, 79
Cloning, subtraction, 437, 439—440
Cograft, of embryonic retinal transplant, 283—284
Color vision defects
   in cone-rod dystrophy, 414, 419
   genetic basis, 520
Cone
   docosahexaenoic acid uptake, 156

   inner segment, see Inner segment, cone
   outer segment, see Outer segment, cone
   perikaryal differentiation, 29
   in retinitis pigmentosa, 365
   in transplanted retina, 266, 267, 281
Cone-rod dystrophy, 409—422
   classification, 409—410
   color vision defects, 414, 419
   dark adaptation, 410—411, 420
   dazzle sensitivity, 412—414, 419
   electrooculogram, 417, 418
   electroretinogram, 411, 414—417, 419
      Ganzfeld, 411
      pattern, 411, 417, 418, 420
   inheritance pattern, 412, 419
   onset age, 412, 419
   oscillatory potentials, 420
   visual acuity, 412, 414, 419
   visual fields, 413
Coronovirus, as retinal degeneration causal agents,
      529, 531—533
Cryopreservation, of embryonic retinal transplant,
      282—284
Cyclic guanosine-binding proteins, in phosphod-
      iesterase activation, 8
Cyclic guanosine monophosphate (cGMP)
   in phototransduction, 6—8
   in *rds* mutant mouse, 9—10
Cyclic guanosine monophosphate-phosphodiesterase
      (cGMP-PDE), in *rd* mouse, 6, 167—172,
      445—454
   α subunit, 456
   α-subunit gene, 460—462
   β subunit, 446, 448—452, 456
   β-subunit gene, 457—460
      alternative splicing, 457—460
      chromosome mapping, 461—462
      mRNA, 461
   calcium accumulation, 168—170
   constant activity, 512, 513
   cDNA, 449—452
   function, 456
   cGMP binding, 167—169
   inhibition, 67
   mRNA, 446, 512
   structure, 445
   δ subunit, 446, 448
   δ-subunit gene, 460—462
Cyclophilin, 524
Cytochrome C oxidase, in blue-light retinal
      degeneration, 186
Cytochrome oxidase, as photochemical retinal
      degeneration chromophore, 183

D

Dark adaptation
   in cone-rod dystrophy, 410—411, 420
   interphotoreceptor matrix in, 228
   photoreceptor protein subcellular localization in,
      503—514